WITHDRAWN

EPIDEMICS

Epidemics

Hate and Compassion from the Plague of Athens to AIDS

SAMUEL K. COHN, Jr.

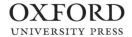

OXFORD

UNIVERSITY PRESS

OXFORD

UNIVERSITY PRESS

Great Clarendon Street, Oxford, OX2 6DP,
United Kingdom

Oxford University Press is a department of the University of Oxford.
It furthers the University's objective of excellence in research, scholarship,
and education by publishing worldwide. Oxford is a registered trade mark of
Oxford University Press in the UK and in certain other countries

Published in the United States of America by Oxford University Press
198 Madison Avenue, New York, NY 10016, United States of America

British Library Cataloguing in Publication Data
Data available

Library of Congress Control Number: 2017954534

ISBN 978-0-19-881966-0

Acknowledgements

This work drew me away from my accustomed haunts, and, as a result, I leaned on the kindness of friends more than usual in the hallways of IASH (Institute for Advanced Studies in the Humanities at Edinburgh), the stairways of numbers 1, 2, 9, and 10 University Gardens, Glasgow, and at the pool table of the American Academy in Rome, among other places. I explored ideas in public lectures at a wide variety of institutions and received helpful advice: in 2011, at the Anglo-American Conference, London (a plenary lecture); the Center for European Studies, Harvard University; the Office of the History of Science and Technology, University of California, Berkeley; a conference on Medical Humanities at the University of Glasgow (plenary). In 2012, at an International Meeting on Infant and Child Growth, Nutrition, and Gastroenterology, Yorkhill Hospital; the Early Modern Workshop, University of Glasgow; the Pybus Seminar in History of Medicine, University of Newcastle; a conference on the emotions at the Villa Le Balze, Fiesole; the 'Healing and Curing: Medieval to Modern' Conference, University of Glasgow (plenary); the 7th Annual 'Search for the Healthy City' Tour (Venice and Padua); the 'ANTIGONE One Health Course', Erasmus MC hospital (Rotterdam); the Pre-Modern Medicine Seminar, Wellcome Library, London. In 2013, at Trinity College Library, Dublin, the Inaugural Lecture of the Medieval and Medical History Lecture Series; Sarah Lawrence College: Florence Program; the Wellcome Unit for the History of Medicine (Oxford); the Early Modern Seminar, University of Warwick; the Annual Early Modern Workshop on Jewish History (College Park, MD). In 2014, three lectures at L'Università degli Studi, Milano (Statale); two lectures at CRASSH (University of Cambridge) Training Course on Visual Representation and the 'Third Pandemic'; Explorathon, Science Centre, Glasgow; Royal College of Physicians, History of Medicine Lecture Series; CRASSH Conference: 'Visualizing Plague during the Third Pandemic'. In 2015, at the Glasgow Syphilis Conference; the Medieval Seminar, University of Glasgow; the Socialist Theory and Socialist Movements Lecture Series, University of Glasgow; three lectures at Universiteit Antwerpen; a workshop on 'Fear of the Foreign: Pandemics and Xenophobia', Bellagio, Rockefeller Foundation; the '800 Years of Riot and Protest' Conference, University of Winchester (on cholera riots in Britain); Strathclyde Early Modern Seminar; the Second Annual CRASSH Conference: 'Corpses, Burial, and Infections'; the Conference on 'Comparative Approaches to Hazards and Shocks', Utrecht, (plenary). In 2016, at Syracuse University (Florence) Lecture Series; 'Religion and Medicine Conference', Birkbeck University (plenary); International Relations Workshop, Leeds University; Institute for the Study of Societal Issues (ISSI), University of California, Berkeley; two lectures, Duke University, Center for International and Global Studies and Department of History; Centrum voor Stadsgeschiedenis, Universiteit Antwerpen. In 2017, at All Souls, Oxford Medieval

Seminar; 'The Idea of Violence' Workshop, Kent State University, Florence; the Medical History lecture series, Royal College of Physicians and Surgeons of Glasgow; and three works-in-progress lectures at IASH in 2014, 2015, and 2016.

In addition, friends from different disciplines and areas of historical research read chapters at various stages. On antiquity, David Konstan, David Purdie, and Matteo Zaccarini; the medieval or early modern chapters, Stephen Bowd, Guido Alfani, William Caferro, Mona O'Brien, John Henderson, Monica Azzolini, and Hamish Scott. On cholera: David Konstan, Martina King, Gordon Johnston, Louise Jackson, and John Foster; smallpox: Lawrence Weaver, David Konstan, and Martina King; India: Miles Taylor and Nicholas Evans; Russia, India, and China: Christos Lynteris; yellow fever: David Konstan, Martina King, and Simon Newman; influenza: Lynn Abrams, Andrew Prescott, and Martin Sanchez-Jankowski; HIV/ AIDS: Bernard Wasserstein, Rebekah Lee, and Lukas Engelmann; introduction and conclusion: Genevieve Warwick. Hannah-Louise Clark read sections on the Middle East. Davide De Franco drafted the maps, and I thank the anonymous readers for Oxford University Press: their close readings went beyond any call of duty and forced me to cut the manuscript. Of the above, I thank doubly Martina King and David Konstan, who endured a special test of patience reading a number of chapters in the early stages, and finally Lauro Martines, who read an early draft of the entire manuscript.

A number of institutions contributed to this work, first in Scotland, the National Library of Scotland and libraries of the universities of Glasgow and Edinburgh; the Wellcome and British Libraries in London; the libraries of the Vatican; the National Libraries of Rome, Florence, and Milan and Mediateca (Milan). In US libraries I read microfilm and online newspapers unavailable in Europe, at Widener Library (Harvard University), Eisenhower Library (Johns Hopkins), Lilly Library (Duke), Doe Library (Berkeley), the Mervyn H. Sterne Library (University of Alabama, Birmingham), and the Library of Congress (Washington, DC). During this project, I enjoyed three two-week periods at the American Academy in Rome and throughout was a fellow of IASH. I thank the directors of the AAR, Chris Celenza and Kimberly Bowes, and Jo Shaw, Donald Ferguson, Jolyon Mitchell, Peta Freestone, and Steve Yearley at IASH. At Oxford University Press, Stephanie Ireland and Cathryn Steele shepherded this work along with patience, encouragement, and expertise, and I thank Jess Smith, the copy editor: certainly no future reader will read this book as carefully as she has. This project was generously funded, first on a two-year Pilot Programme Grant from the Wellcome Trust (09415858/z/10/z), then a three-year Major Research Fellowship from the Leverhulme Trust (MRF-2013-068).

Contents

PART V. MODERNITY: PLAGUES OF COMPASSION

List of Figures and Maps

FIGURES

MAPS

Abbreviations

Aphrodisiacus	Gruner, Christian Gothridus, *Aphrodisiacus sive De Lue Venerea*
ASI	*Archivio Storico Italiano*
AUM	*Annali universali di medicina*
BAV	Biblioteca Apostolica Vaticana
BHM	*Bulletin of the History of Medicine*
BS	*Bibliotheca sanctorum*
Creighton	Creighton, Charles, *History of Epidemics in Britain*
Gomme	Gomme et al., *A Historical Commentary on Thucydides*
Horrox	*The Black Death*, ed. Rosemary Horrox
IOR	India Office Records
LCL	Loeb Classical Library
Livy	Livy, *History of Rome*
Luisini	*De Morbo Gallico*, ed. Luigi Luisini
MGH	Monumenta Germaniae Historica
NSW	New South Wales
Proksch	Proksch, J. K., *Die Geschichte der venerischen Krankheiten*
RIS	Rerum Italicarum Scriptores
SHM	*Social History of Medicine*
The Great Pox	Arrizabalaga et al., *The Great Pox: The French Disease*

Introduction
Hate, Politics, and Compassion

Thoughts for this book arose during the pandemic scare of 2009, the so-called Mexican swine flu. The spectra of racial, class, and religious prejudice clouded newspaper headlines with anticipated acts of violence; yet no riots ensued.[1] I was asked to write a short piece for a New York paper comparing the present pandemic threat to the Black Death's immediate aftershocks. Rather than repeat the story of the mass extermination of 1348–9, predicting the same awaited Mexicans in America, I reflected that I knew of no past influenzas to have spawned massacres of minorities or of anyone else. As a corrective, I concluded that the spread of hatred and blame, especially when it spurred collective violence, was rare in history, no matter how gruesome the disease or how high the body counts. The editor rejected the article, explaining this was not what his readers wanted to hear.

Given the reigning historiography on epidemics and blame, the editor was justified. A scholarly consensus persists. Across time, from as early as the fifth-century BCE Plague of Athens to AIDS and now Ebola, epidemics are thought to have normally provoked hatred, blame of the 'other', and violence towards victims of the disease. As the late Enlightenment Danish-German statesman and scholar of antiquity Barthold Georg Niebuhr (1816) proclaimed: 'Times of plague are always those in which the bestial and diabolical side of human nature gains the upper hand.'[2] In a famous article in 1952, René Baehrel reasoned that epidemics induced 'class hatred'; such emotions were a part of our 'structures mentales...constantes psychologiques'.[3] With the rise of AIDS in the 1980s and into the twenty-first century, such pronouncements became more frequent. According to Carlo Ginzburg, 'the prodigious trauma of great pestilences intensified the search for a scapegoat on which fears, hatreds and tension...could be discharged'.[4] Dorothy Nelkin and Sander Gilman claimed, 'Blaming has always been a means to make mysterious and devastating diseases comprehensible'.[5] Roy Porter concurred with Susan Sontag: 'deadly diseases' especially when 'there is no cure to hand'

---

[1] For a pithy summary of this scare, see Honigsbaum, *A History of the Great Influenza*, 227–9.
[2] Cited by Nohl, *The Black Death*, preface.   [3] Baehrel, 'La haine de classe'.
[4] Ginzburg, 'Deciphering the Sabbath', 121–38.
[5] Nelkin and Gilman, 'Placing Blame', 40. The article has had an authoritative impact; see Craddock, *City of Plagues*, 101; Echenberg, *Black Death, White Medicine*, 130; Eamon, 'Cannibalism and Contagion', 21.

and the 'aetiology...is obscure...spawn sinister connotations'.[6] Recently, from earthquake-wrecked, cholera-stricken Haiti, physician, anthropologist and Harvard University Professor Paul Farmer concluded: 'Blame was, after all, a calling card of all transnational epidemics'.[7]

These judgements, however, have relied on a handful of examples at best and often fewer, which include the Black Death of 1347–51, the Great Pox of the sixteenth century, several cholera riots in the nineteenth, and AIDS, centred almost entirely on the US experience. This book argues that even these canonical examples of disease-infused hatred need qualification. More importantly, from thousands of descriptions of epidemics as early as a 'great pestilence' of Pharaoh Mempses' First Dynasty, *c.*2920 BCE, surviving sources uncover only a minority of epidemics that spurred hatred and violence against outsiders or insiders. Moreover, from antiquity to the twentieth century, epidemics' tendencies to provoke hate and blame were not much the same across time, as the citations above suggest; nor did these reactions prevail when diseases were mysterious, without effective preventive measures or cures to hand, that is, mainly before the late nineteenth-century 'laboratory revolution'. History instead flips this trajectory on its head. With the colossal exception of the Black Death, with its massacres of Jews, beggars, and others, it was the nineteenth and twentieth centuries which produced the major outbreaks of disease-provoked violence and blame, and they did so when diseases such as smallpox and cholera no longer posed great mysteries. While not turning a blind eye to the fantasies and conspiracies that spread at certain times with certain diseases to deadly effect, I also examine epidemics' more usual side effects over time: their power to unite societies and inspire individuals and communities to extraordinary feats of compassion and abnegation.

*   *   *

To write a synthetic volume that cuts across long swathes of time and spans fields of specialization, one of two approaches can be followed. The normal course is to plough voraciously through mountains of published books and scholarly articles to draw new connections and raise new theses. The more risky and time-consuming journey is sampling primary sources. I have chosen the latter. In the main, these have been published sources. For antiquity, the Middle Ages, and the early modern period, they include histories, works of imaginative literature, chronicles, saints' lives, diaries, and medical tracts. For the nineteenth century and later, I have relied on medical journals but predominantly on newspapers of various sorts. Ever-growing resources available online have made this endeavour more feasible than was imaginable even a decade ago.

In addition to new possibilities, reliance on such sources presents new questions and problems for historical research. Especially with the great mass of historical

---

[6] Porter, 'The Case of Consumption', 179.

[7] Farmer, *Haiti after the Earthquake*, 191. Similar remarks are easily found; for instance, Irwin, 'Scapegoats': 'Throughout history, societies have created scapegoats...the innocent...to rationalize and explain the origins and course of disease outbreaks and epidemic disease' (618); and Shah, *Pandemic*, 116 and ch. 6.

newspapers streaming online daily across much of the world, history has become more than before a moving target. Definitive statements such as that foreign papers failed to report a mass demonstration at Juma Masjid in Mumbai in 1897 must be qualified: at the moment of accessing various online newspaper databases with specific sets of keyword searches and given present problems of optical character recognition (OCR), I did not find any. But such long-winded qualifications need not be repeated at every turn. After all, history has always been a moving target, enjoining scholars to search for exceptions and make new discoveries.

This book proceeds roughly chronologically but also topically. Part I concerns antiquity, the Middle Ages, and early modernity, yet these chapters make forays into modernity, such as changes in notions of the scapegoat; leprosy in antiquity and the Middle Ages compared with its nineteenth-century social consequences; naming and blaming; the Great Pox of the sixteenth and seventeenth centuries compared with venereal disease and persecution of prostitutes and young girls in the late nineteenth and early twentieth century; and disease-fuelled massacres of Jews and other minorities in 1348 compared to Nazi blame of them for typhus. Parts II to IV begin with cholera riots in the 1830s, but are chronological only in the sense of concentrating on the nineteenth and twentieth centuries. Here, epidemics are divided by their dominant socio-psychological tendencies, starting with hatred, then politics, and finally compassion. For modernity, I have concentrated on cholera, smallpox, plague, influenza, and yellow fever, but not from any preordained decision. Rather, my research uncovered these as the diseases that have unleashed the most sustained and dramatic collective reactions, whether of violent acts or of compassion, even though other diseases might have inflicted greater misery and higher mortalities.

Finally, before the nineteenth century, this book concentrates on Europe, and then branches out to the US, Canada, India, Australia, the Middle East, China, Latin America, and Africa, even if the focus remains on the West. Overwhelmingly, the examples I present from the nineteenth and twentieth centuries have yet to be reported by historians. This book is an ethnography of epidemics' social toxins and stimuli for compassion and self-sacrifice from antiquity almost to the present.

PART I

ANTIQUITY AND THE MIDDLE AGES

1

Epidemics in Antiquity
The Moral Universe and Natural Causes

Does the historical record confirm the conclusions of historians, social scientists, and public intellectuals: that epidemic disease normally provoked social and ethical tensions, with blaming and violence towards 'others'? Did this violence intensify when diseases were mysterious, that is, mostly before 'the laboratory revolution' of the late nineteenth century? As Oliver Wendell Holmes, Senior, quipped in 1860, 'if the whole *materia medica*, as now used, could be sunk to the bottom of the sea, it would be all the better for mankind—and all the worse for the fishes'.[1] While overstated, as Holmes himself later admitted,[2] most epidemic diseases were without effective cures and preventive measures before the twentieth century.[3] Thus, given current expectations, epidemics' power to spark hatred and blame should have been all the more likely in antiquity, the Middle Ages, and the early modern period.

The most famous of ancient plagues—the Plague of Athens in 430–429 BCE and its recurrence in 427—might suggest such a supposed pre-modern proclivity for blame. It was one of the few epidemics from antiquity to be reported with any detail on symptoms, modes of transmission, demographic effects with variations between regions or peoples, or notions about the origins and movement of the pandemic. More important for our purposes, its principal text, Thucydides' *History of the Peloponnesian War*, focused on its social and psychological consequences, dedicating twenty-five chapters (in part or in their entirety) to it.[4] Thucydides felt obliged to trace its origins and describe its symptoms so if it broke out again, it would be recognized.[5] From Ethiopia,[6] it spread into Egypt and Libya and 'over the greater part of the [Persian] King's territory', before invading Athens' port of Piraeus and then Athens.

---

[1] Holmes, 'Currents and Counter-Currents', 467.   [2] 'Reflections on his Annual Address'.
[3] Wooten, *Bad Medicine*, argues that medicine remained statically more harmful than helpful until Joseph Lister's antiseptic surgery in the 1890s. For advances in surgical practices, understanding of diseases, and cures in antiquity, see Nutton, 'Medicine'. For the development and effectiveness of plague measures in early modern Europe, see Cohn, *Cultures of Plague* and idem, 'Changing Pathology of Plague'.
[4] Thucydides, *History of the Peloponnesian War*, 1.23; 2.47–54, 57–60, and 64; 3.13 and 3.87.
[5] Ibid., 2.48.   [6] Gomme, II, 147, translates its origins as Sudan.

Thucydides claims that the inhabitants of Piraeus 'even said that the Peloponnesians had put poison in their cisterns'.[7] However, no more is heard of these accusations when the plague reached the densely populated upper city of Athens and 'mortality became much greater'.[8] Here, Thucydides begins his detailed account, first of the disease's characteristics and symptoms, then its social, political, and psychological consequences—general lawlessness of the city and the inhabitants' resolve to satisfy bodily and material lust. Seeing their days numbered, Athenians lost their fear of the gods and law; 'their piety and impiety came to the same thing'.[9] He claimed that they 'would satisfy their lusts, regarding their bodies and their wealth alike as transitory'. Believing they had already paid 'the penalty', they felt they might as well reap the pleasures of the moment.[10] Later, Black Death chroniclers—Florence's Matteo Villani, Siena's Agnolo di Tura il Grasso, the English friars John of Reading and Henry Knighton, and others—said much the same of their pandemic but attributed this last-ditch extravagance to the poor, artisans, and labourers. By contrast, Thucydides drew no such class divisions.

Not only was Thucydides an eyewitness, he caught the plague and survived.[11] From his description, it appears to have been completely new to Athenians, and as a result, inhabitants possessed little, if any, innate immunity to it: 'no constitution, as it proved, was of itself sufficient against it, whether as regards physical strength or weakness, but it carried off all without distinction, even those tended with all medical care.'[12] Although he does not use the word, Thucydides describes the disease as highly contagious: those nursing the ill 'died like sheep'.[13] This aroused fear and efforts of self-preservation: 'restrained by fear', Athenians began to refuse 'visiting one another' and 'the sick perished uncared for'. This reaction, however, was short-lived. Unlike the abandonment chroniclers described across Europe during the Black Death,[14] Thucydides emphasized the opposite:

> But still it was more often those who had recovered who had pity for the dying and the sick, because they had learnt what it meant and were themselves by this time confident of immunity; for the disease never attacked the same man a second time, at least not with fatal results.[15]

---

[7] Thucydides, *History of the Peloponnesian War*, 2.48; Longrigg, 'Epidemic, Ideas', 21–2. Gomme, II, 147, translates it as 'wells and cisterns'. Hornblower, *A Commentary of Thucydides*, I, 319, calls it 'a surprising suspicion' but then suggests that it was similar to the Black Death accusations against Jews that led to their slaughter.

[8] Thucydides, *History of the Peloponnesian War*, 2.48.

[9] Ibid., 2.53.   [10] Ibid., 2.53.

[11] Ibid., 2.48. According to Gomme, II, 148, Thucydides drafted this section after recovering from the disease, and his clinical descriptions were based on notes made at the time. Hornblower, *A Commentary of Thucydides*, I, 321, notes it as a rare autobiographical statement.

[12] Thucydides, *History of the Peloponnesian War*, 2.51.

[13] Ibid., 2.51. Also, in his opening lines on the plague, Thucydides claimed the mortality was 'greatest' among physicians, 'because they were the most exposed' (2.47).

[14] See Chapter 2.

[15] Thucydides, *History of the Peloponnesian War*, 2.47. According to Longrigg, 'Epidemic, Ideas', 33–4, Thucydides was the 'first to enunciate clearly the doctrine of contagion and to describe acquired immunity'. Also, see Hornblower, *A Commentary of Thucydides*, I, 317 and 325.

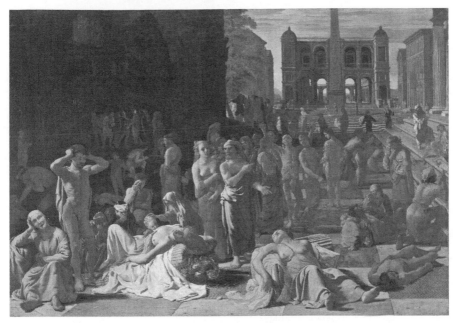

Figure 1.1. Plague in an Ancient City, Michael Sweerts, *c.*1652.

The absence of blaming foreigners or others for the disease as mortalities mounted and morality, law and order, and traditional beliefs declined is all the more surprising given that it devastated Athens but not 'Peloponnese [the land of their Spartan enemies] to any extent'.[16]

The following year, the plague continued with disastrous force against the Athenians, contributing to Peloponnesian military success, first with the Athenian fleet, then on the mainland. For the first time, blame arose among the Athenians. But no hints of enemy poisoning of cisterns resurfaced. Rather, the Athenians now blamed their own leader, Pericles, because of the disastrous war with the Spartans (Lacedaemonians) and his failure to negotiate.[17]

Thucydides' *History* is our only surviving contemporaneous source for the Plague of Athens[18] and appears to have been the major one later ancient writers reflected upon—Lucretius (*c.*99 BCE–*c.*55 BCE, *De rerum natura*), Dionysius of Halicarnassus (60 BCE–7 BCE, *The Ancient Orators 5. Thucydides*), the first-century CE poet and astrologer Marcus Manilius, Plutarch (46 CE–120 CE, *Life of Pericles*),

[16] Thucydides, *History of the Peloponnesian War*, 2.53. Gomme, II, 147, cites George Grote's twelve-volume *A History of Greece* (1846–56) on his surprise that Thucydides supplies no evidence of 'cruel persecutions' against plague spreaders as occurred against *untori* at Milan in 1630. Both authors assume such persecutions were common across time, but neither supplies a case of it in antiquity.

[17] Thucydides, *History of the Peloponnesian War*, 2.59. Gomme, II, 166–84, contains a long section on attacks against Pericles but does not refer to Athenians blaming him for the plague. The same goes for Hornblower, *A Commentary of Thucydides*, I, 330.

[18] Longrigg, 'Epidemic, Ideas', 28.

Galen (130–200 CE), and Ammianus Marcellinus (*c*.325/330–391/400, *Rerum Gestarum*). The first-century BCE historian Diodorus Siculus, who relied partially on a now lost universal history by the fourth-century Greek historian Ephorus, may have been an exception.[19] In recounting detailed developments of the Peloponnesian War, Diodorus mentions the plague only in passing, that 'many Athenians were being slain in the assaults and by the ravages of the plague',[20] but explained the plague's causes arising from natural conditions—overcrowding in Athens and a very wet winter. By contrast, Thucydides refrained from pinning the plague on any specific causes but turned immediately to its course and symptoms.[21] Ammianus Marcellinus reports this pestilence only as an example of how plagues begin through an 'excess of cold or heat, or of moisture or dryness' and then cover vast spaces by air or waters, 'polluted by the stench of corpses'.[22] Marcus Manilius describes the horrors of the disease—'no place was there for a doctor's skill, no prayers availed; duty fell a prey to sickness, and none were left to bury, none to weep for the dead . . . hardly was an heir to be found in that nation once so vast'.[23] Galen drew parallels between the signs and symptoms of the Plague of Athens and the one of his own time, the Antonine Plague, 165–180 CE, drawn from his clinical practice, but did not comment on the Plague of Athens' epidemiology or moral and social consequences.[24] Extrapolating from Thucydides, Lucretius expanded on the psychology of fear and desire.[25] But none of these authors raised any suspicions of blame or even repeated the supposed poisoning at Piraeus.

By contrast, Dionysius and Plutarch centred their attention on blame; yet they too failed to mention any poisoning. Instead, they focused on the Athenians' final reaction[26]—censure of Pericles. According to Dionysius, Pericles had persuaded them to go to war and had caused 'their falling into such misfortunes'.[27] Plutarch, on the other hand, strove to protect his hero. The plague 'had weakened them [the Athenians] in body and in spirit', driving them 'altogether wild against Pericles'. 'In the delirium of the plague', they attempted to harm him as with the madness that leads the patient to attack a physician or the son a father.[28] Yet, instead of imagining plague as caused by diabolic scheming, hatched in a moral universe

---

[19] See Gomme, II, 148–9. Also Lloyd, *In the Grip of Disease*, 218, suggests that Lucretius may have relied on other sources but mentions none.

[20] Diodorus, *The Library of History*, 12.46.4.

[21] Thucydides, *History of the Peloponnesian War*, 2.48. See Gomme, II, 148–9.

[22] Ammianus Marcellinus, *Rerum Gestarum Libri*, 23.24.

[23] Marcus Manilius, *Astronomica*, lines 874–97.

[24] Galen's only epidemiological observation on this pandemic was that it erupted among troops at Aquileia in the winter of 168/9 CE. See Europius, *Breviarium ab urbe condita*, 228 (editor's note), and Littman and Littman, 'Galen', 246 and 249.

[25] Commager, 'Lucretius' Interpretation of the Plague'. According to Gomme, II, 156–7, Lucretius's 'rhetorical method' lacked entirely the 'scientific interest' seen with Thucydides.

[26] Thucydides, *History of the Peloponnesian War*, 2.48.

[27] Dionysius of Halicarnassus, *The Ancient Orators*, 5.14.

[28] Plutarch, *Lives, Pericles*, XXXIV.

where gods employed disease to punish acts of evil, these commentators' reasoning was naturalistic. By Dionysius' account, the plague:

> was caused by the crowding of the rustic multitudes together into the city, where, in the summer season, many were huddled together in small dwellings and stifling barracks, and compelled to lead a stay-at-home and inactive life, instead of being in the pure and open air of heaven as they were wont.[29]

According to Plutarch, no one then turned against this 'rabble from the country...penned up like cattle, to fill one another full of corruption'. Rather, they held their leader responsible.[30]

*   *   *

Thus far, the most systematic investigation of epidemics and their reactions in the ancient world has been R. P. Duncan-Jones' study centred on the Antonine Plague.[31] However, to chart epidemics mostly in the Roman world to the end of the second century CE, he reached back to the fifth-century Plague of Athens. Despite the fragmented survival of early registers and written sources, epidemics fill the annals of antiquity. He calculates that from 490 BCE to 292 BCE Livy alone records an epidemic every eight years, and from 212 to 165 BCE, the rate doubles.[32] Unfortunately, Duncan-Jones gives few details of these epidemics: what they may have been (even in the vaguest terms, as with those confined to army camps or ones that spread through cities and the countryside), when and where they occurred, and, for our purposes, their socio-psychological reactions: did they stir blaming, divisions across social classes, persecution of foreigners or outcasts? Nonetheless, he asserts that blaming others was the usual consequence of ancient plagues: 'Societies with no effective medical explanation for plague', he argues, 'could easily blame it on human agency' (and by this he means poisoning).[33] He mentions, however, only a handful of such cases, and when one turns to the texts, they all appear problematic.

His first case is his best: Thucydides' report from Piraeus, that some may have thought that the Plague of Athens was spread by poisoning cisterns. Even here Duncan-Jones' claim is misleading, that Thucydides 'at first blamed it [the plague] on the Peloponnesians having poisoned wells'. As Thucydides makes clear, the disease spread from distant Ethiopia, not nearby Piraeus. Further, he merely reports that 'the people there *even said* that the Peloponnesians had put poison in their

---

[29] Ibid.

[30] Ibid. In addition, the second-century CE geographer Pausanias, *Description of Greece*, Attica, 3.4, describes a temple erected by the fifth-century BCE sculptor Calamis, dedicated to 'the other Apollo, called Averter of evil', who received his name by ending the Plague of Athens in 430 BCE.

[31] He does not include the possible recurrence of this plague in 189 CE as a part of this pandemic. Also Nutton, *Ancient Medicine*, 24, thought it was a different disease.

[32] This would amount to about thirty-six epidemics mentioned by Livy. According to Duncan-Jones, 'The Impact': 'Major epidemics are so frequent in Roman Annalists that contemporaries must have found them relatively commonplace' (109). This impression centres on one work, Livy's, with only thirty-five of 142 books surviving.

[33] Duncan-Jones, 'The Impact', 115.

cisterns'. More importantly, as emphasized earlier, such suspicions did not lead Athenians to blame Peloponnesians or any others once it reached upper Athens, where it wreaked its greatest havoc.[34]

Duncan-Jones' second case comes from Livy, 331 BCE.[35] That year 'gained an evil notoriety, either through the unhealthy weather or through human guilt', and a strange illness afflicted 'the foremost men of the state...with the same fatal results'. A maidservant of one of the city magistrates (*curule aediles*) gave state's evidence to avoid prosecution, claiming wealthy Roman matrons concocted poisonous drugs to kill off members of the ruling class. Eventually, 170 upper-class ladies were tried and executed. Livy, however, adds that the stories were inconsistent about events that had happened three centuries before his time and for which no earlier records survive. Moreover, he was sceptical of any connection between any poisoning and these deaths, much less believing that the poisoning was an epidemic disease. Until that time, he remarks, there had never been an investigation of poisoning in Rome. Even if it had been an epidemic caused by a pathogen, it was certainly not the usual sort. It began not within a besieged military camp nor concentrated among the poor, nor like the Plague of Athens and the Antonine Plague, originating from foreign lands. Had it been a disease, the 331 incident would also have been unique to ancient history in that it was limited to Rome's ruling class. As Livy comments, even those who considered the mortalities resulting from the 'matrons' poisons' thought them 'to be an act of madness rather than deliberate wickedness'. Memory of this incident endured through antiquity[36] and was related at least twice in the late fourth century CE. Paul Orosius (380–420) embellished Livy's report, claiming it was a 'horrible pestilential year in Rome with bodies of the dead piled high on all sides'. Writing almost seven centuries after the facts, he said that some believed that the disease derived from contaminated air, but he concluded that its true source was with the Roman matrons, 'inflamed with an incredible madness and love of crime'. In his version, the condemned rose to 370, and the victims were no longer confined to Rome's male ruling classes.[37] Writing around the same time, Augustine of Hippo (354–430) used the event as yet another datum to catalogue his condemnations *contra paganos*, but he was more circumspect. Truer to his source (Livy), Augustine questioned the magnitude of the supposed pestilence, but he went beyond Livy in pinning the blame on the general degeneration of pagan society, concluding that the matrons' immorality was 'worse than any plague'.[38]

Duncan-Jones' third case also derives from Livy,[39] when Roman rulers (principally Quintus Naevius) attempted in 184 BCE to crush conspiracies by shepherds around Rome, accusing them of mass poisoning. In two references to these accusations (39.41 and 40.43), Livy, however, never refers to disease or plague, or hints that an epidemic accompanied the elites' charges to justify their onslaught of the

---

[34] Ibid., 115.
[35] Livy lived from 64 or 59 BCE to 12 or 17 BCE; Syme, 'Livy and Augustus'.
[36] See, for instance, Valerius Maximus, *Memorable Doings*, 2.4.
[37] Orosius, *The Seven Books of History*, 3.10.   [38] Augustine, *The City of God*, III, 340–1.
[39] Duncan-Jones, 'The Impact', 115.

shepherds. Finally, Duncan-Jones cites two references from Dio Cassius's *Roman History*, arguing that contemporaries understood criminals' use of poisoned needles as having instigated the 'plagues' in Rome during the reigns of emperors Domitian (81–96 CE) and Commodus (180–192).[40] The first of these, around 90, does not, however, refer to any plague, saying only that 'some persons made a business of smearing needles with poison' and pricked 'whomsoever they would'.[41] The second reflects on the earlier crimes, alleging that they had not completely disappeared. In 189, however, a pestilence —'the greatest of any' the author had known, with as many as 2000 dying 'in Rome in a single day'—ran alongside the criminals' prickings. Yet, despite the parallel courses, neither Dio nor any other ancient author suggests that Romans took the terrible pestilence as derivative from these criminal activities.[42]

Finally, the centrepiece of Duncan-Jones' analysis, the Antonine Plague of Marcus Aurelius's reign, shows no waves of blame or persecution reported by him or others, past or present, even though the disease was new, mysterious, and had originated beyond the Empire's borders. Once thought to have inflicted low levels of mortality from 1 to 2 per cent or around one million within the entire Empire, estimates of its mortalities (now believed to have been from smallpox) have increased, first, to over ten million (7 to 15 per cent of the population).[43] Using surviving tax records and considering sudden increases in wages driven by extreme labour shortages comparable to those after the Black Death and to changes in legislation, Duncan-Jones' estimates reach higher, to a quarter of the Empire's population levelled.[44]

For this plague a larger number of eyewitness reports survive than for any previous epidemic and include medical, Christian, and pagan sources—Galen, Aelius Aristides, Lucian, Jerome, Marcus Antoninus—along with Egyptian sources. Yet, instead of blame, they point to charity and tolerance. The emperor provided funerary statues for prominent members of the nobility with state subsidies granted to celebrate the funerals of the poor.[45] Further, the one plague story related by the anonymous author of Marcus Aurelius's life—to be sure, a eulogy—stresses forgiveness, not hate or retribution. A madman prophesied fires falling from heaven to create further pandemonium during the plague. When he was brought to justice, the emperor intervened after hearing his story and pardoned him.[46] Given that the same Marcus began his reign by inflicting 'the third persecution' on Christians,[47]

---

[40] Ibid., 115. The passages are 67.11.6 and 72.14.3–4; the second one should be 73.14.3–4. Early modern chroniclers of Milan's plague of 1630 (Tadino, *Raguaglio*, 120 and Somaglia, *Alleggiamento*, 495), considered the Roman matrons and needle murders of Commodus' and Domitian's reigns as plague spreaders (*untori*). Also, see Manzoni, *I promessi sposi*, ch. 32, 620.

[41] Dio Cassius, *Roman History*, 8.11.　　[42] Ibid., Epitome, 73.14–15.

[43] For these estimates, see Littman and Littman, 'Galen', 252–5, which revised claims as high as 50 per cent, based on narrative evidence, and as low as 1 to 2 per cent hypothesized by Gilliam in 1961 (ibid., 243). The Littmans' estimates are based on qualitative comparisons with smallpox epidemics in early modern Mexico City and Western Prussia, not from any figures of antiquity. For the disease as smallpox, derived from Galen's case histories, see Nutton, 'Medicine', 965 and Harper, 'Pandemics', 223.

[44] Duncan-Jones, 'The Impact', 118–36.　　[45] *Historia Augusta*, 4.13.

[46] Ibid.　　[47] These begin with Nero.

'crowning many saints with martyrdom',[48] he might have blamed the plague on the Christians or his enemies, since it had spread along with warfare, but he did not. Instead, when the disease reached the Empire's Germanic provinces, where war was raging, Marcus 'acted with extreme restraint and consideration'.[49] No accusations arise of enemy foreigners having caused the plague.

*   *   *

To estimate how often epidemics were blamed on malicious human agency or how normal it was to attack 'the other' for allegedly inflicting such suffering on a population, I have searched for pandemics, plagues, pestilences, and epidemics in antiquity to the first century CE, using the Perseus Digital Library, Lacus Curtius website, and the recently released Loeb Classical Library online.[50] I have uncovered 265 descriptions of epidemics from the seventh century BCE to the sixth-century CE Justinianic Plague. These include mostly outbreaks that can be easily dated, but others which linger in the mists of mythology or are hypothetical cases, which may have occurred but are not dated.[51] From the datable ones, epidemics do not mount in number over time, as might be expected with the greater availability of sources (despite the absence of Livy's books for much of the first century BCE).[52] Instead, the narrative evidence corresponds closely with results from osteoarchaeology in antiquity (although mainly for Greece, found long ago by John Angel): the seventh and sixth centuries BCE appear healthy. With increased migration, population, and 'civilization', the fifth century, however, became more disease-ridden and of reduced human longevity.[53] From my initial sampling, the fifth century also records the highest frequency of epidemics (41). Livy is a major source of them, containing almost a quarter (58 of 265). As a consequence, the epidemics cluster in the City of Rome or within its surrounding countryside (99 of 265 descriptions). Others, however, are found in Spain, Gaul, Sicily, the Lipari islands, Crete, Cyprus, Greece, various Greek islands, Macedonia, and as far east as Armenia, together with unspecified parts of Asia and India. Nonetheless, from these sources, if the ancient Greeks 'were plagued by plagues' as G. E. R. Lloyd has quipped,[54] it appears to have been even more the case among ancient Romans.

Rarely do classical authors give hints about the epidemiology, symptoms, signs, or course of epidemics—far less than in medieval sources, even before the Black Death but especially after it. The two most often cited sources on ancient pandemics,

---

[48] *Orosius: Seven Books of History*, 7.15.4.   [49] Ibid., 174–5.

[50] Perseus 4.0, last updated in 2007 at <http://www.perseus.tufts.edu/hopper/>, accessed 3 August 2011. I used keyword searches (epidemic, pandemic, plague, pestilence, pestilential, disease, poison, and variants of these words). Individual deaths, metaphorical usage, and legendary plagues that are difficult to establish chronologically, such as ones in the Bible, were discarded from my tallies in note 51. I also searched the Brepols Library of Latin Texts (A), finding six further epidemics (<http://clt.brepolis.net/llta/Default.aspx>, accessed 26 April 2012), and have added two from Orosius, *Seven Books of History*.

[51] Eighth century BCE (6) seventh (6); sixth (8); fifth (41); fourth (36); third (21); second (28); first (10); first century AD (15); second (14); third (18); fourth (7), fifth (9). For several others, the dating is difficult to determine.

[52] The summaries of Livy's lost books produces only one plague I did not find elsewhere.

[53] Grmek, *Diseases in the Ancient World*, ch. 3.   [54] Lloyd, *In the Grip of Disease*, 1.

one near the beginning of antiquity, Thucydides' description of the Plague of Athens, and the other at the end, Procopius' of the sixth-century CE Justinianic Plague, are striking exceptions. In between them, no pandemic or epidemic received such attention to a disease's origins, course, epidemiology, morbidity, mortality, susceptibility, signs, and symptoms, not even from Galen, who treated patients at Aquileia in 168 during the Antonine Plague. Thucydides concentrated an entire section (Book II, 49) of over 400 words on the Plague of Athens' signs and symptoms. People in perfect health were attacked suddenly. Extreme headaches, and redness and inflammation of the eyes were the first symptoms. Then, the victims' throats and tongues became bloody; their mouths 'exhaled an unnatural and fetid breath', followed by sneezing, hoarseness, and severe coughing. The disease soon turned downward through the body, 'settling in the stomach' with vomiting 'of bile of every kind named by physicians', causing violent convulsions. In addition, victims' bodies became pale and reddish, breaking out in small blisters and ulcers. The lightest covering of linen sheets irritated patients, who yearned to throw themselves into cold water. No matter how much they drank, unquenchable thirst tormented them. Throughout their suffering, restlessness and sleeplessness overwhelmed them until the seventh or ninth day, when most died. Those who survived the crisis developed acute diarrhoea. Thucydides also described the long-term effects on the survivors: marks on fingers, toes, and genitals, and some lost these bodily parts. Others became blind; others lost their memory, failing 'to recognize themselves or friends'.[55]

Similarly, Procopius traced the Justinianic Plague's origins, from its first known appearance at the port of Pelusium (Egypt), where it forked in two directions: one to Alexandria, the other to Palestine, and from there 'over the whole world', reaching Byzantium by the middle of spring, two years later. According to Procopius, the plague left neither islands nor mountain ridges untouched. Humans also appear to have acquired some immunity to the disease. Procopius sketched in detail the disease's signs and symptoms from a sudden fever to the development of 'a bubonic swelling' a few days later that 'took place not only in the... "boubon", that is, below the abdomen, but also inside the armpit, and in some cases also beside the ears, and at different points on the thighs'.[56]

Procopius described a diversity of clinical patterns. Some died straight away. Others sank into a deep coma, seemed to sleep constantly, and were unable to recognize their friends. Others were seized with delirium, suffered insomnia, suspected others out to kill them, cried at the top of their lungs, struggled to escape from their beds and homes, resisted those nursing them, had difficulties eating, and many died of hunger. Unlike the plagues of the 'Second Pandemic', some died immediately but many others persisted for 'many days' before succumbing. Similar to bubonic plagues from 1347 to the early nineteenth century, 'black pustules

---

[55] Thucydides, *History of the Peloponnesian War*, 2.49. In other places, Thucydides discusses epidemiological aspects of the plague: that it was highly contagious as evinced by infecting those nursing patients, and a notion of acquired immunity—'the disease never attacked the same man a second time, at least not with fatal results' (2.51).

[56] Procopius, *History of the Wars*, 2.22, cit. 22.22.13.

about as large as a lentil' formed on the bodies of some victims and were a sure sign of death: victims failed to survive 'even one day'. Like the Black Death, the Justinianic Plague manifested pneumonic symptoms—vomiting of blood, which, as with the pustules, brought death straight away—and physicians were thrown into confusion. Different treatments led to different consequences with different patients: 'no device was discovered by man to save himself', and 'no cause came within the province of human reasoning'.[57] Procopius could draw only a few conclusions about the disease or its victims: afflicted pregnant women and newborn infants almost invariably died. If the swelling obtained an unusual size and discharged pus, the victim had a better chance of survival than if the swelling failed to grow or to suppurate. Finally, Procopius reported a long-term physical aftereffect, one not observed by late medieval or early modern chroniclers and physicians: a number of the survivors 'lived on with speech impediments, lisping or speaking incoherently'.[58]

The signs and symptoms described by the other two most often cited authors of the Justinianic Plague—John of Ephesus and Evagrius Scholasticus—stray further from the characteristics seen in bubonic plagues of the 'Second Pandemic' and further still from those of the 'Third'—1894 to the present. Evagrius' account, based on his own affliction as a young boy and witness to three further waves at Antioch that took his wife, children, servants, and residents on his estates, appears the more credible of the two. While he was afflicted with the large glandular swellings, the buboes (in the plural[59]), others had 'different ailments' such as bloodshot eyes and swollen faces and pain running down the throat.[60] John's first mention of the plague signs, while laconic, are roughly consistent with those of the other two historical pandemics: 'with this plague of swellings in their groins...which they call boubones'.[61] But later his description changed: 'three signs became visible in the middle of the palm of a man's hand in the form of black pocks which did not depart (from the skin) but (remained) deep (in it), like three drops of blood deep within'.[62] No clinical description from the 'Second' or 'Third Pandemic' reports anything remotely similar: was he simply being allegorical?

As for tracing an epidemic's origins and trajectory, the accounts of Thucydides and Procopius again are unusual.[63] Another exception was the Antonine Plague of 165–180, which the *Historia Augusta* claimed originated in Babylonia.[64] In addition, Livy points vaguely to a pestilence that arose from 'the great number of

---

[57] Ibid., 2.22.18–35.   [58] Ibid., 2.22.30–9.

[59] From late nineteenth-century hospital reports of the Presidency of Bombay, those with more than one bubo comprised less than 5 per cent of cases; see Cohn, *Cultures of Plague*, ch. 2.

[60] Evagrius, *Ecclesiastical History*, 4.29.   [61] *Pseudo-Dionysius of Tel-Mahre: Chronicle*, 87.

[62] Ibid., 88.

[63] Other chronicles charted this plague's progress. According to *The Chronicle of Pseudo-Zachariah*, it 'spread out from Kush that is on the border of Egypt, and from Alexandria, Libya, Palestine, Phoenicia, Arabia, Byzantium, Italy, Africa, Sicily, and Gaul, and arrived in Galatia, Cappadocia, Armenia, Antioch, Osrhoene, Mesopotamia, and eventually the territory of the Persians, and the nations of the Northeast, devastating them' (10, 9, 414–15). Also, see Evagrius, *Ecclesiastical History*, who, despite four encounters with the plague, supplies few details of the plague's spread—only that it originated in Ethiopia—and he insisted it had no fixed seasonality (4, 29).

[64] *Historia Augusta*, 5.8.

locusts and the masses of them that were killed' in Africa and which may have found their way to Rome around 126 to 121 BCE.[65] When ancient commentators described epidemics by natural causes (investigated later in this chapter under that heading), the diseases' traits pertained to conditions incurred during military sieges and overcrowding, abrupt changes in climate, extreme heat, an inability to exercise, or consumption of unaccustomed food because of drought, poor harvests, or warfare.

Military sieges created further inconveniences, which ancient authors took as the epidemiological springs of disease. Most prominent was the inability to bury the dead or remove corpses from cities and camps, giving rise to putrid smells and poisonous vapours, as happened, according to the second-century historian Appian of Alexander (*c.*95–*c.*165 CE), within Carthaginian camps during the Second Punic War (218–201 BCE). Overcrowding of 'a great multitude of men, enclosed in a camp, exposed to the heat of an African summer' were the epidemic's preconditions, but vapours from unburied bodies were the trigger.[66] During the civil war between Julius Caesar and the Roman senate, led by Pompey in the mid-first century BCE, Lucan's epic poem, *Pharsalia*, describes an epidemic that ran through military camps: death was swift, 'no interval of sickness divided death from life', because of 'the press' of unburied bodies among the living.[67]

Occasionally, Livy describes other epidemiological traits such as a plague in 174 BCE, which began with cattle and spread to humans, who 'seldom survived to the seventh day', and those who did, suffered 'a long and tedious illness, generally taking the form of a quartidian [quartan] ague'. The victims were principally slaves.[68] According to Livy, dogs and vultures would not touch the contaminated corpses. In a few instances, he showed an awareness of certain diseases as being highly contagious and noted human adaptation as with an epidemic among Romans and Carthaginians in the region of Syracuse in 212 BCE. Although he saw the epidemic springing from deprivation caused by war and spreading 'by putrefaction and the pestilent odour of corpses', later he claimed the disease spread beyond the camps to civilians and cities, 'carried by those who had cared for the ill': contagion spread the disease (*postea curatio ipsa et contactus aegrorum volgabat morbos*).[69]

Except for the three pandemics (and especially with Galen's case histories at Aquileia), classical authors were sparing in their clinical descriptions even when mentioning dysentery or diarrhoea.[70] Lucan's epic poem of the mid-first-century BCE civil war was one of the few to describe any epidemic symptoms:

> Now the skin grew tight and hard, causing the straining eyes to start out, and the fiery plague, inflamed with erysipelas, moved to the face; and the heavy head refused to carry its own weight.[71]

---

[65] Livy, *Summaries*, LX.

[66] Appian, *Roman History*, 8.1.10: 'Living in the stench of putrefying corpses' ignited the pestilence that annihilated 'the greater part' of their army.

[67] Lucan, *The Civil War*, 6.75–117.   [68] Livy, 41.22.

[69] Livy, 25.26. On immunity, also see Ovid, *Metamorphoses*, 7.453.

[70] Herodotus, *The Persian Wars*, 8.15, reports that Xerxes' army was forced to eat grass, bark, and leaves and was afflicted with dysentery that killed many. On the prevalence of dysentery in antiquity, see Stannard, 'Diseases', 266–7.

[71] Lucan, *The Civil War*, 6.93–6.

During the Parthian wars between Romans and Armenians, the third-century CE Christian bishop and church historian Eusebius of Caesarea reported an epidemic among the Romans: ulcers, called anthrax, spread over entire bodies, but it targeted the eyes 'for special attack', blinding 'numbers of men as well as women and children'.[72]

These, however, are the exceptions from my harvest of 265 literary and annalist reports of epidemics from Hesiod and Homer in the seventh or eighth century BCE to Procopius. Moreover, with Livy, Tacitus, Diodorus, and the Egyptian historian and priest Manetho, these epidemics reach back into mythological and biblical time, as well as datable reigns, the earliest being the 'great pestilence' of c.2920 BCE.[73] Were these writers of much earlier epidemics simply reflecting on diseases of their own times? Were the 'details of all pestilences' described by Livy, for instance, 'certainly later reconstruction', fictions to fill space when little else seemed worth reporting?[74] Without independent descriptions from the earlier epidemics, it is difficult to judge. But indications of change can be delineated, as between mythological time and periods grounded in the datable political history[75] and between periods of ancient history and late antiquity and early Christianity.

THE MORAL UNIVERSE OF DISEASE

A prominent historian of early modern Britain, Keith Thomas, has pronounced: 'The search for a scapegoat sprang from the conviction that every natural disaster must necessarily have a moral cause.'[76] From the examples that followed, his generalization pertained to a longer time span than Puritan religiosity in seventeenth-century England. Thomas did not mention the ancient world, which gave us the concept of the scapegoat (*pharmakos*).[77] But the pestilence that frames the *Iliad*,

---

[72] Eusebius, *Ecclesiastical History*, 9.8. For two authors not covered by my online sources who described the signs and symptoms of epidemics, see Cyprian's description of the plague of c.249–c.275 in Chapter 2, note 71, and Harper, 'Pandemics', 229. In addition, Rufus of Ephesus describes a plague in Libya, Egypt, and Syria in the second century CE characterized by non-suppurating buboes, which formed 'not only in the ordinary places but also in the groins and the neck'; cited in Stannard, 'Diseases', 264.

[73] Manetho, *History of Egypt*, 34–5. For problems of a simple dichotomy, legendary or mythical time versus historical time, see the elaborate divisions in Fontenrose, *The Delphic Oracle*—'Fictional', 'Legendary', 'Quasi-Historical', and 'Historical'. Yet his analysis remains principally binary. Also, see Hughes, *Human Sacrifice*, 71–3. My distinction between datable and non-datable (or difficult to date) history differs slightly from theirs.

[74] Drummond, 'Rome in the Fifth Century', 138.

[75] Fictional works such as Sophocles' *Oedipus Tyrannus*, written at the time of the Plague of Athens, can be placed in historical contexts; see Lloyd, *In the Grip of Disease*, 84–5. I have, however, placed these works in mythological time. Lloyd makes a similar distinction between ancient works of fiction and those of historians (Herodotus and Thucydides). The former 'had nothing to do with real events, however much verisimilitude they could command', while the latter were 'at pains to justify their claim to record what actually happened' (84).

[76] Thomas, *Religion and the Decline of Magic*, 96; and other places: 'whenever disaster struck, the preachers and pamphleteers were quick to indicate its direct origin in the moral delinquencies of the people' (84); and note 162.

[77] Lloyd, *In the Grip of Disease*, 11.

the opening of Sophocles' *Oedipus Tyrannus*, the Minotaur story, and many others might suggest that the ancient world's mental constructs for understanding pestilences were fixed in a universe governed by moral forces. Certainly, ancient literary and historical texts record some pestilences springing from gods' displeasure with mortals' deeds within a moral universe, which paid little heed to physical or biological worlds.[78] In contrast to early Christianity, these misdeeds did not centre so much on individual sin—prostitution, adultery, sexual infidelity, or blasphemy—as on political events—leaders' betrayals, treachery, unjust wars, violations of peace, and breaches of justice. But was such a moral framework the overriding context for explaining epidemics in antiquity, and, if so, did it then induce societies to blame outsiders for them?

The earliest of these stories, shrouded in Greece's mythological past, was also 'the most influential text of all, a work that every educated Greek of the classical period would know', etched in their minds when encountering pestilence in any subsequent work of literature.[79] Homer's *Iliad* described an 'evil pestilence' that Apollo brought on Agamemnon's Greek armies because of the 'dishonour' done to Apollo's priest, Chryses, when he attempted to ransom his daughter from Agamemnon but was refused.[80] Chryses prayed for vengeance, and Apollo answered with the plague. Agamemnon's own death, murdered according to the *Odyssey* (11.409–11) by his wife's lover Aegisthus, and in later versions by his wife Clytemnestra (usually in cahoots with Aegisthus), also fomented a plague.[81] As Lloyd explains, this plague appears in the most prominent position in the best-known text of Greek literature and established that 'gods are responsible for diseases and for their relief'.[82] Yet, as we will see, even these motifs in Greek literature could be remoulded, stripped entirely of divine causation.

About the same time, the early eighth- or late seventh-century Greek writer Hesiod recalled in his *Works and Days*—a predecessor of the Farmer's Almanac in verse—a pestilence coupled with famine, which Zeus inflicted on mortals. Suggesting a slow-killing pathogen or an epidemic that became endemic, it affected the long-term growth and reproduction of society by women failing to give birth. For Hesiod, the affliction had nothing to do with natural causes but arose because of crimes committed by the mortal son of Cronos, himself the son of the god of the universe, Uranus. This unnamed son had destroyed Greek armies, their city walls, and had attacked their ships at sea. Hesiod then expands on the moral message of plagues for rulers:

> For among human beings there are immortals nearby, who take notice of all those who grind one another down with crooked judgments and have no care for the gods' retribution. Thrice ten thousand are Zeus' immortal guardians of mortal human beings upon the bounteous earth, and they watch over judgments and cruel deeds.[83]

---

[78] Lloyd, *In the Grip of Disease*, makes a similar distinction, concentrating on endemic diseases and mental disorders but has less to say about epidemics. He discusses only two, the plague in the *Iliad* and the Plague of Athens.

[79] Ibid., 15–16, 84–6.   [80] Homer, *Iliad*, 1.8–13.

[81] *Remains of Old Latin*, II. Pacuvius, *Tragedies*, no. 137.

[82] Lloyd, *In the Grip of Disease*, 16.   [83] Hesiod, *Theogony. Works and Days*, 106–9.

A further pestilence explained by a criminal act sets the stage for the most famous mythological story post-Freud, the Oedipus myth. The 'hateful Pestilence'[84] that consumed Thebes, and which the Oracle of Delphi proclaimed would not end until the murderer of the former King Laïus was apprehended, was not only explained by moral causes fixed in a long history of human crimes and infidelities, but also produced history's most famous scapegoat, King Oedipus, banished from Thebes to end a pestilence of otherwise perpetual pollution.[85]

But my searches reveal that the most prominent of ancient myths to explain plague determined by human misdemeanour were versions of the Minotaur story, when King Minos of Crete demanded tribute from Athens because his son Androgeos had been 'treacherously murdered' within Attica.[86] The second-century BCE version by the Athenian Apollodorus (born *c.*180 BCE), reworked sometime in the first or second century CE, provides the most widely reproduced version of the tale from Ovid to Dante. When Minos could not conquer Athens, he prayed to his father, Zeus, to take vengeance on the Athenians by inflicting them with famine and pestilence. The Athenians first obeyed their oracle and slaughtered the four daughters of Hyacinth who were from Lacedaemon (Sparta) but lived in Athens. When this solution failed to lift the plague, the oracle added that the Athenians should give whatever Minos wanted. He ordered seven male youths and seven damsels to be sent to him as fodder for the half-bull–half-man monster, the Minotaur, trapped in Daedalus' labyrinth.[87] Here is a classic story of human sacrifice in Greek mythology with scapegoats to benefit the wider community. Yet, as with Oedipus, neither the daughters of Hyacinth nor the yearly sacrifice of seven young men and seven damsels resemble our notions of scapegoating—a venting of anxiety, fear, or anger aroused by epidemic terror to blame and attack the 'other', a religious or ethnic minority, foreigners, and most often the impoverished. The daughters of Hyacinth were of noble heritage. Hyacinth, the beautiful youth, was the son of the king of Macedonia or of Sparta (according to different versions of the story), and was Apollo's lover, hardly an impoverished outsider. Nor is there any reason to believe that the noble youth and damsels chosen for the Minotaur's feasts derived from any underclass. We will return to ancient scapegoats.

Renditions of the Minotaur human sacrifice began to soften by the first or second century CE, when the biographer Plutarch scripted his version. It begins with the treacherous murder of Minos' son Androgeos in Attica, in some versions after winning athletic prizes at the Panathenaic Games. Not only did his father avenge the murder by war against the Athenians, the Heavens also 'laid waste' their country and 'smote it sorely' with pestilence. Athens' own gods demanded that they appease Minos. The Athenians agreed to send him seven youths and seven maidens no longer annually but only every nine years. By 'the most dramatic' version,

---

84   Sophocles, *Oedipus Tyrannus*, lines 24–8.
85   On scholars' view of Oedipus as scapegoat, see Lloyd, *In the Grip of Disease*, 88–9.
86   Plutarch, *Lives. Theseus*, XV.
87   Apollodorus, *The Library*, III, 118–21. Harris, 'The Family', 11–35, argues that into the fourth century BCE, Greeks believed wrongful homicide created societal pollution. With the Minotaur these survived at least into the second century CE.

according to Plutarch, the Minotaur either destroyed the youth in the Labyrinth or they struggled to escape but eventually perished. However, citing Aristotle, Plutarch said he did not believe the youths were put to death; instead, they spent their lives enslaved in Crete.[88] In a later version (from fragments of the third-century BCE 'atthidographer' Philochorus), the labyrinth was only a prison, the man-eating Minotaur no longer played a role, and Minos held funerary games to honour his son with participating Athenian youth eligible to win prizes, as Theseus eventually did, triumphing over Minos' arrogant and cruel general, Tauros, in a wrestling match.[89]

To illustrate the moral causes of pestilence, Apollodorus provides another story from Greek mythology. After the death of Eurystheus, king of the Mycenaean city of Tiryns, the tribe of the Heraclids (i.e. the Dorians associated with the return of the sons of Heracles) invaded Peloponnese and took all their cities. A year later, plague spread throughout that country. An oracle explained the misfortune as resulting from the Heraclids' invasion. 'They had returned [to their homeland] before the proper time'—so the Heraclids left the country.[90] Plutarch also finds a further two tales from mythology to illustrate pestilence's moral causation. First, in the story of Icarus, Saturn taught him the use of wine and viniculture, which Icarus passed on to his neighbours, who became drunk and, on awakening from their stupor, thought they had been poisoned. Retaliating, they stoned Icarus to death, and in despair, his grandchildren hanged themselves. Shortly thereafter, a plague spread among the Romans, which would not cease until they appeased the wrath of Saturn. A Roman noble (Lutatius Catulus)[91] built a temple for Saturn near the Tarpeian Rock, an early place of Roman execution behind the Capitoline Hill.[92]

Plutarch's second story concerned the foundation of Rome and legends surrounding Romulus: a plague overwhelmed the new Roman territory, bringing sudden death, afflicting crops with unfruitfulness and cattle with barrenness; rains of blood filled the city. At once, Plutarch asserted, all agreed that Tatius' execution and the slaying of the city's ambassadors had been a miscarriage of justice, rousing the gods to punish the Romans. Once the murderers had been apprehended and the city purified by lustral rites, the plague ceased.[93] The second-century Greek geographer Pausanias tells another story from mythological time. As a sacrifice to a god, a community in the region of Boeotia (Attica) got drunk on wine, became violent, and murdered the priest of Dionysus. Immediately, a plague struck. To 'cure it', the oracle at Delphi commanded them to sacrifice a young boy annually, but after a few years, the god substituted a goat for the boy.[94]

In datable, historical time, Diogenes Laertius, the third-century biographer of Greek philosophers, reports a pestilence that struck Athens in the period of Solon at the time of the forty-sixth Olympiad, *c.*600 BCE. To end the plague, the

---

[88] Plutarch, *Lives. Theseus*, XVI: Aristotle's Constitution of Bottiaea is lost.
[89] See the texts and commentary of *Philochorus* in ibid., XXVI.
[90] Apollodorus, *The Library*, 218–19.
[91] At least three prominent Roman noblemen were so named. The earliest was a consul in 242 BCE.
[92] Plutarch, *Moralia*, 4.9.   [93] Plutarch, *Lives. Theseus*, XXIV.
[94] Pausanias, *Description of Greece*, Boeotia, VIII.

Pythian priestess at Delphi—Apollo's mouthpiece—told them to purify the city. Black and white sheep were allowed to roam; where they laid down marked the spot to offer a sacrifice to the local divinity. Others declared that the plague had been caused by pollution brought on the city by Cylon, when in 632 BCE he attempted a *coup d'état*. To remove it, the Athenians executed two young men, Cratinus and Ctesibius.[95]

In the *History of the Peloponnesian War*, book I, Thucydides anticipated the coming of the Plague of Athens, then seeing earthquakes, 'great droughts with resultant famines', and the 'noisome pestilence' as explained by politics and morality: the violation of the truce between Athenians and Peloponnesians that had established a thirty-year peace brought on these natural disasters.[96] Yet, as we have seen, when he concentrated on the plague in book II—the longest treatment of an epidemic by any ancient writer—his moral prelude had been forgotten.[97]

Livy recounts a plague that afflicted Rome soon after the trial and execution of [Marcus] Manlius, who earlier had saved Rome's temples from destruction during a siege by the Gauls in 390 or 387 BCE.[98] 'A great many people' thought the gods had infected the Romans to punish them for Manlius' execution, and that 'the Capitol . . . had been polluted by the blood of its saviour'. Livy, however, was sceptical, reporting that this moral explanation arose because no natural cause could be found.[99] He chronicled another plague fifty-two years later (332 BCE) that arose from another political decision. The Roman senate appointed a dictator, Publius Cornelius Rufinus, and then resigned their posts because of 'a religious difficulty' concerning the nomination. 'It seems as though' the defect in formalities led to the plague.[100] With an earlier pestilence in 398 BCE that afflicted city and countryside, Livy agreed with his sources scripted two centuries or more before his birth ('discovered in the books of fates'). Romans, overawed by the social status of those seeking election as military tribunes with consular power at the Etruscan city of Veii (16 km north-west of Rome), affronted the gods by 'prostituting' themselves, choosing only patricians and men from the highest echelons. These patricians achieved 'absolutely nothing' noteworthy and employed all their strength to rob those they ruled, carrying off 'huge spoils' and leaving 'nothing untouched that iron or fire could destroy'. The devastating plague was the gods' response to the Romans' cowardice and their new rulers' treachery.[101]

---

[95] Diogenes, *Lives*, 1.10. By some sources, Cratinus sacrificed himself.

[96] Thucydides, *History of the Peloponnesian War*, 1.23. Gomme, I, 151, questioned whether Thucydides believed the explanation; he may have been reflecting popular opinion. For other natural disasters, such as a later destructive tidal wave, he did not connect natural events with human actions. By contrast, Hornblower, *A Commentary of Thucydides*, I, 317–18, argued Thucydides put stock in portentous events and eclipses of the sun, while with other events he was 'sober and scientific'.

[97] Towards the end of the plague's first phase, Thucydides, *History of the Peloponnesian War*, 2.54, deciphers a line of verse equating a 'Dorian war' with 'pestilence', and reflects on popular expectations from the verse and oracles. It is not clear if Thucydides treated the connections as nonsense.

[98] On Manlius, see Hooper, *Roman Realities*, 53. On Thucydides' naturalism as indebted to Hippocratic writers, see Lloyd, *In the Grip of Disease*, 120–7.

[99] Livy, 6.20.   [100] Ibid.   [101] Livy, 5.14.

Others after Livy continued to explain epidemics within a moral universe. The first-century BCE historian Dionysius of Halicarnassus, who relied heavily on Livy, mentioned a strange pestilence in 471 BCE that attacked women, especially pregnant ones, causing them to die in greater numbers than ever before. During the plague, a slave of the Vestal Virgins revealed that one Vestal, Urbinia, had lost her virginity. Tried and convicted, she was carried through Rome in a solemn procession, while whipped with rods, and then buried alive. One of two men who had slept with her killed himself; the other was 'scourged in the Forum like a slave' and executed. Once the three had been disposed of, the plague ended.[102]

According to Appian of Alexandria (c.95–c.165), the Autarienses joined Molostimus and the Celtic people called Cimbri and went to destroy the temple of Delphi during the Ilyrian Wars of 105 BCE. Most were killed by storm, hurricane, or lightning before they could commit the sacrilege, but Apollo pursued the remaining Autarienses by inflicting a plague of frogs on them, 'which filled the streams and polluted the water, giving rise to pestilential vapours'. The Autarienses left their homes, and from fear of disease, none would help them.[103] The first-century CE Jewish historian Josephus relates several historical plagues, which he explains were not so much caused by transgressions of justice or cruel persecution but were proof of the Jewish God's superiority. He records the story from 2 Kings 17, when the Chūthaioi or Samaritans migrated to Chūtha in Persia. Each tribe brought with them their own god to worship. As a punishment, the Jewish 'Most High God' sent an incurable pestilence on them. An oracle dictated that their only deliverance was to worship the Jewish God. The tribes sent envoys to the king of Assyria, asking him to send them Hebrew priests captured in his war to instruct the Chūthaioi on Judaism. Worshipping the Jewish God ended the plague.[104]

Two further plague stories found in Josephus turned within a moral universe but rested in datable historical time. Shortly after the malicious execution of Mariamme, the beautiful Jewess and wife of King Herod, in 27 or 29 BCE, a disastrous plague killed 'the greater part of the [Herod's] people and the king's most honourable friends'. 'All' suspected the plague was God's reply to Mariamme's unjust murder, but Josephus does not reveal his opinion.[105] During the first Jewish–Roman War (66–70 CE), the brutal murder of the gallant Jewish military leader, Niger of Perea, by the Jewish sect, the Zealots, who refused to grant him his last wish of a grave, brought God's wrath on them with pestilence, famine, war, and 'to crown all', 'internecine strife' among the Jews.[106]

Finally, early Christianity developed Old Testament moral reasoning to explain pestilence: God restored justice to Christians by unleashing plagues on tyrants and their nations, which had persecuted them. Plagues were now seen positively as God's means not only to punish persecutors but to mend their ways. By Orosius' account, the Romans understood the plague of 253 as God's fury against their

---

[102] Dionysius of Halicarnassus, *Roman Antiquities*, 9.41; later elaborated on by Orosius, *The Seven Books of History*, 128–9.
[103] Appian, *Roman History*, 10.4   [104] Josephus, *Jewish Antiquities*, 9.288–90.
[105] Josephus, *Jewish Antiquities*, 15.6.   [106] Josephus, *The Jewish War*, 4.360–5.

wrongs, prompting an about-face in Roman policies, ending their half-century of persecuting Christians.[107] Eusebius, bishop of Caesarea (*c.*260–*c.*339), listed the torments God inflicted on the Romans during the ten-year persecution of Diocletian, but which became especially intense in its final stage with the tyrant Maximinus Daia, from 308 to Constantine's victory at the Milvian Bridge (313). First, famine hit the Romans, then 'worst of all', pestilence

> battened upon every house…in every alley and marketplace and street; there was nothing to be seen but funeral dirges… Thus waging war with the aforesaid two weapons, pestilence and famine, death devoured whole families.… Such were the wages received for the proud boasting of Maximin and for the petitions presented by the cities against us.[108]

Not only did the plague punish and hinder the state's will to persecute Christians, it gave Christians the opportunity to prove their moral superiority 'in every respect…to all the heathen':

> alone in such an evil state of affairs [Christians] gave practical evidence of their sympathy and humanity: all day long some of them would diligently persevere in performing the last offices for the dying and burying them (for there were countless numbers, and no one to look after them); while others would gather together in a single assemblage the multitude of those who all throughout the city were wasted with the famine, and distribute bread to them all, so that their action was on all men's lips, and they glorified the God of the Christians, and, convinced by the deeds themselves, acknowledged that they alone were truly pious and God-fearing.[109]

The pious bishop, however, did not end his account with charity but with more vengeance, celebrating 'God, the great and heavenly Champion of the Christians', who displayed his wrath 'against all men by the aforesaid means, in return for their exceeding great attacks against us', making it 'manifest to all that God Himself had been watching over our affairs continually'. On the other hand, God showed 'mercy and goodwill to those who fix their hopes on Him'.[110] Similarly, the fifth-century church historian Sozomen interpreted the pestilence of 363 as the 'manifest token of God's displeasure brought down against Julian the Apostate's persecution of the church', and in 409 a plague following Alaric's siege of Rome was 'Divine wrath sent to chastise [Romans] for their luxury, debauchery, and manifold acts of injustice'.[111]

But by the first century CE and into late antiquity, other writers began to question and even mock the oracles and others who explained plagues by moral causes. One late pagan scholar to question the moral universe of causation was the fourth-century CE publicist and teacher of Greek paganism at Antioch, Libanius (314–393). He pointed satirically to the unequal exchange between the numbers who had to die from plague for the sins of the few: 'It is an old habit of theirs [the gods] to show their displeasure over persons foully wronged. The vengeance for the misdeeds of individuals often extends over the whole community.' He then ridiculed

---

[107] Orosius, *The Seven Books of History*, 316–17.   [108] Eusebius, *Ecclesiastical History*, 9.8.
[109] Ibid.   [110] Ibid.   [111] Sozomen, *The Ecclesiastical History*, 7.2 and 9.6.

the plague imposed on the Athenians because of the single murder of Minos' son; and the plague that butchered Thebes caused by Oedipus alone.[112] Even in stories premised on moral injustice to gods or men, ambivalence tempered any certainty that human punishment could cure plague.

NATURAL CAUSES

If extended to other natural disasters such as earthquakes, storms, hurricanes, and especially famines, or to endemic diseases,[113] the assemblage of moral exempla would expand, along with increases in the number of disasters explained by natural causes. However, from the 265 descriptions of epidemic diseases I have found, only twenty-five of them—eight from mythological time, twelve from datable history, and five from early Christianity—were framed within a moral universe. Overwhelmingly, ancient authors across different genres either did not hazard a guess as to why a pestilence had infected a community, or they explained it as arising from natural causes, even if the ascribed causes might not now accord with our notions of aetiology or transmission. Furthermore, these naturalistic explanations were not then cobbled together with ones engrained in moral worlds of injustices or indiscretions against gods. These I counted as moralistically determined. To be sure, short annalistic jottings of epidemics, such as Manetho's listing of a 'great pestilence' during the reign of Mempses nearly 5000 years ago with no commentary at all, do not prove that Egyptians priests in Mempses' or Manetho's time (the third century BCE) understood epidemic disease naturalistically or moralistically. But, as seen above, authors who described signs, symptoms, and modes of transmission—Thucydides, Livy, Julius Caesar, the anonymous author(s) of the *Historia Augustus*, the poet Lucan, and others—understood epidemics by turning to the physical world: climate, physical weakness caused by famine, bad food, unaccustomed diets, or vapours from unburied corpses were the determinants.

In contrast to epidemics explained by moral causation, those pinned to the natural world derived almost exclusively from datable history. Only two of the natural ones appear from an undatable past, both from Diodorus. He recounts a story from the 'most learned' men of India[114] to explain a sickness that overcame Greek soldiers led by the god of wine, Dionysius, when invading India 'in the earliest times', before the subcontinent had 'notable cities'. A pestilence arose from oppressive heat. Dionysius, 'conspicuous for his wisdom', led his troop from scourged plains into the hill country, 'where cool breeze blew and the spring water flowed pure', which cured their affliction.[115] Diodorus' second example regards the

---

[112] Libanius, *Oration*, 24.31.

[113] Herodotus, for instance, records 'a female sickness' among Scythians that endured until his time, which he attributed to robbing the temple of Aphrodite at Ascalon. This was not, however, an epidemic; see Lloyd, *In the Grip of Disease*, 117.

[114] On the earliest contacts between Greece and India, see Napier, *Foreign Bodies*, 90–1 and Rawlinson, 'Early Contacts', 421–41.

[115] Diodorus, *The Library of History*, 2.38.

islands of Chios, Samos, Cos, and Rhodes, from a distant past. 'In those times', floods created famine, and pestilence prevailed in the cities of the mainland, 'because of the corruption of the air'. Refreshed by sea breezes, the islands, however, were unaffected: their inhabitants enjoyed wholesome air, good crops, and accumulated great abundance.[116]

The rest can be dated. Weather was a principal factor. In 463 BCE Livy describes an epidemic in Rome caused by 'oppressive heat', made worse by overcrowding from those in the surrounding countryside seeking protection from raids. They entered with their animals, bringing 'unaccustomed' stench to the city. Personal contact in 'ordinary intercourse' helped spread the disease.[117] Lucretius saw the Plague of Athens caused by the earth's atmosphere: 'beat by rains unseasonable and suns, | Our earth hath then contracted stench and rot'.[118] In the first year of the Plague of Athens, Rome suffered from a severe drought. Rivers and springs dried up, causing cattle to die and become infected with mange. The disease spread to herders, then to slaves and farmers, and from them entered the city.[119] In 399 BCE Livy described a pestilence in Rome arising from 'the unhealthy weather', when a pestilential summer followed a severe winter that proved fatal 'to man and beast'.[120] Seven years later, famine, 'excessive heat, and drought' brought another pestilence around Rome.[121] In the thirteenth year of Herod's reign (25/24 BCE) Josephus, who often saw plague as God's vengeance, now pointed to pestilence ignited by droughts that led to drastic changes in diet and famine.[122] Around 100 CE Heraclitus, defender of Homer against detractors such as Plato, used allegory to reinterpret the plague in the *Iliad*. Instead of deriving from Agamemnon's crimes, by Heraclitus' account, it was a 'spontaneous disaster',[123] derived from patterns of the sun that produced scorching heat and 'unusual changes in the atmosphere'. This 'condition of the air', not God's wrath, caused Homer's plague.[124]

Even Christian writers such as Eusebius, who saw pestilences as God's vengeance against pagans, could also explain them as arising from natural causes. The so-called plague of Cyprian that struck Rome in 251 he reported as arising 'from the rivers and mists from the harbours'. The dews were discharges from corpses 'rotting in all their constituent elements', the air, 'made foul by the vile exhalations'.[125] He also explained a plague of anthrax around 310 CE that 'visited Christians' not by any sins they may have committed but from a winter's drought that led first to famine, then plague.[126] The sixth-century Christian historian Evagrius Scholasticus described an epidemic of 451 CE without relying on moral causes, even if afterwards, he thanked God for providing relief from famine to the survivors: 'bodies became bloated from excess of inflammation', victims 'lost their sight, coughing supervened', and on the third day they died. The plague was caused by a drought

---

[116] Ibid., 5.82.   [117] Livy, 3.6.   [118] Lucretius, *On the Nature of Things*, 6.1090.
[119] Livy, 4.30.   [120] Ibid., 5.13.   [121] Ibid., 5.31.
[122] Josephus, *Jewish Antiquities*, 15.299–304.   [123] *Heraclitus: Homeric Problems*, VI.
[124] Ibid., VIII–XI.
[125] Eusebius, *Ecclesiastical History*, 7.22. Also, Harper, 'Pandemics', 227, argues that it was first noticed in Alexandria in 249 and lasted to 275.
[126] Eusebius, *Ecclesiastical History*, 9.8.

covering large parts of modern-day Turkey ('Phrygia and Galatia and Cappadocia and Cilicia'). These disasters created food shortages and 'harmful nourishment' led to plague, 'for which no remedy could be found'.[127]

The strains and consequences of war were another factor which ancients saw as sparking pestilence. Like the weather, it was seen not in isolation but as igniting a chain reaction of natural causes. For Thucydides, war's hardships explained the return of the Plague of Athens in 427 BCE. In 390 BCE, Livy described a famine in Gaul arising from siege warfare between Romans and Gauls that soon spawned plague. His explanation was grounded in natural preconditions: their camp was on low-lying ground and had been scorched by fires filling the air with ashes. Unaccustomed to the wet and cold, the Gauls could not bear the heat and 'died off like sheep'.[128] Explaining the difficulties of Alexander the Great's campaigns in 330–328 BCE, the first-century CE rhetorician Quintus Curtius pointed to non-combatant consequences of war. When entering 'the remotest parts of the Orient', Alexander's troops became overextended; dwindling supplies necessitated slaughtering their draught animals and horses for sustenance, and the poisonous juices from this unwholesome food led to famine, then pestilence.[129]

In the winter of 73 BCE, during the Mithridatic Wars, Appian recounted that the Roman army had cut off supplies by sea to the king of Pontius and his soldiers in northern Anatolia ('Armenia Minor'). Suffering from hunger, they ate entrails and herbs; many became sick and died; their unburied corpses ignited plague.[130] In 49 BCE Julius Caesar recalled a pestilence among the Marseillians after they were beaten in battle. They had been forced to eat rancid meal and barley from emergency stores collected long ago.[131] As seen in Lucan's poem on the civil war between Julius Caesar and the senate, rotting of unburied bodies killed in war 'infected the stagnant air' and polluted the water, sparking pestilence in Rome, and volcanic eruptions in the Bay of Naples worsened the 'deathly atmosphere'.[132] About the same time, Plutarch in his life of Caesar reported a similar plague among Caesar's troops, arising from his men being old and weakened by long marches, frequent encampments, siege warfare, strangeness of diet, and night watches.[133]

As these various examples suggest, notions of contagion were implicit in ancient explanations of epidemics. Thucydides saw the Plague of Athens' mortalities soaring once it reached upper Athens, because it had struck 'the densest population'.[134] Diodorus also noted demographic factors and contagion in explaining Athens' extraordinary mortality: 'a vast multitude of country immigrants' had streamed into the city; their 'cramped quarters caused them to breathe polluted air'.[135] The same factors influenced Josephus' description of a plague on the eve of the siege of Jerusalem during Passover, 70 CE: many entered the city 'from every corner of the

---

[127] Evagrius, *Ecclesiastical History*, 2.6.   [128] Ibid., 5.48.
[129] Quintus, *History of Alexander*, 9.8–16.   [130] Appian, *Roman History*, 12.76.
[131] Caesar, *Civil Wars*, 2.22.   [132] Lucan, *The Civil War*, 6.83–105.
[133] Plutarch, *Lives, Caesar*, XL.   [134] Thucydides, *History of the Peloponnesian War*, 2.54.
[135] Diodorus, *The Library of History*, 12.45. He also attributed it to climatic conditions. See Gomme, II, 149 and 158, who attributes Diodorus' explanations to reliance on a lost fourth-century work of Ephorus.

country' to celebrate the feast of unleavened bread, overcrowding the city, which produced pestilence before the siege began.[136] Overcrowding caused by migration was also the reason the plague of 189 CE was more severe in Rome than elsewhere, according to Herodian of Antioch (*c.*170–*c.*240).[137] As we have seen, humans were not the only ones to propagate disease in these authors' reasoning. According to Livy, a pestilence in Sardinia in 174 BCE, when few survived beyond a week, derived from a cattle plague of the previous year.[138] From one of his lost books, covered by his summaries, Livy reported a pestilence in Africa in 126 BCE that stemmed from 'an extraordinary multitude of locusts', rotting on the ground.[139]

Classical authors pointed to other natural factors explaining epidemics. In his biography of the early fifth-century Greek philosopher Empedocles, the third-century CE Diogenes Laertius reported a pestilence among inhabitants of Selinus (Selinunte), a Greek colony near Sicily's south-westernmost tip. 'Noisome smells' from a nearby river caused citizens to perish, especially women in childbirth.[140] In 126 BCE, Livy noted an eruption of Mount Aetna, which spewed 'fire far and wide', causing seas around the Liparae Islands to boil, burning ships, and killing large quantities of fish. The islanders consumed them at their feasts, causing an unheard-of plague of stomach poisoning.[141] In a case difficult to date but not a part of mythological time, Plutarch mentions a plague near Boulis, east of Anticyra on the Phocian Gulf, caused by the rotting of a beached whale.[142] In his life of Nicias, a general during the Peloponnesian War, Plutarch claimed the Plague of Athens resulted from Athenians' change of abode and their unwonted manner of living.[143] Moreover, humans were not solely acted upon by these external factors; humans could also adapt. According to Livy, Romans tolerated a pestilence that ran through Roman garrisons and Carthaginian camps around Syracuse better than Carthaginians, not because of the gods or lessons governing morality, but because they had spent more time in the region, becoming accustomed to the weather, water, and 'foul and deadly miasma emerging from the bodies' of the afflicted and unburied.[144]

Finally, it is difficult to know whether the Hippocratic corpus should be included in this sample of ancient epidemics. The compilations called *Epidemics*, meaning 'visitations' either of the diseases or doctors' rounds through Thessaly, Thrace, and the island of Thasos from the end of the fifth to the mid-fourth century, mostly concerned the patient cases of individuals. The three 'constitutions' in *Epidemics*, book I, however, pertained to diseases afflicting communities, and for these, no moral considerations arise. Instead, similar to Thucydides' Plague of Athens, causes are hardly discussed. Rather, the 'constitutions' concentrated on the course of a disease or a bundle of diseases occurring in different seasons, the condition of

---

[136] Josephus, *The Jewish War*, 6.420–34.   [137] Herodian, *History of the Empire*, 1.12.
[138] Livy, 41.21.   [139] Livy, *Summaries*, LX.
[140] Diogenes, *Lives*, Empedocles, 8.2. On Empedocles' mixed character as a dispenser of *pharmaka* and charms and spells, see Lloyd, *In the Grip of Disease*, 25–6, but here Empedocles clearly saw the disease rooted in the natural world.
[141] Livy, *Summaries*, Julius Obsequens, *A Book of Prodigies*, VI.
[142] Plutarch, *Moralia*, 12.31.   [143] Plutarch, *Lives*, Nicias, 6.3–4.   [144] Livy, 25.26.

patients, the traits of those who succumbed, who recovered, and especially the diseases' signs and symptoms. If there were any explanations for these diseases, they derived from the present or preceding climatic conditions.[145]

*   *   *

A moral universe to explain epidemic disease was hardly omnipresent in antiquity even from the earliest writers, Hesiod and Homer, or later with Christian polemicists into the sixth century. Instead, the majority turned to natural causes, without reflecting on previous human misdeeds (thirty-two cases versus twenty-three). Moreover, over a third of the epidemics explained within a moral universe derived from shadowy and temporally indeterminate worlds of mythology, while those explained naturally derived almost exclusively from datable historical time. In addition to the effects of war, scarcity of supplies, famine, abrupt changes in diet, and climate, ancient commentators also saw epidemics spreading by human contact and contagion, as well from animals to humans, and in one instance from humans to animals.[146]

In addition to explaining the rise of epidemics by natural causes alone, ancient writers occasionally attacked directly moral explanations of epidemics. Reflecting on Rome's distant past (*c.*672 to 640 BCE) just after the death of its second king, Numa Pompilius (*c.*753–673 BCE), Livy accused early Romans of becoming filled with 'all sorts of superstitions great and small' because of the spread of a pestilence in the city. The superstitions included the belief that 'the only remedy left for their ailing bodies was to procure the peace and forgiveness from the gods'.[147] Dionysius of Halicarnassus reported a pestilence that began with cattle and spread to people. Some thought it erupted because the Heavens had grown angry with the Romans for having banished their most deserving citizens, but others maintained that these and other human events were due to chance.[148] In his life of Nero, Suetonius (*c.*69–*c.*130 CE) distinguished between disasters caused by the prince and ones that were accidents of fortune, such as a plague, which in a single autumn had killed 30,000 people.[149]

Fragments from Greek mathematical works poke jibes at the oracles' advice on how to end plagues. To end a fictional one in the period of Plato, an oracle demanded that a community build a new altar 'double the existing one'. The community would have to compute how to double the space—the duplication of the cube. The fragment's oracle was a reproach to Athenians for neglecting mathematics and their supposed contempt of geometry.[150] The second-century CE satirist Lucian mocked the oracles and their cryptic verses. Such amulets could even prove counterproductive, as with a verse placed over doorways to ward off the plague.

---

[145] On the three constitutions, physicians' visitations at Thasos, see Hippocrates, *Epidemics*, 1.1–26. Similarly, Hippocrates, in the opening of *Airs, Waters, Places*, establishes that the determinants of disease were naturalistic. At the same time, as King ('Comparative Perspectives', 85) has shown, the Hippocratic doctors saw prayer benefitting healing and sponsored the cult of Ascelpius.

[146] Herodian, *History of the Empire*, 1.12.   [147] Livy, 1.31.

[148] Dionysius of Halicarnassus, *Roman Antiquities*, 7.68.

[149] Suetonius, *Lives of the Caesars, Nero*, 6.39.   [150] *Greek Mathematical Works*, 9.1.

In fact, the houses worst afflicted were the ones with the verses. Lucian pondered if the verse had instead been an unlucky curse, but reasoned that the inscriptions had no magical effect. Rather the negative consequence arose from believers' false confidence in the verses, leading them not to take precautions.[151] In the first century CE, Plutarch reported that numerous oracles had lost their authority to ward off plague, as at Orchomenus in Boeotia.[152] Around the same time, the satirist at Nero's court, Petronius Arbiter, saw any belief in oracles as absurd. His example turned on 'oracles in time of pestilence'—the demand for 'the blood of three virgins or more, honey-balls of phrases, every word and act besprinkled with poppy-seed and sesame'.[153] This survey of epidemic explanations in antiquity challenges the widespread assumption that societies up to the laboratory revolution saw 'spirits, witches, sorcery, and other magico-religious forces' as causing disease and that this was the reason why they sought scapegoats and resorted to collective violence in times of plague.[154] Chapter 2 further explores these scapegoats and blame for disease in antiquity, exposing a world far removed from modernity but not in the direction we might have expected. It also sketches another moral universe, one that stretched across the long duration of antiquity and the Middle Ages, spawning individual and community compassion in the face of pestilence. This culture of pestilence has yet to be explored.

---

[151] Lucian, *Alexander the False Prophet*, XXVI.   [152] Plutarch, *Moralia*, 5.44.
[153] Petronius, *Satyricon*, 2–3.
[154] See, for instance, the medical sociologist, Rushing, *The AIDS Epidemic*, 132, who cites a number of authorities for his claims, including Ackernecht, *Medicine and Ethnology*, 121–3.

2

Ancient Epidemics
What the Oracles Had to Say

Before the end of the first century CE, the oracles' remedies to end plagues lend insight into the socio-psychological reactions to epidemic disease in antiquity.[1] We begin with those remedies that involved human sacrifice and antique notions of the scapegoat. As seen in Chapter 1, most prominent of these was the Minotaur story. Over time, the oracles appear to have changed their minds from the original ghoulish sacrifices, demanding the flesh of Hyacinth's daughters, and afterwards, an annual supply of seven Athenian youths and seven damsels to satisfy the man-bull's appetite. As early as the fourth century BCE, versions of the myth required no human sacrifice, and by the third century BCE, if not before, both the Minotaur and human sacrifice had vanished. The annual Athenian tribute to King Minos had become one of games, honouring his murdered son, in which Athenian youth could win prizes. Other examples of 'scapegoating' to end epidemics chart similar trajectories from human sacrifice to substitution of animals to no sacrifices by killing at all. Instead, the oracles and Rome's Sibylline books demanded the opposite: charity and ending civil strife between classes or wars among nations.

THE SCAPEGOAT

First, oracles certainly did not invariably ask for human sacrifice to arrest pestilence. Of thirty-five cases that I have found of communities or their leaders going to oracles, their priestesses, or sacred books to end plagues, ten demanded human sacrifice. Yet, as we shall see, several of these did not materialize, and for others the oracles or communities' interpretations of them changed the demands over time. The majority of these stories of human sacrifice occurred in mythological time. Apollodorus tells the story of when the Locrians regained their country in central Greece only to be stricken three years later by plague. An oracle demanded that they placate Athena at Ilium (Troy) by sending her two maiden suppliants for a thousand years. But the command seems never to have been implemented. Even the first chosen, Periboea and Cleopatra, escaped to Troy, where they took refuge in a sanctuary. Here, they swept and sprinkled the floors, cropped their hair, wore simple garments and no shoes, but they were not sacrificed.[2]

---

[1] On oracles, see Fontenrose, *The Delphic Oracle*.
[2] Apollodorus, *The Library*, II, *Epitome*, 266–7. Also, Hughes, *Human Sacrifice*, 168–9.

According to fragments from the sixth-century BCE poet Hipponax of Ephesus, the *pharmakos* was a purification ritual performed when a famine, pestilence, or other natural disaster struck a city. Supposedly, the ugliest man in town was sacrificed to purify the city and remedy the illness. He was given cheese, barley, and dried figs, while they flogged his penis seven times with squills and wild fig branches. Then they burnt him alive and scattered his ashes in the sea and to the winds.[3] In a surviving fragment of a play by Euripides, King Athamas of Boeotia sent a servant to Delphi because his kingdom was stricken by famine and plague. His wife Ino intercepted the servant and told him to bring back a false oracle, proclaiming that if Athamas sacrificed Phrixus, one of his twin sons sired by another of his three wives—the goddess Nephele—Zeus would stop the plague. The father refused to obey the oracle and bound his son for the sacrifice. Out of pity for the boy, the servant revealed the plot and exposed the culprit. Athamas handed Ino and one of her sons over to Phrixus for execution. But they too were saved: in this case by Dionysius, who happened to have been nursed by Ino. The dramatic fragment never reveals the actual oracle delivered at Delphi, but in the play, no human sacrifice occurred.[4] Another myth of human sacrifice linked to plague comes from the same region. As we have seen, the murder of Dionysius' priest caused a plague. To end it, the Delphic oracle demanded the sacrifice of a boy 'in the bloom of youth'. But within a few years, Dionysius changed the oracle, substituting a goat for the boy.[5]

Another oracle from Greek mythology commanded a human sacrifice to end a plague at Syracuse (Sicily), but it differed from those above: it was a death sentence against an individual who had disturbed the moral universe by dishonouring the gods rather than the sacrifice of an innocent child, youth, or animal. An oracle at Syracuse demanded that the community 'sacrifice the "impious man"' (without naming Cyanippus) who had angered the gods and then violated his own daughter. Only that daughter, Cyanê, knew the guilty one. She cut his throat, then her own; so in the end, the oracle reaped an innocent's death, but the death of the innocent one was unintended.[6] Plutarch presents two further plague stories calling for human sacrifice. With a pestilence raging at Sparta, an oracle decreed the epidemic would not cease unless a noble maiden was sacrificed yearly. Helen of Sparta (also known as of Troy), daughter of Zeus, was to be the first victim. When led to her sacrifice, an eagle swooped down, snatched the executioner's sword, carried it to a field, and dropped it on a heifer. Spartans then knew not to sacrifice their maidens.[7] A similar fate awaited the innocent when a plague afflicted the ancient Etruscan city of Falerii (in the province of Viterbo). Here, however, the eagle was late arriving. To end the plague, an oracle advised the city to sacrifice a maiden yearly to Juno (which Plutarch called 'superstitious'). Many perished from the practice, until a noble damsel, Valeria Lupera, was drawn by lot. An eagle then swooped down,

---

[3] *Greek Iambic Poetry*: Hipponax, *Fragments*, V. On this ritual, see Hughes, *Human Sacrifice*, 141–3, who suggests it was an annual custom with probably nothing to do with plague or famine.

[4] Euripides, VII: *Dramatic Fragments*, 436–7.

[5] Pausanias, *Description of Greece*, Boeotia, 8.1–2.   [6] Plutarch, *Moralia*, 4.9.

[7] Ibid., 9.35; also Hughes, *Human Sacrifice*, 82–3.

stole the sword, and dropped it on a heifer. Understanding its significance, the girl grabbed the sword and sacrificed the heifer, ending the human sacrifice.[8] Another reference to human sacrifice comes from the first-century CE satirist Petronius. While it does not derive from Greek mythology, it comes from an undatable past, a supposed custom of 'the people of Massilia [Marseille]'. When pestilence struck that city, one of the poor would volunteer (not chosen by lot as in Attica). From public funds, the volunteer was fed for a year 'on food of special purity', clothed with sacred herbs and sacred robes, and led through the streets, cursed by the people, 'in order that the sufferings of the whole state might fall upon him; and so he was cast out'.[9]

A final case of an oracle calling for human blood to stop plague was also of a sort different from mythology. This one derived from hypothetical cases invented to teach law students around the second century CE by a rhetorician of the school of Quintilian. The exemplum hardly venerated oracle wisdom. It ridiculed the archaic rites of human sacrifice even more than Plutarch's of a century earlier. 'A people suffering from pestilence' (it is not stated who or where) sent a legate to an unspecified oracle, which informed the official that his own son was to be sacrificed. The legate announced the required sacral procedures to the citizens without revealing the targeted person but confessed the truth to his son. The plague continued. The son came to an assembly and killed himself. After the plague ended, the legate was tried for treason.[10] By the late second or third century BCE, even the sacrifice of animals to end plague appears to have become a dim memory. The *Historia Augusta* (*c.*117–284 CE) refers to

> an emperor's sacrifice, a hundred lions, a hundred eagles, and several hundreds of other animals of this kind. The Greeks, it is said, at one time used to do this when suffering from a pestilence, and it seems generally agreed that it was performed by many emperors.[11]

Yet none of our sources ever mentions an oracle commanding the mass slaughter of exotic animals.[12]

Against these oracles' commands for human sacrifice from mythology, hypothetical cases, or vague notions of past customs, I have thus far found only four connected with epidemics within historically dated time, despite dated references to pestilences being far more numerous than ones from mythological time. Moreover, of the four, one may have been an invented story; another was not exactly a ritual sacrifice of the innocent but an execution of persons judged to have committed grave crimes; and the third was from a philosopher, not an oracle. This last example, mentioned in Chapter 1, reached back to a plague in seventh-century BCE Athens, and was in its more prominent version an animal sacrifice at Areopagus, north-west of the

---

   [8] Ibid.
   [9] Petronius, *Fragments*, I. In other versions, he was stoned to death outside the city; Hughes, *Human Sacrifice*, 158–9.
   [10] [Quintilian], *The Lesser Declamations*, no. 326.   [11] *Historia Augusta*, 21.11.
   [12] According to Livy, 22.10, it was exceptional in 217 BCE, when 300 oxen and 300 white oxen were sacrificed to Jupiter, but these were not exotic animals.

Acropolis. In Diogenes' version, a sacrifice of two young men replaced the sheep to deliver Athens from the pestilence.[13]

A second story appears in the distant past from an author's perspective, the first-century CE commentator Valerius Maximus. A serious Roman plague that can be dated through Livy's *History of Rome* to 364 BCE prompted citizens to prepare a banquet (a Lectisternium), the third in its history, to appease the gods.[14] Unlike Livy, Valerius tells a story of human sacrifice that may have been his invention. A wealthy man of rustic ways called Valesius had two sons and a daughter dying from the plague. He prayed for the gods to transfer the disease from them to himself. A voice told him to take his children down the Tiber to Tarentum to refresh them with water from the altar of Dis Pater and Proserpine, but no altar was found; so Valesius ordered his men to dig on the spot. Twenty feet down, they found the original altar. Saved from buying a new one, he decided to sacrifice black victims called 'duskies'. In addition, he spread out the couches for banquets and held games at Tarentum for three consecutive nights, and his children were cured.[15]

A third story occurs more than two centuries later and this one without any of the ambivalences seen in Solon's time or even for several of the mythological ones. In 181 BCE, Livy reports a pestilence that spread through market towns and villages around Rome, which was so severe that funerary materials became scarce. Alarmed by its deadliness, the city fathers decreed that the consuls sacrifice full-grown victims (*hostiis maioribus*) to whatever deities they deemed proper.[16] The next plague that caused Romans to execute humans was not a sacrifice, nor had any oracle advised it, and perhaps it should be excluded from our list. It was the execution of those guilty of the impious defilement of the Vestal Virgin Urbinia that to end plague resulted in her flogging and burning, the suicide of one of her lovers, and the ceremonial execution of the other.

In summary, ritualistic sacrifices of humans to end pestilence were rare in antiquity. The majority, moreover, are fixed in legendary time or invented to ridicule the practice and belief in oracles. Additionally, authors relate that several of these never occurred or ended after a short spell without enduring for a thousand years as first commanded. But more to our historical point, the scapegoating in these ancient and archaic sacrifices was categorically different from the nineteenth-century notion of the term that continues today: that the sacrificed were minorities, the poor, or some other despised group held responsible for bringing about an epidemic. First, the sacrificed in antiquity were individuals, not distinct groups, and were often drawn by lot or could even volunteer. On first sight, three cases may appear as exceptions. The probably concocted story of the ugliest man in town was not in any case an attack against a distinctive group of ill-favoured uglies, and the chosen one was not an outsider but a member of the community. Petronius' satire about the sacrifice of a poor man was again one individual, not an attack on the poor, and he had volunteered. Even the case (again, probably concocted) of the rich rustic

---

[13] Chapter 1, note 95. Hughes, *Human Sacrifice*, 155, called this version fictional.
[14] Livy, 7.2.   [15] Valerius Maximus, *Memorable Doings*, 2.5.
[16] Livy, 40.19.

sacrificing 'duskies' at Tarentum casts no racial shame on blacks for causing the plague. These three cases, however, were exceptional in another sense: unlike the other stories of human sacrifice, the victims were not drawn from the elites. In antiquity, the rule was different: for a sacrifice to be worthy, the victims represented a community's future at its highest and included the most beautiful noble youths and maidens, even Helen of Troy or the king of Thebes.

At the end of the first century CE, the earliest surviving epistle in Christianity after the New Testament, the letter of Clement, bishop of Rome (*c.*96), gives further insights into pagan sacrifices in Roman history linked to plague. Paragraph 54 of this book-length letter asks who among you is noble, compassionate, or filled with love. And who have performed their civic duties to God? In contrast to early Christian writers such as Orosius, Eusebius, and Augustine, Clement begins his exempla by applauding the Gentiles:

> Many kings and rulers, [who] after receiving instruction from an oracle, have handed themselves over to death during the time of plague, in order to deliver their fellow citizens by shedding their own blood. Many left their own cities to avoid creating more factions.[17]

Even in the pagan realm, this Christian recognized that human sacrifice had transformed into charity and abnegation. Certainly, Christianity had not created this tradition.

BLAME

In the hundreds of stories of pestilence in ancient societies—historical, exemplary, and mythological—only three exceptions by two authors, all three reinterpreting the same Old Testament story, cast blame for creating pestilence. Two of these condemned and targeted the outsider, and in these cases, the outsider was a distinct social group or groups. Surprisingly, recent historians wishing to argue that ancient societies blamed outsiders for epidemics have failed to mention these exceptions. All three inverted the Exodus story of Moses, the Hebrews' liberation from Egyptian bondage, and their forty years in the desert before entering Judaea. For the first-century BCE Diodorus and for Tacitus, writing in the second half of the first century CE, the Jews' exodus was instead their expulsion. Their stories, however, differ. According to Diodorus, because of pestilence native Egyptians cast out not only Jews but aliens of all sorts. The 'common people' ascribed the troubles to divine agency and found their own rites, sacrifices, and traditional religious practices under threat because of the numbers of foreigners living in their midst. They included those led by Danaüs, who as a consequence would found Argos in the Mycenaean Peloponnese, and others led by Cadmus, the celebrated founder and first king of Thebes. But the greatest number expelled were the Jews led by Moses, 'outstanding both for his wisdom and for his courage', who founded cities and

---

[17] *The Apostolic Fathers*, 1.54–5.

most importantly, 'the colony' of Judaea. From this expulsion, Moses 'established the temple that the Jews hold in chief veneration, instituted their forms of worship and ritual'.[18] Thus, by Diodorus' first rendition, the Egyptian expulsion enabled these foreigners to found their own civilizations; ultimately, they became stories of liberation.

In recounting the later siege of Jerusalem by King Antiochus (VII Euergetes [the Benefactor], nicknamed Sidetes) in 134 BCE, Diodorus reflected again on Moses and the subsequent trajectory of Jewish civilization. His view now changed from praise to anti-Semitic condemnation, or at least these are the sentiments the Sicilian ascribes approvingly to those who advised the second-century BCE king. They urged him 'to take the city by storm' and wipe out completely 'the race of Jews', since 'they alone of all nations avoided dealings with any other people and looked upon all men as their enemies'. To back their claims they returned to the Jews' exodus from Egypt, arguing that they had been driven, not liberated, from Egypt because they were 'impious and detested by the gods'. In this version, plague was not the impetus for assembling and driving out foreign peoples. Now, the Jews along with other aliens were purged from Egypt because of their 'curse' by leprosy.[19] Moreover, once they occupied the territory around Jerusalem, they organized a nation that made 'their hatred of mankind into a tradition'. They 'introduced utterly outlandish laws: not to break bread with any other race, nor to show them any good will at all'.[20] The wise and courageous Moses of book XL was now transmogrified into 'the man, who ordained for the Jews "their misanthropic and lawless customs"'.[21]

Tacitus' retelling of Exodus adds further details. While earlier authors of the Exodus expulsion story had emphasized leprosy as the cause, Tacitus pinned the blame on plague (*tabes*) for causing the Jews' bodily disfigurement that threatened to spread the ailment among the Egyptians. To rid the country of the threat, the eighth-century BCE king of the Egyptians, Bocchoris,[22] approached the oracle of Ammon at the Siwah oasis (Libya) and was instructed to purge 'the race' of Hebrews from his lands because they were 'hateful to the gods'. He searched them out and banished them into the desert. In their new lands of conquest, Tacitus sketched their 'new religious practices', concluding they were 'opposed to those of all other religions. The Jews regard as profane all that we hold sacred' and 'permit all that we abhor'.[23] Finally, in the first century CE, Alexandrian scholars harked back to the third-century BCE Egyptian priest Manetho, whose histories no longer survive. In their versions, the disease justifying the Jews' expulsion was not an epidemic but chronic leprosy imagined as a genetic component of the Hebrew race. Once the Jews reached Judaea, they plundered and set fire to the inhabitants' temples.[24]

---

[18] Diodorus, *The Library of History*, 40.3.   [19] Ibid., 34/35.1.
[20] Ibid.   [21] Ibid.
[22] The biblical Exodus had traditionally been dated to 1450 BCE but now to the eighth century BCE.
[23] Tacitus, *Histories*, 5.3–4.
[24] See van der Horst, 'From Liberation to Expulsion', 389–94; and Bar-Kochva, *The Image of the Jews*, 316–26, which reflects on other versions of the story. According to Manetho (*History of Egypt*, 120–5, 134–5, 138–9, 142–5), the lepers cleansed from Egypt included Egyptians and Jews, and

Yet these exceptions, all based on reinventing one story almost a millennium after the events, do not alter the general pattern. Of the many pronouncements of the oracles—the ones already discussed and others to be investigated in this chapter—the inverted Exodus story is the lone exception and Ammon the lone oracle that advised a ruler to purge any minority or 'race' to end pestilence.

BONES

As the examples suggest, oracles, priestesses, and Sibylline books bade communities to do more than sacrifice humans or animals when pestilence threatened. They proposed a variety of remedies: some were practical; some mysterious; some simple. For instance, in recounting the trials and tribulations of Aeneas and the Trojans, Virgil (70–19 BCE) describes a pestilence that caused them to flee Pergamum. Urged on by his father, Aeneas consulted the oracle of Ortygia, which confirmed his father's advice to re-cross the sea.[25] Valerius Maximus recalled a pestilence that afflicted Rome for three years, for which 'neither divine pity nor human aid' was of any use. The priests inspected the Sibylline books and discovered the only remedy was to call on the famed physician from Epidarus and god of Medicine, Aesculaprius (Ascelpius).[26] In other instances, the oracles' replies to their plague-stricken communities were more mysterious. In two regions of Greece at two different times, the oracle at Delphi's response was a call for bones. In the first story, 'many years after the Battle of Troy', a fisherman from Eretria arrived at Delphi at the same time as an envoy from the region of Elis: the fisherman asked what he was to do with human bones he had just found, and the Eleans, suffering from pestilence, asked how to rid themselves of the disease. The priestess ordered the Eleans 'to recover' the bones of Pelops, a king of their region at the time of the Trojan War, and the fisherman to give to them those he had found (which happened to be the old king's scapula). The fisherman obeyed; the plague ended, and the Eleans appointed him and his descendants as guardians of the bone.[27] The second bone story is much the same. A pestilence of cattle and humans struck the region around the sanctuary of Orchomenus (in Boeotia). An envoy went to Delphi to find a cure and was told that the 'one and only remedy' was to recover the bones of Hesiod,

Moses was an Egyptian god, not a Jew. However, Manetho's works are known from citations by others, and for this section, Josephus. On Josephus' attack on the story concocted by first-century CE Alexandrian scholars, see *The Life. Against Apion*, 1.229–37 and 1.304–11. In the version of the Alexandrian Lysimachus, King Bocchoris consulted the oracle of Ammon because of a drought and crop failures. The response triggered another reversal of the biblical Exodus: the command was to purify the temples and the land by drowning lepers and those afflicted by scurvy in the Red Sea and sending other 'unclean' people into the desert. Parts of this Exodus/expulsion story were repeated in the early sixteenth century in connection with another expulsion story, that from Spain in 1492, when Jews were afflicted with syphilis because of their supposed disposition for leprosy; see Chapter 5.

[25] Virgil, *Aeneid*, 3.121–46.
[26] Valerius Maximus, *Memorable Doings*, 1.2. On the enduring importance of Aesculaprius, reaching his pinnacle of success in the second century ce, see Nutton, 'Medicine', 956; Napier, *Masks*, 80–2, 234–5; Lloyd, *In the Grip of Disease*, 40, 53, 57, 85, 237.
[27] Pausanias, *Description of Greece*, Elis 1.13.

their ancestor, and bring them back from the land of Naupactus.[28] So what do we make of these stories: were they just matters of magic? As seen in these examples, of which more shall shortly follow, the advice of oracles and sacred books had an overriding theme—unity. In the face of pestilential adversity, the command was not to purify by expelling any 'other' or despised foreign body but to mend societal divisions. As Joseph Fontenrose argued, the recovery of heroes' bones protected communities against defeat from antagonistic cities.[29] The stories emphasized the themes of unifying the community against any adversity and also with their own ancestors.

GAMES, THEATRE, BANQUETS, AND VOWS

Similar to processions, commissions for votive shrines, and celebrations of thanksgiving during or immediately after plagues in late medieval and early modern Europe, antique oracles and priestly interpretations of sacred books also called on societies to bind together when pestilence threatened. In 399 BCE a cold winter followed abruptly by summer heat produced a severe pestilence.[30] Failing to understand the disease's cause or find a cure, the senate commanded their priests to consult the Sibylline books. The resolution was to invent a banquet, the 'lectisternium'. Three couches were spread out for Apollo, Latona, Diana, Hercules, Mercury, and Neptune, 'with all the splendour then attainable to honour the gods'. The banquet lasted eight days. It was no modern 'gala' exclusive to elites but instead embraced the entire population, including outsiders, foreigners, even prisoners:

> It is stated that throughout the City the front gates of the houses were thrown open and all sorts of things placed for general use in the open courts, all comers, whether acquaintances or strangers, being brought in to share the hospitality. Men who had been enemies held friendly and sociable conversations with each other and abstained from all litigation, the manacles even were removed from prisoners during this period, and afterwards it seemed an act of impiety that men to whom the gods had brought such relief should be put in chains again.[31]

The lectisternium became a tradition repeated at least three times during the fourth century BCE, called on when a pestilence was particularly mysterious and severe as in 364 BCE, 'with neither human wisdom nor the help of Heaven able to mitigate the scourge',[32] and again in 347–6 BCE.[33] To end other plagues, the sacred books called on Roman governments to bequeath largesse on the population in the form

---

[28] Ibid., Boeotia, XXXVIII.
[29] Fontenrose, *The Delphic Oracle*, 73–5. For another multilayered story of bone recovery, see Zaccarini, 'The Return of Theseus'.
[30] Curiously, the editor translates 'gravis pestilens' as 'distemper'.
[31] Livy, 5.13. Here, I follow the translation in Perseus by Rev. Canon Roberts.
[32] Ibid., 7, 2.
[33] Ibid., 7, 27. The lectisternium continued into the second century BCE, but after 347–6 BCE, I have found it connected with war, not epidemics, and it had lost its original character of opening homes to strangers and ending litigation; see ibid., 8.25, 98–9 (326 BCE); 21.62,186–7 (218 BCE); 22.1, 202–3 (217 BCE); 22.9, 230–1 (217 BCE); 22.10, 234–5 (217 BCE).

of extended work-free holidays as in 181 BCE, when the keeper of the Sibylline books decreed that a special intercession should be offered at all the shrines for a day with work suspended for three days throughout Italy.[34]

Severe epidemics also sparked other new and communal forms of piety and entertainment, which did not always receive praise from later commentators. Livy describes a pestilence lasting two years, 364–3 BCE, which could not be 'alleviated by…men or gods'. The lectisternium of 364 BCE had failed and people's minds, according to Livy, had become 'completely overcome by superstitious terrors'. To placate heaven's wrath, Romans invented another ceremonial performance, a type of musical theatre with 'scenic representations', in which characters danced to the measures of the flute and practised graceful movements in the Etruscan fashion. The ritual 'became an established diversion and was kept up by frequent practice'. Yet Livy was ambivalent: not only did it reflect 'superstitious fears', it was 'a novelty to a nation of warriors who had hitherto only had the games of the Circus'. Young Romans imitated the Etruria dance 'to the strains of the flautist…exchanging jests in uncouth verses, and bringing their movements into a certain harmony with the words'. The professional actors were called 'histriones, fromister', Etruscan for player.

Looking back on these practices of pagan entertainment to placate the gods during plague, Augustine was more scathing. He saw the performance as a sham, a craft of profane spirit. Foreseeing that pestilence had run its course, soon to end, the players took the opportunity 'to infect…their moral nature with another, far more serious, plague' of the mind.[35] Moreover, he repeated this invective several more time in his *City of God*.[36] Yet, despite his frequent tirades against the Romans, he does not reveal any pagan practices to end plague that created social or political divisions or led to persecuting foreigners or any groups within Roman society. Instead, his criticism was the opposite: to his chagrin, these performances created 'delight' in unifying Romans in the face of their pestilential adversities.

Plague and the priestly interpretations of the sacred books also spurred celebrations at the statues of gods, public religious vows, new festivals of thanksgiving, and further work-free holidays. These too produced public gatherings at places such as the Forum to unite social classes. In 208 BCE 'a serious pestilence' struck Rome, which was usually not fatal but inflicted long illness. To still the epidemic, prayers were organized at street corners, and the city Praetor proposed a bill that games should be vowed in perpetuity on a fixed date. Three years later, it was approved, and the chosen day became a holiday.[37] In 174 BCE, because a plague continued to linger, the senate advised consulting the Sibylline books and decreed a day of prayer, in which 'the people' would assemble in the Forum. When the disease ended, collectively, they promised to celebrate a festival of thanksgiving for two days.[38] The following year, portents and plague prompted further intercessions along with a repeat of the

---

[34] Livy, 40.19.   [35] Augustine, *The City of God*, 1.32, 132–3.
[36] Ibid., 3.17, 340–1; and 2.8, 168–9.   [37] Livy, 27.23.
[38] Ibid., 41.41.

previous year's public vows at the Forum.[39] Yet, the most dramatic of these cross-class, cross-gender, and cross-age assemblies among the Romans appears much earlier, during a plague of 462 BCE. 'Finding no help in man' to stop or cure the pestilence,

> the state summoned the people of Rome with their wives and children to supplicate Heaven for forgiveness. They crowded the shrines, and everywhere were prostrate matrons, sweeping the floors of the temples with their hair...[40]

Furthermore, ancient authors describe plagues easing class tensions, intrigues, and conflict between the plebeians and senatorial classes. In 433–2 BCE, a plague provided a respite from struggles over elections between the tribunes of the plebs and patricians. The two classes allied to build a temple to honour Apollo 'for the health of the people'. Moreover, to avert impending famine, with so many farmers afflicted, the government intervened, sending for grain from Etruria, Pomptine, and Sicily to be paid for from its reserves.[41] Two decades later, another plague rescued Rome from another threat of class war. The leader of the plebeian tribuneship, Lucius Icilius, had been stirring sedition through legislating new and radical agrarian reforms. The outbreak of pestilence thwarted his designs. Men's minds turned from the Forum and political strife 'to their homes and the care of the sick'. As in 432 BCE, 'considering the great number...who had fallen ill', political factions unified to ensure famine would not follow pestilence, dispatching emissaries to purchase grain.[42] Evidence of plague averting civil strife did not pertain solely to Rome or to class struggle. Around the mid-fifth century BCE, after the death of the famous Olympian Theagenes of Thasos, pestilence erupted at Thasos. Unable to remedy it, the islanders consulted an oracle and were instructed to 'restore the exiles'.[43] Interpretations of this story were complex and we shall return to them, but its first meaning was straightforward. The message was unity: instead of expelling rival groups, plague called on them to reunite.

Not all natural disasters, however, were alike. In contrast to pestilence, famine could provoke accusations and incite protest against the senate and theatre-going elites,[44] and often led to violent sedition, as Peter Garnsey has shown for Rome from the fifth century BCE to the end of the fourth century CE and Dionysios Stathakopoulos for all the major cities of the Roman Empire, east and west, from the fifth to the seventh century CE.[45] Furthermore, in his life of Caius [Gnaeus] Marcius Coriolanus, Plutarch records class tensions arising within Rome in the early fifth century BCE from a famine at the conclusion of a war with the Volscians.

---

[39] Ibid., 42.2.   [40] Ibid., 3.7.   [41] Ibid., 4.25.   [42] Ibid., 4.52.

[43] Dio Chrysostom, *Discourses*, 31.95–9. After the Thasoians had restored their exiles, the plague, nonetheless, continued. The oracle offered a second cryptic message, in which 'exiles' was interpreted to mean one exile in particular, the island's deceased Olympian hero, Theagenes, whose statue had fallen, killing one of his former opponents; the criminal courts sentenced the statue to be thrown into the sea.

[44] See Garnsey, *Famine and Food Supply*, 206.

[45] For ancient Rome, see ibid., 29, 206, 207–8, 226, 240–3. Garnsey maintains that no food riots occurred in democratic Athens (30). For food riots in Constantinople, Rome, Antioch, Alexandria, and Thessalonica in late antiquity, see Stathakopoulos, *Famine and Pestilence*, I, 73, II, 30, 42, 59.

With a scarcity of market supplies and 'the people' without money to buy them, leaders of the plebeians 'assailed the rich with slanderous accusations of purposely arraying the famine against them, in a spirit of revenge'. Pestilence, however, soon ensued and ended the slanders and threats of sedition. In neighbouring Velitra, a serious pestilence left 'hardly a tenth of their population alive',[46] convincing the Romans to end their social antagonisms. Hot-headed citizens from the populace were elected as Consuls and ordered forth as colonists to assist their enemies—the crippled Velitrae—while others were enlisted in a campaign against the Volscians. In Plutarch's words, now there was 'no leisure for intestine tumults, and believing that when rich and poor alike, plebeians as well as patricians, were once more united in military service and in common struggles for the public good, they would be more gently and pleasantly disposed towards one another'.[47] Later in the fifth century, another epidemic showed the force of plague to mitigate class struggle. In 435–6, pestilence caused 'fears and ravages in city and country', which led plebs and patricians to abandon 'any thought of waging war'. According to Livy, a tribune of the plebs, Spurius Maelius, 'tried to stir disturbances against the patricians', but failed: 'the people paid less attention to these accusations... now they were much more concerned about the increasing virulence of the epidemic'.[48] Ancients from biblical times to at least the time of Josephus thought pestilence was the least likely disaster to induce blame. Josephus relates the biblical parable, 2 Samuel 24. Angry with David, God offered him a choice of punishing his people by one of three disasters—famine, war, or pestilence. After tortured deliberation and procrastination, he chose plague, reasoning that for that disaster he would appear the least blameworthy.[49]

Back to Rome's fifth-century war against the Velitrae and Volscians, plague also ended external hostilities. In this case, it changed Roman sentiments towards at least one of their enemies. The Romans answered the Velitrae's request to send them a large colony of emigrants to replenish their catastrophic demographic loss. According to Dionysius of Halicarnassus, Rome's plebeians under periodic threat of famine were at first pleased with this prospect of gaining new lands in a fertile country, even if they began to fear the dangers of contagion. According to Plutarch, the Velitrae's request came at a propitious moment. Rome could rid itself 'of its burdensome numbers', and the elites could dissipate the threat of sedition.[50]

PUBLIC WORKS AND CHARITY

As we have seen in the previous section, plagues moved ancient governments at least temporarily to end hostilities and hatred and commit to benefiting the poor by purchasing cereals with public funds. Rulers' ameliorative actions, however,

---

[46] According to Dionysius of Halicarnassus, *Roman Antiquities*, 7.13, this pestilence hit the Volscians the worst.

[47] *Plutarch's Lives, Coriolanus*, 9.12.   [48] Livy, 4.21.

[49] Josephus, *Jewish Antiquities*, 8.2–3.

[50] Dionysius of Halicarnassus, *Roman Antiquities*, 2.54; and Plutarch, *Lives. Coriolanus*, XII.

went beyond supplies of grain, as suggested in a mythological story told by Valerius Maximus. When Rome was afflicted by a particularly mysterious pestilence, the Sibylline books instructed its leaders to bring Aescelpius, the god of medicine, to their city, a task requiring embassies and expenditure. Other stories praise the behaviour of leaders at specific moments in historical time. Except for the first of these listed below, the accounts derived from contemporaries or near-contemporaries of the leaders they praised. As cited in the first section of this chapter, the third-century Diogenes described a plague in the Greek colony of Selinus, probably during the fifth century BCE, which colonists believed had been caused by smells emanating from a nearby river. At his own expense, the philosopher Empedocles conceived a plan to converge two neighbouring rivers, calculating that their confluence would sweeten the waters. The plan worked, and the city praised him as a god.[51] Suetonius praised Emperor Titus (39–81 CE) for his service during a plague, when he employed 'every kind of sacrifice' and sought to procure 'all kinds of medicines'.[52] The *Historia Augusta* extolled Marcus Aurelius for his charity from his own estates during the great pandemic named after him. For the nobility who perished during the decade-and-a-half-long plague, he erected statues for their commemoration, and for the poor, he celebrated their funerals at public expense.[53] His strategy for maintaining stability during the plague was not to blame any social group or foreigners. Instead, he opened new occupational opportunities for them. Addressing the decline of his soldiers and guards because of the pandemic, he trained slaves for military service and called them 'volunteers' (*voluntarios*). He armed gladiators and recruited 'even bandits of Dalmatia and Dardania', converting them into soldiers and hired troops from the Germanic tribes to fight against other Germanic tribes.[54]

For the next pandemic that swept Europe, northern Africa, and the Middle East, the Plague of Justinian, its principal historian, Procopius, paid similar tribute to an emperor and his administration. With mounting plague deaths in Constantinople ('Byzantium') from a trickle to 'five thousand…even ten thousand a day', and with 'confusion and disorder everywhere', slaves, destitute without masters, and men previously very prosperous 'deprived of their domestics', Justinian stepped in, sending the military to assist civilians and to distribute money to them.[55] His announcer of imperial messages, Theodorus, took over the relief, coordinating petitions, communicating the emperor's decisions, and allocating public funds for assistance. In addition, he gave from his own purse to ensure that piles of the plague dead would be buried.[56] Procopius' praise was all the more remarkable given his previous disposition towards the emperor as revealed in his *Secret History*, which lambasted the emperor for his greed, corruption, cruelty, and especially his support of the circus of the Blues[57] with their harassment and murder of rivals, fanning division

---

[51] Diogenes, *Lives: Empedocles*, 8.2.   [52] Suetonius, *Lives: Titus*, 8.2.
[53] *Historia Augusta*, 4.13.   [54] Ibid., 4.21.
[55] Also see editor's note 86, 233, in Evagrius, *Ecclesiastical History*, and 4.30; and 4.32, for Evagrius' berating of Justinian.
[56] Procopius, *History of the Wars*, 2.22.
[57] On circus factions, see Cameron, *Circus Factions*, esp. ch. 1.

throughout the city. The longer account, more apocalyptic, more repetitive, and more sparing of specific facts about this plague—that of John of Ephesus—makes one comment of praise: the 'merciful emperor' and his 'referendarius' Theodorus, 'also zealous in good deeds', judiciously spent the necessary monies to rid the streets and houses of corpses, supervised these matters, and encouraged people not to be negligent but to dig large ditches and to fill them by piling up the corpses.[58]

Emperors, administrators, and philosophers were not the only ones ancient authors acknowledged for charitable deeds and self-sacrifice in time of plague. Following an epidemic in Rome in 451 BCE, and the senate's public sacrifices of thanksgiving and games to alleviate the hardships, private merchants contributed to replenishing supplies of grain.[59] Plutarch in the first century CE supported what Thucydides had said earlier about the Plague of Athens: 'those who had the highest claim to virtue perished with their friends who were ill; for they did not spare themselves in going, as they did, to visit those who had claims on their friendship'.[60] As with the sympathy spurred by pestilential disaster shown by Romans to their enemies, cross-border sympathies also flowed Rome's way. Plutarch retells the story of the fourth-century BCE origins of 'histriones' from Livy, but Plutarch's has a different twist: the 365 BCE plague destroyed to a man all the stage actors in Rome. To revive their theatre, the Romans requested new actors from Etruria, and 'many excellent artists' came.[61]

Adding to Livy's account of the plague of 399 BCE, which introduced the first lectisternium, Dionysius of Halicarnassus used the now largely lost *Annals* of the mid-first-century CE plebeian tribune and consul Lucius Piso, 'the ex-censor'. In addition to the Roman elite preparing 'most magnificent banquets', 'entertaining the strangers who were sojourning in their midst', and liberating their slaves 'previously kept in chains', Piso's account recognized a reciprocal turn of gratitude and charity coming from the poor, freed slaves, and strangers:

> though the city was filled with a throng of strangers, and though the houses were open day and night and all who wished entered them without hindrance, yet no one complained of having lost anything or of having been wronged by anyone, even though festal occasions are wont to bring many disorderly and lawless deeds in their train because of the drunkenness attending them.[62]

At the end of the third century, by the account of the zealous bishop of Caesarea, plague advantaged Christians, affording them an opportunity to exhibit 'sympathy and humanity', 'charity and self-sacrifice' by 'performing last rites to the plague

---

[58] *Pseudo-Dionysius of Tel-Mahre: Chronicle*, 94–107, for the plague (mixed with other matters such as persecutions, earthquakes, and sins that prefigured the plague); and 91 for Justinian and Theodorus. Even when departing from stories of demons and prophecies, his stories appear far-fetched, as with daily plague deaths of 16,000 in Constantinople (86) and plague signs of three black pocks in the palm of the hand (88). For this plague's longer-term consequences, see *Plague and the End of Antiquity*.
[59] Dionysius of Halicarnassus, *Roman Antiquities*, 9.54. Livy mentions this plague only in passing, 3.32.
[60] Plutarch, *Moralia*, 2.7.   [61] Ibid., IV. *Roman Questions*, no. 107.
[62] Dionysius of Halicarnassus, *Roman Antiquities*, 12.9.

infected, burying the dead, and distributing bread to all'.[63] Some 240 years later, with the next pandemic, the picture was mixed, at least initially, as depicted by Procopius: while the corpses mounted, individuals at first

> were unwilling even to give heed to their friends when they called to them, and they shut themselves up in their rooms and pretended that they did not hear, although their doors were being beaten down, fearing, obviously, that he who was calling was one of those demons.[64]

But when the plague reached Constantinople, the story changed. Now, he praised physicians and others 'who were constantly engaged either in burying or attending the sick' and 'held out in the performance of this service beyond all expectation'.[65] Just as Livy, Dionysius of Halicarnassus, Plutarch, and others had done in pagan times, Procopius observed the ameliorative powers of plague in Christian times. Those who formerly had been members of factions (circus parties)[66] abandoned their hatred and allied to bury and honour the dead, carrying 'with their own hands' the bodies of those with whom they had no previous connections. 'Nay, more, those who in times past used to take delight in devoting themselves to pursuits both shameful and base shook off the unrighteousness of their daily lives'. Yet, as suggested earlier with the ancients, these noble habits and attitudes could be short lived. As soon as the terror of imminent death lifted, the same individuals turned 'once more to their baseness of heart, and now, more than before…altogether surpassing themselves in villainy and in lawlessness of every sort'.[67] Moreover, economic catastrophes accompanied pestilence, ending 'work of every description'. Yet Procopius' final assessment of his fellow-citizens in the capital remained positive. Neither he nor any other eyewitness of this plague described the searing Black Death horrors of abandonment by family members or of trusted priests, notaries, and doctors that rang through chronicles from Ireland to Poland 800 years later. Instead, at Constantinople:

> all who had the good fortune to be in health were sitting in their houses, either attending the sick or mourning the dead. And if one did succeed in meeting a man going out, he was carrying one of the dead.[68]

*   *   *

For late antiquity, historians have asserted that the Pestilence of Cyprian, *c.*249–*c.*275, coincided with tense relations between the Roman emperor and the emerging Christian community and that the epidemic sparked their persecution.[69] But the sources show little evidence of it. For a variety of reasons, Cyprian may have been threatened with being fed to the lions in the circus,[70] but his two letters on the plague

---

[63] Eusebius, *Ecclesiastical History*, 9.8.
[64] Procopius, *History of the Wars*, 2.22.12–17.   [65] Ibid., 2.22.24–9.
[66] See Stathakopoulos, *Famine and Pestilence*, 152.
[67] Procopius, *History of the Wars*, 2.23.   [68] Ibid.
[69] Stathakopoulos, 'Plagues of the Roman Empire'.
[70] See his epistle 59.6.1, cited in Clarke, 'Third-Century Christianity', 637.

do not relate persecution of Christians as due to the plague named after him.[71] By Orosius' account, the Romans understood the plague of 253 as God's fury against their persecutors, prompting an about-face in their policies, ending, not sparking, persecution.[72]

Instead, the 'Great Persecution' of Christians by the Roman emperors came half a century later, after a long period of toleration initiated by the plague of 253, during the rule of the emperor Valerian and then his son Gallienus. Moreover, no epidemic triggered the bloody decade of the 'Great Persecution', beginning with the edict against Christians in 303, with 'no end to the burning of churches, the proscription of the innocent, and the slaughter of martyrs',[73] orchestrated by Diocletian in the East and Maximian Herculius in the West.[74] Instead, a plague erupted towards the end of this decade-long slaughter, terminating the persecution, according to Eusebius, by God's punishment of the tyrants.[75]

Hundreds of epidemics can also be drawn from the sources of the early and central Middle Ages. For the period 541–767, Jean-Noël Biraben has found sixty-one episodes of plague alone in Europe, principally in the Mediterranean region, and more recently Dionysios Stathakopoulos has increased the number to 124.[76] Yet, none reports incidents of mass ethnic violence in this ethnically charged world or class hatred arising from these plagues. Moreover, such violence or accusations of intentional plague spreading remain rare for any epidemic before the Black Death of 1347–51. Agobard, bishop of Lyon, chronicles a story that circulated around 810: Grimoald IV, duke of the Beneventans, had supposedly sent some of his people to spread a special dust on fields, mountains, meadows, and springs of northern Europe to kill the cattle of his enemy, Charlemagne. Many were apprehended and confessed to have scattered the poisonous dust.[77] But this was an epidemic of cattle, not of people, and was a matter of economic warfare, not of internal anxieties leading to supposed diabolic acts or persecution of outsiders living within the affected society. In 1172, the army of Emperor Emanuele of Constantinople in conflict with the Venetians over possession of the island of Chios (Scio) in the Aegean

---

[71] His plague tract, *De mortalitate*, describes the signs and symptoms of the disease and claims that 'Many of us died from it', but says nothing about any ensuing persecution. Clarke, 'Third-Century Christianity', 637, nonetheless, conjectures: 'One can imagine orders for a public expiation against the plague, at a ceremony in the circus from which the notable figure of the leader of the Christians [was] popularly blamed for the visitation of the plague through their failure to worship "Roman gods"', but he supplies no evidence of any such persecution. Cyprian's 'Ad Demetrianum' was a defence against a local pagan who blamed Christians in general for war, drought, famine, and plague but relates no attacks against Christians in Carthage for the plague; see Harper, 'Pandemics', 229.

[72] Orosius, *The Seven Books of History* (Deferrati translation), 316–17.　　　[73] Ibid., 7.25.13.

[74] Clarke, 'Third-Century Christianity', 649–52. The later Christian chronicle of ten persecutions from Nero to Constantine in 313 does not allude to any provoked by plague. The relationship was the opposite: God's vengeance by plague ended the Roman persecutions; see *Orosius: Seven Books of History*, 7.26.

[75] According to Sozomen, *The Ecclesiastical History*, 6.2 and 9.6, the pestilence of 363 also ended Julian the Apostate's persecution.

[76] Biraben, *Les hommes*, I, 27–32; and Stathakopoulos, *Famine and Pestilence*.

[77] Dutton, *Charlemagne's Moustache*, 170–1, 185. I thank Jennifer Davis for this reference. In addition, Muratori, *Del Governo della peste*, 126–7, retells the story to condemn 'fantasies' provoked by pestilence.

Sea poisoned wells to kill off the Venetian soldiers. As a result, of one hundred galleys that returned to Venice, sixty-four were 'full of the afflicted and were half empty'. But the chroniclers made no claims of the poisoning leading to an epidemic or that it infected any in Venice.[78] Better known is the 1321 slaughter of lepers in southern France, instigated principally by the king on grounds that they had poisoned wells. Although this massacre may have provided a blueprint for the Black Death mass murder of Jews in 1348–51, no new epidemic or sudden increase in leprosy sparked the atrocities. Nor have any other mass riots against lepers appeared for the Middle Ages.

In antiquity, treatment of lepers may have been more pernicious, with lepers cast out of cities or tribes, ordered to wear torn clothes and to yell 'Unclean! unclean!' when anyone approached.[79] By Josephus' elaboration on Leviticus 13, the banished leper was 'to have [social] intercourse with no man', for in no way did he differ 'from a corpse'.[80] As writers such as Philo suggest, the disease was not only physical but possessed moral implications. In his *Allegorical Interpretations of Genesis*, he cites biblical authority to associate the leper's banishment with:

> everyone who is unclean in soul, both male and female (Numb. v. 2), and eunuchs with the generative organs of the soul cut away, and fornicators, deserters from the rule of One, to whom entrance into the assembly of God is absolutely forbidden (Deut. xxiii. 2).[81]

According to Demosthenes, 'the utterly wicked' were called 'moral lepers'.[82] Likewise, in early Christianity, the word could be applied metaphorically to a person's spirituality.[83] Following the Old Testament, St Basil the Great (330–79 CE), Archbishop of Caesarea, attributed Giezi's leprosy to covetousness (4 Kings).[84] More striking and paradoxical is the clause from Leviticus 13:12, that captured Philo's attention in two of his works and which he interpreted morally: 'complete leprosy is clean',[85] 'whose body is no longer particoloured, shewing a variety of hues, but has turned white all over from head to foot'.[86] Philo inferred that the first condition was 'involuntarily immoral and therefore innocent', while the particoloured, partially afflicted leper showed 'partial enlightenment, by which the soul knows that it is sinful but does not amend'.[87]

However, even as Moses' harsh laws in Leviticus make clear, the decision to mark a man or woman a leper was complex and not taken hurriedly. From detailed instructions, a priest was charged to examine the course of precise skin disorders over time before an individual could be declared a leper. And if the scars disappeared, the individual could return to the camp reunited without penalty or stigma. Even

---

[78] Sanuto, *Vitæ Ducum Venetorum*, col. 501. Corradi, *Annali delle epidemie*, I, 115, claims that Doge Vitale Michele II said that the posioning 'was born from the discontent of the islanders for the taxes imposed on them'. Sanuto makes no such allegations.

[79] Leviticus 13:45–6.   [80] Josephus, *Jewish Antiquities*, 3.261–4.

[81] Philo, *Allegorical Interpretation*, 3.3.

[82] [Demosthenes], *Orations*, III. *Against Aristogeiton*, 1.94–6.

[83] Prudentius, *Crowns of Martyrdom*, 2.225–60.   [84] Basil, *Letters*, XLII.

[85] Philo, *On the Unchangeableness of God*, IV.   [86] Philo, *Concerning Noah's Work*, XXVI.

[87] Philo, *On the Unchangeableness of God*, IV (cit.) and XXVI–XXVII.

honoured kings so afflicted were isolated because of their medical condition, as Josephus illustrates with his story of the king of Jerusalem, Uzziah, in 2 Chronicles 26. As a consequence of his smitten face, he was forced from the city, no different from any other man or woman with the characteristic white marks and white body hairs.[88] Certainly, this king was no persecuted 'other'.

The Jews were not alone in promulgating such harsh laws. Herodotus maintained that the Persians prevented any 'citizen' with leprosy or white sickness from coming into town or mixing with other Persians. Here the moral implications were more explicit: 'They say that he is so afflicted because he has sinned in some wise against the sun.'[89] In Samaria too, those with 'leprosy and whose bodies were not clean from such diseases' were banished from their cities.[90] However, except for the inverted Exodus story, reinvented a millennium after the supposed historic facts, lepers were not isolated in mass as a measure to purify a nation against 'foreigners' or any 'other' minority; nor was the leper's isolation expressed as a punishment, even in Herodotus's version of the disease as a moral affliction. Instead, the disease itself, and not the community's measures against it, was the gods' punishment against the sinner. As seen, according to Moses' law, once the bodily scars disappeared, the victim was reunited with the community without any religious or moral conversion.

Finally, despite the Old Testament's heavy influence and Greek literature's interaction with it, it is questionable just how significant leprosy and its modes of expulsion might have been in antiquity. From Roman history no incidents of it appear in my survey of sources, and Pliny the Elder maintained it was an Egyptian disease, not present in Italy before the time of Pompeius Magnus (106 BCE–48 BCE), and soon it died out. By Pliny's time (23–79 CE), one name given to it in Italy (*gemursa*) had become obsolete.[91] But even if the isolation of lepers was as severe as seen in Leviticus, the disease remained confined largely to an individual's physical affliction and had not become, as it would in the nineteenth century, a social disease attached to nations or races who were blamed for spreading it. Finally, ancient histories record no massacres of lepers, except for the imagined first-century CE reinvention of the Exodus, when supposedly Pharaoh Rameses drowned all Egypt's lepers in the Red Sea. We now turn to the Black Death: did it end epidemics' altruism and unifying force?

[88] Josephus, *Jewish Antiquities*, 9.224–8.   [89] Herodotus, *The Persian Wars*, 1.138–40.
[90] Josephus, *Jewish Antiquities*, 9.74–81.
[91] Pliny the Elder, *Natural History*, 26.5. From the paleopathology, Grmek, *Diseases in the Ancient World*, argues that leprosy did not become endemic in Greece 'until the end of antiquity' (133).

3

Black Death Persecution and Abandonment

BLACK DEATH SOCIAL TOXINS

The Black Death of 1347–51 has cast a long shadow over how big epidemics are seen to shape socio-psychological reactions, not only with regard to plague or the Middle Ages, but to epidemics across time and place.[1] As this chapter will argue, the burning of Jews and the flagellant movement were not the only acts of cruelty, or even the principal ones, to have astonished contemporaries. To be sure, the Black Death unleashed waves of persecution against beggars and priests in regions such as Narbonne (Spain)[2] and Carcassonne and Grasse in southern France,[3] against pilgrims in Catalonia, Catalans in Sicily, and most viciously Jews across German-speaking regions of Central Europe, down the Rhineland, and into Spain, France, and the Low Countries. The volumes of the *Germania Judaica*, painstakingly amassed from archives in Germany, Austria, and other Central European countries by several generations of German and Israeli scholars, provide accounts of mass persecution against at least 235 Jewish communities immediately before or during the Black Death.[4]

Yet in other regions of Europe, no evidence of such massacres occurred, as in England, where Jews had already been expelled, or in Italy, which contained ancient Jewish settlements in cities such as Rome and Spoleto.[5] Besides, not all inhabitants, even in the worst-affected regions—cities and castellans of the Rhine—partook in this mass hysteria, if it was in fact 'mass hysteria'. As I have argued previously, the primary sources do not support the standard story that artisans, labourers, and peasants concocted myths of the Jews having created the plague 'through their poisons of frogs and spiders mixed into oil and cheese' deposited in streams and wells to destroy Christendom, or that the lower classes perpetrated the hundreds of massacres to destroy Jewry that took place from 1348 to 1350.[6] Instead, elites—castellans, patricians, and bishops—were the perpetrators, with numerous German chroniclers from the higher echelons of the Church justifying the Jews' fate.[7] For many, 'Jews deserved to be swallowed up in the flames'.[8] Nor did elites as a rule

---

[1] See Delumeau, *Rassurer et protéger*, esp. 571–2.   [2] Horrox, 223.
[3] Biraben, *Les hommes*, I, 59.   [4] Voitgländer and Voth, 'Persecution Perpetuated', 1348.
[5] According to Roth, *The History of the Jews*, 142, Jewish communities in Mantua and Parma were attacked during the Black Death, but he does not elaborate or cite sources; and I know none to refer to them.
[6] *Die Weltchronik des Mönchs Albert*, 109.   [7] Cohn, 'The Black Death', 16, esp. note 31.
[8] Ibid., 16–17, and for the poems of Michael de Leone, Arnold, 'Pest', 368.

intervene to protect the Jews. Pope Clement VI was an exception: his *Sicut Judeis* of 26 October 1348 argued that Jews were dying of plague in as great numbers as Christians, and he ruled that anyone joining or authorizing the persecution would be excommunicated. The Middle Ages' other superpower, Holy Roman Emperor Charles IV of Bohemia, was on the other hand the principal architect of the persecutions in several northern German cities, where he arranged to dispose of Jewish property even before the massacres began, and encouraged leading burghers, bishops, and knights at Nuremberg, Regensburg, Augsburg, and Frankfurt to murder Jews, granting them immunity from punishment and afterwards cancelling their debts to Jews.[9]

Few contemporaries placed the blame for these atrocities on artisans, peasants, the poor, or even vaguely on citizens. I know of only one source to have made the allegation, a chronicle that continued into the fifteenth century, scripted by monk Albert of Cologne, who died in 1456. It maintained that Jews in 1349 'across all of Germany (Theutoniam) and many other provinces' were cruelly 'consumed in flames' by a popular insurrection (*tumult furente populari et in sedicionem concitato*) of those incensed by the Jews' enormous wealth, their ruthless usurious exploitation of

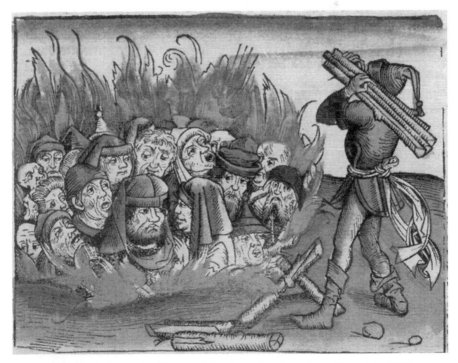

Figure 3.1. Burning of Jews *c.*1348, from the Nuremberg Chronicle, 1493.

9 On Charles IV's pivotal role in the massacres, see Haverkamp, 'Die Judenverfolgungen', 65; and Müller, '*Erez gererah*', 257; for earlier works, see Cohn, 'The Black Death', 15.

nobles and many others, including the poor and indigent, and especially because of the Jews' 'iniquitous and malicious poisoning of sources of water and spread of the pestilence then infecting the world'.[10] But this was not a contemporary chronicle, and monk Albert was mistaken about Jews of the mid-fourteenth century making loans to the 'many' including 'the poor and indigent'. Instead, such trends for lending in German-speaking regions had only begun to evolve towards the end of Albert's life. As German scholars have shown over the past several decades, Jewish creditors of the fourteenth century did not fit the stereotype of the pawnbroker lending to impoverished peasants or artisans. Instead, well into the fifteenth century, their loans served elites and for the most part rural ones.[11]

In Strasbourg, where a Jewish community of several thousand was eventually annihilated, the relationship between those seeking to blame the Jews and those wishing to defend them is clear. Responses to letters sent by that city's guild government in the autumn of 1348 to other cities and regions down the Rhineland and into present-day Switzerland allow the historian to go beyond the chroniclers. Strasbourg, then governed by an artisan-guild council, differed from most other cities; it resisted calls to destroy its Jewish community. Nevertheless, by August 1348, under pressure from the region's aristocratic bishop, Berthold II von Bucheck, its city council began sending letters to city mayors, patrician councils, rural castellans, and territorial rulers, such as Duke Albrecht of Austria and Lord Amedéo VI, Count of Savoy, to ascertain proof of Jews spreading plague.

Nineteen responses survive, which also refer to now-lost letters sent from other cities and regions, reporting interrogations of Jews and their testimony derived from 'due legal process' (including torture). Almost invariably, these trials ended in mass public burning—men, women, and infants. Yet not a single letter mentions any accusations by or involvement of workers, artisans, or peasants. The lowest rung of those pressing charges or committing the violence was that of the notary. Instead, patricians, castellans, and major European dignitaries were the instigators. The replies, moreover, often named the Jews arrested and their supposed accomplices. Of fifty named, not one was a usurer. Instead, they were doctors, women, students, cantors, and, most often, rabbis.[12] Yet still Strasbourg's guildsmen resisted Berthold's pressure. As a result, on 8 February 1349, he organized an assembly at Benfeld, attended by 'all the feudal lords of Alsace' and patrician representatives of three imperial cities.[13] Staging a revolt from above, they ousted the artisan government, and immediately, the new oligarchic government massacred its ancient Jewish community, burning them alive on an island in the

[10]　*Die Weltchronik des Mönchs Albert*, 272.

[11]　Kisch, *The Jews in Medieval Germany*, 225. For more recent research: Ziwes, 'Zum jüdischen Kapitalmarkt'; Mentgen, 'Herausragende jüdische Finanziers', esp. 331–2 and 345–6. For Speyer: Voltmer, 'Zur Geschichte der Juden im spätmittelalterlichen Speyer', 102. For lower Bavaria, Toch, 'Geld und Kredit', esp. 509–13; and idem, 'Between Impotence and Power', 242. For Würzburg, Jenks, 'Judenverschuldung und Verfolgung'. Only in the fifteenth century did indigenous bankers force Jews from markets of elites.

[12]　Cohn, 'The Black Death', 25–6. One merchant was named, not for his economic dealings, but because he was a community leader.

[13]　*Chronik des Jakob Twinger*, ii, 759–65.

Rhine. That the blind fury of 'mobs' comprised of workers, artisans, and peasants was responsible for the Black Death annihilation of Jews derives from modern historians' musings, not medieval sources.[14]

Nonetheless, the Black Death unleashed hatred, blaming, and violence on a more horrific scale than any epidemic in world history. Historians, however, have failed to notice how quickly plague disappeared as a trigger of violence. I have found only one further incident of mass persecution of Jews or other minorities sparked by plague or any disease from the Black Death to the early modern period, and historians, even Joshua Tractenberg and Séraphine Guerchberg, who argued that later plagues spurred a new regime of persecutions against Jews across Europe, have missed it.[15] The *Annales Mechovienses* reported the plague of 1360 as having been caused by Jews who poisoned wells in the region of Krakow and, as a result, were burnt alive in Krakow 'and other places'. But should this report be believed? The chronicle ends in 1434 and was probably written several generations after the Black Death. Moreover, it seems to have confused the second plague with the first, claiming that in 1360 plague 'spread through all of Christendom, especially through the Kingdom of Poland: only a third of "Christians" survived it with even less in Krakow'.[16] No other chronicle mentions these massacres in 1360, including the more detailed one for the same region by Krakow's contemporary canon Johannes Dlugossi.[17] On the other hand, the first plague of 1348 may have skipped over southern Poland altogether. The *Annales Mechovienses*, in its entry for 1349, describes the plague in Hungary but not in its own region of Krakow, and for 1348, Dlugossi reports the Black Death ravaging the Kingdom of Poland as well as in 'Hungary, Bohemia, Romania (Dacia), France, Germany, and almost universally through Christendom and Barbarian kingdoms', but says nothing about his home town or region.[18] So even if Jews were burnt at Krakow in 1362, it would have been during that region's first plague.

LEPROSY AND MASS VIOLENCE?

Before 1348, no epidemic or pandemic had spurred such mass violence. As we have seen, the mere blaming of a people for a disease in antiquity and the early Middle Ages was extremely rare, the Plague of Athens included. The most significant exception was the 1321 slaughter of lepers in southern France.[19] But no new epidemic or sudden increase in leprosy sparked it. Instead, as Zachary Gussow was the first to stress and which the more detailed research of François-Olivier Touati, Carole

---

[14] For assumptions that anti-Semitic violence originated from the lower classes provoked by Jewish lending, see Nohl, *The Black Death*, 116, 122; *Jew in the Medieval World*, 49–50; Breuer, 'The "Black Death" and Antisemitism'; Foa, *The Jews of Europe*, 16; and others summarized in Cohn, 'The Black Death'.

[15] For Tractenberg, see Chapter 6; for Guerchberg, 'La controverse'.

[16] *Annales Mechovienses*, 671; and *Rocznik Miechowski*, 886.

[17] *Annales...Joannis Dlugossii*, IX, 301.

[18] Biraben, *Les hommes*, I, 104, maintains that no source mentions plague in southern Poland in 1348.

[19] The historiography on this massacre of lepers is large; see Barber, 'Lepers'.

Rawcliffe, and Luke Demaitre has recently and authoritatively underscored, medieval persecution of lepers was largely a myth created in the nineteenth century by politicians and governments to justify their own brutal segregation and treatment of lepers.[20] As Rawcliffe has summarized: 'Armed with a conviction that the West faced an epidemic of devastating proportions [in the late nineteenth century], leprologists needed ammunition to support a campaign for segregation and thus constructed a medieval leper to serve their purpose.' By contrast, leprosy in the Middle Ages could be regarded as a mark of election and 'did not lead automatically to segregation or vilification'.[21] Official segregation of lepers tended to arise in times of crisis, 'when concerns about epidemic disease, disorder and vagrancy were running high', as during the early fourteenth century with rising population, cattle plagues, and food shortages and with human plague from 1348.[22] At such times, certain towns, such as Bristol in 1331, attempted to remove lepers from their city walls, 'voicing fears about infection'.[23] On the other hand, in normal times, lepers were 'deserving objects of Christian compassion'.[24] Even in periods of crisis, scholars have yet to document incidents of mass or small vigilante violence against lepers or their hospitals beyond the French case of 1321, often imagined as typical of mass hysteria against lepers in the Middle Ages. In England the only severe legislation against them was Edward III's ordinance of 1346 excluding them temporarily from London; similarly in France, the only ordinance banning them from the capital was in 1488.[25]

The Black Death was different. In the nineteenth and early twentieth centuries, when hundreds of riots comprising thousands of people, fuelled by waves of cholera, plague, and smallpox, broke out around the world (as Part III of this book will describe), none produced any massacres on a scale approaching the Black Death's. In this regard, the Black Death was unique. The only possible exception

---

[20] Gussow, *Leprosy*; and Gussow and Tracy, 'Stigma', 425–49. I have yet to find further cases of mass slaughter of lepers in the Middle Ages. Nor do such atrocities surface in recent exhaustive studies by Touati, *Maladie et société*; Rawcliffe, *Leprosy*; and Demaitre, *Leprosy in Premodern Medicine*. Touati combats the old myth that authorities and the general population despised and ruthlessly segregated lepers throughout the Middle Ages and shows the rise of a positive attitude towards lepers in eleventh- and twelfth-century France. Their communities flourished economically and were held in esteem as exemplars of sanctity by the populace and religious authorities. However, as early as the mid-thirteenth century, in works such as the *Summa pastoralis*, learned attitudes towards lepers changed: they became perceived as a moral and pathogenic threat to the healthy and with the ecological disasters from the late thirteenth-century and later plagues, enforced isolation of lepers became more common. Yet Touati supplies no evidence of riots or mass persecution by the state or any social group against them, except in France, 1321. As he states, this incident was 'unique' to medieval and early modern Europe. More recently, Rawcliffe, *Leprosy*, has shown no such transition in attitudes to lepers in England. In places such as Nuremburg, charitable sentiment towards them even became more favourable from 1395 into the early modern period. After a plague of 1394, its mayor enacted beneficial measures towards lepers, and by the 1490s the city transformed its annual inspection of lepers 'into a grand celebration to shower the leprous poor with gifts'; see Boeckl, *Images of Leprosy*, 64–5. For the rarity of prejudice against lepers in the Middle Ages, see also Creighton, I, ch. 2, 69–113.
[21] Rawcliffe, *Leprosy*, 43.   [22] Ibid., 253 and 255.
[23] Ibid., 282 and 285.   [24] Ibid., 259 and 267. Also see idem, *Urban Bodies*, 321–3.
[25] Creighton, I, 103, 104, and 437. However, in Scotland such ordinances of exclusion were more frequent: in 1242 and 1269, canons ordered their isolation; in 1427, the Parliament of Perth ordered minsters to search out lepers; and in 1283–4 statutes of the Merchants of Berwick prohibited their admission into the borough but also organized collecting alms on their behalf; ibid., I, 106.

might have been the Nazis blaming Jews for spreading typhus, in part to justify the enforced ghettoization of Jews[26] and ultimately the wholesale use of Zyklon B, originally developed to eradicate typhus-spreading lice, to annihilate the supposed carrier of the disease Nazis called 'Judenfieber'.[27] The Ottoman state may have anticipated the Nazis' ideological connection between typhus and hatred of a people by branding Armenians as typhus carriers during the massacre of 1915–19.[28] But in neither case was typhus the trigger or the essential spark leading to these genocides. Instead, it only buttressed trends that were well on course, engendered by other causes and ideologies. In the case of Nazi Germany, no epidemic of typhus then lurked on Germany's horizons or in other regions to the east, as had been the case in parts of Russia during the famines of the 1920s. Instead, typhus was steadily on the wane and by 1940 had virtually disappeared from Western Europe.[29]

ABANDONMENT

Back to the Middle Ages: while the Black Death may not have unleashed pogroms against Jews, Catalans, or beggars everywhere in Europe or extended across social classes, it triggered other anti-social consequences that were more pervasive. These have received far less attention than the flagellants of 1349–50 or the burning of Jews. While in German-speaking regions, the supposed vicious deeds of Jews to end Christendom and their mass executions were central planks of Black Death chronicling, it was not the case beyond these regions. Out of 128 chronicles covering the Black Death written across the Italian peninsula from Savoy to Sicily, I know of none to have reported these supposed plots and executions. Similarly, of forty-two contemporary French chronicles, only two referred to accusations against the Jews or to the atrocities that followed.[30] Of fifty-eight British and Irish chronicles, none reported these accusations or massacres, and of twelve from the Low Countries, three alluded to them: a short one by the Avignon court musician Louis Heyligen [Sanctus],[31] one by Gilles li Mussit, abbot of Tournai,[32] and a third

---

[26] Roland, *Courage under Siege*, 120 and 125.

[27] Weindling, *Epidemics and Genocide*, esp. 70–1 and 106–7.

[28] Dadrian, 'The Role of Turkish Physicians', esp. 178 and 182; and idem, *The History of the Armenian Genocide*, 219–300, which does not repeat the accusations against Turkish physicians; nor have I found them in later works. Instead, Turkish authorities were accused of purposefully exposing Armenian deportees to typhus, causing thousands of casualties; see Kaiser, 'Genocide', 380 and 384.

[29] Weindling, *Epidemics and Genocide*, 426–7 and appendix.

[30] While Lescot (*Chronique de Richard Lescot*, 83) believed the charges against Jews, Jean de Venette (*Chronique latine*) was sceptical and reported Christians also being so charged. The country friar then raised the obvious point that curiously no one else mentioned: 'even if these things really happened, [they] could not have been solely responsible for so great a plague that killed so many people' (translation from Horrox, 56). Several French chroniclers reported the flagellants, such as *Les Grandes Chroniques de France*, IX, 323; and *Chronique de Jean le Bel*, I, 222 and 224.

[31] Welkenhuysen, 'La peste en Avignon (1348)', text on 465–9; and *Breve Chronicon Clerici Anonymi*, 5–30. These tallies are taken from an earlier survey in my *The Black Death Transformed*, 251–73.

[32] *Chronique et annales de Gilles le Muisit*, 222–3.

by an anonymous chronicler of the dukes of Brabant, saying only, 'in that year [1349] Jews were murdered'.[33]

The more widespread message heard in the sources for 1348 was a direct consequence of the disease's rapid contagion, considered by chroniclers and physicians as unprecedented. Fear of contagion and almost certain death fractured societies to their core—the family. Most famously, Giovanni Boccaccio in his Introduction to the *Decameron*, completed around 1355, elaborated on this reaction. This 'unheard of contagion':

> caused various fears and fantasies to take root in the minds of those who were still alive and well. And almost without exception, they took a single and very inhuman precaution, namely to avoid or run away from the sick and their belongings....It was not merely a question of one citizen avoiding another, and of people almost invariably neglecting their neighbours and rarely or never visiting their relatives...this scourge had implanted so great a terror in the hearts of men and women that brothers abandoned brothers, uncles their nephews, sisters their brothers, and in many cases wives deserted their husbands. But even worse, and almost incredible, was the fact that fathers and mothers refused to nurse and assist their own children, as though they did not belong to them.[34]

More than most, Boccaccio elaborated on these themes of fear, flight, and abandonment along with the refusal by physicians, notaries, clergy, and gravediggers to render essential services. He was not, however, the *Urtext* of these opinions or obervations. As early as October 1347, when the plague first arrived in Western Europe at Messina (Sicily), the Franciscan friar Michele da Piazza observed: 'Neither priests nor sons, nor fathers nor any other kinsmen dared enter [to bury them]'. The living did not enter houses of the dead even to collect their goods or money.[35] At Catania, those who fled Messina were treated with contempt; the Catanesi persuaded their ecclesiastic Patriarch to enact an ordinance prohibiting the Messinesi being buried within the city 'or indeed outside it'. Even worse, 'the timorous and abhorrent ones of Catania' refused to associate with the Messinesi but 'fled at their sight'.[36]

A wide variety of authors in literary letters, chronicles, histories, and monastic annals reported fear of any human contact that led to the widespread familial abandonment. The German chronicler Mathias de Nuwenburg claimed that the contagion was such that plague victims perished without last rites; parents refused to care for their children; friends, for one another; household servants for their masters. 'Such things', he concluded, were 'too horrible to write or tell!'[37] The Netherlandish musician Louis Sanctus marvelled at the same sudden disappearance of care and affection by loved ones and trusted professionals. However, he was unusual in explaining it with a modicum of sympathy. People quickly recognized two essential characteristics of the new disease—its high mortalities and contagion. As a result, 'men dare not speak with anyone whose kinsman or kinswoman has died: as often observed, when one family member dies, almost all the rest

---

[33] *Chroniques des Ducs de Brabant*, II, 683.   [34] Horrox, 28–40, 50–8.
[35] Michele da Piazza, *Cronica*, 82.   [36] Ibid., 86.
[37] Mathias de Nuwenburg, *Chronica*, 262.

follow': no doctor visited the sick; the father the son, the mother the daughter, the brother the brother; the son the father, the friend, the friend, the acquaintance, the acquaintance—

> unless, that is, they wished to die suddenly. . . . And thus an uncountable number of people died without any mark of affection, piety or charity—who, if they had refused to visit the sick themselves, might perhaps have escaped.[38]

In the north of France, the aristocratic canon Jean le Bel, the anonymous chronicler of the *Grandes Chroniques*, and the Carmelite Jean de Venette also saw fear of contagion splitting societies when plague first struck: 'one did not dare help or visit the ill; nor could anyone find a priest who would agree to hear confession'.[39] The Carmelite friar condemned priests as cowards but claimed that those in religious orders stood their ground and assumed the duties abandoned by priests, hearing confessions and performing last rites and funerals.[40] Similar descriptions circulated in Eastern Europe. The Krakow canon Dlugossi witnessed the reaction arising from the plague's 'contagion'—that it spread 'from mixing with others', 'by breath', and even 'by a mere glance (aspectu) from the infected. So horrified, parents fled from curing their offspring, and children fled their parents'.[41] A chronicler on Italy's borders with Eastern Europe at Aquileia also marvelled (*Mirabilior tamen hujus pestilentiae qualitas*) that the disease spread so fast it seemed to be transmitted by sight. As a result, 'as soon as the father or son became ill, the other fled, while the afflicted nearly fell from bed with hands outstretched for affection'.[42] An Olivetan monk in Poland with different words drew the same relation between ferocious contagion and the plague's consequences: physicians refused to visit the sick and fathers and mothers, their own children.[43] A chronicler from Salona on the Dalmatian coast was equally horrified: 'The raging plague slayed men, women, the old, and the young all together before their own eyes; yet none of any age bothered to show mercy. Boys and girls left their parents and vice versa, and brothers did the same without any sense of pity'.[44] The English, Scots, and Irish hinted at the same without refrains of family relations. According to Geoffrey le Baker, 'Hardly anyone had anything to do with the sick'.[45] The chronicle attributed to the Scot John of Fordun (*Gesta Annalia*) condemned the 'horrific' behaviour of his countrymen, 'because of the fear of contagion with sons fleeing their parents on their death beds and vice versa, as though confronted by lepers or serpents, and dared not to visit'.[46] According to the Dublin friar John Clyn, because of fear of contagion, hardly anyone could be found to visit the sick or bury the dead.[47]

Such evidence comes not only from chronicles and imaginative literature but from medical writing as with Guy de Chauliac's famous tract on surgery, completed in the 1360s but whose section on *apostemes* reflected on 1348.[48] Moreover, following

---

[38] Horrox, 43.   [39] *Chronique de Jean le Bel*, I, 222.

[40] *The Chronicle of Jean de Venette*, 55.   [41] *Annales. . . Joannis Dlugossii*, 252.

[42] De Rubeis, *Monumenta Ecclesiae Aquilejensis*, Appendix X: 'Necrologio deprompta', 42–4.

[43] *Chronica Olivensis*, 310–50.   [44] *Ecclesia Spalatensis*, 324.

[45] *Chronicon Galfridi le Baker*, 99.   [46] In Bower, *Scotichronicon*, VII, 272–3.

[47] *Annalium Hiberniae*, 36–7.   [48] Cited in Archambeau, 'Healing Options', 538–9.

papal instructions, the Bishop of Bath and Wells addressed his congregation in January 1349 not with fiery exclamations but with practical advice:

> because priests cannot be found for love or money to take on the responsibility of visiting the sick or administering the sacraments...we understand that many people are dying without the sacrament of penance...Therefore, if...they cannot secure the services of a properly ordained priest, they should confess their sins...to any lay person, even to a woman if a man is not available.[49]

Such Black Death reports of abandonment and neglect by doctors, notaries, and clergymen to service those in need in 1348 abound through Italian city-states, presenting a rich tapestry of expression and a diversity of explanations. A chronicler of Cremona pointed to the high rates of mortality, especially with those 'spitting blood, when not one in a hundred survived', to explain why 'the father dared not visit his strickened son or the son, his father'.[50] A Rimini chronicler noted that just by mixing with the ill the healthy became 'lethally spotted', and soon afterwards, 'the father shunned the child; the brother his brother; the wife her man; and later the healthy also began to avoid one another', along with priests and doctors, 'who fled from the ill'.[51] Writing later in the fourteenth century, Pisa's principal chronicler of the Black Death, Ranieri Sardo, began by pointing to the plague's arrival at Pisa's Piazza dei Pesci, spread by sailors disembarking from two Genoese galleys. Their chattering with locals (*chiunqua favellava loro*) unwittingly transmitted the disease instantly. As a consequence, 'the father wished not to witness his son dying; nor the son the death of his father; nor one brother, the other; nor the wife her husband. Everyone fled from death....'[52] However, during the Black Death's brief four-month terror, things began changing, and they began with fathers:

> seeing the death of his child, abandoned by everyone, without any daring to touch him, care for him, or carry him, the father now unafraid to die, laid out his son for burial, placed him in a wooden casket, and with help carried him to the grave....And God instilled charity from one to another, and people started saying, 'let us help and bring the dead to their graves so that we might be carried to ours'.[53]

Other Italian commentators were not as optimistic. More than the disease's gruesome signs or spitting blood, a chronicler of Trent stressed its lightning contagion which 'created such fear among people' and led the clergy to flight, mass burials without chants or processions, and, worst of all, the abandonment of family members. By his account, familial relations also became violent:

> the father and mother turned against the child and vice versa; the sister against the brother...out of fear parents did not attend the burial of their children...and almost no priest carried the sacraments, unless they were twisted (*torquebantur*) by a craving for money.[54]

---

[49] Horrox, 271–2. Prelates' flight during the plague continued haunting the Franciscan John of Rupescissa until 1350, when he scripted a letter expressing outrage over this cowardice; Casteen, 'John of Rupescissa's Letter', 160 and 181 (text).

[50] De Bezanis, *Cronaca Pontificum et Imperatorum*, 102.

[51] *Marcha di Marco Battagli da Rimini*, 54–5.   [52] *Cronaca di Pisa*, 96–7.   [53] Ibid.

[54] *Cronica inedita di Giovanni da Parma*, I, Appendice, 50.

Florence's principal Black Death chronicler, Matteo Villani, was disgusted with his countrymen's behaviour in 1348:

> early on men, women, and children saw that the disease could strike simply by touch, even by sight, and could be recognized by the tell-tale traits of the swelling (*enfiatura*). As a consequence, many were abandoned and a vast number died who could have survived had they been helped. Such inhumane cruelty began with the infidel—that of mothers and fathers abandoning their children, and children, their fathers and mothers, and one brother, the other, and other kinsmen and women.

Villani exclaimed that this cruelty was 'of the habits of barbarians', to be despised by the faithful. Yet, like Ranieri, he observed a change over the course of the plague, and, for Villani, it went beyond burial. Once Florentines saw that some could be cured, they began helping others in a variety of ways, including nursing the plague-stricken, which Matteo conjectured helped to end the plague.[55]

In appraising the Black Death, the Florentine poet Antonio Pucci turned his attention entirely to the theme of abandonment and neglect by trusted professionals. Like Villani, he compared these responses to those of the infidel, but for Pucci the cruelty of his Christian compatriots may have even been worse. On describing 'blood brothers, fathers, and children' abandoning one another, 'because the disease provides no cure', he alleged:

> Not even Saracens, Jews, or turncoats deserve such treatment!
> And for God's sake, you doctors, priests, and friars, you might try acting
>   with some piety towards those who plead for help!
> You might act for the wellbeing of your souls instead of just seeking profit!
>   As for the rest of you, relatives, neighbours, and friends
> For love of God, when you see someone in pain, overcome your fears
> And show a little courage to provide some comfort.[56]

According to the *Storie Pistoresi*, deserting loved ones was most distinctive at Pisa but was widespread through Italy, spreading with plague from Avignon through Provence and Tuscany. Those willing to aid the sick or carry the dead to the grave could not be found; neither friar nor priest dared approach the ill.[57] Finally, the lawyer Gabriele de' Mussis, who chronicled Europeans' first contact with the Black Death at Kaffa, continued the story once it reached his home town, Piacenza, detailing citizens' reactions. Unlike Boccaccio and others, de' Mussis did not bother explaining why friends, relatives, and professionals abandoned the ill. Instead, he dramatized their reactions through imagined dialogues:

> Listen to the tearful voices of the sick: 'Have pity, have pity, my friends. At least say something, now that the hand of God has touched me. Oh father, why have you abandoned me? For you forget that I am your child? Mother, where have you gone? Why are you now so cruel to me when only yesterday you were so kind? You fed me at your breast and carried me within your womb for nine months.'

---

[55] Matteo Villani, *Cronica*, I, 11.   [56] Pucci, 'Delle crudeltà della pestilenza', 413.
[57] *Storie Pistoresi*, 235.

'My children, who I brought up with toil and sweat, why have you run away?'
Man and wife reached out to each other, 'Alas, once we slept happily together but now are separated and wretched.'
And when the sick were in the throes of death, they still called out piteously to their family and neighbours, 'Come here. I'm thirsty; bring me a drink of water. I'm still alive. Don't be frightened. Perhaps I won't die. Please hold me tight, hug my wasted body.'[58]

A generation later, chroniclers continued to reflect on these reactions in 1348. The Florentine merchant Marchionne di Coppo Stefani (Baldassarre Bonaiuti) writing in the 1380s, who was a child in 1348, lived through three further plagues with devastating consequences; yet for none of these later ones did he repeat the collective memory of the Black Death's first appearance. His descriptions of abandonment fill more space than even Boccaccio's and contain details not seen in other surviving sources. I translate a small portion of it.

> Those in cities fled for the countryside. Doctors could not be found. They had died along with the others. But those who could be found, demanded extortionate fees to enter the homes of the afflicted.... Fathers abandoned their children, husbands their wives; wives their husbands; one brother the other; one sister the other. Throughout the entire city, one could do nothing other than carry the dead to their graves. Many died without confession or other sacraments. And more died without anyone witnessing their death; many died of starvation since no one would bring them food. Those occupying the same household, would promise, 'I am going for the doctor' ... [they] then locked the front door [without leaving food, water, or medicine] not to be seen again.[59]

Unlike Boccaccio and others who explained the cruel desertions by referring to the plague's extraordinary contagion and lethality, Stefani made no such link explicit. Instead, like de' Mussis, he scripted stories, perhaps heard from childhood, of abandoned relatives left locked in their homes to starve. By contrast, no such stories are found in the greatest storyteller of them all, and from Stefani's long chronicle, he appears not to have known the *Decameron* or heard of Boccaccio, despite both being Florentines. Of hundreds of Florentines cited in his chronicle, including several from the Boccaccio family, Giovanni was not mentioned.

ABANDONMENT AFTER THE BLACK DEATH

Were these stories of abandonment from Scotland to Krakow simply a matter of one author copying another with little basis in Black Death realities, as some insist?[60] If so, how could the topoi have been conveyed so quickly across widely dispersed societies, traversing thousands of kilometres and cutting across social and professional divides in a matter of months without the internet or printing? More importantly for our analysis, why did this literary device (if it were only that) suddenly fall from grace with successive plagues, running through the early modern period, even

---

[58] Horrox, 22–3.   [59] Stefani, *Cronica fiorentina*, 230.
[60] See notes 97 to 100.

within works by the same author, as with Stefani or Giovanni di Pagolo Morelli? Almost without exception, descriptions of the callous abandonment of family members and flight and neglect by professionals disappeared from hundreds of chronicle entries, physicians' tracts, and other literary works describing plagues from 1357 to the end of the 'Second Pandemic' in the nineteenth century. When the second wave of plague struck England, John of Reading commented that 'the greatest cause of grief' was the behaviour of women: 'Widows, forgetting the love they had borne towards their first husbands, rushed into the arms of foreigners or, in many cases, of kinsmen, and shamelessly gave birth to bastards conceived in adultery. It was even claimed that in many places brothers took their sisters to wife.'[61] But this abandonment differed from that of 1348. Reading did not repeat the Black Death refrains of one relative abandoning another while alive. Now, the outrage was one over sexual mores, not of loved ones fleeing in times of need. As Marco Lastri showed at the end of the eighteenth century, plagues throughout the Renaissance and early modern period consistently spurred populations to replace lost numbers by reproducing at higher rates immediately following an outbreak.[62] Plague became a mechanism for new family unions, not separations.

For subsequent plagues, others pointed to other forms of abandonment. A chronicler of Tournai claimed that during 'the terrible pestilence' of 1400, 'many abandoned their work', some to go on pilgrimages and 'some to do nothing of use', but he did not repeat the Black Death laments: refusals to attend the stricken; parents abandoning their children, and vice versa.[63] A closer parallel, however, comes with Ser Luca Dominici's initial description of plague at Pistoia in 1399–1400, which he estimated from parish and tax records eventually killed just under half Pistoia's population,[64] comparable to Black Death levels. He lamented: 'they locked their houses and shops, and fled here and there. The dead and afflicted could find no assistance and remained behind. A more astonishing thing had never been seen.'[65] Clearly, Ser Luca, a highly educated notary, residing less than 40 km from Florence's walls, knew nothing of the Black Death abandonment and had not read Boccaccio. Soon, however, his tone changed. The bulk of his chronicle charted the charitable activities of the 1399–1400 mass movement called the Bianchi that crossed central and northern Italy and into Provence. Instead of abandonment, the remainder of his chronicle repeatedly shows the opposite: communal solidarity with families assembling together in city- and country-wide processions, shouting 'Pace e misericordia', pleading to individuals and city governments to end their grievances and make peace. He chronicles the spread of this interregional movement spurred by plague as terminating longstanding factional strife in Pistoia (at least temporarily) and uniting peoples across sex, class, and city and countryside in a new and optimisitc zeal for mutual assistance. No more is heard of abandonment or neglect as this plague intensified.[66]

---

[61] Horrox, 87.   [62] Lastri, *Ricerche sull'antica e moderna popolazione*.
[63] *Chronique des Pays-Bas*, III, 332.   [64] *Cronache di Ser Luca Dominici*, I, 233, 238.
[65] Ibid., I, 232.   [66] For Fermo and Florence, see *Cronaca Fermana*, 27.

For early modern plagues further instances of chroniclers stressing cruel abandonment are difficult to find. A Perugian chronicler notes it in 1448.[67] With plague at Padua in 1504, the Venetian Girolamo Priuli held that so many citizens left for the countryside that hardly any were left in the city. But he did not suggest the exodus had splintered families as in 1348.[68] Later still, during the plague of 1575–7 the merchant Olivero Panizzone Sacco wrote a pamphlet on his discomfits when detained in Milan against his will, unable to return to his family and friends in Alessandria. Among his many attacks against the Health Board and its regulations, he accused barbers and physicians of 'abandoning' him but not the population at large.[69] During the same plague, Marcantonio Ciappi claimed that 'men became cruel, and losing all humanity, wives came to abhor, then to abandon their husbands, and vice versa'.[70] But his was a theoretical work, constructing a general premise without citing specific instances or places. Besides, by pointing only to husbands and wives, he may have been expressing moral regrets similar to John of Reading's earlier raging.[71]

In 1629, a particularly disastrous plague at Digne in Provence reduced its population from 10,000 to 1500. The late Enlightenment historian Jean-Pierre Papon attributed its fate to a foolish political decision to place a 'cordon of troops' around the city. Foodstuffs and other supplies were not allowed to enter the city and the Dignois could not leave even to bury their dead or construct huts ('cabanes') outside the city to isolate the afflicted, as had become general practice since the sixteenth century.[72] He then sounded laments reminiscent of the Black Death, although with language, examples, and reasons not copied or borrowed from any medieval writer: 'domestic servants abandoned their masters', and 'neighbours became deaf to their neighbours' pleas for help'; 'everyone was preoccupied with their own fears, without concern for anyone else and offering no one any help'.[73] Yet he did not repeat the cries of close relatives fleeing the dying; instead, because of the absence of gravediggers, sons buried their fathers; fathers, their sons; husbands, wives, etc. even if they did a bad job of it, 'digging shallow graves that exposed bodily parts after a windy day'. Moreover, for his detailed accounts of Lyon and Montpellier, and mentions of plague at Aix, Marseille, and Milan, he made no references to abandonment or neglect.[74] In fact, the abundant chronicles, letters, and administrative sources for Milan's plague of 1629–32 express no evidence of abandonment, and this despite pictures of horror, distrust, and cruelty penned by writers such as Giuseppe Ripamonti, who decried the internecine suspicions that split Milan to its core—'the matrimonial bed and the dining table'—because of the recriminations and rumours against suspected *untori* purposefully spreading the plague.[75]

---

[67] *Cronica della città di Perugia*, 600.   [68] *I Diarii di Girolamo Priuli*, 384.

[69] Cohn, *Cultures of Plague*, 112–15.   [70] Ibid., 273.

[71] Another claim of abandonment comes with a plague in Istanbul of 1467. According to the chronicler Kritovoulos, *History of Mehmed the Conqueror*, 220–1 'For some, fearing plague, fled and never came back, not even to care for their nearest relatives, but even turned away from them, although they often appealed to them with pitiful lamentation, yet they abandoned the sick uncared-for and the dead unburied' (220).

[72] Papon, *De la peste*, I, 200–2.   [73] Ibid., 202–3.

[74] Ibid., 165–93, 206.   [75] See Chapter 6.

Nonetheless, in other places in northern Italy, with mortalities rebounding to Black Death heights, glimpses of family abandonment returned during this plague, even if they remained rare. Modena's chronicler, Giovan Battista Spaccini, commented that 'it was certainly with great sadness that many of the stricken were abandoned by their own fathers and mothers, by brothers and sisters, and by other relatives'.[76] He then showed his unawareness of Black Death sources, adding 'such terrible cruelty had never before been heard of'.[77] But he does not repeat these tales for any other city;[78] although, for the plague, he concentrated more on Mantua and Milan than on his home town. A second description of abandonment comes from the Florentine Giovanni Baldinucci, even though plague mortalities here were relatively low for this epidemic:

> because of the fear of death and plague the husband abandoned his wife; the wife, her husband, her son and daughter; and fathers and mothers, their children, and vice versa. The poor died alone like animals without the sacraments or medical care.[79]

Yet for Italy's diastrous seventeenth-century plagues—1624–5 for Sicily, the 1630s for Northern Italy, and 1656–7 for the regions of Genoa, Rome, and Naples with numerous texts describing them, these are the only two exceptions I have found. Finally, during the Barcelona plague of 1651, Miquel Parets scorned judges and the secular clergy who abandoned their parishioners, but he also praised monks, who remained at their posts, caring for parishioners and sacrificing their lives while serving in pesthouses.[80] Finally, there was mass flight from Marseille during France's last major plague in 1720–2. These included desperately needed civil servants of the municipality, especially the police, and at least one commentator, the cleric père Giraud, claimed 'the father did not stay to assist his son, nor the husband his wife'.[81]

Moreover, chroniclers and physicians during the late Middle Ages and early modern period often repeated the classical cliché *scilicet cito, longe, et tarde* (leave quickly, go far away, and stay away a long time) as the best remedy against plague. To a great extent, elites along with wealthy artisans continued heeding this advice during plague seasons, whether or not plague struck. With Florence's third plague, in 1374–5, so many city councillors (which included shopkeepers and artisans), had left town that no quorum could be obtained from 11 April to 23 August, and the councils shut their doors again during Florence's fourth plague in 1383.[82] Although the humanist chancellor Leonardo Bruni had scorned his compatriots for fleeing the city in 1383, he changed his tune in 1400. Because of that plague's severity, flight was then the only remedy.[83] Lucca's chronicler, Giovanni Sercambi, also reported that a great many citizens left his town during this unusually virulent

[76] Spaccini, *Cronaca di Modena*, II, 108.   [77] Ibid.
[78] He comments that Turin and Vercelli were 'greatly abandoned by the plague', but does not mention any family members abandoning one another; ibid., 89.
[79] Baldinucci, *Quaderno*, 78. I thank John Henderson for this reference.
[80] Amelang, *A Journal of the Plague Year*, 22.
[81] Beauvieux, 'Expériences ordinaires de la peste', 76–7, 127, 134–5, and 363–4.
[82] Cohn, *The Black Death Transformed*, 125, 146–7.
[83] Bruni, *Historiarum Florentini*, 236 and 280.

plague, and added that the disease spread so swiftly through the countryside that citizens now fled further afield: 'some to Bologna, others to Genoa, others to Savona and to the Riviera', leaving few behind, at least 'among those who mattered (*persone da facti*)'. Yet he mentioned nothing about husbands and wives abandoning one another, their children, or of other kin. Sercambi instead praised a 'small band' among the laity who remained, sacrificing themselves for Lucca's 'security'. These were young men of Lucca's ruling 'House of the Guinigi and their friends'. They remained, though fully aware of this plague's disastrous death rate (*smisurata moria*).[84]

Flight from cities was no longer the same as in 1348. Already during the plague exodus of 1374–5, Florence's Stefani made it clear: citizens now moved together 'with their children and wives',[85] despite the plague continuing to be highly contagious with deaths clustering in households.[86] Moreover, chroniclers did not describe these new seasonal departures as selfish or cruel, leaving the sick unattended without medicine, food, or care, and few accused physicians, notaries, priests, or friars of shunning their flocks to save their skins. By the end of the fourteenth century, the debate had instead shifted full circle. Florence's chancellor, Coluccio Salutati, was in the distinct minority when he berated fellow citizens for fleeing the city. Others, such as the Bolognese humanist and jurist, Pellegrino Zambeccari, questioned his judgement in failing to observe caution, especially regarding the safety of his three young children. At the very least, Zambeccari advised, he might ensure their health by allowing them to escape and invited them to stay with him in Bologna.[87] At the same time, cities were not left abandoned by trusted officials or priests. During the plague of 1526–7 in Ragusa on the Dalmatian coast, its worst since the Black Death, 'most priests remained faithful to their calling and cooperated fully with the authorities to curb the spread of the disease'.[88] During the disastrous plagues of 1603, 1625, and 1665 in London, writers such as Thomas Dekker, John Taylor, Thomas Brewer, and (later) Daniel Defoe crafted vignettes of cruelty concerning the reception by villagers of Londoners who had fled the capital with their families. But these plague authors praised mayors such as Sir John Lawrence, aldermen, councillors, their deputies, surgeons, and apothecaries, who remained at their posts, with many dying as a consequence.[89]

Plagues post-1348, even before the deadly ones of the seventeenth century, could be almost as destructive as the Black Death, at least within certain cities and localities, and in a few instances were more vividly remembered by their chroniclers than the Black Death. Such was the case of the 1405 plague at Padua, recorded by the Gatari chronicles. War in the countryside had sparked crop failure and malnuitrition

---

[84] *Le Croniche di Giovanni Sercambi*, III, 4–5: only by November 1400 did a few citizens begin to return to the city; ibid., II, 11.

[85] Stefani, *Cronica fiorentina*, 289.　　　　[86] See Cohn and Alfani, 'Households and Plague'.

[87] *Epistolario di Coluccio Salutati*, II, 226, for Salutati's letter to Zambeccari, on 2 August 1390; and ibid., IV, part 2, 293–7 for Zambeccari's reply, 13 August 1390.

[88] Tomič and Blažina, *Expelling the Plague*, 224. Also see Benadusi, *A Provincial Elite*, 95, for the small Casentino town of Poppi, where the wealthy during the disastrous plague of 1631 remained at their posts, exposing themselves to contagion, and died in proportions equal to the poor.

[89] Creighton, I, 481–4, 512, 517, 666–7. On hostility towards Londoners who fled to the country during the plague of 1665; also see Wear, 'Fear, Anxiety, and the Plague', 343.

that drove peasants into the city. Overcrowding and worsening sanitary conditions produced stench and putrification, triggering a 'ferocious plague' with the tell-tale signs and death within two or three days. From these contexts, the Gatari then described mass burials:

> And you the reader should note the way in which people were buried. In the morning, carts gathered the dead, each carrying sixteen to twenty bodies. At the head was only one priest with a cross fitted on the cart's rudder and a lighted lantern. Every day a large ditch was dug in the churchyard and in every ditch two hundred or even three hundred were thrown, one over the other, covered little by little with dirt. And these were citizens... Some carried their fathers on their shoulders to the grave; others, their sons in their arms; husbands, wives; wives, husbands; brothers, sisters, with such anguish, screams, and cruel cries that could be heard in heaven.[90]

On first sight, Padua's anguish of 1405 may recall the horrors of 1348, but it differed profoundly: no descriptions are given of cruel abandonment splintering families or of doctors, notaries, and priests abjuring their duties. Now, at the head of the carts collecting the dead, was a priest followed by fathers, sons, husbands, wives, brothers, and sisters, who, despite fears of contagion, carried the dead on their shoulders. Instead of callous indifference without tears, treating loved ones as no more than 'dead goats' (as Boccaccio had put it), Paduans' anguish and screams over lost loved ones now reached the heavens.

Finally, despite the Black Death fuelling a new satirical literature, mocking priests and especially friars for their gluttony, cupidity, and petty desires for worldly gain, as seen in stories by Boccaccio, Giovanni Sercambi, Franco Sacchetti, Gentile Sermini, William Langland, Geoffrey Chaucer, Agnolo Firenzuola, and others,[91] I know of only one chronicler who criticized the clergy's lack of involvement or profiteering during a later plague. According to the anonymous 'bourgeois of Paris', probably a clergyman, the plague of 1418 was the worst anyone had seen in three hundred years! So many priests had died that they adopted economies of scale, singing one grand burial mass (*une messe à notte*) for 'four or six or eight heads of households (*chefs d'hôtel*)'. In addition, priests bid up their prices for these services.[92] But this was no repeat of the accusations of cowardice made in 1348. Instead, it was the opposite: priests toiled 'night and day', transporting Eucharists to the thousands dying in Paris and its environs.[93] Moreover, I know of no reports in later plagues claiming that notaries fled or refused to redact testaments of the plague-infected. Again, the opposite was reported, as at Ivrea in 1585 during its worst plague of the sixteenth century[94] or at Aix-en-Provence during the plague of 1580, when, because of the demand for wills, notarial business became frenetic.[95] Butchers and bakers might have threatened to leave Aix because of suppliers' refusal to enter the plagued city, but the horrors of abandonment had not returned. Soldiers and

---

[90] Gatari, *Cronaca Carrarese*, 559–60.
[91] See for instance the fifteenth-century stories in Martines, *An Italian Renaissance Sextet*.
[92] *Journal d'un bourgeois de Paris*, 134.   [93] Ibid., 133.
[94] Alfani, *Il Grand Tour*, 155.
[95] Dolan, *La notaire*, 25–35; also Wrightson, *Ralph Tailor's Summer*.

young artisan and merchant volunteers maintained law and order and guarded the city; churchmen continued their services; and families, anxious over catching plague from pall-bearers, carried their children or parents to the cemeteries with their own hands. According to Claire Dolan, the 'exceptional situation' of plague in 1580 'revived family solidarity'.[96]

CONCLUSIONS AND COMPARISONS

Shona Kelly Wray has argued that the pictures painted by Boccaccio and chroniclers of family abandonment, mass burials, and of priests, notaries, and neighbours shunning their vital duties during the Black Death were literary topoi, copied from one writer to the next, and should be cast aside.[97] Instead, these professionals and especially family members in 1348 unflinchingly supported neighbours in their hour of death. She bases her conclusions on a study of last wills and testaments in one city, Bologna, and argues that citizens stricken by plague continued drawing the requisite number of neighbours, kin, and friends to witness wills, and notaries readily drafted them. Trust and social bonds remained secure.[98] But even in Bologna, where testaments were copied for tax purposes and survive almost intact (*I Memoriali*), those of 1348 represent no more than 5 per cent of the city's population dying that year, assuming a conservative estimate of half the population succumbing to the Black Death. In fact, the wills represented a significantly lower ratio of the dying in 1348 than in the only non-plague year Wray analysed (1337, about 20 per cent of the dying).[99] We simply have no way of viewing the vast majority of those who died during the plague months without making wills: had they died too quickly to redact one? Had their deaths been invisible as chroniclers claimed? Had priests, notaries, loved ones, or neighbours abandoned them, refusing to enter their homes even to take precious possessions, as in fact chroniclers across Europe attested?[100]

---

[96] Dolan, *La notaire*, 34.

[97] Wray, *Communities and Crisis*. Before her, Smail, 'Accommodating Plague', 22, argued that the abandonment tales in Boccaccio and chroniclers were 'tropes', 'literary constructions' to heighten the drama of the plague. His conclusion rested entirely on surviving notarial contracts in one place—Marseille—and not on an analysis of texts in 1348 or over time. To show that relatives and servants stayed by the bedside in vigils for the dying, he cites two cases from the notarial records (21). Yet he also shows that efforts to find notaries to draft last wills were not always successful (21).

[98] Wray, *Communities and Crisis*; and see my critical but favourable review in *Speculum*.

[99] Emery, 'The Black Death', 617, argued that despite the 1348 spike in testaments, the numbers represented a small proportion of those who died during the plague; yet he concludes that the presence of testaments showed the afflicted had not been abandoned.

[100] From ten witness testimonies at Apt from the canonization of Countess Delphine de Puimichel, Archambeau, 'Healing Options', 544 and 558–9, supports Wray and Smail: the ill could seek 'healing' (559). Again, the fact that not everyone ran and not all institutions collapsed does not prove that abandonment was not widespread, as is also seen with cholera at Sligo in 1832, Garfagnana in 1884, and occasionally in India during the Third Pandemic; see Chapters 7 and 10. As Hatcher, 'England in the Aftermath of the Black Death', has argued, on certain matters impressions from chroniclers and other commentators are more reliable than medieval statistical evidence. In addition, archival evidence points to the flight of professionals; see Bowsky, 'The Impact', 18, regarding the notarial books of Siena's Ser Francesco di Pietro di Ferro, who fled Siena for the coastal village of

Nor has Wray or others examined texts to determine the extent that one author may have copied another: was there some *Urtext?* Certainly, it was not the *Decameron*, as Wray seems to suggests, finished around 1355 but circulated later—a text which from remarks by Stefani and Ser Luca does not appear to have been known even by learned Tuscans thirty or fifty years later. Nor has she or others explained how such texts could have circulated so quickly across Europe, in a matter of days, from country friars such as le Beauvaisis Jean de Venette to merchant writers such as Siena's Agnolo di Tura.[101] Finally, if simply a topos without grounding in social realities, why did it virtually disappear with later plagues, when texts such as the *Decameron* would have become better known, with time now to copy?

One later chronicler to admit that his source for 1348 came from Boccaccio— the only one I know to have cited the *Decameron*—was the early fifteenth-century Florentine merchant Giovanni di Pagolo Morelli.[102] While he mentions the tale of two pigs eating paupers' rags, his account shows no slavish copying. He dwells on matters not mentioned by Boccaccio, such as elaborations on the haemorrhagic and pneumonic symptoms of the plague and Florence's population before and after the Black Death. Like Boccaccio, Morelli reports the abandonment of family members in 1348, but here too Morelli's description is wholly different. He is the one chronicler to reflect on testaments.

> Then there came something truly amazing: many died in the street and on benches, abandoned without help or comfort from anyone, and left there unburied, because their neighbours had fled from the stench ... The afflicted received no services; no one came to bury them, and if you had desired a witness for your last will and testament you could not procure one. Quite simply there was none to be found, or it'd cost you 6 or 8 florins.[103]

Furthermore, Morelli lived through and commented on seven further plagues in Florence, but without repeating any stories of abandonment.

Morelli's account along with the other texts examined here show a wide variety of expression and interpretation. Boccaccio was unique in describing a certain sector of society who 'took a single and very inhuman precaution' of running away from the sick, but who also bonded together in small groups of trusted ones, to 'entertain themselves with music and whatever other amusements they were able to devise' to avoid and forget the lugubrious scenes of death back in the city. The hundred stories to follow curiously place his witty, noble, and sophisticated storytellers in a none-too-favourable light. True to what Boccaccio described as the 'callous ones', his merry band followed suit, isolating themselves in the hills of

---

Talamone early in the plague and did not return until 19 January 1349. Bowsky concludes, 'those who could flee probably did'.

[101] See *Cronaca Senese*, 555.

[102] Several physicians in plague tracts mentioned Boccaccio from the sixteenth century on, but for his descriptions of plague signs and symptoms, not abandonment; see Cohn, *Cultures of Plague*, 33, 39, 70, 72, and 93.

[103] Morelli, *Ricordi*, 208–9.

Settignano, delighting themselves without once mentioning the Black Death or those they left behind facing the carnage back in Florence.[104]

Boccaccio was hardly the only one to make unique pronouncements about Black Death abandonment. Louis Sanctus expressed sympathy with those who refused to visit the plague-afflicted, explaining that such close proximity would almost certainly lead to sudden death. Matteo Villani, on the other hand, was the only one to suggest that had citizens not abandoned the sick in such numbers, the mortalities would have been lower, and with his fellow Florentine, the poet Pucci, he went to the other extreme. Citizens who fled had violated Christian tenets and aped the habits of infidels. For the German Mathias de Nuwenburg, 'such things' were just 'too horrible to write or tell', even though he had just recounted the burning alive of entire Jewish communities. Only the Pisan Ranieri shared the same view as Villani that towards the end of the Black Death, citizens recovered their humanity by assisting the afflicted, but he had not copied Villani and did not draw the same conclusion that the change of heart had ended the plague.

The anonymous *Storie Pistoresi* and the chronicle of the abbot of Cremona were the only accounts to suggest that abandonment was more common when the dying relative or friend was stricken with pneumonic plague. By contrast, the chronicler of Rimini and Villani pointed to buboes as the signs that made relatives run. Both Michele da Piazza and Jean de Venette, separated by over 2000 km, one in Messina, the other in rural Beauvaisis, castigated 'the cowardly priests' (de Venette's words) but absolved the regular clergy for not abandoning their flocks. According to Pucci and the *Storie Pistoresi*, neither friar nor priest dared to approach the ill. By contrast, the abbot of Tournai alone defended a town's clergy, priests, and friars: they heard confessions, administered the sacraments, and visited the afflicted.

As we have seen, many attributed the unusually 'cruel' behaviour of neighbours to the plague's lightning contagion, with some seeing it transmitted by sight. Yet Florence's Stefani and Piacenza's de' Mussis gave no explanations. Instead, they spun stories of abandonment with invented dialogues, which no one bothered copying. Even the litany of fathers, abandoning sons; sons, fathers; brothers, sisters, etc., varied in language and kinship from one author to another. Boccaccio was alone in mentioning uncles abandoning nephews; Louis Sanctus, alone in mentioning acquaintances; and the English, Irish, and Scots rarely specified the blood relations. Finally, describing the hostility received at Catania by those who had fled Messina, Michele da Piazza is the only medieval chronicler I know to recount the experiences of the departed.[105] For cruel receptions, the next stories come from the fiction writer Thomas Dekker during a plague of 1603: one fleeing London became ill forty miles from home and sought help in an inn. Assistance came only once a fellow Londoner arrived, but by then it was too late. The victim

---

[104] In the stories, Boccaccio mentions the plague on Day Nine—*gli animali, sì come cavriuoli, cervi e altri, quasi sicuri da' cacciatori per la soprastante pistolenzia*, but it comes from his introductory commentary, not the noble interlocutors. I thank Timothy Kircher for this reference. Stefani, *Cronica fiorentina*, also mentioned small bands of trusted friends forming to render support for one another (*le genti si ragunavano in brigata a mangiare per pigliare qualche conforto*, 232).

[105] Michele da Piazza, *Cronica*, 82–4; and Horrox, 37–41.

was carried to die on a straw heap in a field, where the village parson and clerk had refused him a proper Christian burial, and was left in the hole where he died.[106] For the plague of 1625, storytellers depict those fleeing London confronting more direct violence: 'They are driven back by men with bills and halberds', and were forced to 'sleep in stables, barns and outhouses, or even by the roadside in ditches and in the open fields. And that was the lot of comparatively wealthy men'.[107]

Back to Black Death: more important than particularities from one writer to the next—variations in language, stories, and explanations of fear, flight, and neglected duties—was an abrupt change after 1348. With numerous successive waves of plague and hundreds, if not thousands, of accounts of them, little more than a handful of abandonment stories seep into accounts of later plagues, and none fills page-plus descriptions as they did for 1348. If the 1348 descriptions of abandonment, flight, and neglected duties were empty phrases for dramatic affect, literary topoi without relevance to realities, then why did authors suddenly cease repeating them for successive plagues, especially those who had recorded them in 1348 but lived through and recorded later ones? As with the mass slaughter of Jews in 1348 and its cessation with future plagues, so too with abandonment, sentiments changed: denying one is as absurd as denying the other. While the Black Death tore societies asunder to their very core—the family—later plagues, even when unusually deadly, united inhabitants across city walls, factions, class, and gender, as happened in 1400 in central Italy, 1536 in Ragusa, and 1580 in Aix. A reason for the change can be seen as early as the last stages of the Black Death itself. As reports by Matteo Villani and Ranieri Sardo suggest, people began realizing that flight and abandonment were counterproductive; for self and community preservation, charity and sacrifice proved more efficacious. We now turn to further ways in which the Black Death divided communities, while plagues post-1348 united them.

---

[106] Dekker, *The Wonderfull Yeare. 1603*; cited in Creighton, I, 483.
[107] Brewer, *The Weeping Lady*, cited in Creighton, I, 517. Also, see Taylor, *The Fearfull Summer*, who at Hampton Court described the 'Welcome' given to London plague fugitives 'like dogs into a church' and those in the surrounding towns as 'Uncharitable hounds, hearts hard as rocks'.

4

Mechanisms for Unity
Saints and Plagues

Unlike stories from Livy, Procopius, and others in antiquity, the history of plagues in the late Middle Ages and Renaissance reveals few incidents where authors point explicitly to the spread of epidemic disease as ending warfare or social strife between factions or classes. Moreover, into the eighteenth century, chronicles and other narrative sources—saints' lives included—reveal few examples of martyrs, who struggled against the plague to save their cities or to alleviate the suffering of strangers and the poor. Instead, for 1348, the opposite was heard. Chroniclers, writers, even the preambles to new legislation ranted about greed, increases in litigation,[1] selfishness, and charity gone cold. According to Jean de Venette, in 1348,

> the world was not changed for the better but for the worse...For men were more avaricious and grasping than before, even though they had far greater possessions. They were more covetous and disturbed each other more frequently with suits, brawls, disputes, and pleas.[2]

Such antipathy, the Carmelite claimed, was played out not only in market squares and country lanes but interregionally between vying political powers: 'the enemies of the king of France and of the Church were stronger and wickeder than before and stirred up wars on sea and on land.... Charity began to cool.'[3] Certainly, increased warfare afflicted regions beyond the battlefields of the Hundred Years War, as seen with papal aggrandizement of power in central Italy under the command of Cardinal Egidio Albornoz (1310–67), consolidation of Church control over several major city-states, intensification of war between Florence and Milan, and the emergence of territorial states steadily absorbing once-independent cities such as Prato, Pistoia, and later Arezzo, Cortona, and Pisa.

Studies grounded in administrative archives have argued that violence, criminality, and especially controversies over inheritances and dowries increased during and immediately after the Black Death. Best studied remains Siena examined over forty years ago by William Bowsky.[4] He pointed to the breakdown of police enforcement and suspension of civil courts from 2 June until 1 September 1348, and of the city

---

[1] See Bowsky, 'The Impact', 28. Palmer, *English Law*, 3, shows that cases brought before certain courts stalled because of plague and did not return to pre-1348 levels until 1365; he does not, however, evaluate these statistics based on population. For increased litigation with plague in 1636 in Newcastle upon Tyne, see Wrightson, *Ralph Tailor's Summer*, ch. 11.
[2] *The Chronicle of Jean de Venette*, 51.   [3] Ibid., 51.   [4] Bowsky, 'The Impact', 27–8.

council from 2 June to 15 August. During these plague months and into the early 1350s, the *Comune* lamented the increase in violence and ease with which criminals evaded justice. After the plague, the government attempted to stem the tide of illegal seizures of inheritances, dowries, and other property, and to protect orphans and widows by creating special courts, judges, and commissions.[5] To address the breakdown in law enforcement and the increase in violence, the city council created a new magistrate, 'the Official for the Custody of the City'.[6] During plagues in early modern Italy, Alessandro Pastore and others have found that criminality also increased, at least during the last disastrous outbreaks in Bologna in 1630 and Genoa and Rome in 1656–7.[7] Moreover, for the late Middle Ages, perceptions of epidemics sparking conflict and beastly behaviour were not unique to 1348. Against the backdrop of an epidemic at Mainz in April 1367, a local chronicler decried that acts of human evil and insolence by members of the clergy or rustics multiplied. 'Commoners lived like beasts, were contemptuous of spiritual matters and created fear for all travellers throughout Germany and especially within the Rhine valley . . . the evil of thieves, adulterers, usurers, law enforcers, and men who disgracefully sought out sexual favours grew in strength'. The disease in question appears not, however, to have been plague but a disease (*morbida pestis*) with influenza-like symptoms of coldness, coughs, an unheard-of tightness of the chest, and expectoration from which many died.[8] It was a remarkably rare instance, when a medieval chronicler commented at all on a population's reactions to any epidemic that was not plague.

LAWS

After the Black Death, however, chroniclers' reports on law and order did not usually point to beastly behaviour or anarchy. With Florence's third and fourth plagues in 1374 and 1383, its chronicler, Stefani, expressed none of the hysteria about his countrymen heard in 1348. In 1374 the plague heralded the passage of new ordinances concerned with funerary customs—prohibitions against ringing bells, handing over of funerary coins, carrying more than four torches, and dressing in black anyone who was not the child of the deceased. Further laws were drafted against those who fled town, failed to appear in town councils, or had not attended other political duties after a ten-day absence. Instead of rousing conflict, the laws, he comments, were mostly obeyed: 'no one complained'.[9] In 1383, Stefani repeats his rubric of 1374—'How because of the plague (*mortalità*), Florence promulgated many laws and ordinances'. Now, matters differed slightly.

---

[5] Ibid., 27–8. Also, see idem, 'The Medieval Commune', 15.   [6] Ibid., 15.

[7] Pastore, *Crimine e giustizia*, chs 6–7; and for crimes of theft, violations of quarantine, and violence in Florence's lazaretto, see Calvi, 'The Florentine Plague of 1630–33'. Others such as Langer, 'The Black Death', claimed that the Black Death, subsequent plagues, and all big epidemics provoke lawlessness, but his proof rests on a single undated citation from Wycliff (117).

[8] *Chronicon Moguntinum*, 173.   [9] Stefani, *Cronica fiorentina*, 289.

Laws were passed preventing citizens leaving the city because of the plague, because it was surmised that the lower classes (*la minuta gente*) would not leave but would take the opportunity to revolt, and would be joined by other malcontents. Seeing that only the rich were leaving, the government would allow only those with special permits to depart, but the measures did not work.

Rather than resort to more Draconian measures, the councils adopted a mixture of appeals to self-interest and leniency, asking those who had already left and those desiring to leave for a fee, and no revolt erupted.[10] Even during the Black Death, city-states passed legislation to preserve their populations and alleviate suffering. Most famous were those of Pistoia, north-west of Florence. Unlike many city-states whose legislative assemblies did not convene during the summer months because of plague deaths and the flight of citizens, Pistoia not only passed decrees early in the plague (2 May 1348), but amended them on 4 June, when mortality rates were approaching their peak. These decrees largely comprised restrictions. They prohibited the entry of goods and people from two cities—Pisa and Lucca—which Pistoia's councillors saw as staging posts for the spread of the disease through Tuscany. Citizens would be heavily fined for showing any hospitality to these people. It passed restrictions against ringing funeral bells, sharply limited funerary attendance, and imposed numerous prohibitions on tanning and butchering to prevent polluting the air. Given prevailing notions about miasmas and also because they saw the disease spreading rapidly from person to person, such laws made sense. At the same time, however, they caused divisions between the citizens of Pistoia and between those within the city and those outside the walls, and offered no assistance to the afflicted. The statutes' revisions on 4 June may have pointed in a more charitable direction. Perhaps from observing epidemiological trends, as seen with Ebola today, where unburied cadavers of diseased victims create dangerous nodes of transmission, the city appointed sixteen men from each quarter to remove corpses from homes to carry them to church and then for burial. The provision attached a punitive clause that may have justified family members abandoning their loved ones: 'no one shall dare enter a house...where a person has died or carry the body to burial...'.[11]

Pistoia was not the only city to initiate plague legislation during the Black Death. Far less mentioned are Siena's laws, which can be glimpsed only in the work of its principal chronicler, Agnolo di Tura. They differed from Pistoia's restrictive clauses as well as laws introduced in Orvieto and Florence in 1348. Siena's governors elected citizens, granting them a thousand gold florins to be distributed to the afflicted and those too poor to bury their dead.[12] But Siena seems to have been the exception. For the most part, plague legislation up to the fifteenth century did not grant sustenance to the poor, despite commerce being blocked and employment curtailed, nor aid to provision new facilities, medicines, and care. Instead, these laws imposed restrictions, dividing populations by locking houses and imposing other internal

[10] Ibid., 427.   [11] 'Gli Ordinamenti sanitari'.   [12] *Cronaca Senese*, 555.

quarantines and barriers against any wishing to enter from outside, as with Ragusa's 'Trentino' in 1377, those of Bernabò Visconti in Milan in the 1370s, those in Mantua in 1374, and Venice's famous 'quarantine' of 1422. These barred inhabitants from re-entering their cities, prevented travel, and embargoed goods. In 1399, Milan ordered the fumigation of homes and destruction of property. As Ann Carmichael argued almost thirty years ago, plague controls became social controls.[13]

Moreover, Black Death legislation passed in Provence early in 1348,[14] which soon appeared across monarchies, city-states, and other regions, blamed portions of the population—generally the poor, peasants, workers, and artisans—supposedly for exploiting shifts in supply and demand created by the demographic catastrophe and charging extortionate wages or demanding higher prices for basic commodities. Best known are England's Ordinances and Statues of Labourers enacted in 1349 and 1351. In addition to fixing prices and wages, they restricted labourers' freedom of movement. Writers such as Giovanni Boccaccio, William Langland, Matteo Villani, Agnolo di Tura, Marchionne di Coppo Stefani, and Henry Knighton scorned labourers for their post-plague sloth, dissolute behaviour, arrogance, lack of obedience, and, above all, greed. The laws prompted conflict and division by branding artisans and labourers as the guilty ones.[15] Although mainly created soon after the Black Death, not all these laws vanished quickly, as happened in Provence or the Ile de France. Others changed their face fundamentally instead. With the second plague of 1361–3, new labour decrees in Italian city-states now accepted the new market realities, no longer blaming or penalizing labourers with heavy fines or imprisonment. Governing elites competed for these rare resources and passed decrees to encourage movement. During its second plague in 1363, Florence's labour legislation shifted abruptly from the stick to the carrot, granting farm labourers tax exemptions of up to fifteen years to settle and work within its territory.[16] England was the exception: its wage and price limits with restrictions on labour movement continued into the fifteenth century. Amendments to the original laws of 1351, in fact, became more restrictive and Draconian in 1360–1, 1388, and 1406, although low monetary fines replaced flogging and branding violators' foreheads.[17] Yet even in England, a shift occurred in the opposite direction. Cases coming to court declined sharply after 1352, a *modus vivendi* developing between labourers and lords;[18] both paid low fines to ensure labour stability and rising nominal wages, and popular riots against these laws disappeared by 1357.[19]

---

[13] Carmichael, *Plague and the Poor*, 108–18.

[14] See Braid, '"Et non ultra"'; and idem, *Peste, prolétaires et politiques*, 577.

[15] Boccaccio, *Decameron*, 15–16; Langland, *Piers the Ploughman*, 127–8; Matteo Villani, *Cronica*, I, 15–17 and 392; Stefani, *Cronica fiorentina*, 232.

[16] See Braid, '"Et non ultra"', 437–91; idem, *Peste, prolétaires et politiques*, and its exhaustive bibliography. For the shift in labour legislation in central and northern Italian city-states, see Cohn, 'After the Black Death'. As early as 1350, Siena began abandoning its punitive measures so as to attract labourers from other city-states; Bowsky, 'The Impact', 32.

[17] Cohn, 'After the Black Death'.

[18] Poos, 'The Social Context', 48; Penn and Dyer, 'Wages', 359; and Cohn, 'After the Black Death', 461.

[19] Cohn, *Popular Protest in Late Medieval English Towns*, 126–8.

RELIGIOUS PROCESSIONS: THE BLACK DEATH

Another change in reactions that followed the Black Death through successive waves of plague was the organization and prevalence of processions to fight against it. Such initiatives by the Church, city councils, and the populace, despite epidemiological dangers, brought societies together in penitent devotion and at a plague's end in joyous celebration and public works to fulfil promises to the saints. Only at the end of the sixteenth or seventeenth century might they have also sparked division. However, I know of only one case to have been cited.[20]

Nonetheless, despite awareness by physicians, municipal governments, the populace, and the Church of the dangers of contagion, communities across class and professions agreed that a two-pronged attack was needed to arrest plague—quarantine and appeals to God's mercy with public prayers, litanies, and above all, processions. Even during Italy's peninsula-wide plague of 1574–8, when people were paying increased attention to the networks of carriers who were transmitting the disease, no conflicts arose between Church and State. Instead, in places such as Palermo, Mantua, Milan, and Venice, the Church cooperated with Health Boards and concurred with the latest findings on contagion. New forms of piety and devotion were invented, such as prayers and litanies at precise hours of the day when, from the confines of quarantined homes, all could participate.[21] Church leaders such as Milan's archbishop, Carlo Borromeo, were cognizant of the dangers and devised new rules to protect the clergy, demanding that they carry long sticks to prevent worshippers coming within breathing distance and building barriers within churches to separate the clergy from congregations.[22] Even in Ragusa (Dubrovnik), which led the way with new regulations on quarantine and other plague laws from 1377 to its last disastrous plague in 1526–7, the patrician ruling class not only tolerated religious processions, they 'used them to their advantage to inform the citizens about plague control measures and impose new plague control regulations'.[23]

By contrast, evidence of collective devotion was rare for 1348. Giovanni Boccaccio, Matteo Villani, and Siena's Agnolo di Tura argued that those who survived the Black Death horrors formed two groups—the few who understood the plague as God's wrath against sin and thereby attended to mending their ways, and the majority who turned their backs on God to indulge in pleasurable pastimes—gaming, gambling,

---

[20] Cipolla, *Faith, Reason, and the Plague*, 5–6, claims 'conflicts between the health authorities and the men of the Church were an everyday occurrence in times of epidemics', but he mentions only one case at Montelupo in 1630, 75–9. Henderson, 'The Black Death', argues that in 1348 'no conflict' arose between Church and State on approaches to curtailing plague but they 'occurred in later centuries' (144). Yet, based on his earlier work, he references only one such later conflict—in Florence in 1523 (149). However, that earlier study showed no conflict between Church and State, even though its government had locked churches, stopped preaching, and prohibited public celebrations of the city's principal feast days—Corpus Christi and San Giovanni. Instead, by its own volition, the government mollified its ordinances; idem, 'Epidemics in Renaissance Florence', 182. Later, state restrictions on processions were one factor that triggered the Moscow riots in September 1771; Alexander, *Bubonic Plague*, ch. 7.

[21] Cohn, *Cultures of Plague*, 288–90.   [22] Ibid., 288–90.

[23] Tomić and Blažina, *Expelling the Plague*, 224.

and feasting off the newborn wealth bequeathed by the high mortalities. Except perhaps for small street parties or groups of trusted friends who escaped societal responsibilities, both tendencies were individual, not collective, actions. Of course, according to chronicle reports, the major collective form of devotion was the flagellant movement that crossed Europe from Hungary to London. While this movement brought people together to calm God's wrath, chroniclers attest to the ways it ripped communities apart, fuelling conflict between the flagellants on the one hand and Church and State on the other, leading to the flagellants' excommunication.[24] In places, chroniclers also maintained that these bands contributed to the persecution of the Jews. Flagellants were not the only new pious movement to sprout in the plague's wake. Yet I know of only one chronicler to describe them and for one city alone—Tournai. Here, penitent groups such as the feet washers competed for public space to perform their rituals and recruit followers. According to its abbot, Gilles le Muisit, these groups came to blows with one another as well as with the Dominicans, who at Tournai jealously guarded their square against the new competitors.

Beyond the flagellant movement, descriptions in chronicles of processions or other communal acts of devotion organized by the Church or town councils appear rarely in 1348, and I know of no festivals of thanksgiving to celebrate the end of plague, as became common in the Renaissance and early modern period.[25] For 1348, Jean le Bel said the people (*les gens*) thought the plague resulted from God's vengeance and the only solution was to demonstrate 'great and various forms of penance by grand devotion', but he did not clarify if these pertained to individual acts of piety or were communal acts of penitence or processions.[26] An exception occurred in Barcelona, in mid-May, when its citizens 'made a beautiful and grand procession', that included 'many clerics' across the hierarchy (*sedis*) to the parish churches, along with 'many of the laity' (*pluribus gentibus*).[27] Another comes in a brief note from le Muisit of a procession by those in Tournai (*Tornacensis*).[28] Writing in the late sixteenth century, a Perugian chronicler maintained that 'all the people of the city and the outlying villages (*e de castella e de ville*) joined in processions that included acts of flagellation (*in discipline*) and the recitation of the litanies'.[29] If he were using sources now lost for 1348 and not reflecting expectations from his own time, it would be the only reference to flagellation during the Black Death anywhere in Italy.

In contrast to these rare, brief, and hazy descriptions of communal acts of piety in 1348, the Sicilian friar Michele da Piazza devotes considerable space to attempts to organize public devotion to placate God's wrath in two Sicilian cities. As in

---

[24] See Louis Sanctus's chronicle in 'La Peste en Avignon (1348)'; on the flagellants, Cohn, 'The Black Death', 11–12 and Graus, *Pest—Geissler—Judenmorde*, 38–59.

[25] A possible exception may have been Siena's decision to build a chapel adjoining the Palazzo Comunale, dedicated to the Virgin Mary, begun in 1354, completed in 1376; Bowsky, 'The Impact', 15. However, there is no evidence of celebrations of thanksgiving at the plague's end.

[26] *Chronique de Jean le Bel*, I., 222.   [27] *Cronica del Racional de la Ciutat*, 119.

[28] *Chronique et annales de Gilles le Muisit*, 248.

[29] *Cronica della città di Perugia*, 148. In addition, an entry in Siena's government accounts, the Biccherna, contains a payment for candles for one man on 30 June 1348 to process to the sacristy of a church but describes no collective processions; Bowsky,' The Impact', 15.

Barcelona, they occurred early on during the plague. More importantly, they did not unify communities but split them further apart. In November 1347, several people from Messina who were residing in Catania appealed to the Patriarch to carry the relics of Agatha back to Messina to save their city from plague. Citizens of Catania, however, saw these plans as a cunning plot by new immigrants to steal her relics, and marched en masse to the cathedral, where they shouted and abused the Patriarch, wrested his keys to the church containing Agatha's relics, and threatened to kill him if he allowed her bones to escape. Meanwhile, the fate of the immigrant Messinesi worsened along with others who had sought refuge from the plague at Catania. They were so loathed that no Catanese would befriend, speak, or shelter them. They could find lodging only if a Messinese already established in town would 'secretly' take them in. The Catanesi fled at their sight.[30]

Citizens of Messina who remained at home also participated in a procession; in their case, to a village six miles away to capture and bring to the city another sacred object—a statue of Santa Maria della Scala—to miraculously heal plague-stricken citizens. This venture also proved disruptive. Before arriving at Messina, the Virgin Mary intervened, refusing to let her bones enter the city. What civil conflict this miraculous resistance concealed is difficult to know. But after the statue finally passed through Messina's gates to its principal church, Santa Maria la Nuova, and women had adorned it with silk and jewels, the results failed to arouse communal devotion, heighten morale, or remedy the plague. Michele disapproved of his townsmen's actions, commenting dryly: the statue performed no favours; the mortality grew worse.[31]

Only one example of communal masses and processions shows a positive response from a population during the Black Death of 1348, and it came towards the plague's end. Stefani, twelve at the time, leaves us with material not seen in any earlier account. Processions with *orlique* (relics) now took place, and one carrying the painting of the Madonna of Santa Maria dell' Impruneta,[32] chanting 'Misericordia', marched through Florence's streets to the Ringhiera dei Priori on the Palazzo della Signoria's south side. Unlike the Messinesi's attempts at communal devotion, Florence's efforts succeeded. According to Stefani, 'the people' drew up peace pacts (*paci*) resolving disputes of indebtedness, physical injuries, even murder. He then pointed to another change in sentiment: the terror and fear had led people to gather in small bands of trusted friends of about ten (*brigate*) to eat together and comfort one another, suggesting that the *Decameron*'s frame was not a literary invention.[33] As with impressions left by Matteo Villani, the Pisan Ranieri Sardo, and Gilles le Muisit, Stefani's narrative appears to chart a change over the Black Death's brief course. With the plague becoming perceived as a pandemic with no place to run, individuals and governments began to see mutual aid as more efficacious than flight, abandonment, or cruel self-interest. However, from

---

[30] Michele da Piazza, *Cronica*, 83–4.   [31] Ibid.
[32] Stefani, *Cronica fiorentina*, 231. On this image, Trexler, 'Florentine Religious Experience', 11–13, who appears not to have known this chapter in Stefani, claims the cult began later.
[33] Stefani, *Cronica fiorentina*, 232.

searching over 300 chroniclers who cover the Black Death, 1347–51, Stefani's description of this procession is unique in clearly unifying a community faced by plague in 1348.

PLAGUE PROCESSIONS POST-1348

Not only did communal forms of piety organized by the Church and municipalities become more common; often they became the centrepieces of chronicle descriptions for later plagues. The continuator of the *Gesta archiepiscoporum Magdeburgensium* makes one observation only for the plague of 1363: Magdeburg's archbishop led a 'general' procession against 'the disaster of the plague, then viciously spreading through the region'. With his prelates, canons, and those from religious orders, along with the people (*populo*), each carrying candles, he performed a high mass that involved the devotion of 'the entire congregation' and included an office, instituted by Pope Clement VI to end the plague. On foot, the archbishop visited all the city's churches to deliver special prayers.[34] Nothing is said about pustules, estimates of mortality, or the plague's spread.

For the same plague, 'the people' of Ragusa displayed 'great devotion', praying to God and giving charity to the poor, churches, and monasteries, and in the next plague, 1374, they also engaged in *gran devotione*. For these plagues, these were the chronicler's only comments.[35] His report of 1348 differed: estimates of the numbers killed were divided by categories, 'gentlemen and gentlewomen', 'the people who counted' (*povolo de conto*), and the lower classes (*povolo menudo*). He claimed the plague lasted a year, calling it the 'wrath of God' but said nothing about any *gran devotione* or communal acts by the citizenry.[36] For the third plague in 1374, a chronicler of Trent reported citizens' behaviour in a radically different light from the 1348 hysteria, fright, neglect, and violence he reported earlier: 'Those convalescing and those on their deathbeds conducted themselves with great discretion and devotion, requesting indulgence from those around them.'[37] For the 1375 plague in Barcelona, the only one other than the Black Death reported by the *Cronica del Racional de la Ciutat*, the entry was devoted solely to the city's 'big procession' at the end of June.[38] In Paris the clergy organized the celebration of litanies, in which clergy of every rank joined the laity to calm God's anger and end the plague of 1387.[39] Because of the great number killed during the plague of 1399, and to prevent further alarming citizens, the municipal government prohibited public announcements of plague victims' names and the usual funerary processions. Nonetheless, 'numerous gatherings of men and women from the lower classes (*plebe*), processed, most of them barefoot, weeping, genuflecting before the Lord, with contrite hearts pleading for deliverance from the plague'.[40] During the same

---

[34] *Gesta archiepiscoporum Magdeburgensium*, 440. [35] *Annales Ragusini*, 41–2.
[36] Ibid., 39. [37] *Cronica inedita di Giovanni da Parma*, Appendice, 52.
[38] *Cronica del Racional de la Ciutat*, 150.
[39] *Chronique du religieux de Saint-Denys*, I, 475. [40] Ibid., II, 694–5.

disastrous plague in Pistoia, Ser Luca Dominici, one of the few to report familial abandonment for a plague after 1348,[41] now described his citizens on 11 July 1399 as united, processing with the relics 'in love' to end the pestilence.[42]

For the next Europe-wide plague of 1438–9, citizens again united with communal masses and processions. In Basel, in quick succession, at least three processions were directed to end 'this big plague'. The initiative for the first came from the city. 'From its own expenses', it sponsored a procession with twenty-two priests and a thousand from the laity, with each granted a five-year indulgence for crimes of corruption (*venialium*), five for other criminal offences, and ten bottles of sweet wine (*carenas*). Nine days later, Basel's sacred council organized a 'solemn procession through the city against the plague', again with major indulgences. And on 3 July, its chaplains organized a procession involving 1400 people, performed with 'great devotion'.[43] These communal acts comprised the whole of this chronicler's plague entry. The same was true of Bologna for the same plague: 'seeing the cruelty of this massacre', its senate organized three *divote processioni*.[44]

A decade later, during the plague of 1448 that swept through central and northern Italy, the number, duration, and organization of communal processions involving clergy and laity became more extensive. Between the end of March and September in Perugia, at least six processions were organized. On 27 March, 'all the religious of Perugia along with the Monsignor and the city's Priors, all the gentlemen and women, and generally every person, including children (*fina alle rede*)' formed a procession. Congregating outdoors and dressed in white, they sang 'all the time the litanies, the laude and prayers, and marched to Saint Peters, where they prayed to God to end the plague'. On 28, 29, 30, and 31 March, chroniclers described similar processions with the clergy and laity marching, singing, and praying together and each procession ending at a different church.[45] On 14 September Perugia's rulers and religious orders organized three days of processions and fasts.[46] During the next big plague (1476), they held processions for five days, carrying holy images and banners. When these failed to end the plague, a longer series of processions ensued, lasting eighteen days, including three days of fasting.[47] In southern France, the people of Puy made a procession with their painting (*ymage*) of Our Lady of Puy 'to receive a remedy from God' to end the plague in 1480.[48]

Such special supplications proliferated in the sixteenth century, with cities staging numerous communal and ecclesiastical prayers, litanies, and processions,[49] as happened in Frankfurt-am-Main at the beginning of the century. These were often 'general processions', with clerics and the people (*cleri et populi*) assembling and

[41] See Chapter 3.
[42] *Cronache di Ser Luca Dominici*, I, 233. For the same plague at Tournai and its plague processions, see *Chronique des Pays-Bas*, III, 332.
[43] *Die Chronik Erhards von Appenwiler*, III, 251.
[44] *Historia di Bologna*, 53.   [45] *Cronica della città di Perugia*, 600.
[46] Ibid., 607, from another contemporary chronicle, the *Annali Decemvirali*.
[47] Bornstein, *The Bianchi*, 22. In 1486, plague turned church and government again to community-wide processions.
[48] *Le livre de Podio*, I, 194.   [49] Cohn, *Cultures of Plague*, ch. 9.

marching together *propter epidemiam*.[50] Other forms of procession further unified urban populations. These were votive celebrations that officially declared the end of a plague, with festivities freeing parishioners from quarantine onto streets and bridges for songs and fanfare, for which city governments commissioned artists to create banners, paintings, floats, triumphal arches, ephemeral works of art, fireworks, and ultimately promised construction of grandiose monuments in praise of God's redemption, most famously in Venice, where the churches Il Redentore and Santa Maria della Salute were commissioned by plague survivors, with annual processions that continue to this day.[51] These celebrations of thanksgiving, however, were hardly unique, as Santa Rosalia's numerous communal votive offerings from Sicily and then across Europe, India, Africa, and the New World will shortly reveal.

Instead of arousing blame and violence, plagues post-1348 could stimulate the opposite, peace movements and new organizations to succour the poor and infirm, as Magdeburg's archbishop achieved during its second plague in 1362 by organizing special masses and prayers sung and 'charity for peace and against plague expanded'.[52] More significantly, the next transregional religious movement after Black Death's flagellants was the 'Bianchi', which accompanied the plague of 1399–1400. According to its legend, a disguised Christ, seeking vengeance against mankind for his crucifixion, ordered a peasant to throw three pieces of bread into a spring, each piece condemning a third of humanity to annihilation. The peasant followed orders and threw one into the water, whereupon the benevolent Virgin miraculously intervened, convincing him to hold fast to the other two. The piece that was thrown referred to the Black Death's devastation and the present need for compassion, human and heavenly, to ensure humankind's survival. Laced through the journeys of the Bianchi were processions organized to end the plague (*per amore della pestilenza cessare*), such as one in mid-September 1399[53] that beseeched Christ, the Virgin Mary, and all the saints to bring 'peace, unity, and concord' and thereby 'protect all from the pestilence'.[54]

In contrast to the violence and conflicts in cities such as Tournai by the flagellants of 1349, the Bianchi with their hallmark cry 'Pace e misericordia' was a peace movement. It sought to placate God's anger by ending human anger and division, from petty disputes over debts among peasants to interregional military rivalry with the ongoing feuds, murders, and vengeance of Pistoia's aristocratic clans—the Panciatichi, Cancellieri, and Lazzati[55]—that fed wars between Florence, Milan, and their allies.[56] Unlike the flagellant movement of 1349, this one was joyous and devotional, stressing songs of praise (*laude*) over whipping (*disciplinati*) and spilling

[50] Latomus, *Acta aliquot*, 423.

[51] At the end of the 1574–8 plague, entire pamphlets were devoted to describing these festivities; see Cohn, *Cultures of Plague*, ch. 9.

[52] *Gesta archiepiscoporum Magdeburgensium*, 440.

[53] *Cronache di Ser Luca Dominici*, I, 238.

[54] Ibid., 171; see also the procession in Pistoia at the plague's height on 11 July 1400; ibid., 233.

[55] Ibid., 67. For the Bianchi boosting individuals' peace agreements in Siena, see Kumhera, *The Benefits of Peace*, 161–2.

[56] Florence supported the Panciatichi; Milan, the Cancellieri; *Cronache di Ser Luca Dominici*, 8.

blood, accompanied by visions of the apocalypse.[57] Further, the Bianchi provoked few, if any, conflicts with established churches or the state.[58] As Daniel Bornstein concluded, the Bianchi was a movement of 'popular orthodoxy' that exalted approved beliefs and traditional practices of the Church.[59] Beside figures at the top of Church hierarchies, secular leaders such as the merchant of Prato, Francesco di Marco Datini, and Duke Giangaleazzo Visconti of Milan, staffed or endorsed the movement, despite its egalitarian dress of white linen and red crosses that strove to blur distinctions and achieve unity between clergy and laity, men and women, city and countryside.[60]

SAINTS

The creation of saints and blessed ones (*beati/ae*) and the telling of their lives mark another divide between the Black Death and later plagues. In this case, however, the change appears more gradual and comes later. In the vast literature of saints' lives, and in contrast with contemporaneous chronicles, the Black Death hardly figured at all. In the rare instances when it is mentioned, it appears merely as a marker, indicating the death of someone within a saint's narrative or the date of a gift made to a church. No Black Death martyrs appear; nor are the sacrifices acknowledged of men or women from 1347 to 1351, who risked their lives to aid the plague-afflicted, spiritually or corporeally. Yet as historians, such as Richard Emery, William Bowsky, Daniel Smail, and Shona Wray, have emphasized, not everybody ran, despite an early and clear recognition that the disease was highly contagious and lethal. Societies continued to function and quickly reinstated institutions of government, even if these were suspended during the worst summer months with crime and greed on the increase. Everyday religious and civic practices, such as making wills, notarizing contracts, baptisms and funerals, continued, though wills dwarfed other notarial business during the plague months of 1348.[61] As we have seen, although chroniclers charged prelates with abandoning their flocks, others such as Michele da Piazza and Gilles le Muisit praised the clerics who stayed, visiting the afflicted and administering the last rites, though this proved fatal to thousands of them.

---

[57] Bornstein, *The Bianchi of 1399*, 46; see *Cronache di Ser Luca Dominici*, I, 64, 67, 125, 203–4, 220, and esp. 172, for flagellation that spilled blood: it was more prominent than Bornstein alleges. Moreover, the Bianchi performed other forms of penitence (*grandissima penitenzia, astinenzia, digiuni*).

[58] Among the movement's early leaders were Genoa's archbishop and Fiesole's bishop; *Cronaca Fermana di Antonio di Niccolò*, 132.

[59] Bornstein, *The Bianchi of 1399*, 7.   [60] Ibid., 115.

[61] For instance, during the eight years preceding the Black Death (1340–7), 136 legal contracts (land transactions, loans, dowries, etc.) and three testaments were notarized within the dependent villages of the monastery of San Salvatore in the mountains of Monte Amiato, south of Siena, 27.5 contracts per annum vs 0.38 testaments. By contrast, when the Black Death struck the region, mid-June to September, twelve testaments were notarized, compared to zero contracts; Archivio di Stato di Firenze, Inventario delle pergamene, Abbadia di San Salvatore, Spoglio, vol. 16. I know of no work to analyse changes in contractual activity during or immediately after the Black Death.

Without using the word, authors sketched pictures of martyrdom of those following religious and humanitarian convictions. But unlike newspapers in late nineteenth-century America, which explicitly glorified individual 'martyrs' who sacrificed their lives to comfort Yellow Fever victims, neither Michele, Gilles le Muisit, nor any other contemporary commentator used that word or named any of the thousands they claimed sacrificed their lives for plague victims. The massive compilation of saints' lives in the Bollandists' *Acta Sanctorum*, with stories of holy men and women from the earliest Roman martyrs to the eighteenth century, sketched for hagiographic glory in sixty-eight weighty volumes, failed to mention even in passing the Franciscans at Messina, curates at Tournai, or others who faithfully performed their duties caring for the sick and dying in the Great Plague. Hagiographers blotted the Black Death from their pages, and historians have failed to realize it.

With later plagues of the fourteenth into the fifteenth century, hagiographic attention, however, began to shift slowly and subtly. Later stories of saints risking their lives to save the plague-afflicted remained rare, and when their intercessions increased in the later sixteenth century, these were overwhelmingly risk-free works by saints, who had been long dead before the Black Death. Even for the few holy ones, who attended plague victims during their lifetimes, these acts rarely emerged as their iconic traits or became central to their cultic remembrance.

The first holy one to intervene during his or her lifetime to rescue a plague victim did not occur until the fourth wave of pestilence in 1374. The figure was Saint Catherine of Siena, but her acts were of no importance to her later cult. Looking back from 1390, ten years after her death, her confessor and teacher, blessed Raymond of Capua, recollected her miraculous deeds. She intervened on four occasions in 1374, first, for Matteo di Cenni di Fazio, rector of Siena's hospital of the Misericordia. A nobleman and close friend of Raymond, Matteo was more than an administrator removed from mundane hospital chores; he was engaged in the dangerous care of plague patients, working the wards, attending to pilgrims, the poor and sick, and in so doing caught 'the contagion in the groin'. When his lay brothers carried him to his room, 'like one dead', Catherine heard the news and raced to his bedside. She did not, however, nurse him, nor even touch him. Instead, uttering an angry incantation against the plague, she cured him. He rose to his feet, enjoyed a festive meal with the brothers, and immediately returned to attending Misericordia's plague sufferers.[62]

Her next two interventions followed similar magical suits. Another of Raymond's friends, the hermit Santi, who led an exemplary life of poverty, was stricken. Catherine arrived at his bedside, now accompanied by her companions (unnamed), and whispered he would recover. Words again worked the miracle. No nursing, toil, emptying of bedpans, or acts of abnegation were required: 'Nature had obeyed God through the mouth of the virgin'.[63] In a third miraculous act, she brought

---

[62] Raymond of Capua, *The Life of St Catherine*, 222–4; and *Acta Sanctorum* (hereafter *AS*), 1. Apr. III, 914–16.
[63] Raymond of Capua, *The Life of St Catherine*, 224 and 228.

the Sienese friar Bartolommeo di Domenico back to life from death's throes.[64] Finally, the virgin cured Raymond, after he had attended plague victims for weeks, 'always leaving the monastery, hardly with any time to eat and sleep or even to breathe'.[65] Placing her hand on Raymond's forehead and praying silently, the virgin finally touched a plague victim. Once he recovered, she ordered him to return to his non-miraculous risk-prone chores working the plague wards.[66] Catherine returned home.

In contrast to Catherine's plague experience, Raymond's biography for 1374 became more his autobiography, heralding his own sacrifices, working to exhaustion for his flock until succumbing to the disease. He was fully cognizant of the risks he ran, but from duty, with so many dying, exposed himself to death, 'obliged' to love his neighbours' souls more than his own body.[67] He 'made a firm decision... to visit as many of the sick' as he could. Raymond was there caring for his friends, nursing them, taking their pulses, bringing their urine samples to his trusted doctor, and exposing himself to contagion, before Catherine arrived on the scene. Yet, in his life and process towards beatitude, this sacrifice played no part. Instead, he won his fame in this world and beatitude in the next as Catherine's confessor and hagiographer.

The next holy person whose Life describes any charitable deeds undertaken while living through a plague comes again from Siena but not until the city's sixth plague in 1400. As chroniclers and burial statistics from Florence suggest, this plague was particularly virulent and reversed the steady downward trend in plague mortalities since 1348. According to Bernardino's hagiography, the governor of Santa Maria della Scala, Siena's principal hospital, almost single-handedly tended to the overflowing numbers of pilgrims, drawn by the papal jubilee, and the indigent who had fallen victim to the plague. Bernardino, aged nineteen, heard the governor's call for assistance and arrived with twelve companions from his confraternity (who are never named). Unlike Catherine's, Bernardino's plague interventions were this-worldly and practical. Immediately, he was given keys to the hospital with responsibilities for its administration, taking over from its exhausted, now sickly director. Bernardino organized and allocated the workloads to treat the sick, accepted and rejected pilgrims, and distributed alms. He procured vinegar and strong fumigations to purify the air and cover the stench. He made sure priests were called to administer sacraments and that all were given decent burials. As death tolls mounted, he recruited more from his confraternity (again unnamed). Several died performing their charity. Bernardino's contribution was not limited to possibly safe administration; rather, he assisted the sick 'day and night', providing food and medicine, applying plasters, cleansing wounds, washing feet, preparing beds, and listening to their troubles. He assumed any task 'with delight' no matter 'how loathsome or vile'. His ardour and seeming lack of concern for his own life in treating patients raised suspicions from relatives, who called him mad.[68]

---

[64] Ibid., 231.   [65] Ibid., 230.   [66] Ibid., 231.   [67] Ibid., 229–31.
[68] *The Life of S. Bernardine of Siena*, 21–6. *AS*, Maii V, Dies 20, 'S. Bernardinvs Senensis', 299–301.

But as with Catherine's plague work in 1374, Bernardino was not alone in his abnegation. Before his arrival, the aristocratic rector had worked himself to exhaustion and illness. Nor was Bernardino the first to heed the rector's call. Instead, he followed the footsteps of his cousin Tobia (*sequens vestigia Tobiæ consobrinæ*), who had served as one of his two pious mentors when he first arrived as an orphan in Siena, aged six.[69] Yet neither the rector nor Tobia received any lasting Church recognition beyond brief mentions in Bernardino's life. The same was true of Bernardino's confraternal companions who devoted themselves to the stricken over the plague's four-month devastation, most paying a higher price than Bernardino. Yet the Church named none of them. Even this, Bernardino's one narrated plague experience (he lived through several others), made little impact on his cult or on the Church's ideological message. Of the many pictorial representations of his life—preaching to masses in front of numerous churches, chasing demons, and especially haggardly posed before his 'IHS' insignia—none illustrates his risks at Santa Maria della Scala (see Figure 4.1). Modern surveys of saints, such as the *Bibliotheca Sanctorum* and various editions of *Butler's Lives*, have followed, devoting no more than a phrase or two to his plague experience.[70]

The third saint who worked in his lifetime for the treatment and salvation of plague victims became pictorially the most important plague saint of the Renaissance—San Rocco (Roch). He is also the most difficult to pin down historically. According to André Vauchez, the various versions of his life 'consist of legends entirely without ascertainable basis in fact'.[71] The account that contributed most to his cult dates his birth to 1290 and death to 1327. Vauchez questions these dates because no signs of his cult appear until the fifteenth century. More to the point, according to these narratives he died before the Black Death happened, and in the interval, 1290–1327, no transregional epidemics of any sort spread through central and northern Italy, where Roch worked his miracles. Furthermore, the most detailed plague in which he intervened struck Acquapendente, Cesena, Rome, Rimini, and Novara severely, while the major cities and ports, so hammered in 1348 and in the later fourteenth century—Florence, Siena, Messina, Genoa, Pisa, Venice—are not mentioned, suggesting that the plague was probably not the Black Death nor any of the major ones of the second half of the fourteenth century. In addition, Roch visited the pope in Rome during this plague, but no post-plague pope resided there until 1367.[72] According to Vauchez, speculation presently points to Roch's plague being either one which began in 1414 at the Council of Constance, or a plague in Ferrara in 1439. But why date it then and not to the more widespread plague of the previous year, and why have historians not sought to check when early fifteenth-century plagues struck places such as Acquapendente,

---

[69] *AS*, Maii V, 301; and Origo, *The World of San Bernardino*, 15–16 and 68.
[70] *Butler's Lives* (hereafter *BLS*), May, 107–8. The *Bibliotheca sanctorum* entry (Korosak, 'Bernardino da Siena') is equally brief on Bernardino's plague experience. Similarly, Origo, *The World of San Bernardino*, 18, spends less than a paragraph on it.
[71] Vauchez, 'San Rocco'.   [72] Ibid.

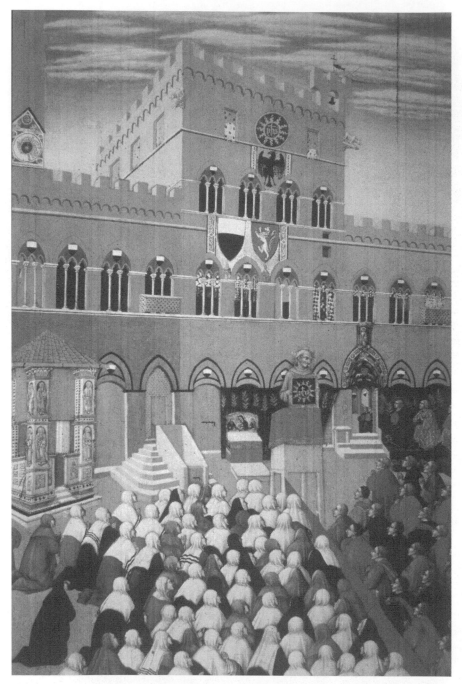

Figure 4.1. San Bernardino preaching in Piazza del Campo, Siena. Sano di Pietro, 1440s, Museo del Duomo.

Cesena, Rome, Rimini, and Novara with particular force?[73] As with other aspects of the chronology of Roch's ragged life, perhaps these plagued cities formed a collage of multiple plagues in the fifteenth century. Given the sequence of events, Roch was converted to treating plague victims later at Piacenza, where he was inspired by the patrician Gottardo Pallastrelli's self-sacrifice in the city hospital. But Roch's charitable conversion would then appear *after* he had already travelled from Rome to Novara, serving the plague-afflicted.

Nonetheless, the interventions Roch made during his lifetime were more direct and risky than Catherine's but not the equal of young Bernardino's changing of bedpans and sheets, washing patients, and administering medicines. Roch cured his patients mostly miraculously but did more than whisper incantations. At least he touched them and at Piacenza worked in the hospital alongside Pallastrelli. Ultimately, Roch caught the plague and retired to the wilderness to die before being cured by a dog licking his pestilential wounds. No matter how vague or absurd Roch's story may appear, finally with the curing cur by his side and a suppurating bubo on his thigh, a graphic iconography of a plague saint arrived in Western art in the fifteenth century (Figure 4.2). Yet, as with the rectors of the Misericordia and Santa Maria della Scala, Bernardino's cousin, and his many companions, Pallastrelli, Roch's exemplar and mentor, received no holy recognition.

Francesca Romana (Francesca Bussa dei Ponziani, 1384–1440) unites various strains of the few plague saints already discussed, who, while alive, risked their lives. Unlike Roch, her life is well grounded in political facts, precise chronologies, and specific institutions of social welfare, which she founded and which have left lasting marks.[74] Unlike Catherine, her intervention was not even partially miraculous, and Francesca paid the price of her care in 1414 when she became afflicted. Unlike the two Sienese saints, plague figured in her future cult, recognized by later painters and scholars. From a wealthy background, she married into the Ponziani family, one of late medieval Rome's most powerful dynasties. With the Great Schism and civil war between the Roman *Comune* and the papacy, the *Comune* ended in defeat in 1398. After several invasions and eventual occupation by Ladislao di Durazzo, king of Naples, combined with famine and plague, Rome reached its late medieval nadir. The Ponziani paid dearly for these disasters with their family fortunes and their lives.[75] During the famines and plagues of 1402–1414, Francesca worked in Rome's hospitals—Santa Cecilia, Santo Spirito in Sassia, and, above all, Santa Maria in Cappello in her neighbourhood of Trastevere—and converted her husband's palace into a plague hospital. She foraged in the outlying suburbs and on her husband's estates for firewood and food to comfort her patients. Yet, just as in the other stories, she was not alone or even extraordinary in her

---

[73] Also, see Marshall, 'Manipulating the Sacred', 502–4; and Worcester, 'Saint Roch vs. Plague'. Neither speculates on the plagues he confronted.

[74] It is not true that saints' lives were indifferent to precise dates and events as apologists for Roch's life insist; see for instance Terry-Fritsch, 'Introduction', 24–6.

[75] Esch, 'Processi medioevali', 39–40.

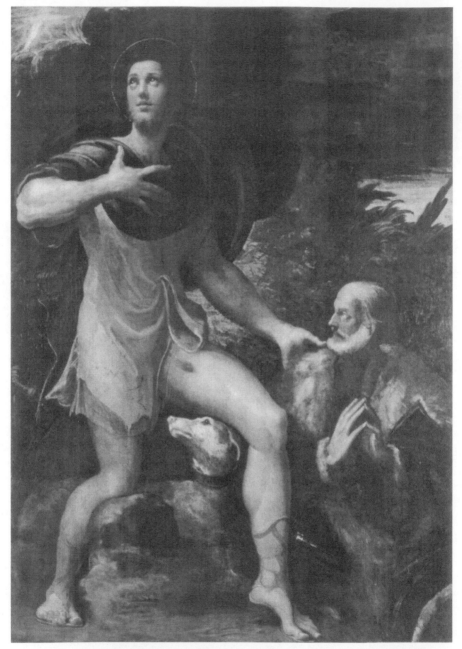

Figure 4.2. San Rocco, Il Parmigianino, 1527, Basilica di San Petronio a Bologna.

endeavours. For thirty-eight years, her sister-in-law Vanozza worked alongside her without receiving any blessed status.[76]

More extraordinary, however, is the complete absence of anyone, anywhere in Europe, obtaining holy status for real-life sacrifices or charity performed during the Black Death itself, and the absence of anyone achieving holy status whose iconography reflected hands-on care, before Francesca in the mid-fifteenth century. (She was not elevated to sainthood until Pope Paul V's canonization in 1608.)[77] Moreover, Francesca did not mark a watershed. While many men and women followed in her footsteps, caring for plague victims in hospitals across Europe, I know of no others to receive holy awards for such deeds before the sixteenth century and these remained rare for the next two centuries. Saint Aloysius might count as an exception. He died at twenty-three, after months dedicating himself to the physical and spiritual needs of the indigent and ill in Rome's streets and hospitals, sweeping floors and cleaning filth from beds during the famine and plague (*lues*) of 1591— the century's worst food shortage and, by some accounts, the worst ever faced by Italians.[78] That 'plague', however, was not the bubonic one. Perhaps it was typhus or dysentery combined with other ailments associated with starvation, even if it spread to members of the papal court and included the pope himself, Sixtus V.[79]

Even the intervention of San Carlo during the Italian plague of 1574–7, named after him, was different from Bernardino's, Roch's, and Francesca's. His cult focused largely on administration, drafting statutes to protect his clergy, inventing new communal forms of prayer for Milanese citizens still under quarantine, and cooperating closely with the city's Health Board to achieve the duchy's spiritual and physical well-being. While Carlo Borromeo may have visited the sick, he was careful to keep them at a distance. Not even his most sympathetic supporters nor his later iconography pictured him emptying bedpans.[80] In addition, before the seventeenth century, plague saints actively intervening in their lifetimes appeared to be exclusively from Italy. Even the largely legendary Roch, who by all accounts was born in Montpellier and returned there to die, after being imprisoned as a foreign spy, was in effect an Italian saint: his endeavours to cure plague sufferers occurred solely on Italian soil from Rome to Novara.

Such was not the case with Europe's most prominent contagious disease (at least culturally) before the plague: leprosy. Except for Saint Francis of Assisi, its best-known saints came from beyond the Alps—Saint Elizabeth of Hungary and Thuringia, Saint Louis IX, king of France (1214–70), and Saint Martin of Tours (†397).

---

[76] *AS*, 2. Mar. II, Dies 9, 179, 186–7; Vaccaro, 'Francesca Anna-Francesca Romana', 1011–28; *BLS*, rev., March, 'St Frances of Rome', 79–82.

[77] Picasso, 'Introduzione'.

[78] Alfani, 'The Famine of the 1590s', 34. On the climatic, economic, and psychological factors of this three-year epidemic, see idem, *Il Grand Tour*, 96–109.

[79] *AS*, June, IV, 1009–10 and 1018. No descriptions of buboes or quick death appear with the diseases of 1591. It took the already sickly Aloysius fifty days to die from the disease. I know of no work that examines medically the 1591 epidemic.

[80] Among other places, see my *Cultures of Plague*; Jones, 'San Carlo Borromeo'; and Sannazzaro, 'Note sull'immagine agiografia', 33–47.

More strikingly, along with Italian leper saints such as the Florentine Philip Benizi (1233–85), their curative interventions occurred during their lifetimes and their later iconography illustrates them engaged in risky charitable deeds, donating their cloaks, holding lepers' hands, washing their feet, administering medicines, and nursing them in *leprosie*.[81]

Nonetheless, from the mid-fifteenth to the seventeenth century, holy interventions during plagues increased exponentially. These saints and blessed ones differed from the few plague saints already examined. These later ones had died centuries before the Black Death, and many show no evidence during their lifetimes as healers, no matter what the disease. The plots of their miracle tales remain largely the same from 1348 to the eighteenth century. After physicians had tried their remedies, with all hope lost while the patient awaited the last rites, a relative, usually the mother, went to the grave of a local saint, prayed, and offered a votive gift—a candle, a wax figure, occasionally a painting. The earliest to succeed in one of these post-mortem acts was the blessed Giovanna da Signa (1266–9 November 1307), at Signa, a market town 12 km west of Florence. As a young girl, she had herded sheep and cows for her father, and learnt to cherish solitude, becoming a hermit in Signa's foothills, where she performed miracles and at the end of her life walled herself into a gate. She was the only holy person miraculously to save a plague victim in 1348,[82] and did it that year only once. Even these post-mortem miraculous interventions remain extremely rare throughout the fourteenth century, despite the great numbers felled by plagues across Europe.

By the fifteenth century, plague interventions by saints increased. The mid-thirteenth-century Saint Rosa of the Franciscan tertiaries at Viterbo became active in the plague of 1449 to 1451, miraculously curing seventeen individuals after relatives made votive offerings.[83] In the late sixteenth and seventeenth centuries, post-mortem plague miracles finally fanned from Italy across Europe, from Ireland to Poland, and then to the New World. The intercessions, moreover, show new trends, becoming more communal than earlier ones centred on individual sufferers. Now, those who were to become blessed inspired community-wide processions. Such was the call of the blessed Franciscan tertiary Columba of Rieti (1467–1501) in Perugia during the pestilence of 1494. On receiving posthumous advice from Saint Bernardino and Catherine of Siena, she encouraged the Church and Perugia's municipality to organize public processions and create a fund for the poor afflicted by plague. At the holy altar in one of Perugia's churches, she made known to the populace that she was present to cure any who became afflicted: 'many' came to benefit from her miracles. She then travelled to outlying villages, beseeching Catherine to intervene to end the plague, and, as in Perugia, had monasteries open their doors to sufferers, where she erected a bed to perform hands-on

---

[81] Boeckl, *Images of Leprosy*, 45, 52, 81, 83–90.

[82] Canonization inquests could produce further examples; however, the testimonies for canonization of Apt's local saint, which stretched across the first and second plagues, indicate no plague miracles in 1348; Archambeau, 'Healing Options'.

[83] *AS*, Rosa virgo tertii Ordinis S. Francisci, Viterbii in Italia, 4 September.

miracle cures.[84] On her advice, the University of Perugia built a monastery from their own and public expenses and commissioned a painted banner to be kept in the city's archives, ready to lead the populace in processions to end future plagues.[85]

During a 'big plague' in Monza in 1521, citizens walked in procession with paintings of the Roman martyrs and commissioned a painting of Saint Gerard the dyer, their twelfth-century patron and founder of the town's hospital. Afterwards, no one from Monza died in this plague. To protect the town from future plagues the procession, like a communal vaccine, was instituted annually on Gerard's anniversary, ending in his church with songs, masses, and offerings of wax and money.[86] Saint Torpes, a courtier of Nero, beheaded for his conversion during 'the first persecution' of 68 CE, was the most ancient saint to intercede in a later epidemic. During the last plague of Pisa in 1630, the city organized various processions. But the plague was not calmed until a Pisan magistrate presented the head of the martyr to lead a procession through all the squares and streets of the city.[87]

Such community-wide actions also occurred beyond the Alps. However, the only one that I have found before the second half of the sixteenth century took place in Perpignan in 1384, where a plague which reputedly killed 8000 people between November and March was extinguished by a procession organized by the local monastery with the relics of the ninth-century Occitan peasant, Gualdericus (Guaderico).[88] The next collective enterprise to end a plague outside of Italy as recorded in the *Acta Sanctorum* appears almost two centuries later, in rural Portugal near Várzea. Shepherds tending their flocks came upon a painting of the fifth-century virgin martyr, Saint Quiteria. They happily handed it over to a local monastery, which built a church around it. In 1568, many years after the church had fallen into ruins (*decursu longioris temporis*), with the plague raging through Portugal, the community restored the church. In return, Quiteria interceded, and afterwards no villager was infected.[89] From the late sixteenth to the eighteenth century, such general processions illustrated in saints' lives multiplied, with the faithful carrying paintings or holy insignia to end a plague or protect a city or village from getting it in the first place. In the seventeenth century, the thirteenth-century Polish saint and virgin queen Kinga (Kunga, Cunegundis, or Cunegonda[90]) performed sixty-seven post-mortem miracles to help dispel plagues. Several were collective endeavours that bound communities together during or immediately after a plague, first to hold processions and make votive offerings beseeching Kinga's intercession, then with festivals of gratitude to make good their promises. In 1624, plague hit Neumarkt (Novum Forum) in Silesia. Twice, its inhabitants processed to Kinga's grave, where they offered prayers for deliverance from the epidemic. They carried a silver icon of

---

[84] *AS*, Maii V, Dies 20, B. Columba Reatina, Virgo tertii Ordin. S. Dominici Perusii in Vmbria; *BLS*, May, 110–11; Blasucci, 'Colomba, da Rieti'.

[85] *AS*, Maii V, Dies 20, another life of Beata Columba.

[86] *AS*, Jun. I, Dies 6, S. Gerardus Tinctorius, Modoetiae apud Insubres in Italia, miracles 20 and 21.

[87] *AS*, 1. Maii IV, Dies 17, De S. Torpes Martyr, Pisae in Hetruria, 18.

[88] *AS*, Oct. VII, Dies 16, S. Gualdericus agricola in Occitania, 1116.

[89] *AS*, Maii V, Dies 22, S. Quiteria Virgo, Martyr in Adurensi Vasconiae dioecesi.

[90] Naruszewicz, 'Cunegonda (Kinga, Kunga)'.

the saint (*argentea tabula*) with the inscription: 'the inhabitants of the royal city of Neumarkt because of the plague devote themselves to Beata Cunegundis with their prayers'.[91] Two years later the community assembled and staged another procession, commemorating Kinga's liberation of their town.

Sicily, however, was the region par excellence of these communal plague rituals. In 1525, 1575, and 1625, inhabitants of Licata on Sicily's southern coast, marched barefoot in multiple processions with relics of their thirteenth-century patron saint, the martyr Angelo, a priest of the Carmelites, who 300 years earlier had combated the Cathars. While nothing in his hagiography suggests any involvement with any disease during his lifetime, suddenly, in the second half of the seventeenth century, he defended his city against plague, but now with a new twist: no plagues were threatening.[92] In 1662, Licata's citizens exhumed their patron and buried him in a new votive church, constructed for him out of gratitude for protecting them over the previous thirty-nine years from plague.[93]

SANTA ROSALIA

The most prolific of miracle-makers as regards plague was another Sicilian, Rosalia, born of a mid-twelfth-century Norman aristocratic family resident at Palermo. Like Licata's Angelo, her moment of glory did not arrive until much later, during Palermo's last plague in 1624, when a peasant woman supposedly discovered her bones in a cavern (*spelunca*) atop Monte Pellegrino, 606 m above Palermo. For this plague alone, she interceded over 200 times, miraculously curing at least 101 persons individually (forty men, thirty-seven women, and twenty-three infants undistinguished by sex). Most often, her cure was the waters taken from her grotto. In addition to sex, these victims were often identified by age, place, and occasionally profession, with the course of their illness and date of recovery recorded. Further, the plague miracles detail whether the waters were mixed with stones at the shrine or her bones, and how or where the solution was applied. A thirty-year-old fisherman from Palermo, attacked by plague in 1624, for instance, suffered from high fever and horrendous tumours. The doctors gave up hope, 'having never heard of any in his condition surviving'. When priests came to perform the last rites, a Capuchin suggested fetching water from Rosalia's grotto for him to drink and to bathe his pestilential wounds. The fever subsided, the swellings healed, and he recovered.[94]

Her plague miracles, however, point to trends rarely seen, if at all, earlier. First, she not only cured young innocents whose mothers happened to summon the long-dead saint, but several of her intercessions recognized the sacrifices of those

[91] *AS*, 252. Jul. V, Dies 24, S. Kinga seu Cunegundis virgo, Poloniae ducissa, Ord. S. Clarae, apud antiquam Sandecz, in palatinatu Cracoviensi.

[92] *AS*, Maii II, Dies 5, 'S. Angelus, Presbyter Ordinis Carmelitani, Martyr Leocatae in Sicilia, miracles', 6, 7, 9.

[93] Morabito, 'Angelo da Gerusalemme', 1240–3.

[94] *AS*, September, vol. 2, S. Rosalia, 4 September, Appendix Miraculorum ac Beneficorum, no. 19.

working in hospitals or outside them, such as the Jesuit Father Francesco Marino, who became infected while serving plague sufferers.[95] After his doctors had given up hope (*a medicis esset derelictus*), he accepted Rosalia's waters and in twenty-four hours was restored to health.[96] Another, Domenico of Messina, also caught the plague while caring for the plague-infected in Palermo's hospital. Once recovered, he returned to his duties and caught it again, now left to die until Rosalia's waters cured him.[97] These miracles celebrated the virgin but also, for the first time in the *Acta*'s plague miracles, the charitable work and sacrifices of the non-saintly: seven men and two women—nurses, doctors, and surgeons—working the men's and women's wards of Palermo's *valetudinarium*, infected during the 1624 plague.[98] Saved by her waters, all returned to their duties caring for plague sufferers.

More significantly, nearly two-thirds of Rosalia's intercessions were collective. Several were multiple miracle cures for groups of afflicted, as during the 1625 plague in Corleone, when with collective votive gifts the town's inhabitants implored her to save them from the disease: four men and one woman were named along with their 'two or three' children and another thirteen unnamed infants.[99] More numerous, however, were those who organized and brought forth entire communities into collective acts of veneration with processions, communal prayers, and contributions for votive gifts, ranging from roadside shrines, paintings, and statues to extravagant artistic ephemera and the construction of new churches to celebrate a pestilence's end. From the plague of 1624 on, Rosalia became a turbine of artistic production in Sicily. These works of art included a painting of Rosalia commissioned by Palermo's senate during the plague in 1624.[100] When that plague ended, the senate organized much more, spending at least 15,000 gold coins (*aureorum*). It received contributions from Palermo's principal nations (*gens*) of foreign bankers and merchants—the Catalans, Florentines, Genoese, and Neapolitans—to construct four well-buttressed triumphal arches, decorated 'at the highest expense' (*maximo sumptu*) with paintings, insignia, epigrams, verses, forty-eight columns draped with painted silk interwoven with gold and silver and other decorations, a large building, preciously attired with long curtains, four new open spaces in the city (*aere*), thirty-three altars, decorated with insigne and vases 'ingeniously crafted in gold and silver' and erected at each of the city's major street crossings, and 'innumerable other ornaments' 'exciting the highest admiration' in thanksgiving to the saint for ending the plague. According to her life, this collective giving turned the entire city into 'a gigantic temple' in her honour.[101] Collective gifts and acts spread to smaller Sicilian towns. The following year, the inhabitants of Bivona commissioned a church

---

[95] Ibid., cap. II: Prosecutio eorundem miraculorum ex Cascino, cap. 12, no. 40.

[96] Ibid., no. 46. The hospital is not identified but was probably Palermo's lazaretto. As the hagiographer expressed it, Francesco 'was damned because of the services he paid to the plague-infected in the hospital'.

[97] Ibid., no. 49.   [98] Ibid., nos 34, 36, 40, 42, 43–6, 49.

[99] Ibid., cap. XXXIV, no. 361.

[100] Ibid., XX. Cura archiepiscopi: Vota Panormi contra pestem, no. 208.

[101] Ibid., XXII Corpus S. Rosaliae solemni pompa per urbem circumlatum finis pestilentiae ejus beneficio impetratus, no. 235.

and shrine with a painting of Rosalia,[102] and in Noto, another ex-voto painting of the saint.[103] In 1626, the hilltop town of Modica (Motucae) constructed a new church next to its hospital in her honour.[104] In 1630, a monumental marble tomb (*Arca marmorea*) for Rosalia was erected at her grotto of Monte Pellegrino.[105] In September 1743, when Messina's most disastrous plague since the Black Death came to an end, the city's senate commissioned a painting of the saint for a chapel in their chambers.[106] When the plague was declared officially over, 'all its citizens' in gratitude adopted Rosalia as their patron and promised to build a temple to her.[107]

While these works of art, paintings, shrines, and churches clustered in Sicily and primarily Palermo, gifts promised to her to end plagues spread to other parts of Italy, such as Cremona in 1633 and Sezza, near Rome, in 1716.[108] Moreover, such gifts, commemorations, and celebrations in her honour fanned across Europe: to Paris in 1628,[109] Gau (Molinenses) in Germany in 1631,[110] and for the construction of a church at Cilley (Celia) in Austria, where 60,000 (according to the saint's life) had perished in the plague of 1649.[111] Her fame then crossed continents to infected Portuguese Goa, where 'an elegant votive church' was built during or immediately after a plague in 1666.[112]

Beyond votive commissions, Rosalia brought communities together in plague time by other means—processions through cities, towns, and villages, with inhabitants bearing her relics. Within Sicily, these relics came on loan from Palermo, extending that city's networks of solidarity across Sicily, but her cult reached beyond Italy. In the late seventeenth century, she was active in Mela in Brabant and Antwerp, where she became that city's patron saint. With commissioned paintings and a shrine during the plagues of 1668 and 1678, its citizens collectively invoked her intercession at least seven times during plagues in 1629, 1665, 1668, and 1678.[113] Her cult travelled west to Nice in 1633,[114] south to Malta in 1676,[115] east to Warsaw in 1630,[116] south-east to Transylvania in 1737–8,[117] and across the ocean to the New World, 'to all of Brazil' and Peru at unspecified dates, Durango, Mexico (Nova Biscaia) in 1716,[118] Lima in 1746, California in 1701, although the disease now was smallpox,[119] and Africa (*in regno Tunetano*) in the early 1700s.[120]

---

[102] Ibid., Vita Brevis, Octavio Caietano S.J., no. 2.

[103] Ibid., XXXVII. Cultus, reliquiae & miracula in diocesibus Catanensi & Syracusana, no. 398.

[104] Ibid., no. 397.

[105] Ibid., Vita Altera, Jordano Cascini S.J.: II. Miracula post corpus inventum; no. 22.

[106] Ibid., no. 151.   [107] Ibid., Appendix: Miraculorum ac beneficiorum, no. 152.

[108] Ibid., Commentarius Praevius: XXXIX. Cultus, reliquiae & beneficia S. Rosalia in Italia, nos 420 and 422.

[109] Ibid., XL. Gallia, Hispania, Germania & Hungaria, no. 429.

[110] Ibid., no. 431.   [111] Ibid., no. 437.

[112] Ibid., XLI. Cultus, reliquiae & beneficia S. Rosaliae in Belgio & praesertim Antverpiae: item Polonia & in insula Melitensi, no. 468.

[113] Ibid., XLI, nos 445, 478, 450–3.   [114] Ibid., no. 427.

[115] Ibid., nos 456–7.   [116] Ibid., no. 455.

[117] Ibid., XL. Gallia, Hispania, Germania & Hungaria; post votum S. Rosalia, no. 441.

[118] Ibid., XLIII. America & Africa: variola, no. 472.

[119] Ibid., XLIII. America & Africa, no. 472–6; and XXXI. Missa propria pro regno Siciliae, no. 326.

[120] Ibid., XLIII, no. 447–8.

Increasingly during the second half of the seventeenth and early eighteenth century, she operated not only when plagues struck, but, like Licata's martyr, was called to keep communities plague-free. To insure her cover, citizens made processions with her relics, engaged in collective prayers and litanies, offered votive gifts, and when the danger passed, celebrated her success with city-wide festivals. In 1645, a second shrine was promised in fields outside Bivona,[121] where no plague had struck (or for that matter anywhere else I know of in Italy).[122] In 1649, a plague case arose in Palermo's hospital but spread no further. The city's mayor (*praetor*) attributed Palermo's immunity to Rosalia's intercession and ordered a public festival.[123] When Italy's last plague pandemic in 1656–7 struck Genoa and Naples at levels not seen since 1348, a Florentine merchant smuggled goods into Palermo, breaking its quarantine. The goods, however, failed to ignite the pandemic in Palermo or elsewhere in Sicily. In return, Palermo's citizens held a procession in thanksgiving, and its senate voted to erect a monument and a statue 'in her likeness'.[124] Nonetheless, plagues continued to threaten Palermo, coming from Coversano (Conversanum) near Bari in 1691,[125] Marseille (Massaliam) in 1720,[126] Messina in 1743,[127] as well as from unnamed places in 1710[128] and 1744.[129] Despite contraband goods slipping through its docks, Palermo escaped them all, thanks they thought to their votive gifts, fasts, and barefoot treks to Rosalia's cave. Instead of stirring blame and hatred, dividing classes or targeting minorities, these acts, despite epidemiological dangers, unified inhabitants across social classes and city walls into the countryside. With the expansion of her cult and free exchange of her relics, Rosalia's intercessions via the Jesuits extended Palermo's connections beyond Sicily, Italy, and even Europe.

In conclusion, the Black Death sparked conflict, hatred, and violence from 1347 to 1351, and not just incidents that involved flagellants and the burning of Jews. Evidence from chronicles reveals that the cruel abandonment of loved ones and the refusal of trusted professionals to perform vital duties horrified contemporaries across Europe. In addition, laws fixing prices and wages also made artisans and peasants the targets of violence, blamed for greedily exploiting their masters. The current historiography has failed, however, to notice how short-lived these Black Death reactions were. Successive plagues ceased to spur pogroms against Jews or any other 'others'; claims that afflicted loved ones were being abandoned all but disappeared; and plague decrees regulating wages turned about-face to reward rather than punish those who moved.

Another indication of post-plague mentality is more enigmatic. The Church failed to recognize the thousands who faced the violent contagion and sacrificed

---

[121] Ibid., Vita Brevis, Octavio Caietano S.J., no. 2.

[122] Gigli, *Diario Romano*, 270, reports a 'Mortalità' of a malignant fever that killed 'a good part of the Popolo' in July that year, with live worms found in the corpses that could be killed only with wine.

[123] *AS*, Appendix III. Alia miracula, relata a Cascino, no. 138.

[124] Ibid., Appendix Miraculorum ac Benediciorum, XXXIX. Cultus, reliquiae & beneficia S. Rosalia in Italia, no. 138; and Appendix: Miraculorum ac beneficiorum, no. 168.

[125] Ibid., no. 139.   [126] Ibid., no. 141.   [127] Ibid., no. 142.   [128] Ibid., no. 140.

[129] Ibid., no. 139.

their lives to comfort plague-afflicted neighbours. The Church acknowledged no Black Death martyrs or others succouring plague victims until 1400 and thereafter only faintly—a fact that neither religious nor art historians have confronted. With successive plagues, the Church slowly began rewarding a few who in their lifetimes assisted the plague-stricken. Yet overwhelmingly, the increasing numbers of plague saints were long-dead figures, resurrected to save the afflicted risk-free, when votive gifts were on offer. By the seventeenth century, the miraculous deeds of plague saints began to shift from saving individual supplicants to unifying communities through collective acts of penance and festivals of thanksgiving. These produced public works, from ephemeral objects to major ecclesiastical constructions, with charitable offerings to the poor and infirm. Previous understanding of socio-psychological reactions, not only to the Black Death but to epidemic disease across time, has emphasized the negative, highlighting violence, blame, and division, while being blind to epidemics' powers to unify and strengthen societies in past times.[130]

---

[130] Recently, art historians have changed an earlier view that plagues shrouded Europe in fear and doom from 1347 to the Enlightenment; see, for instance, essays in *Hope and Healing*.

PART II

EARLY MODERNITY

5

Syphilis

Naming and Blaming?

With Charles VIII's invasion of Italy and siege of Naples during the winter of 1494–5, a new disease exploded in pandemic proportions, quickly circulating through Western Europe and beyond, reaching corners as distant as Aberdeen by April 1497,[1] Poland by 1499, Russia and Scandinavia, 1500, India, 1498, and Canton, 1505.[2] It combined three aspects that have led recent scholars to regard it as the perfect antecedent of HIV/AIDS: it was new, mysterious, and sexually transmitted.[3] Of course, all three characteristics can be qualified. Almost immediately, a central debate emerged on whether the 'new' disease was new to Europe— imported from the New World or tied to leprosy described since biblical times. Even today, with tools for detecting ancient DNA and comparison of European and pre-Columbian bone specimens, the riddle remains.[4] Second, compared with other diseases before the laboratory revolution, this 'new' disease was less mysterious than many. Almost immediately, physicians and the laity understood that it spread principally by being transmitted sexually.[5] Third, although most agreed about its connection with sexual activity, a variety of other factors were believed to have caused it. The disease was placed in the usual schema of late medieval/ Renaissance causation: God's punishment of sin; confluence of stars and constellation of planets; and medieval Galenic notions that contaminated food often sparked it. Into the nineteenth century, those at the cutting edge of medicine continued to believe that it was transmitted by various means. Although the city of Nuremberg in its earliest statutes (1496 and 1497) banned those infected from its

---

[1] Creighton, I, 417; Fabricius, *Syphilis*, 54; and Jillings, 'Plague, Pox', 71. Aberdeen town council issued an ordinance to prevent the spread of syphilis on 21 April 1497—the earliest record of the disease in Britain.

[2] Bollet, *Plagues*, 70–1.

[3] For an argument stressing the parallels, see Gilman, 'AIDS and Syphilis'.

[4] Berco, 'Syphilis, Sex, and Marriage', 226–7; and Bollet, *Plagues*, 70. As of 2016, molecular phylogenetic approaches have yet to solve the riddle; Gall, 'Quarantine', 2.

[5] See Arrizabalaga, 'Medical Responses': 'all agreed that coitus was the easiest and most frequent way' (53). Doctors at Barcelona treating Columbus's sailors with 'las Bubas' understood the disease as sexually transmitted. In addition, by the end of the fifteenth century, most chroniclers and doctors described the disease as venereal, even if they believed it was communicated by other means. See Bloch, 'The History of Syphilis', I, 12; Quétel, *History of Syphilis*, 66. Proksch: the chronicle by Doge Johannes Baptista Fulgosi, I, 318; the physician Antonio Benivieni II, 31; the Spanish physician, practising in Bologna, Juan Almenar, II, 33; the Paduan professor and physician, Alessandro Benedetti, II, 41–2; the canon-chronicler of Orvieto, Tommasi di Silvestro, II, 154, all writing at the end of the fifteenth or early sixteenth century, pointed to the disease's sexual transmission.

public baths, suggesting that they understood it as sexually transmitted, they also thought it could be contracted by eating bad pork.[6] In 1596, the Paris-trained surgeon and founder of the Royal College of Physicians and Surgeons in Glasgow, Peter Lowe (1550–1610), argued it was spread by breath and 'sitting on the privie after use by one infected'.[7] In the seventeenth century, some believed Brussels sprouts triggered it.[8] At the end of the eighteenth century, Edinburgh's surgeon Benjamin Bell argued correctly that syphilis[9] and gonorrhoea were two distinct diseases with different agents, thirty-six years before the medical establishment began to accept the distinction. Yet Bell thought syphilis could also be 'communicated by eating and drinking out of the same vessel, or drying with the same cloth'.[10] Finally, as John Henderson has argued, throughout the early modern period, miasma continued as the theoretical framework for explaining plague and the Great Pox. Yet physicians and health boards saw fundamental differences in the contagiousness of the two: because of plague's capacity to spread 'by distance', its lazaretti were extramural, while Pox hospitals were mostly placed in city centres.[11]

WHAT'S IN A NAME?

It would be fair to assume that in the main Europe understood syphilis as new, mysterious, and sexually transmitted. In addition, particularly for the first generation of sufferers until the 1520s, its symptoms were extraordinarily painful and seen as disgusting, as described in excruciating detail in works repeatedly reprinted such as Von Hutten's *De guaiaici medicina et morbo gallico*, Fracastoro's *De Contagione*, and others to be explored later. So what has been historians' evidence of syphilis's social violence and power to stigmatize the 'other'? Much of the argument centres on one factor alone—the naming of the disease.[12] More than with any previous disease, contemporaries were obsessed with what to call it and recorded the names given to it by fellow physicians as well as by commoners. Because of the long-repeated presumptions about the naming and its social implications, and because no previous

---

[6] Sudhoff, 'Die ersten Maßnahmen', 5 and 17. I thank Mona O'Brien for this reference.

[7] Fabricius, *Syphilis*, 63.   [8] Berco, 'Syphilis, Sex, and Marriage', 235.

[9] Throughout this chapter, I use various names for venereal disease, despite syphilis's causative agents being unknown until 1905, and gonorrhoea and syphilis being generally thought to be the same disease until 1838.

[10] Bell, *A Treatise on Gonorrhoea*, I, 38. Syphilis can be transmitted non-sexually through skin contact; see Gall, 'Quarantine', 3.

[11] See Henderson, 'Coping with Epidemics', 176, 178, 185, 187–8, 193.

[12] The assumption that naming meant blaming is found across the literature, even with the most sensitive handling of the topic—*The Great Pox*. The authors strenuously refrain from treating the pox in transhistorical terms, insisting that it cannot be assumed to have been *Treponema pallidum*. Nonetheless, they assume the standard truism that naming equals blaming: 'As during epidemics of plague, it was convenient to find a scapegoat to blame for the epidemic [the Great Pox]' (166) ... 'It is a truism of such societies that bad and new diseases come from somewhere else ... generally brought by people with bad habits, especially your neighbours. Thus the Italians so effectively blamed the invading French ...' (279). Also, see Nelkin and Gilman, 'Placing Blame', and more recently Raimond-Waarts and Santing, 'Sex: A Cardinal's Sin', 169.

disease in history had been so troublesome to name, this chapter takes pains to unearth these concerns from 1495 to the seventeenth century.

To understand the socio-psychological significance of the Great Pox, recent historians such as William Eamon have begun with the great pandemic of our day. At the outset, he proclaimed that 'new diseases bring out a culture's deepest phobias';[13] AIDS' targeting of 'marginalized groups'—'gays, IV drug users, and Haitian immigrants'—'was depressingly reminiscent of medieval Europe's response to Black Death, when Jews...were rounded up and exterminated'.[14] Eamon then turned to the Great Pox, calling it the great disease of 'otherness' that spread blame across the nations of Europe and beyond.[15] But despite doctors' 'bewilderment', syphilis's gruesome symptoms, stench, and torture of the joints[16] that produced sleepless nights, crippling, loss of noses, lips, hair, eyes, and penises as recounted by chroniclers, physicians, and most harrowingly by writers inflicted with the disease— Joseph Grünpeck, Ulrich von Hutten, Ser Tommaso di Silvestro, the Sienese poet Niccolò Campani, and an Olivetan canon[17]—Eamon could do little more than point to various names given to the disease as evidence that minorities were being blamed. Certainly, many before Eamon assumed the same: asserting that those outside France called it the 'French disease' ('morbus Gallicus', 'mal francese', 'Malafranzcoso', 'Franzosenkrankheit', etc.); the French, 'mal de Naples'; the Poles, the German disease; the Germans, the Polish disease. Later, the Japanese called it the Portuguese disease; the Persians, the Turkish disease, and other names designating other peoples, who were thereby supposedly responsible for it.[18] Yet, neither Eamon nor others have discovered pogroms against Jews or other minorities, accused directly or indirectly of spreading syphilis because of differences in religion, lifestyle, or morality. Still more surprising, no one has pointed to the persecution of foreign communities in an inflicted city—soldiers or prostitutes—despite these two groups, even before the siege of Naples, being seen as spreading the disease. The absence of popular rioting or harsh and cruel edicts against foreigners and the rarity of new legislation targeting prostitutes or blaming them for outbreaks of the pox during the sixteenth century is all the more perplexing given that the disease erupted during moments of heightened hatred, fear, and insecurity—in times of war with invading foreign armies, especially throughout the Italian peninsula between 1494 and 1559.[19] Commoners, physicians, and bureaucrats rightly perceived invading armies as spearheading this gruesome disease. A town ordinance of Aberdeen in 1497 may be the earliest that blamed women for spreading it—'all licht weman be chargit and ordaint to deciest fra thar vicis and syne of venerie'.[20] But these laws did not shut houses of prostitution or chase 'dishonest women' from town because of their moral pollution as often happened with plague.

---

[13] Eamon, 'Cannibalism', 1.   [14] Ibid., 1.   [15] Ibid., 2 and 5.

[16] In Guicciardini's words 'sottoposti a cruciati quasi perpetui'; *Storia d'Italia*, 233.

[17] Von Hutten, *De guaiaici*; Quétel, *History of Syphilis*, ch. 1; and *The Great Pox*, 25–7. On Campani, see Alonge, 'Campani', 404–6.

[18] See Nelkin and Gilman, 'Placing Blame', 43; Farmer, *AIDS and Accusation*; and McGough, *Gender, Sexuality, and Syphilis*, 6 and 48, who cites other recent examples.

[19] See Mallet and Shaw, *The Italian Wars*.   [20] Cited in Creighton, I, 417.

The current stereotype, that one nationality called the disease after another, needs investigation. Although physicians normally called the disease 'morbus Gallicus' into the second half of the sixteenth century, numerous medical tracts such as Nicolai Leoncini's on the 'French Disease', published in 1497, to the vast compilations of treatises, letters, and *consilia* published in 1566–7, with additions to them in the eighteenth century by Jean Astruc[21] and Christian Gottfried Gruner (1744–1815),[22] show a wide diversity in naming. Except for variations on the French disease (which declined rapidly by the late sixteenth century), naming the disease after other nationalities (other than the French) was rare, especially in common parlance.[23]

One of the most frequent questions physicians posed from the end of the fifteenth century was whether this pox was new or had been around since biblical times, commented upon by Hippocrates, Pliny, Galen, or others. Many thought the disease a form of leprosy or possibly other known skin disorders. Physicians cited Pliny the Elder's *Natural History*, book 26, as proof of its earlier appearances and attempted to ferret out information from various antique sources to identify the disease currently sweeping through Europe—'Lichenas, Mentagram, Asaphati, Elepjantiasin, et igne Persicum'.[24] Others returned to Old Testament descriptions,[25] even to Homer's *Odysseus*, as with one of Germany's earliest syphilis tracts.[26] Some located later Arabic sources, such as Pope Alexander VI's physician Petrus Pintor, who claimed the disease's signs matched those of a rarely mentioned variant of *variola* (smallpox), described by Rhazes and Avicenna, and should be called 'aluhumata'.[27]

The notion that a disease could be new was anathema to physicians and deemed a misconception of commoners. Worse still was calling it by a vernacular name—such as 'mal francese' or 'mal de Naples'—or even a translation of these terms into Latin.[28] Nonetheless, the suitability of various ancient terms to describe the present pandemic created heated debate. In 1504, the physician-poet Peter Crinitus scoffed: 'to say that the similarities in the skin disorders between the new disease and "elephantis" were the same was not only absurd; it was downright ridiculous'.[29] Physicians who considered the disease new, such as Gaspar Torella, bishop

---

[21] Astruc, *De Morbis Venereis.*   [22] *Aphrodisiacus*; and Gruner, *De Morbo Gallico scriptores.*

[23] On Luisini (or Luigini), see *The Great Pox*, 4–5. They count 'no less than 59 authors'. Also, see ibid., 4–18, on the tradition of compiling sources and summaries of diseases.

[24] Luisini, 72; and Leonicini, *Librum de Epidemia*, 15. Neither Pliny, Galen, nor other ancient physicians saw these diseases with various skin disorders as the same disease; on their differences, see Scheidel, 'Germs for Rome', 169–70: lichen or mentagra was 'a pustulous lichen on the chin, transmitted by kissing, confined to the upper classes, while, ' "elephant disease" poses no difficulties'; it was caused by *Mycobacteriun leprae*, common in Egypt in antiquity but almost unknown in Rome until the second century, when it spread slowly. Whether the venereal disease was lichens led to heated debate: in support of Leoniceni, Symphorianus Champerius, a Lyonnais physician also used Pliny's, *Natural History*, book 26, ch. 1, to stress the disease's survival since antiquity; *De lichen seu mentagra*, 128. Leonardo Fuschsii, *De Morbo Gallico*, 137–8, agreed with Von Hutten, claiming 'morbus Gallicus' was a new disease. Another Lyonnais physician opposed Fuschsii's claim, siding with his compatriot Champerius; Montuus, *De morbo gallico*, 139–40.

[25] See for instance Corradi, 'Nuovi documenti', 355–6, and note 35.

[26] 'Martin Pollichs von Mellerstadt', 44.

[27] Pinctor, *Tractatus de morbo foedo*; and *The Great Pox*, 117–19.

[28] On physicians' arguments rejecting the disease as new, see *The Great Pox*, 71, 74, and 95.

[29] Crinitus *De poetis latinis*, 119.

of Santa Giusta, another of Alexander's physicians, sometimes refrained altogether from calling it by variants of 'mal francese'. Throughout his four tracts on the disease, Torella consistently called it 'de pudendagra', the disease of genitals.[30] His term for it, moreover, influenced later medical nomenclature. Forty years on, a Bolognese physician, Giovanni Battista Theodosius, and a Spaniard, Leone Lunensis de Zuccano, maintained that physicians in Rome continued calling it 'pudendagram'.[31] Others refused to name it after the French or any other people and referred instead to the disease's physical signs—'mala pustularum' or 'turgentium pustularum', as with Heidelberg physician Conrad Schellig and Ioannes Trithenmius[32]—or just the pustules, as with the Spanish physician Marcellus Cumanus, active at Navarra in 1495, even though he described soldiers returning from war in Venice and Milan as carrying it to his home town.[33] In the earliest tracts edited by Karl Sudhoff (1853–1938), German doctors such as Thomas von Hochberg, writing in 1503, called it 'morbum Gallicum', but also after its signs, 'morbus pustularum', and, like other physicians, thought it originated not with the French, Spanish, or Indians but from the ancient disease described by Pliny, 'mentagram'. In his tract of 1503, Joseph Grünpeck called it 'de mentulargra'.[34] Joseph von Hochberg speculated that its origins were earlier, described in Deuteronomy, chapter 28, as 'plaga egipciaca'.[35]

As Pintor's manual suggests, physicians revealed not only the terms they used for the disease, but also those used by the laity, even commoners. Consalvo Ferrandi,[36] a doctor of Orvieto, and the Genoese Giovanni da Vigo, who was surgeon to Pope Julius II (a victim of the disease[37]), said the Spanish called it 'de las Buas'.[38] Others in the Iberian peninsula called it 'Patursa', after the ugliness of Saturn that matched the disease's filth ('feodus').[39] According to the Modenese surgeon Gabriel Falloppio, who held a chair at the University of Padua, the Spaniards adopted this term when first encountering it in the New World, because it was 'big, disgusting, and violent (*magnus, foedus, & violenus*)'. These names did not, however, implicate Indians as the disease spreaders.[40] Furthermore, da Vigo maintained that the term 'mal francese' was hardly universal in the Italian peninsula. In his native region, Genoa, it was called 'lo male de le Tavelle'; in Tuscany, 'lo male de le Bulle'; and in Lombardy, 'lo male de le Brosulae', names describing skin disorders and not carriers or origins.[41] The Genovese chronicler Agostino Giustiniano concurred: 'we *Genossi* call it *tavelle*'.[42]

---

[30] Torella, *De pudendagra*; *De dolore in pudendagra*; *De Ulceribus in Pugendagra*; and *Adversus Pudendagram*. On Torella and Pintor, see Proksch, II, 378–9.

[31] Theodosius, *Medicinales Espistolae* (1553); its dedication, however, was dated 1541, in *Aphrodisiacus*, 140–1; and de Zuccano, *De Morbo Gallico*.

[32] *Consilium breve contra malas pustulas*; and *Ein Syphilis-Consilium*.

[33] Cumanus, *Observationes Medicae*, 52: 'Pustulae sive vesicae epidemiae'.

[34] *Libellus Iosephi Grunbebkii de mentulargra*.   [35] *Ein Syphilis-Consilium*, 138.

[36] Neither this work nor its author is found in Edit 16.

[37] Raimond-Waarts and Santing, 'Sex: A Cardinal's Sin', 171–2, 174–6.

[38] In Luisini, I, 308–9. On da Vigo, see Proksch, II, 44–7.

[39] [Joannes Almenar] *Libellus ad evitandum et expellendum*, 203r (BAV pagination).

[40] Falloppio, *De Morbo Gallico*.   [41] In Luisini, 386.

[42] His *Castigatissimi Annali* was published in Genoa in 1537; see Corradi, 'Nuovi documenti', 362–3. According to Serra, *La storia della antica Liguria*, III, 291, 'tavelle' was Genoese for the disease, citing a contemporary Genoese chronicle by Bartolomeo Senarega not noted by Corradi.

In German-speaking regions, people named it 'Blattern', pustules or pox. Sebastian Brant called it 'the grievous sickness of the pustules and warts (*der schweren Kranckheit der Blattern und Wartzen*)'.[43] In an entry for 1495, the chronicle of the Austrian monastery of Melk claimed people of that region—the Danube valley—were calling it 'Bös Blatern und Lembt der Glider' ('the evil poxes and pain in the joints').[44] Other German speakers also called it by names pertaining to signs and symptoms: 'wilde Warzen' (wild or furious warts) or just warts ('Warzen') or scabies ('Krätze'). Later, it was even called 'pestis inguinalis' ('the plague of the groins'), no doubt leading to confusion with plague.[45] Finally, the papal doctor Pintor said that those in his native Valencia did not call it 'morbus Gallicus' but by another name, which he did not remember. In other Spanish regions, people used other names, which Pintor again failed to mention. But he was emphatic: they did not call it 'the French disease'.[46]

Nor did the French typically call it after Italians or Neapolitans. Perhaps the earliest French chronicler to comment on the disease, an anonymous Lyonnais writer in 1501, entitled his section, 'Remede contre la grosse verolle', and not of Neapolitans. Only later, after adding that some called it 'la grant gorre', others, the 'grosses veroulle', did he add that some also called it 'la maladie de naples'.[47] Strangely, one of the few places where a name referring to Neapolitans surfaces is in the 1506 municipal ordinances of Aberdeen—that 'strange seiknes of Nappillis' and at Linlithgow in 1500 as 'Spanyie pockis'. Yet in Scotland, as elsewhere, there is no evidence that Neapolitans, Spaniards, or the French were victimized in connection with the disease.[48] Moreover, until the seventeenth century, when across Europe the common medical term had become 'lues venerea', which endured into the nineteenth century, the usual name in Scotland was 'Grandgor' as seen in a 'Proclamation of King Iames IIII' found in the records of Edinburgh's town council of 22 September 1497.[49] Other French sources added further names which were unconnected with Naples or Italy and thus no tit-for-tat retaliation. In Lyonnais and Parisian ordinances it was called 'Verolle'.[50] The popular poem first published in Lyon in 1539, 'Le Triomphe de très haulte et puissante dame Verolle', never once mentions 'mal de Naples', although the poet reported in detail Charles VIII's conquest of Naples, where 'that pox' first erupted with epidemic force. Instead, he said no one was sure what to call it and referred to a wide variety of names, of which only one named a

---

[43] Brant, in *Aphrodisiacus*, 54. Also, early sixteenth-century Swiss commentators called it the 'bösen Blatteren'; see Proksch, II, 371–2; and Gall, 'Quarantine', 3.

[44] *Chronicon Monasterii Mellicensis*, in *Aphrodisiacus*, 46. Also, see Stumpf, *Löblicher Eydgenossenschafft Chronik*, 62, who called it 'Plaag, die bösen Blattern'.

[45] Proksch, II, 4; and II, 150–1.   [46] Pinctor, *Tractatus de morbo foedo*, 86.

[47] Proksch, II, 5, is the only scholar I know to have recognized that the French rarely called it after Neapolitans.

[48] Creighton, I, 418–19.   [49] In *Aphrodisiacus*, 71.

[50] See the Parisian ordinances of 1497 and 1498: *Arreste du Parlement de Paris* and *Ordonnance du prevost de Paris*, in *Aphrodisiacus*, 71. Only once did scribes use 'Malades de Naples'. The next Parisian decree concerning the disease (1498; ibid., 71) mentions only the term 'la Grosse Verole'. Other French names depicted skin disorders or the disease's patron saint without implicating supposed carriers or origins: 'les grosses pocques', 'la grande gorre', 'la pancque denarre', 'les fiebvres Sainct-Job'; see Quétel, *History of Syphilis*, 11.

people: the Lombards (and here he clearly means those of northern Italy, not all Italians) called it '*le mal francoys*'. On the other hand, by his account, the Neapolitans called it '*le souvenir*'; in Arabic, it was '*Sahaphati*'; in Latin, 'it should be called *Mentagra*'; 'the Flemings and Picards called it *gore* and *verole grosse*'; the Germans, '*groitre blatre*' (*grotte blatte* or big poxes); the Spanish, '*lesbones*'; and 'the Savoyards said *la clavela*'.[51] Later, the poem focused on one name alone, and it pertained to 'one of the most renowned of French cities (*Sur toutes villes renom*)': Dame Pox entitled herself 'la Gorre de Rouen'.[52] In addition, names of the disease after other French cities and regions sprouted in French sources. These were places reputed to have been the worst hit: 'peste de Bordeaux', 'mal de Niort' (the second city of Poitou), and 'mal du Carrefour de Poitiers'.[53] Again, no evidence points to any animosity towards the inhabitants of these supposed syphilitic hubs. Sixteenth-century doctors' tracts published in France could even be entitled 'morbus Gallicus'.[54] In one case, a tract published in Provence (which had been incorporated into France in 1481) and presented to its Estates General, was entitled 'Mal François', and this by an author whose pro-French political sentiments were patent: he supported France's Catholic king against Huguenot threats and the 'enterprinse' of Geneva.[55]

After the disease had spread 'thoroughly' through Germany and 'invaded (*invasit*)' the 'tough people (*robustissimas gentes*)' of Eastern Europe and Russia (*Sarmatiae regiones*), the early seventeenth-century chair of medicine at Padua, Eustachio Rudio, reported that these people were not calling it after origins or peoples 'who may have carried it to them' but after the disease's strange appearances. Because of loss of hair, they named it 'the illness of the curly tuffs or of the skinheads (*morbus Cirrorum sive Plica*)'.[56] In 1546, Fracastoro observed (as had others) that the disease had changed over the past twenty years: pustules now appeared 'in very few cases, and with hardly any pains', but one's hair falls out, making 'men look ridiculous'.[57] Two generations later, the Breslau physician Daniel Sennet said the same.[58]

Finally, Italian chroniclers referred to the disease by other names that failed to reflect origins or foreign places, but rather invoked the disease's patron saint, Job ('mal di Santo Giobbe'; 'la lebbra di S. Giobbe', 'la lebra de san Jobe').[59] In Bologna, an anonymous chronicle from 1496 to 1513 called it 'el male frazoxo overo el male de sam iob', as did another Bolognese and a civil lawyer of Ferrara: 'la lebra de san Jobe' and 'il male de S. Job'.[60] The physician Giovanni Battista Fulgosi from Piacenza (?) did not call it after Saint Job but said that others did: 'Alii autem aliter,

[51] 'Le Triomphe de très haulte et puissante dame Verolle', 242.　　[52] Ibid., 258.

[53] Quétel, *History of Syphilis*, 13.

[54] According to the 'Universal Short Title Catalogue' (USTC, St Andrews), twenty works (including re-editions) were published in France (either Paris or Lyon) with 'de morbo Gallico' or 'Morbus Gallicus' in their titles from von Hutten's (1519) to Mattioli's (1598). Two were by Frenchmen, Auger Ferrier, from Toulouse, *De lue Hispanica*; and the Montpellier physician Guillaume Rondelet's, *Methodus curandorum*, but in the text, he calls it 'morbus Italicus', BNF pagination, 37–8, 39, 40, and 91.

[55] *Remede tres salutaire contre le mal françois*, 3–9.　　[56] Rudio, *De morbo Gallico*, 1v-2r.

[57] Fracastoro, *De Contagione*, 138–9.　　[58] *The Great Pox*, 276.

[59] See cases in Corradi, 'Nuovi documenti', nos 6, 7, 12, 21; for chroniclers outside Italy as with an early sixteenth-century chronicler of Cologne, see *The Great Pox*, 52; and Berlerus, *Chronicon*, 125.

[60] Corradi, 'Nuovi documenti', nos 4, 7, 8.

nonnullique Iob Sancti aegritudinem esse dicebant'.[61] Also, Saint Job appears in one of the earliest references to the disease in a German chronicle, christened in 1496 by the Cologne Chronicler of Hilligen as 'Sent Iobs Krenkde'.[62] And a chronicle from Zeeland, first published in 1551, said that when the Spanish invaded the Low Countries, they carried with them 'a disease never heard of before', which was 'commonly called the plague of Saint Job, or the pox from Naples, or the Spanish pox'.[63] New confraternities and hospitals in Bologna, Ferrara, and Modena,[64] dedicated to syphilitic care, also took Job's name and special prayers and masses were addressed to him to relieve the sufferers' pain, as with the 'Missa Beati Jobi' composed by Paciudi.[65] Common sufferers invoked his name and took him as their guiding example, as seen in the long, blackly comic poem 'Lamento di quel tribulato' by the Sienese rhymester Niccolò Campani, where the speaker pleads with himself to exhibit the same patience:

> Udito ho dir che quello antiquo Iobbe
> In questo mal fu molto patiente.[66]

Finally, as early as 1527, the French physician Béthencourt christened the disease 'Morbus venereus', and by the end of the century the territorially neutral term 'lues venerea' replaced 'morbus Gallicus' in medical texts.[67]

STORIES OF BLAME

Even among those calling the new disease after other peoples or places, only one of over 250 texts I have examined from 1495 to the seventeenth century linked such naming explicitly with blame. With his third name for the disease—'la maladie de Naples'—the anonymous Lyonnais chronicler explained the reasons for it. Here, the term did not exactly fit those blamed. According to his story, not in Naples but after leaving the city, the French encountered foul play in Lombardy. The Lombards, 'the inventors of the disease', 'spread it to the French to wreak vengeance on them (*ques les Francoys venant de Naples en estoyent Lombars avoyent esté inventeurs de ceste maladie pour leur venger des Francoys*)'.[68] Only one Italian writer may have suggested that another people intentionally spread the disease. But in this case, not

---

[61] In *Aphrodisiacus*, 116.   [62] *Cronica der Hilligen stat Coellen*, 54.
[63] Van Reygersbergen, *Cronijck van Zeelandt*, 346–8. I thank Inneke Baatsen for this reference.
[64] *Gride Ducali...Modena*, 112 and 125.   [65] Corradi, 'Nuovi documenti', no. 18.
[66] Campani, *Lamento*, np; according to Edit 16, it was published at least twelve times in the sixteenth century: four undated editions and *c.*1511, 1521, 1523, 1529, 1537, 1559, 1564, and 1599. The only recent study to mention Campani is Zanrè, 'French Diseases', 203, but does so only in passing as a possible source for Agnolo Firenzuola's story on 'mal francese'. Earlier, the poem was treated by Luzio and Renier, 'Contributo', 420–4. Also, see 'Le Triomphe de très haulte et puissante dame Verolle', 243: 'Les aultres ont eu recours à saint Job'.
[67] This conclusion derives from a survey of 211 titles on syphilis and venereal disease dating from the earliest *incunabula* to 1820, first compiled by Robert McLean and myself, held in Glasgow's Special Collection, 'The Wellcome Trust Syphilis Project', <www.gla.ac.uk/services/specialcollections/collectionsa-z/syphiliscollection/>. Also see Proksch, II, 151.
[68] 'Was sagen...Chroniken von der Franzosenkrankheit', 155.

only is the reference unclear, the ones spreading the poison were not the Italians' (or at least not the Neapolitans') enemies but their allies—Spanish mercenaries sent by Ferdinand to assist against Charles' siege.[69] From his long tractatus on medicine and surgery, Falloppio claimed that certain cunning Spanish soldiers left their garrisons at night to poison Naples' wells.[70] The surgeon, however, does not suggest that their poisons were concocted from the disease, as Anna Foa claimed,[71] or as would occur with plague by the 1530s, giving rise to fantasies of 'plague spreaders' (see Chapter 6).

Yet Falloppio never used any term for the disease connected with Spain, and, more telling, his charge of contamination during the siege was not limited to the Spanish. He further reported that because of shortages, Italian bakers ('Italos Pistores') mixed gypsum with flour and that practice helped spread the pox.[72] The spread of contagion, he makes clear, had not been intended. Instead, following Galenic logic, the contamination of foodstuffs weakened the population of Naples, thereby indirectly fuelling the epidemic.[73] As we will see, another Italian doctor with Neapolitan connections would incriminate his fellow Neapolitans more sharply for inventing and spreading the new disease. But Falloppio laid greater emphasis on a third reason for pox's spread, and this one was closer to the mark: the terrible socio-economic conditions caused by the siege formed the epidemic matrix. Because of drastic food shortages, the 'contagion took wings', 'propelling' Naples' 'most beautiful girls' into 'secret prostitution'. Otherwise, they would have had to abandon their city. Drawn by their beauty, young French soldiers engaged in unbridled sex and infected them. Because of their extreme poverty, the women acquiesced, and soon, 'the entire French army' became infected, and 'afterwards, all of Europe'.[74] But even here, with sexual licence and promiscuity rife, Falloppio, despite his Counter-Reformation milieu, expressed sympathy for the victims and did not blame the calamity on a sinful, impoverished, indigenous 'other' or the enemy.[75]

Nevertheless, despite great variations in naming the new disease and misgivings about using the vernacular, even if translated into Latin,[76] the majority of physicians and surgeons during the first half of the sixteenth century used variations on 'mal

---

[69] According to Foa, 'The New and the Old', 'Syphilis for Falloppio...originated from poison that Spanish soldiers had put in the wells during the War of Naples' (39). Instead, Falloppio says only that Spanish soldiers poisoned wells.

[70] Falloppia, *Tractatus*, 663; idem, *De Morbo Gallico*, 2r.   [71] Foa, 'The New and the Old', 39.

[72] Falloppio, *De Morbo Gallico*, 662–3; and idem, *De Morbo Gallico*, 2r–v. The Cologne physician, Vochs, *De pestilentia anni presentis*, 120–1, also saw the corruption of badly baked bread as infecting the blood and afterwards, the sin of pride caused the disease's spread in Germany.

[73] Sixteenth-century physicians often saw corruption of foodstuffs as a cause of pestilence and cited Galen; however, Galen saw it as the consequence, not the cause, of plague; see Cohn, *Cultures of Plague*, 216.

[74] Falloppio, *De Morbo Gallico*, 662–3; and idem, *De Morbo Gallico*, 2r–v.

[75] Ibid. On beautiful women and prostitutes as imagined origins of syphilis, see McGough, 'Quarantining Beauty', 211 and *Gender, Sexuality, and Syphilis*, 45.

[76] *The Great Pox*, 21, claimed that 'morbus Gallicus' was 'a designation that most university physicians disliked as inappropriate'; if so, few said so, and most used the label consistently through their tracts. Yet neither von Hutten nor Guicciardini, who argued as strenuously as any that the term was inappropriate, were university physicians. Von Hutten was intensely critical of these physicians.

francese', 'morbus Gallicus', and occasionally the 'French scab (*gallica scabia*[77])'. Because of this name's prevalence, should we then presume they believed the disease originated with the French or held them responsible for it? Doctors and chroniclers alike engaged in debate on the disease's origins. The doctors, in fact, grounded their medical hypotheses more within historical and current events than they had in any previous medical writing, and no medical writings on any other disease would be as attentive to historical and political factors until the spurt in plague tracts during Italy's plague of 1575–7.[78] The majority of the early 'mal francese' tracts began by charting Charles VIII's campaign into Italy in 1494–5, the siege of Naples, and the envoy of King Ferdinand's Spanish mercenaries sent to assist the Neapolitans. Physicians then charted earlier movements of the New World conquistadors, returning from 'the islands' infected with the new disease, who King Ferdinand recruited to fight at Naples. By their sexual intercourse with prostitutes and others, the disease spread to French soldiers and from them to local Neapolitan women, then across Europe when mercenaries of various nations returned home. Despite calling the disease 'morbus Gallicus', authors such as Falloppio, the Veronese Giovanni Battista da Monte,[79] Fracastoro, and many others saw the discovery of the New India of the West and sexual contact with Indians as the origin of the disease, but did not blame the discoverers or the Indians. Nor did they see the calamity as the result of foul play or as a lesson to condemn the Spanish exploration.[80] After describing the disastrous epidemiological consequences ignited by Columbus's voyage, Falloppio vigorously argued that the bravery and ingenuity of his Italian compatriot was worth it. His chapter on 'morbus Gallicus' momentarily broke from the usual citations to Hippocrates, Galen, Arabic philosophers, and contemporary doctors to chronicle and celebrate Columbus's voyages: his itineraries to various islands, and the 'bountiful and most precious metals', 'the gold, silver, pearls' he brought back to Europe.[81]

In their detailed descriptions of the new disease's origins, sixteenth-century physicians and chroniclers, moreover, did not necessarily locate a single site or specific moment for the disease's origin. As with understanding of HIV/AIDS today, there could be ambiguity over the meaning of origins. Doctors in the late fifteenth century were of the view that the disease had been around for some time—either in a dormant state from antiquity or a 'domesticated' one with the Indians. Even after Columbus's sailors returned from their first voyage, physicians saw the disease as limited to certain communities, in hospitals in Barcelona, for example, and not of epidemic force. It was the disease's second origin—described more often and in greater detail—that created the pandemic as the consequence of Charles VIII's

---

[77] For the last term, see Penni, *Chroniche*, 371; Lusitano, *De Morbo Gallico et Gallica scabie*, 560; idem, *Epistola ii*, 'De Gallica Scabie', 560; Falloppio, *De Morbo Gallico*, 662–3; and Tomitano, *De Morbo Gallico*, 65.

[78] Cohn, *Cultures of Plague*. Surprisingly, Siraisi's excellent *History, Medicine* does not consider syphilis tracts.

[79] Montani, *Tractatus etiam utilissimus de Morbo Gallico*, 1v–2r.

[80] Falloppio, *De Morbo Gallico*, 662. Fracastoro, *De Contagione*, attempts to have it both ways: 'This is a new disease, long unknown on our continent...' (134–5).

[81] Falloppio, *De Morbo Gallico*, 663.

invasion of Italy. As with HIV/AIDS, a crucible of mass extra-marital sex was needed to ignite it. The Spanish may have brought the disease back, drawn from their 'commerce' with Indian women, but Charles' invasion, long encampment outside Naples, and entry into the impoverished city transformed the disease. From this melting pot of foreign soldiers and camp followers, the pox raced across Europe. Chroniclers and physicians made clear that the spread from Naples did not depend on one people—Neapolitans, French, or Spanish—and several attributed it to their own homelands, carried by their own soldiers. According to an early German chronicle, because of their sexual appetites, Germans brought the disease to Germany and the Swiss to their cantons.[82] According to the physician Bernardino Tomitano, another chair-holder of medicine at Padua, the disease had a third 'origin' or moment of dissemination, when in the 1530s it spread through Eastern Europe. Although this Italian, in fact Venetian,[83] continued calling it 'morbus Gallicus', neither war nor the French were now needed. By Tomitano's account, its vector was trade and its spreaders, Tomitano's own Venetian merchants.[84]

*   *   *

Anna Foa and William Eamon (relying here largely on her work) have in fact argued that naming did not entirely blame those named: that despite the common term 'mal francese', the blackest, most virulent blame fell not on fellow Christians, whether French or Neapolitan, but on more distant, pernicious, and alien others. First, it was the Jew, who supposedly transmitted it around Europe when expelled from Spain in 1492, but more so, the Indian, in Foa's words, 'the absolute Other', 'the person who had never known Christianity' a 'nonhuman', the 'totally alien'. To put naming and blaming back together again, she alleges that 'mal dell'Indie' had won against the older 'mal francese' by the 1530s;[85] blame for the disease then became 'redirected in the scholarly and ecclesiastical milieu to the most useful scapegoats, the Indians, then the Jews'.[86] But what is the evidence?

To take Jews first, Foa focuses on the Roman chronicler and papal secretary Sigismondo dei Conti da Foligno, who tells the story of Jews or Marranos transmitting syphilis from Spain to Italy with their expulsion in 1492, three years before Charles' capture of Naples.[87] To theorize further, the Roman chronicler then cited Tacitus as his source to claim that just as Jews had been more susceptible to leprosy in antiquity because of their dietary laws prohibiting pork, they now were more susceptible to the new disease, which possibly was not new but leprosy or related to it. Sigismondo's chronicle, however, was not published until 1883. Neither Foa nor Eamon shows that it was copied or even known in the sixteenth century, and I know of no references to it before Alfonso Corradi's in the 1880s. Even Germany's father

---

[82] 'Ein Chronikmarchen', 144.

[83] Tomitano was born and died in Padua (1517–76), part of the Venetian state, and was employed by Venice as a professor at Padua; after 1563 he became a physician in Venice.

[84] Tomitano, *De Morbo Gallico*, 64–5. This work is not listed by Edit 16.

[85] Foa, 'The New and the Old', 31.   [86] Ibid., 33–4.

[87] Ibid., 31, and Eamon, 'Cannibalism', 22; *Le Storie de suoi tempi*, excerpted and commented upon by Corradi, 'Nuovi documenti', 303–4 and 363–4. Also, see *The Great Pox*, 23–4.

of the history of medicine, Christian Gottfried Gruner (1744–1815), who searched far and wide for scraps of evidence linking Jews and syphilis, as his *Aphrodisiacus* attests, and who concocted a vicious anti-Semitic version of syphilis's origin, does not mention Sigismondo. In addition, Foa cites a short passage of Leo Africanus's geography of Africa, written in 1559, which attributed the spread of the disease in part to Ferdinand's expulsion of the Jews, with Jewish women having sexual intercourse with 'Scurrilous Ethiopians', which disseminated the disease through Lybia, Numidia,[88] and Black Africa (Nigritarum regionem).[89] Another short entry from the northern Italian humanist Paolo Giovio, written in the mid-sixteenth century, pointed to the Jews' expulsion from Spain as one (but only one) source of the disease's spread to Italy.[90] Yet, these three sources hardly constitute a new orthodoxy, as Foa and Eamon have claimed. They have shown no evidence that people followed their lead, or called the new disease by some variant of 'mal dei Ebrei' or of the Marranos.

Eamon adds another dimension, claiming that lepers were yet another 'Other' blamed for the disease.[91] But no references to the 'lepers' disease' or any variant of it, that is, to a disease of present lepers, appear in these sixteenth-century texts. As we have seen, physicians early on speculated that the disease was not new but a recrudescence either of ancient leprosy or related to it. Yet only a few, such as Paracelsus (1493–1541), who had no influence until after his death, pointed to lepers of their own time having anything to do with the disease's dissemination—and only then at its origins.[92] No special decrees promulgated by municipalities or princes and no riots ensued against this minority in connection with the pox and certainly none that targeted lepers as willing spreaders of it. Moreover, even by the papal secretary's account (and unlike that of the late Enlightenment Gruner), no vicious attack on Jews is made explicit. Instead, Sigismondo portrays them principally as the victims of Ferdinand's expulsion.

What about the most absolute 'Others', the Indians? By contrast with Jews, chroniclers and physicians of the new disease often mentioned Amerindians, who by the early sixteenth century were being distinguished from Indians of the subcontinent as 'the Indians of the Western Isles'.[93] However, from Edit 16's survey of all known works published in Italy during the sixteenth century or that are presently in any Italian library, not a single title, along with their often paragraph-long descriptive subtitles, records any variant of 'mal d'India', despite numerous authors pointing to New India as the disease's origin. The same holds for the fifty texts published by Corradi in 1884, the seventy-nine tracts, letters, and consilia gathered by Luisini, others added by Jean Astruc, then Gruner, in the eighteenth century, plus writings I have collected at the Vatican Library, the Bibliothèque nationale de

---

[88] The ancient term for the Berber kingdom covering present-day Algeria and western Tunisia.

[89] Leo Africanus, *De totius Africae*, 125. The Genoese chronicler Bartholomaeus Senarega also said that many believed the disease came from Ethiopia but did not attach racial prejudices to this origin; Proksch, I, 318.

[90] Giovio, *Historiae Sui Temporis*, 125.

[91] Eamon, 'Cannibalism': 'Similarly, transmission of *morbus Gallicus*, he claims, was blamed on persecuted minorities at home, notably lepers, prostitutes, Jews, and Marranos' (22).

[92] Foa, 'The New and Old', 39. Also, see notes 182–3.

[93] See Pagden, 'The Challenge of the New', 449–62.

France, or those listed in the Universal Short Catalogue of books published during the sixteenth century in libraries across the world.[94] Moreover, within these texts, physicians, chroniclers, and other commentators rarely referred to such nomenclature. The first exception appears in a tract by a physician of Ravenna published in 1538—'Morbuscue Indicus'; the reference, however, does not appear in the chapter on the disease's names and in no fashion blames Indians.[95] The second, Pietro Rostinio's (or Rostini's) *Trattato del Mal Francese*, published in 1556, claims 'some called it male Indiano'. But instead of a tag of blame, Rostinio explained the disease was so named because 'Indians did not usually suffer much from it'.[96] Later, Prospero Borgarucci, physician to King Charles IX of France, lists 'Indus' among various names for the disease—'morbus Gallicus, Hispanis, Neapolitanus, Indus, vel Catholicus, aut Venerens, sive Meuius'—but no animosity is implied; no more, that is, than for any others he lists, including Europeans themselves as with 'the disease of Catholics'.[97]

While Spanish and Portuguese conquistadors, physicians, and historians, who first saw pox in Barcelona in 1493, called it principally after the skin disorders that characterized it—'las Busas'—occasionally they called it after its geographical origins, 'mal de la ysla Española', but again, without any implication of blame.[98] The religious chronicler Franciscus Lopez de Gomara thought it came from the Indians but called it 'las bubas'. He maintained that many labelled it 'mal Frances', not because people thought it had originated with them or blamed them for it but because it had hit the French 'the worst'. Lopez also called the disease 'el mal de las Indias', but only once and in that instance to praise Indians for their remedy or 'vino' for the disease.[99]

Even commentators such as the nobleman and royal historian Gonzalo Fernández de Oviedo, whose multi-volume *Natural History of the Indians* sought to justify their exploitation and enslavement, did not call the disease after Indians or blame them but consistently called it after its signs, 'del mal de las búas'. Only once does he allude to others, who might have called it 'el *mal de las Indias*'.[100] Neither here nor

[94] USTC, 2015.

[95] Thomae Philologi, *Mali Glaeci Sanandi*, 116r. This tract is not found in Luisini.

[96] I have used the third edition of Rostinio's, *Trattato del Mal Francese* (BAV); he praised Fioravanti's, *De' Capricci Medicinali*; however, the earliest known printing of that book was not until three years later (1568). On Rostinio, see McGough, 'Quarantining Beauty', 211 and *Gender, Sexuality, and Syphilis*, 45, on his reliance on Brasavola's theory of the origins of the French disease, written mid-century (*De Morbo Gallico*) and later published in multiple editions. Edit 16 incorrectly attributes Rostinio's *Trattato del mal francese* to Brasavola.

[97] Borgarutius, *Methodus*, 151. In addition, I have found 'mal'Indiano' in Alessandri, *Trattato della peste*, 8r. Here, 'Catholicus' did not mean the Spanish as it might in other contexts; Alessandri already listed 'Hispanis'.

[98] The Barcelona physician, Ruy Diaz de Isla (1462–1542?), who treated syphilis patients returning from the New World as early as 1493 and wrote a syphilis tract in 1510 (not published until 1534), *Tratado*, called it 'mal de la ysla Española' but did not blame the Indians, and held that the disease's common name was not descriptive of the Indians but of the skin disorders—'Bubas'; see Bloch, 'The History of Syphilis', 12; Proksch, I, 380 and II, 101. The explorers also translated and presumably used names given by the Indians—'Guaynaras, Hipas, Taybas, and Icas'; Bloch, 'The History of Syphilis', 12.

[99] Lopez de Gomara, *Sacerdos Hispanis*, 129.

[100] Oviedo, *Historia*, I, 49 and 53. Also, Proksch, I, 384, argued 'bubas' was the common name in Spain.

elsewhere did he accuse the Indians of any retaliatory tricks to wreak vengeance on the conquistadors. Instead, he describes how 'las búas' became domesticated with the Indians before the Spanish arrived—'así pro la tierra donde tan natural es esta dolencia...Las cuales pasiones son naturales destas Indias'[101]—and for this reason Indians suffered mildly, while the Spaniards, much more cruelly ('e muy crueles dolores e pasión'[102]). To account for the difference, Oviedo does not begrudge the Indians for their natural advantage. In fact, his *Sommario*, the only part of his *Natural History* published in his lifetime, praised the Indians, not only for their sacred wood, but for their medicinal botany and talents as great herbalists ('et in terra ferma con altre herbe, o cose che loro sanno, percho sono molto grandi herbolari').[103] The mid-century historian of the New World and chronicler of Peru, Hieronymus Benzonus, also praised the Indians for their sacred wood and herbs, especially 'Zarzaparillam', gathered in Puno (Peru) and Guasyaquil (Ecuador), and the Spanish learnt from 'their example'. Explorers claimed these plants cured a number of illnesses and were especially notable in alleviating pain caused by the pox.[104]

Not all sixteenth-century writers were convinced that the sacred wood was the miracle cure proclaimed by von Hutten and others. The mid-century Bolognese doctor Giovanni Battista Theodosius had his doubts: 'The Indian concoction seems to me still to be proven...it may only work in hot and dry conditions'.[105] The physician Michael Angelis Blondus, writing around the same time, expressed little 'faith' in the 'Indian wood', claiming it could even lead to infection by 'morbus Gallicus'.[106] More famously, Paracelsus praised and elaborated on the mercury treatment at the expense of the sacred wood, claiming it did nothing.[107] Yet, none of these authors, including Paracelsus with his many prejudices and eagerness to buck orthodox medical opinion at any turn, went on to blame the Indians.

I have, however, found one source that blamed Indians for Europe's new disease, but receives no mention from Foa, Eamon, or other recent historians. The Spanish navigator Albericus Vesputius (Vespucci) savagely castigated the Indian woman for her 'atrocious habit', which he described as 'totally exempt from humanity': her 'insatiable sexual desire' was the cause of the disease's spread, first among the Indians, enabled by their promiscuity and lack of any taboos on incest, such that 'mothers married sons and brothers, sisters'. 'Their indiscriminate libidinal practices approximated that of savage animals', and 'by shameless prostitution of their bodies and their most libidinous zeal, their women of outstanding and salacious beauty spread [the disease], beyond all cruelty, to great numbers of Christians'.[108] But nowhere does Vespucci call the disease after the Indians.

---

[101] Oviedo, *Historia*, I, 49 and 53.   [102] Ibid., I, 54.

[103] Oviedo, *Sommario*, in *Aphrodisiacus*, 133.

[104] Benzonus, *Novae novi orbis historiae*, 141, made his observations in the New World between 1541 and 1556; and de Cieça de Leon, *Chronica del Peru*, 141–2.

[105] Theodosius, *Medicinales Epistolae LXVIII*, 141.

[106] Blondus, *De origine morbi Gallici*, 159.   [107] Paracelsus, *De Morbo Gallico*, 134–7.

[108] *De novo orbe in lingua Hispana*.

Across countries, continents, and time, did 'myths of origins' imply blame, as historians and public intellectuals often assume?[109] According to the fragment of the *Sicilian Annales* of 1498, 'some said that the "mal francese" originated in the Kingdom of Naples', 'brought there' by Spanish soldiers, while 'others claimed the Spanish brought it with them from India'. Either way, the chronicler makes no allusion to the disease's various possible origins as reasons to blame those from where it may have arisen.[110] Later, the chronicler of L'Aquila, Bernardino Cirillo, was more definite about origins: 'mal francese' was a new disease, unknown in antiquity. When French soldiers returned home from Naples, they said that it came from Neapolitan women. But Cirillo denied it: the disease was 'neither *mal di Napoli*, nor that of France'; rather, it came from the Spanish returning from 'new India', several of whom were afterwards sent by their king ('Re Cattolico') to fight in the Neapolitan war. They 'carried the contagious illness' and infected local women. Thus, it was the Spanish soldier, not the Indian, who was at the disease's origin, even though he caught it and brought it back from the Indian islands. Cirillo did not, however, blame his allies, the Spanish, and certainly not Indians. Instead, he praised new India and God for having 'given birth in this India' to the 'sacred wood (*il legno Santo*)', guaiacum or guaicanum, which Europeans also called the Indian wood and imagined from the early sixteenth into the next century as the cure that would deliver them from their new nightmare.[111]

Instead of 'mal' being associated with the naming or blaming of the new India of the West, 'sacred' was the adjective sixteenth-century doctors and chroniclers associated with Indians and pox: 'il legno d'India' or 'Lignum illud quod vulgo Sanctum, alias Indicum appellatur', as the Neapolitan physician Alphonso Ferri elaborated, devoting an entire book to its wondrous cures.[112] These sixteenth-century intellectuals praised the Indians for their discovery and expressed gratitude to them for passing their knowledge to the afflicted Spaniards. In his poem 'Syphilis', Fracastoro describes in detail the Indians' methods for preparing Guaiacum, the doses of the 'divine liquid', and a regime of 'great fasts' to follow that caused 'the plague to vanish into vacant air'.[113] He ends with an ode to the Indians' sacred tree:

Hail great tree sown from a sacred seed by the hand of the Gods, hope of mankind, pride and new glory from a foreign world.[114]

---

[109] See McGough, 'Quarantining Beauty', 213, relying on Farmer: 'Origin myths locate blame for the epidemic within a wider geopolitical and moral framework'.

[110] *Frammenti degli Annali di Sicilia*, 347.

[111] *Annali delle Città dell'Aquila*, 365–6; Bloch, 'The History of Syphilis', 13. According to *The Great Pox*, 100, news of its use reached German-speaking regions between 1506 and 1516.

[112] Ferri, *De morbo Gallico*, 347, published first in Rome, 1537, then in Paris, 1543. Also see Il Grappa, *Cicalamenti*, 3; Campani, *Lamento*, 'illegnio Dindia', np; 'Lettera, Mantova, 1534', 335; Ferrandi, *De Guaiacano Ligno*, 308; *De ligno sancto*, 309; Montani, *Epistola*, 495; Manardi, *De morbo Gallico*: 1; idem, *Eiusdem de ligno Indico*, 518. These may come from his *Epistolae medicinales*, first published in Ferrara, 1521. Brasavola, *De radicis Chynae*, 616–35; Falloppio, *De Morbo Gallico*, 669 (five editions in the sixteenth century, the first in 1563). Fracantiani [Francanzani], *De Morbo Gallico*, 728. Vergesaci, *Liber, ex Enchiridio ipsius Chirurgico excerptus*, 1.

[113] *Fracastoro's Syphilis*, 87–91.

[114] Ibid., 107. His *De Contagio* criticized physicians who prescribed the wood, saying they did so to enhance their authority and profits; see Henderson, 'Fracastoro', 77, 81.

New recipes for preparing a powder and beverage from the sacred wood passed quickly through learned circles across Europe.[115] According to the Modenese physician Alexander Fontana, the Portuguese, 'being sharp-sighted and able men (*viri ingenio perspicaces*)', observed Indians using their sacred wood to treat their own people, suffering with the same signs of the French disease, and learnt from them how to cure themselves and the Spaniards.[116] An anonymous physician writing in Provence at the end of the sixteenth century said the same: 'even if they were barbarians and ignorant of learned medicine, through their experience (*en ceste coustume fondee sur la maistrise de l'experience*), they had found the cure for this illness and faithfully taught us the means and remedies by which they cured themselves of the disease'.[117] The Indian wood not only cured syphilis; according to the doctor Antonio Galli, it could treat any number of pestilential maladies: 'Cum ligni nuper ex India ad nos advecti vis, ac natura curandis Hispanicae luis omnis generis malis'.[118] Fracastoro agreed but not so approvingly: the wood was being applied to various other ailments in Italian hospitals—'for any old and cold complaint of the head, nerves, stomach and joints'.[119] The Neapolitan physician Alfonso Ferri or Ferro went the furthest, dedicating his opening chapter and then the entire second book of his 220-page tract to the sacred wood and its multiple cures—melancholy, insomnia, epilepsy, paralysis, spasms and contractions, ailments of the nose, deafness, ranula, asthma, breathing difficulties, bad breath, kidney and bladder troubles, tuberculosis ('phthisi'), sterility, gout, flux of the uterus, hernia, leprosy ('elephantia'), and more.[120]

Far from blaming it on non-Christians, non-Europeans, even the non-human 'absolute Other', the Catholic Abruzzese chronicler Cirillo was not alone calling the disease after Europeans, the 'Catholic disease'. Writing in the 1530s, the Venetian Tomitano was clearer. He charted its transmission as 'first coming to light' in Italy, then in Spain, followed by England, Germany, Hungary, and Sarmatia (lands of Eastern Europe into Russia). From this dissemination, he concluded, the disease had infected many more than just the French, and should no longer be called after them but should instead be called 'the European disease (*morbum Europaeum*)'.[121] Similarly, the Spanish physician, Rodericus Diacius, felt no compunction stressing the role played by his own people: along with Portuguese sailors, the Spanish had spread the disease from the New World to the Old, with Barcelona as its staging post. He then ridiculed the naming after various regions, attributing the cause in

---

[115] See numerous recipes for it in Luisini and elsewhere.

[116] *Morbo Gallico et ligno indico*, I, 610–15 (does not appear in Edit 16).

[117] *Remede tres salutaire*, 13–14.

[118] Galli, *De ligno sancto*, 3r. For Oviedo, *Historia*, I, 54 and others praising the wood, see Zanrè, 'French Diseases', 200–3. In his 'In lode del legno santo', the Florentine Agnolo Firenzuola pushed aside his usual sarcasm (203).

[119] Cited in *The Great Pox*, 203.

[120] Ferri, *De ligni sancti*, 6–9, 23–4, and 60–136; see Proksch, II, 106–9.

[121] Tomitano, *De Morbo Gallico*. The Florentine physician Beniveni, *De Morbo Gallico*, 345–6, charts a similar spread of the disease from the New World through Europe, although he claims it appeared first in Spain. Even earlier, in 1505, the bishop-physician Torella charted this trajectory from Spain across Europe and then 'the entire world', exonerating the French and Italians without pinning it on any country or people; Torella, *De pudendagra*, 423.

part to air floating between regions, and concluded: if the disease must be named after people, then the names of all the peoples of the globe should be used for it ('quod volet, nomen imponere poterit, ut omnes orbis nationes hactenus fecere').[122] In this vein, a 'medécin ordinaire' of Bordeaux said the 'venereal disease', first called after the French, then the Spanish, must now be called the 'universal' disease.[123]

* * *

In addition to seeing multiple origins of the disease, doctors and chroniclers in Galenic fashion saw multiple layers of causation—remote, near, and immediate. The Bavarian physician practising in Bologna, Vvendelini Hick de Brackenau, believed that 'this disease did not arise solely from contagion; its true cause was the influence of wandering stars... various planetary conjunctions and solar and lunar eclipses'.[124] Other doctors such as Martin Pollichs from Mellerstadt made similar claims,[125] and some located these causative conjunctions well before either Columbus sailed for America or Charles crossed the Alps. The Veronese physician Pietro Maynardi began the first of his two tracts on the 'French Disease' by pointing to conjunctions of Mars and Saturn in 1489 that overwhelmed Jupiter.[126] For Joseph Grünpeck, despite his disparaging and politically attuned remarks against the French and Italians to ingratiate himself with Emperor Maximilian, the disease's rise depended on earlier and more complex constellations, made all the more convoluted by recent astrological charts showing no significant planetary conjunctions during the last decade of the fifteenth century. First, Saturn met Jupiter at 6:04 p.m. on 25 November 1484, a solar eclipse followed on 30 November 1485, and all this by Grünpeck's reckoning depended on Saturn's earlier history of ten revolutions.[127] By Gaspar Torella's calculation, the planetary conjunctions in 1493 occurred closer to the disease's outbreak but this was still before Charles' invasion.[128] These remote events beyond the human plane caused the disease, not actions by Spaniards, Frenchmen, Italians, or Indians.

Even the famous theoretician of contagion, Fracastoro, saw the rise of 'morbus Gallicus' coming from the stars, especially in his famous poem of 1530, though also in his more nuanced chapters of *De Contagione*. In the later work, changes in air, putrefaction, and their production of germs took centre stage, but the stars remained the governing motor: 'As I have shown above, the heavenly bodies can

---

[122] Diacius, *Tratado contro la enfermedad de las bubas*, 162–3.

[123] Briet, *Explication de deux questions*, 15.   [124] Hick de Brackenav, *De Morbo Gallico*, 268.

[125] 'Martin Pollichs von Mellerstadt erste Syphilisthesen', 43. On multiple causation within Galenic medicine, see Arrizabalaga, 'Medical Responses', 33–5 and 52–3, but the essay does not relate this framework to the question of blame.

[126] Maynardi, *Morbo Gallico*, 337.

[127] Hayton, 'Joseph Grünpeck's Astrological Explanation', 91–2 and 100–1. Also see Clementius, in *Aphrodisiacus* (1535), 120, for the importance of these conjunctions in 1484 and 1485.

[128] Torella, *De pudendagra*, 423. Also see the earliest known Syphilis tract of Leonicini, *Librum de Epidemia*, 15, who saw the disease 'born under the influence of the stars'; as did Tomitano, *De Morbo Gallico*, 64, citing Fracastoro's poem. Concerning the nature of causes of venereal diseases, see Fernel, *Ambiani de lue venera dialogus*, 524–8, who saw the disease arising from the stars' 'insolenti constitutioni'. For Almenar, *Libellus ad evitandum et expellendum Morbus Gallicum*, 203r, Saturn caused it, coming within the path of Mars.

bring into play on this earth great and portentous phenomena when several of them are in conjunction'.[129] The conjunction of Saturn, Jupiter, and Mars had 'induced a foul putrefaction, and the germs from it were carried to us'.[130] The disease's contagion followed as a consequence of motion started by stars. Through the sixteenth century and beyond, doctors placed epidemics, plague and syphilis included, in this Aristotelian–Galenic frame of 'intemperances of the air'.[131] Previous changes in the stars or climate induced these changes, which then corrupted the humours, disrupting bodily balances that produced the pustules ('pillulae morbae gallici').[132] For the Ferrarese Leoncini, the preconditions of pox were immediate changes in climate: the warmth and humidity of the Italian summer followed by heavy rains in the winter of 1495–6 and flooding.[133] Such events did not rely on importation by outsiders or human carriers but on atmospheric events beyond human influence. Instead of pinning blame on the peculiarities of Italian or Neapolitan weather in 1494 or 1496, German physicians turned to their own climatic conditions. One known as Linturius argued that the new disease's origins in Franconia ('plaga malum Francigenum') and its spread through the Rhineland (Rheni), Swabia, and Bavaria depended on their hot autumn of 1496.[134] The Heidelberg doctor Schellig also began with the air as this disease's 'Causa primitiva'.[135] The famous Parisian physician, Jean Fernel, pushed aside both theological and astrological determinants and questioned the importance of corrupted food, since magnates and the rich also were catching the disease. But in their place, he emphasized changes in the airs as the principal external cause inseminating the new disease ('ut pestilentiae semina').[136]

The immediate cause of disease in these Galenic frameworks could also concern the individual patient and not outside forces carried by outside agents, whether people or germs. Instead, the disease depended on humoral imbalances, engendered by diet and behaviour—Galen's six non-naturals.[137] According to this model, if anyone was to blame, it was the individual insider, not any 'Other'. In a practical handbook for surgeons, Antoine Chaumette wasted no time with God or stars but delved immediately into procedures for treating pox. It was the patient's obligation first to adopt the proper rules of life ('à l'ordonnance de vie'), selecting a temperate climate and diet to avoid big or viscous humours ('ni deliez ny acres').[138] Another doctor, Michael Angelis Blondus, went further, focusing solely on internal causes, calling astrological explanations 'false opinions' and notions of

---

[129] Fracastoro, *De Contagione*, 48–9.   [130] Ibid., 50–1.

[131] Leonicini, *Librum de Epidemia*; and *De morbo Gallico Petrihaschardi insulani*, 72: the excessive intemperance of the air destroyed the humours, especially after sexual intercourse.

[132] For this chain reaction from stars to air to humours to pustules, see Clementius, 120.

[133] *The Great Pox*, 75.   [134] Linturius, in *Aphrodisiacus*, 119–20.

[135] Schellig, *Consilium breve*, 41. In an earlier letter, the stars are mentioned only briefly, after sin: their 'fluxus' being one cause of the disease.

[136] Fernel, *De luis venereare*, 142–3. Similarly, the Montpellier physician and advisor to the king of France, Rondeletti, *De Morbo Gallico*, denied that stars or corruption of food caused the disease; rather, it came from 'India', where it had been domesticated (78).

[137] Numerous works by Torella, Pinctor, Lobera di Avila, Steber of Vienna, and others used the system of humours and Galen's six non-naturals to explain the rise of the new disease.

[138] Chaumette, *Enchiridion* (a longer edition was published in 1572).

one region spreading it to another as 'ridiculous'. For him, the disease was 'born from corrupt juices within us (*in nobis nascitur ex corruptis succis*)'; only later did it spread person to person, 'corrupting the blood and black bile of others'.[139]

The other fundamental cause of the pox—this one outside of Galen's framework but fundamental to medieval and early modern medicine—centred on God and His 'punishment for our sins'. As with Galen's six non-naturals, it turned inward and not against outsiders. After describing the disease as coming from Saturn, the Valencian physician Joannes Almenar[140] declared that it was not only a matter of our bodies; the disease arose as punishment for our sins.[141] Falloppio said much the same: 'Hinc factum est, quod Deus saepe morbis castigavit peccata nostra',[142] as did the Ferrarese court physician, Corradino Gilino; yet he more specifically pinned the blame on his own, the 'Italian people'.[143] Those outside of the medical profession saw pox's ultimate cause as having the same origins. Like the doctors, Florence's firebrand preacher Girolamo Savonarola looked within, seeing the affliction as God's judgement on the sinful Florentines.[144] Others such as the Duke Ercole of Ferrara saw these causes not as vague or necessarily global. Influenced by Savonarola, he viewed the new disease in combination with other troubles then plaguing Italy as manifestations of God's wrath. To protect his people, he passed an edict on 3 April 1496 'to eradicate all vices' with severe punishments mandated against blasphemy, sodomy, games of chance, concubinage, prostitution, and pimping. These laws, however, did not scapegoat an outsider or marginalized group, such as prostitutes, but affected Ferrara's citizens and inhabitants as a whole.[145] In the same year, the Diet of Worms placed blame for the disease on its own people: their excessive blasphemy had brought it on.[146] Finally, the physician Piero Rostinio maintained that some placed the cause 'of this evil' in God: He had sent it to compel men to put aside their lecherous debauchery ('la lussuria') and recognize their disgusting habits and shame ('cosa sozza & di molta vergogna'). Unlike others, Rostinio then reasoned that if these were God's intentions, 'why was the disease not worse with thieves, assassins, and murderers; why had it killed babies within their mothers' wombs: what had they done?'[147] But he jettisoned his doubts along with any search for a scapegoat, including the thieves, assassins, and murderers.

Most sixteenth-century physicians accepted the interaction of primary or external causes with the internal ones of humoral imbalance, like the French king's physician and consular Hieronymus Montius who argued that 'externally the stars caused excessive air, heat, and intemperate humidity', which upset the body's constitution, causing bodily weakness ('cacochymia') that gave rise to contagion and

---

[139] Blondus, *De origine morbi Gallici*, 157–62.

[140] On Almenar, see Arrizabalaga, 'Medical Responses', 40.

[141] Almenar, *Libellus ad evitandum*, 203r.   [142] Falloppio, *De Morbo Gallico*, 661.

[143] Cited in Arrizabalaga, 'Medical Responses', 37. Grünpeck's first cause was God and blame was directed inwards, although he used the term 'malum de Franzos', see Hayton, 'Joseph Grünpeck's Astrological Explanation', 86.

[144] McGough, *Gender, Sexuality, and Syphilis*, 2; on Savonarola's influence on doctors, see Arrizabalaga, 'Medical Responses', 37. Also, the historian Sigismondo (1497) asserted the disease arose to chastise us for our excessive sins ('i troppi peccati').

[145] *The Great Pox*, 42.   [146] Ibid., 88.   [147] Rostinio, *Trattato del Mal Francese*, 22.

then 'begat thousands of particular pustules to form'.[148] By the beginning of the eighteenth century, however, even in regions of Europe not at the forefront of medicine, this relationship of primary or external and internal causes of pox had changed completely. In a rare tract, with only three copies of a second edition known in Britain (and none of the first), the surgeon Pedro Lopez Pinna from Fuente del Maestre in the province of Badajoz defined 'the primitive or external cause' of the 'morbo Gallico' as venereal contact or sleeping in the bedding or clothing of one already infected with the disease. The 'internal causes' were 'antecedent' conditions of the body, such as the digestive system and other conditions that predisposed the individual to contract the disease; humours and bodily balances were no longer mentioned.[149] By then (at least in this physician's account), the three phases of syphilis had also been anticipated.[150]

*   *   *

Authors who called the disease after the French not only refused to use their texts to cast aspersions against them, but occasionally were explicit in expressing their reserve and displeasure with the term, and not just because of humanist snobbery over the vulgarity of the vernacular or to distance themselves from lowly empirics. Modern historians have passed over these texts without comment, despite two coming from well-known authors. Von Hutten used the name in the title and throughout the text of his *De Morbo Gallico*, first published in 1519, its second edition of 1524 becoming the most popular syphilis tract in Europe,[151] but at the outset he made his sentiments clear:

> in this modest work I shall follow the usage which has prevailed generally, and call it the French sickness; this is most definitely not because I bear any grudge against a most renowned nation which is, perhaps, the most civilized and hospitable now in existence, but simply because I fear that the majority of my readers will not understand me if I call the malady by a different name.[152]

The less-known Sienese poet and papal rhymester, Niccolò Campani, also used 'mal francioso' but similarly exculpated the French: 'El non ci han colpa le genti francisose'. Despite his long and terrible suffering from the disease, which allowed him 'neither to eat nor sleep…only to cry and long for death', his poem ends praising Charles 'the King of France'. Even if his praise is taken as an attack masked in sarcasm, he makes no allusion to Charles bringing, setting off, or being in any way responsible for the new disease that spread with his troops:

Laude del Re de Francia:
Vedrai il Re Francesco, un nuovo Marte.
Come buon difensor, di sancta chiesa,
Mosso daspontanzel per divina arte

---

[148] Montius, *Halosis Febrium*, 163–6.   [149] [Lopez Pinna], *Tratado de Morbo Gallico*, 10.

[150] As the tract shows, Ricord's discovery of syphilis's three phases in 1850 had been anticipated; on Ricord, among other places, see Ackerknecht, *History and Geography*, 126.

[151] On its popularity, translations, and sixteenth-century editions, see Zanrè, 'French Diseases', 202.

[152] Von Hutten, *De guaiaici*, 4r–v, translated in Quétel, *History of Syphilis*, 27.

> Glie questa aspiration dal ciel discesa
> Andunque exurga Dio, e suoi amici,
> E dissipentur eius inimici.[153]

Instead, the targets of Campani's stinging wit were the lovesick youth from his own community. He belittled their complaints by offering them the opportunity of changing places with him:

> Chio per me ho lamor ne le calcagnia
> Ragioni contra de amore: Queste quel che ogni membro ti fracassa
> Questo perturba ogni tanquillo ingegnio
> Si che ti duol tanto de lamore,
> No ha provato il francioso dolore
> Desiderio di tutti li mali amorosi in cambio di questo.[154]

The maverick Bolognese physician and surgeon, Leonardo Fioravanti, who spent much of his medical career at the epicentre of the epidemic—Naples—and therefore might well have held a grudge against the French, invented a novel theory of the 'mal francese' that got the French, along with Spaniards and Indians, off the hook.[155] Emphatically, he maintained the disease was not new, yet disagreed with others who agreed. This disease could not be uncovered from ancient texts. Pliny, Hippocrates, Galen, the Arabs, and the rest had it in their midst but never knew it. As for the recent wave of 'mal francese' to circumnavigate Europe, Fioravanti also saw recent origins, but these he centred squarely on Naples with little, if anything, to do with Columbus's voyage, Hispanic sex with Indians, or Charles' siege in 1495. Instead, it originated in a previous war in Naples, when the young son of Rinato (René), Duke of Anjou, attacked King Alfonse of Naples 'around' 1456. In Fioravanti's tale, no outsider brought the disease to Naples; rather its native butchers unknowingly were guilty. Facing food shortages, especially meat, they carved up humans felled in war and sold their butchered flesh to famished soldiers: cannibalism was the cause; consumption of human flesh gave the pox its characteristic pustules. By his account, the siege of Naples led to more severe shortages, prompting Neapolitan butchers once more to play their old tricks. For proof, he claims to have heard the 1456 experience from a trustworthy old man—'un certo Pasquale Gibilotto di Napoli'—aged ninety-eight, when he first met him on arriving in Naples. Secondly, he claims to have confirmed the old man's story through experimentation, by feeding various animals—a piglet, a small dog, and a bird of prey ('un nebbio')—bits of their own kind, after which all of them broke out with the pox. Yet, despite the popularity of his *Capriccio Medicinale*, which went through at

---

[153] Campani, 'Lamento', np. Since Campani was a courtier to Pope Leo X, perhaps unsurprisingly he praised the papal ally, Charles VIII. Yet anachronistically, the current historiography pictures those across the peninsula, regardless of city-state alliances, as blaming the French. As Machiavelli and Guicciardini stressed, Charles' invasion of Italy depended on divisions within Italy. Perhaps, nineteenth-century nationalism tightened the relationship between pandemic and blame.

[154] Campani, 'Lamento', np.

[155] Fioravanti, *De' Capricci Medicinali*, first published in Venice in 1564. In contrast to Eamon and Foa, Proksch, I, 310, concentrates on the supposed Neapolitan acts of cannibalism in 1456 and 1495.

least five editions in the sixteenth century, his theory does not appear to have caught on, at least in the sixteenth century. Even Rostinio, who praised Fioravanti for treating the subject of 'mal francese' 'better than any who had written on the disease', did not bother repeating the cannibalism thesis.[156] In the seventeenth century, the story—the old man, piglets, and all—enjoyed a revival by Protestant writers across the Alps, in the Low Countries, and in England (although Fioravanti was given no credit; nor have historians seen the connection).[157] But my point here is that despite Fioravanti's use of 'il mal Francesce' throughout his text, he did not hold them in contempt or responsible for the disease. His use of the term appears wholly without blame. The Neapolitan surgeon instead showers them with sympathy, calling the invading French 'li poveri Francesci', describing the conditions of their camp, their suffering from the disease, and maltreatment at the hands of the Neapolitans.[158]

Finally, in his short but insightful chapter on the 'male detto da' francesi', in his *Storia d'Italia*, the famous Florentine statesman-historian Francesco Guicciardini ends by explaining why it is appropriate ('conveniente') to 'remove the shame (*ignomina*)' of the name 'franzese'. He argued that the disease was first brought from Spain to Naples but adds that it was 'not exactly of that nation'. Instead, it came from the islands (West Indies), made possible by the 'otherwise most fortunate (*più opportunamente*) voyages of Christopher Columbus, the Genoese',[159] but he does not then blame this Italian hero or the Indians.

BLAMING OTHERS

More than Indians, Neapolitans, or the French, one group to come under fire for spreading syphilis in the West has gone unmentioned by Foa, Eamon, and other recent historians. These were Catholic priests in Reformation England and Scotland, who could even be ridiculed by Catholics in Scotland. According to James VI of Scotland and I of England, his mother, Mary Queen of Scots, was reputed at his baptism in 1566 to have forbidden the archbishop 'to use the spittle', saying she would not have 'a pokie priest to spet in her child's mouth'. Yet no evidence appears of attacks on or arrests of priests stemming from these anxieties, certainly nothing akin to the mob attacks against foreign clergymen in England in 1231–2[160] or the carnage of the religious wars and massacres of the sixteenth and seventeenth century. According to Creighton, hardly any evidence for the existence of syphilis

---

[156] Rostinio, *Trattato del Mal Francese*, 9.

[157] André du Laurens (1558–1609) and Francis Bacon (1561–1626) tell versions of the story of Neapolitan cannibalism; see Foa, 'The New and Old', 40; and *The Great Pox*, 268.

[158] Fioravanti, *De' Capricci Medicinali*, 49v and 50r. After dwelling on the Neapolitan butchers' sale of human flesh and his experiments with animals, Fioravanti adds in passing: 'I have found reading histories of India that these irrational humans ate one another', and for this reason 'mal francese' afflicted them as well, but the cause of the disease's spread came from within, from Naples' butchers—his central story of cannibalism.

[159] Guicciardini, *Storia d'Italia*, 234.

[160] Cohn, *Popular Protest in Late Medieval Towns*, 283–4.

is found in England (as opposed to Scotland) before William Clowes' treatise of 1579.[161]

The most persistent butt of blame found in continental texts on syphilis, however, was women, though before the 1550s the criticism was usually implicit or else mildly disguised in ironic praise, as with the sonnet by the learned and unidentifiable poet called 'Il Grappa'.[162] Dedicated to a fictitious noblewoman, signora Antea Arcifanfana (Tuscan for arch-braggart or flauntress), from a fictitious place, San Petronio Vecchio, Il Grappa's poem begins by attacking Boccaccio's aggressively misogynist *Corbaccio*, his anti-*Decameron*, and ends by questioning those who call women 'ugly, dirty, fetid, and stinky': 'quelli che dicono che voi sete lorde, sporche, fetide & puzzolenti'.[163] His defence of women may reflect an underlying current of blame of women for the disease. In the tradition of Boccaccio's *Decameron*, the poet presents his sonnet to 'a virtuous band of women (*honesta brigata di donne*)', but in Il Grappa's case 'to prattle on, as was his custom, about things such as the *mal francioso*'. His poem was one of the few works of fiction, medical writing, or poetry to concern a woman afflicted with the disease as opposed to seeing women as carriers and perpetrators. Yet this is where Il Grappa's irony first appears. Signora Arcifanfana is afflicted with 'mal francioso' and called 'un cimitero' of it: women were the fount and deathbed of the new disease. Il Grappa then spends the remainder of his poem rescripting Petrarch's love ode to Laura (*Canzoniere*, 88), now casting Petrarch as syphilitic, the recipient of 'that gift' from his beloved Laura, whose 'Love', quite literally, 'inflames'.[164]

Chronicles and medical tracts also either professed the idea or claimed that others targeted women as the disease's origin. Bernardino Cirillo reported that French soldiers, bringing the disease home from Naples, complained of having been 'attacked' by Neapolitan women, and that because of feminine aggression, the disease was called 'mal Napolitano'. Yet to defend Naples, he refuted not only the soldiers' story but—expressing a view that was rare among sixteenth century writers—saw men as the prime movers: 'some Spanish [men] carried the contagious illness back with them from new India, and when sent by their king to support the Aragonese, they infected women. Little by little, the infection spread to others'.[165] Others treated men and women as equals in the spread of the pox, though men who served as invading troops should be seen as the principal perpetrators, taking booty of all kinds, including women, in an unequal exchange of sex and conquest through rape.[166] After his bizarre explanations of the disease's origin and spread, Fioravanti tacked on another cause—the disease could also be disseminated sexually. His description of sexual transmission was another rare example that did not explicitly or implicitly place a greater blame on woman: '*mal Francese* was nothing more

---

[161] Creighton, I, 415.

[162] McGough, *Gender, Sexuality, and Syphilis*, also sees women as the butt of blame after 1550.

[163] *Il Grappa*. According to Zanrè, 'French Diseases', 193, 'Il Grappa' may have been Antonfrancesco Grazzini, Pietro Aretino, Agnolo Firenzuola, or Francesco Beccuti. Luisini, Corradi, and Gruner do not cite the poem.

[164] Zanrè, 'French Diseases', 187–206.   [165] *Annali delle Città dell'Aquila*, 365–6.

[166] On violence against women in early modern warfare, see Martines, *Furies*.

than a humour corrupted by sexual union between a man and woman, and if one of the two were already corrupted, the other could be corrupted, but it need not always occur'.[167]

Other sixteenth-century writers, however, saw women as directly responsible for the disease's dissemination, such as the Bolognese Dalle Tuatte or Tuade Fileno, writing around 1511: women possessed the disease in their genitals ('lo avevano in la natura').[168] The Ferrarese chronicler dello Zambotti implied the same: at the end of 1496, the disease began spreading through 'commerce with sluts (*donne immonde*)'.[169] The Brescian chronicler Elios Capreolus claimed it began in the groin of women and then infected the glands of men: 'Ab inguine mulieribus a glande viris saepius incepit'.[170] Chroniclers were not the only ones to see women as principally responsible. The legist of Como Francesco Muralti judged women as the prime movers and men as the victims: 'initially, the disease is caught from the woman's vulva; sex with an infected women leads to the man becoming ill: first his penis itches; then he breaks out with scars (*cicatrices*), followed by intense pain in the joints, large pustules in the mouth and throat with the loss of his nose, even his eyes'.[171] The Florentine physician Antonio Benivieni claimed the disease began with women, describing how the disease called 'the Gallicum' left the vulva entirely eroded.[172] Julius II's surgeon, da Vigo, also suggested the disease originated with women: 'For the most part, men developed this pox from intercourse with dirty women with ulcerated vulvas', contracting it from a malignant ulcer or 'from recent menstruation (*vel quia fuerit noviter menstrata*)'.[173] Paracelsus maintained that the 'seat of the disease was in the mouth of the vulva (*et sedem salem habet in matrice vel orificio vuluae*)': 'all venereal diseases were concealed in women'.[174]

The Ferrarese Rostinio went further, concocting an elaborate theory that bequeathed to the female anatomy greater susceptibility and transmission of the pox. As with other early sixteenth-century writers, he did not see the disease as exclusively dependent on sexual activity. Yet on this score, he branded women as the cause. First, women developed the disease through the mouth, their breasts, or by sitting. Men were less prone to pick up the poisonous seed ('il venenoso seme'). Instead, they caught it from women's genitals ('nel seno della matrice'), but usually did not receive the seed unless well bathed in it ('se ben se ne bagna'). For women, however, it was easier.[175] Rostinio then explains that while men can catch it through three routes—the mouth, genitals, and anus—women get it in four, the previous three portals plus the breasts ('le mammelle'). According to Rostinio, you could 'easily pick it up by kissing' and through the ass by sitting, rubbing, from heat, and constipation [?] ('per la confricatione calfaciente & rarefaciente') as well as by anal intercourse ('dall'ano si da al priapo & dal priapo all'ano'), a mode some

---

[167] Fioravanti, *De' Capricci Medicinali*, 51v. [168] Dalle Tuatte, *Historia di Bologna*, 346.
[169] *La cronaca ferrarese dello Zambotti*, 346–7.   [170] Ibid., 116.
[171] *Annali a Pietro Aliosio Doninio*, 361–2.   [172] Benivieni, in *Aphrodisiacus*, 85.
[173] Da Vigo, *De apostemate virgae*, 126.   [174] Paracelsus, *De Morbo Gallico*, 134 and 135.
[175] Rostinio, *Trattato del Mal Francese*, 23r–24r.

sixteenth-century physicians denied.[176] But he emphasized women's mammary glands and lactation as the most prevalent means of transmission: lactation may have been the original mode of dissemination for 'mal francese'. He based his hunch on his friend's 'most chaste wife (*moglie honestissima*)' who reputedly caught 'mal francese' 'through her breasts'.[177]

In addition, Rostinio proposes a 'Patient Zero' story of pox's sexual transmission, not far removed, as Laura McGough relates, from the AIDS myth of Canadian airline steward Gaetan Dugas. According to Rostinio, a 'bellissima' public prostitute achieved much the same at Naples in 1495.[178] Yet, to be fair to Rostinio and the Neapolitan whore, none of the selfish maliciousness of Dugas appears: her initial contact with one man was enough to send 'this illness spreading through all of Italy, France, and Europe'. Its spread depended 'on human nature', on men, women, and their 'great appetite for sex'.[179] As McGough has shown, four years earlier, the Ferrarese physician Brasavola published the story of a 'most noble and beautiful whore (*scortum nobilissum ac pulcherrimum*)', who possessed a putrefied abscess at the throat of her uterus and then had sex with men: 'assisted by the putrid and humid conditions, first one man, then two, three, and a hundred became infected and through public and beautiful prostitutes.... Because human nature is so wanton, these infected men had sex with many women, and the women further communicated the disease to other men'. By Brasavola's account, this event began a decade before the siege of Naples.[180]

Another case of a prostitute as 'Patient Zero' appears in a tract by the nobleman Domini Leon Lunensis de Zuccano. His story places the origins not in Naples or the New World but in Valencia, where on the eve of Charles VIII's expedition a nobleman caught the disease from a certain whore ('quodam scorto').[181] The Paduan professor of surgery, Pietro Mainardi, in 1525, elaborated further, putting the whore in a better light. Before having sex with the nobleman, she had been deceived and for 50 gold coins had sex that night with a leper ('elephantiosus') in the cavalry. After intercourse with the infected prostitute, he had sex with many women, and within a few days, over four hundred had been infected. Some joined Charles VIII's army, thereby exporting the disease to Italy.[182] For the famous Sienese pharmacist and compiler of recipes, Andrea Mattioli, a woman again was the origin, but now she was the leper.[183]

---

[176] According to Hewlett, 'The French Connection', 244, Lucchese authorities thought anal intercourse was syphilis's usual mode of transmission.

[177] Rostinio, *Trattato del Mal Francese*, 23v. Others, such as Galli, *De Ligno Sancto*, saw the mammary glands as a conduit of the disease but only to infants through nursing: 'qui sicut mammarum suctu infantes malum trahunt' (20v); the English surgeon Clowes, *A briefe and necessarie treatise*, 2v, cursed and accused the 'wicked and filthy nurses' for infecting infants.

[178] Rostinio, *Trattato del Mal Francese*, 30 [Special Collection Glasgow, 1556 edition]; McGough, 'Quarantining Beauty', 212–13, and *Gender, Sexuality, and Syphilis*, ch. 2. On Dugas, see Shilts, *And the Band Played On.*

[179] Rostinio, *Trattato del Mal Francese* [1556 edition], 30.

[180] Brasavola, *Examen omnium Loch*, 193v–194r; cited in Astruc, *De Morbis Venereis*, 44.

[181] De Zuccano, *De Morbo Gallico*, 48–50.   [182] Cited in Astruc, *De Morbis Venereis*, 43.

[183] Ibid., 44.

Finally, in contrast to Fracastoro's boy-shepherd 'Syphilis', the Lyonnais poem published in 1539 personified the disease as a lady. The poet, whose mid-nineteenth-century editor speculated might have been Rabelais, placed Lady Pox (Verolle) on a pedestal as queen of the mound of love ('Le Puy d'amour'), praising her as the greatest conqueror of all time: her victories vanquished more than any other military commander, including Alexander the Great.[184] Should we then conclude that the French disease was responsible for the rise of a new phase of anti-feminine prejudice across Europe, or were these sentiments simply reflections of an intellectual and medical milieu already well entrenched from antiquity to early modernity?[185] To repeat, for the late fifteenth or sixteenth century, no one has found any crowd action against women or prostitutes in connection with the disease's arrival or spread. Nor was there a rash of new decrees promulgated by Church or State, blaming and penalizing women, as would occur in Western nations in the late nineteenth and twentieth centuries.[186] A claim by the Bolognese chronicler Dalle Tuatte may stand as an exception: 'many whores were chased from Bologna and Ferrara' (by whom he fails to say). Yet at least for Bologna, where all sixteenth-century 'manifesti', 'bandi', 'gridi', and decrees have been catalogued (3705 of them), he appears to have been mistaken: not a single decree expelled its 'meretrici' because of pox.[187]

In contrast with fear of syphilis in late nineteenth- and twentieth-century America and Europe, when nations organized vice squads to arrest prostitutes, quarantining them in barbed-wire encampments, early sixteenth-century legislation on prostitution could turn in the opposite direction. In his 1884 survey of documents, Corradi may have initially thought the new disease had prompted new legislation against prostitution; instead, he found new decrees such as ones at Lucca in 1532 and 1534 that protected prostitutes from maltreatment and injury. As the preambles make clear, the Republic sought to create a safe haven for prostitutes to combat a greater evil—sodomy ('ut evitetur majora mala'),[188] and established a

---

[184] 'Le Triomphe de très haulte et puissante dame Verolle', 225.

[185] According to Moore, *The Formation of a Persecuting Society*, 97–8, by the end of the Middle Ages, prostitutes were outcasts, excommunicated, and often treated like Jews with red-light districts 'walled like a ghetto'. However, Italian communes in the late Middle Ages established and protected houses of prostitution. More work is needed on popular and state violence against prostitutes in the Middle Ages; for now see Rossiaud, *Medieval Prostitution*; and Karras, *Common Women*. Zanrè, 'French Diseases', holds that before 'mal francese', 'attacks against *puttane* were something of a literary tradition' (197). On the Aristotelian–Thomist natural philosophy and gynophobia current before syphilis, see *The Great Pox*, 52; and Karras, *Common Women*, 134–5.

[186] See Brandt, *No Magic Bullet*, esp. chs 1–2 and 5; and Baldwin, *Contagion*, ch. 5.

[187] However, forty-two decrees across the century prohibited prostitutes living in certain squares near nunneries; yet the first decree regarding prostitutes in this collection does not appear until 1563; *Bononia Manifesta*, doc. nos 345, 410, 488, 496, 529, 531, 571, 721, 726, 1053, 1273, 1440, 1571, 1662, 1663, 1667, 1668, 1696bis, 1813, 1882, 1883, 1996, 2000, 2004, 2008, 2042, 2119, 2352, 2360, 2638, 2700, 2814, 2830, 2863, 2868, 2921, 2922, 3007, 3114, 3144, 3241, and 3238). By 1586, decrees began flushing prostitutes and their pimps ('ruffiani et ruffiane') from larger districts of the city—'vie', 'borghi', 'contrade'—without mentioning nunneries. None of these acts, however, mentions the pox. Moreover, *The Great Pox* pays close attention to chronicle and archival sources from Bologna and Ferrara without reporting prostitutes chased from these cities.

[188] 'La Repubblica di Lucca: Provissioni', no. 46. On these laws, see also Hewlett, 'The French Connection', 256.

new appellate court—the Protettori delle meretrici—to empower prostitutes to prosecute abusive clients. As Mary Hewlett concluded, the Lucchese had 'no particular suspicion' that prostitutes were 'directly blamed' for spreading 'mal francese'.[189] Moreover, after exhaustive combing through published and archival documents, Corradi failed to uncover any decrees that banished prostitutes from cities because of the threat of the new disease.

More recently, Jacques Rossiaud for France and Ruth Karras for England have found the same: social attitudes to prostitution changed slowly during the sixteenth century. Repressive legislation and the closure of brothels came not with the swift spread of syphilis during its first decades but later in the century, and these measures were not tied to pox.[190] For early modern Amsterdam, Lotte van Pol concluded that state regulation or repression of prostitution 'was unthinkable', despite the threat of syphilis.[191] Moreover, as early as 1500, Alexander VI's physician Gaspar Torella proposed novel legislation that would have been progressive by early twentieth-century standards: leaders should send matrons to investigate the disease, especially among prostitutes. If women were found infected, they would be confined temporarily to a place designated for the purpose by the community, where they would be treated by a physician or surgeon paid by the papacy.[192] Slightly later, in Perugia and Valencia, such policies came into force, providing prostitutes with free medical care.[193] This was a far cry from rounding up prostitutes and casting them out of cities to fend for themselves during the sieges, famines, and plagues of the sixteenth century.

By contrast, to dampen the spread of venereal disease during both World Wars, health boards in the US arrested and incarcerated thousands of women, quarantining them in barbed-wire encampments and 'civilian conservation camps'.[194] As Allan Brandt concluded, '[T]he prostitute had become the war's venereal scapegoat, vilified, shunned, and eventually locked up',[195] constituting 'the most concerted attack on civil liberties in the name of public health in American history'.[196] Physicians, health boards, and vice squads saw these women as the cause and carriers of

[189] Hewlett, 'The French Connection', 256. The sixteenth-century decrees in England, Germany, and Italy fail to mention syphilis as justification for closing brothels; Karras, *Common Women*, 42, but see note 190.

[190] Rossiaud, *Medieval Prostitution*, 50–1. An exception appears with legislation passed by Aberdeen on 21 April 1497, demanding prostitutes ('all light women') to 'decist from their vices and sin of venery'. They 'were ordered to shut up shop and seek lawful employment or face branding and banishment' (Jillings, 'Plague, Pox', 70). This was 'the first civic authority in the British Isles to enact such legislation' (70), and she mentions none to follow. Similarly, with Zurich's second decree on 'Böse Blattern' in 1496, foreigners were banished along with prostitutes and loose women; Gall, 'Quarantine', 4.

[191] Van de Pol, *The Burgher and the Whore*, 75.

[192] Torella, *De dolore in pudendagra*, 453; *The Great Pox*, 34; and Arrizabalaga, 'Medical Responses', 53. Unlike sixteenth- and seventeenth-century plague tracts, writings on syphilis did not recommend repressive measures to control prostitutes. For contrasts with the US and Europe, c.1880–1920, see notes 194–8.

[193] Corradi, 'Nuovi documenti', no. 50; *The Great Pox*, 175–6 (for Valencia).

[194] Brandt, *No Magic Bullet*, 72, 86, 89, 167.   [195] Ibid., 87.

[196] Brandt, 'AIDS', 151. In Battle Creek, Michigan, police rounded up and imprisoned women thought to be carrying venereal diseases; *Detroit Free Press*, 8 January 1918, 16.

venereal diseases.[197] As John H. Stokes, who organized and directed a new section of Dermatology and Syphilology in 1916 at the prestigious Mayo Clinic, declared, 'the prostitute was the intermediate host or carrier of the *Spirochaeta pallida*, akin to the mosquito in the spread of malaria'.[198] The US was not alone in promulgating such repressive measures. Despite laissez-faire, non-interventionist policies towards impositions on individuals' behaviour during epidemics, fears of syphilis led Britain to grant the police 'formidable powers', making it one of the most repressive European nations in penalizing prostitutes.[199] Although the French approach to venereal disease was to regulate rather than suppress prostitution, authorities viewed the infected as guilty. Increasingly, before World War I, municipalities from Lille to Marseille intensified their surveillance, and in 1906 changes in the age of penal majority resulted in mass arrests across France of young women.[200] In twentieth-century Germany, fears of venereal diseases provoked growing prejudice against the Eastern 'Other': German troops returning from Russian Poland 'were held to be at particular risk from sexually transmitted diseases', with prostitutes indiscriminately denounced as polluted ('verseucht'), despite the incidence of syphilis and gonorrhoea being far higher in German cities than in rural districts of Eastern Europe and Russia, from where the soldiers had returned.[201]

THE ENLIGHTENMENT'S UNDERBELLY

Nonetheless, something new was happening with the history of hate and disease in early modernity. As Chapter 6 will argue, the leading edge of that connection was not the new disease, pox, but a disease that had become periodic and familiar by the sixteenth century—plague. However, the 'French Disease' had scored a first in its obsessive concern with naming, even if historians have overstated the stigmatization it led to. With this disease, physicians and surgeons expressed a new concern with carriers, tracking trajectories of disease dissemination with new historic attention to human contacts, explorations, mobilization of peoples, and war.

The writings of the late Enlightenment Gruner illustrate that early modern Europe was not divided by two world views: an enlightened one advanced in theories of pathology with new notions of disease entities versus a popular one that viciously blamed outsiders for the suffering of a community or nation, inflicted by diabolical carriers and inseminators of evil. Along with his critical tools of scholarship, his compilations of previously unedited historical medical tracts, and

---

[197] Brandt, *No Magic Bullet*, 21, 29, 32, 25, 37, 72–7, 82, 85, 86.   [198] Ibid., 72.

[199] Baldwin, *Contagion*, 485–6. Also see Walkowitz, *Prostitution*, for the effects of the Contagious Diseases Acts (1864 and 1866) on the lives of working-class women who had to endure torturous examinations, new police powers of surveillance, and public humiliation that divided many from their families and neighbours.

[200] Corbin, 'La grande peur'; and idem, *Women for Hire*, 25–9 and 246–58, 326–30.

[201] Kraut, 'Plagues and Prejudice', 98. For scapegoating of women, especially lower-class ones, for spreading VD across Europe and Asia in the late nineteenth and twentieth centuries and prostitution as the cause of syphilis, see *Sex, Sin, and Suffering*. For syphilis testing to deport Mexicans from California's Imperial Valley in the 1940s, see Molina, *How Race Is Made*, 99–102.

understanding of the latest germ theories, Gruner developed a new myth of the origins of syphilis based on race that targeted outsiders—the Ethiopian, Marrano, and Jew.[202]

In 1793, the myth of the Jews' role in disseminating syphilis surfaced in Gruner's long introduction to his earlier syphilis tracts compiled in 1789. While he copied almost verbatim Leo Africanus's remarks about scurrilous Ethiopians and promiscuous Jewish women, his argument featured new twists and origins, now with clear anti-Semitic and racist theories. He claimed that 'whether Jews or Sabbatines (e.g. the "Marani"), they were all Africans by race and origins'.[203] Like earlier narratives, his version had two distinct origins, yet it diverged from the old plot: Ethiopia and Rome replaced New Spain and Naples. First, the disease originated from Jewish women having 'sexual commerce' with the most disgusting Ethiopians ('scleratissimi Aethiopes').[204] Second, Rome, not Naples, had been Italy's first port of call in this 'plague's' explosive transmission. Copying from Stefano Infessura's Roman diary about plague—not syphilis—Gruner alleged that after their expulsion from Spain, Jews encamped outside the gates of the Appian Way in 1492 and from there 'invaded' the city with their disease—syphilis.[205] Gruner then stirred new anti-Semitic venom into sixteenth-century accounts. Jews were no longer victims; instead, 'The madness of the Maranos's innumerable religions was not enough for them to inflict their injuries' on the rest of the world. With their new disease, 'they despoil all goods and life, spreading infamy, poverty, nudity, and illness'.[206] Even de Oviedo, who described Indians as half-human, liars by nature, lazy, lacking faith, melancholic, cowardly, and 'of low and evil inclinations',[207] did not create new racist myths to blame them for syphilis.

Change, however, was in the wind before the Enlightenment. Already by the first printing of the long treatise on 'morbus Gallicus' in 1579, or what the author preferred to call 'lues venerea', the London surgeon and personal physician to Queen Elizabeth, William Clowes,[208] who had treated pox patients at St Bartholomew's over the past 'nine or ten years', introduced new elements of hate and blame to the discourse surrounding the spread of infectious diseases. Like sixteenth-century physicians and surgeons on the Continent, Clowes emphasized God's wrath and

---

[202] Gruner, 'Morbi Gallici Origines Maranicae', i–xxxvi, *De Morbo Gallico scriptores*, xxv–vi.

[203] Gruner, 'Morbi Gallici Origines Maranicae', xxxii. *The Great Pox*, 14, argues that Gruner grouped Arabs and Jews together, calling them Marrani.

[204] Gruner takes this story of Jewish expulsion from Leo Africanus, *De totius Africae*, 125. Also, the humanist Italian chronicler Paolo Giovio pointed to Jews and their expulsion from Spain as one (but only one) source of the disease's spread to Italy; *Historiarum Sui Temporis*, 125.

[205] Infessura, *Diario della città di Roma*, 38, maintains that the Marranos, expelled from Spain, camped out 'in great numbers' at the gates of Rome with the pope's consent. They 'secretly' entered the city and supposedly but inadvertently spread plague in October 1493.

[206] Gruner, 'Morbi Gallici Origines Maranicae', xxviii–xxx: 'Maranorum, quos non satis erat rabie sub specie religionis innumeris affecisse iniuriis, omnibus bonis vitaque pluribus abhinc abbis spoliasse, sed etiam, ut infames, finibus pauperes, nudos et aegros expellere'.

[207] Brading, *The First America*, 31–44.

[208] Proclaimed as England's 'greatest surgeon': see Siena, *Venereal Disease*, 63–4; Furdell, *The Royal Doctors*, 87–9; and Fabricius, *Syphilis*, 106–12.

vengeance, but he had no desire to pin the blame on Indians, Spanish, French, or Neapolitans.

> First I saye, the disease it selfe was never in mine opinion more ryse among the Indians, Neapolitans, yea in Italie, France, or Spaine, then is at this daye in the realm of England.[209]

Like many doctors and chroniclers examined here, Clowes looked inward and found pox's cause to have come from his own environs. Here, however, discrepancies with continental commentaries arise. Clowes hardly mentions stars or air, and humours take a back seat to the disease's true cause—'filthie lust: a sickennesse verie loathsome, odious, troublesome, and dangerous'. That 'stincking sinne' was 'the originall cause of this infection'. This filth derived not from invading soldiers, foreigners, or any other 'Other' but from within his city of London, creating 'the great daunger to the common wealth and the staine of the whole nation'. He then specified who these Londoners were:

> The causes whereof, I see none so great as the licencious and healthy disorder of a great number of rogues, and vagabonds, the filthy lyfe of many lewde and idle persons, both men and women, about the citie of London, and the great number of leude Ale houses, which are the very nestes and harbours of such filthy creatures.

More than in any of the 250-plus texts I have examined, Clowes turned his scorn against the disease's victims. Except for children, who, he claimed, received the disease from the breasts of their nurses, he showed no mercy for the pox-marked proven sinners, and complained 'the maisters of the hospital [of Saint Bartholomew]', of which he was one, had to endure 'what griefe of mynde...dayly to take in a number of vile creatures, that otherwise would infecte many good and honest people'. Although confident of his procedures and treatments to cure what he and later physicians preferred to call 'lues venerea', Clowes was not eager to relieve these miserable sinners from their deserving misery. Anticipating the pleas of Christian fundamentalists in the US of the 1980s, who protested against funding HIV/AIDS research, he feared his cures would 'encourage those wretches that wallow in this sinne, to continue in their beastly lyfe'. He promised not to 'helpe at all' these victims, whom he called 'those leude and wicked beastes...except they be at defiance with this sinne, and who he bend themselves to walke in the obedience of Gods holes laws'. Unlike earlier writers on the pox, Clowes saw God's wrath and punishment as insufficient. He called on city magistrates 'in the love of their countrie' to become in effect a vice squad against extra-marital sex:

> to have a watchfull eie, to finde out the offenders in this behalf. To execute upon them such condign punishment, as may be a terror to the wicked, the rather to abstaine and abandon themselves from such abhominable wickednesse, so filthie in the sight of God and man...and that the magistrates doe with great care, seeke correction & punishment if that filthie vice, as also for the reformation of those places above mentioned. And except the people of this lande do speedily repent their most ungodly lyfe, and leave

---

[209] Clowes, *A briefe and necessarie treatise*, 1r.

this odious sinne, it cannot be but the whole land wil shortly be poisoned with this most noisome sickness.

Clowes had created an 'other', deserving blame and punishment. It was an enemy that threatened his beloved commonwealth but was not the outsider—the Jew, the Indian, or foreigner (despite his pleas for national pride). Instead, Clowes' 'other' was an internal moral and class 'other', one of vagabonds, the sort who drank in alehouses.

Clowes was not an isolated exception. In 1599, the governors of London's St Thomas's Hospital institutionalized a ritual of publicly flogging patients diagnosed with the 'foul' disease once they had been 'cured', but before being discharged, to ensure they would not wish to return.[210] As the seventeenth century progressed, less charity and fewer hospital beds were made available to the syphilitic destitute.[211] By the eighteenth century, at the Parisian hospital of the Bicêtre, flogging was also instituted but for more than a parting ritual. Now it became part of syphilitic treatment, a cure by 'moral purification'.[212] Earlier on the Continent, when pox was spreading rapidly, I know of nothing akin to these practices mixing cure with punishment. As Claudia Stein shows, the poor vigorously petitioned to be admitted into the Blatterhaus and Fuggerei of Augsburg, and after their release, they generally resumed their former lives without difficulty.[213] In Rome, the mid-sixteenth-century popes were spending enormous sums treating over a thousand indigent syphilis patients annually for free, constituting 1.3 per cent of their total expenditure.[214] In Modena, the ducal government extended treatments with the luxurious 'l'acqua del legno' to indigent syphilitics at two of its hospitals twice yearly until 1569, when the 'grandissima' expense became too grand and free treatment was reduced to a single annual dose with less costly remedies offered to foreigners.[215] Such heavy subsidies from governments and charities of noblemen and women to hospitalize and care for the pox are also seen in sixteenth-century Genoa, Florence, Venice, and Verona.[216]

By the end of the eighteenth century and into Victorian England the subjection of these patients, especially women, to separation, stigmatization, social policing, and new programmes of moral discipline intensified within English lock hospitals

---

[210] Siena, *Venereal Disease*, 10 and 90. While *incurabili* hospitals at Rome were concerned with moral 'education', patients were not flogged for possessing the disease; Henderson, 'Fracastoro', 89.

[211] Ibid., 105. Also see, Merians, 'The London Lock Hospital': as the eighteenth century progressed, increasingly, women were blamed for spreading venereal disease and charity for their hospitals declined, even if care of prostitutes in lock hospitals could be sympathetic and compassionate (130).

[212] Conner, 'The Pox', 21. After the revolution, the Hospice des Vénériens replaced the Bicêtre and provided more humane care to carriers, especially prostitutes, and their survival rates improved dramatically (27–8). But by 1802 a new regime of police surveillance of prostitutes targeted them as the cause of venereal disease; Norberg, 'From Courtesan to Prostitute'. By the 1820s, hospitals across the US, as with Boston's Massachusetts General refused admission to venereal sufferers (Brandt, *No Magic Bullet*, 43–4).

[213] Stein, *Negotiating the French Pox*, 125–6. Also see Jütte, 'Syphilis and Confinement', for a positive view of syphilis patients in these publically funded and free Blatterhausen. For hospitals and the care of the syphilitic principally in northern Italy, see *The Great Pox*, chs 7 and 8.

[214] *The Great Pox*, 189–90.   [215] *Gride Ducali*, 125–6.

[216] Henderson, 'Fracastoro', 82, 84; and idem, 'Coping with Epidemics', 87–9.

and asylums.[217] The victimization of those infected by syphilis begins in the late sixteenth century at the very moment when the disease's accepted medical nomenclature had changed from the 'French' to the 'venereal disease'. Against the assumptions of Sontag, Farmer, and many others, naming a disease after its supposed carriers or origins did not necessarily spell blame or scapegoating. In the case of syphilis, naming and blaming in fact moved in opposing directions.

To repeat, a disease–hate connection which blamed epidemics on the 'other' was not a timeless element of our psyche or the product of a pre-scientific, pre-Enlightenment world that would vanish in the West with progress in medical comprehension, only to arise again when new, mysterious diseases such as HIV-AIDS bewildered medical communities. Rather, it was more the other way around. When Clowes wrote, the Great Pox was no longer considered a disease of the 'incurabili'. As early as the second decade of the sixteenth century, Europeans thought they had discovered their 'magic bullet' with the decoction of the Indian's sacred wood. Physicians such as Fracastoro by 1546 saw the disease changing: by then, it had 'entered old age'. Optimistically, he concluded it had become 'domesticated' in Europe as it had been in the West Indies.[218] Doctors had grown confident in their remedies, as Clowes sought to prove by his patient case histories. Stripped of antique and medieval theories of stars, climate, and airs, his 'lues venerea' focused blame on individuals' willingness to sin. Hate certainly was not modernity's invention, but increasing awareness of epidemics' dependence on individual and trackable carriers opened possibilities for hate to become more pervasive in times of pestilence.

---

[217] Siena, *Venereal Disease*, 89–90, ch. 5, and 261–3.   [218] Fracastoro, *De Contagione*, 154–7.

6

Plague Spreaders

This chapter opens with an earlier question: as far as the persecution of Jews and other minorities goes, to what extent did the Black Death cast a dark shadow over Europe that endured by some historians' reckoning until the Enlightenment?[1] We then grapple with a related question: to what extent were the trials and executions of plague spreaders during the sixteenth and seventeenth centuries across regions of Europe evidence of disease-inspired hatred of outsiders and marginal populations—Jews, foreigners, and the lowest of plague workers, who almost invariably came from outside the communities they served?

Certainly Europe's most deadly and devastating disease, the Black Death of 1347–51, unleashed mass violence: the murder of Catalans in Sicily, clerics and beggars at Narbonne, and especially pogroms against Jews, with communities entirely annihilated through the Rhineland, into the Austrian Archduchies' territories, Spain, and France.[2] Yet subsequent strikes of plague in late medieval Europe into the sixteenth century failed to spark waves of violence against Jews or any other minorities—a trend historians have yet to reflect upon.[3] Instead, scholars often assume that the Black Death either set in course a new excuse for persecutions or continued a process that had been a feature of epidemics since antiquity. Yet I know only two historians to have pointed specifically to incidents during plagues post 1348 that sparked persecutions of Jews or any 'others' before the sixteenth-century trials against plague spreaders—*untori* or *engraisseurs*. First, Joshua Tractenberg, in remarkable research, published in 1943, gathered eleven incidents of accusations against Jews for plague spreading before 1541 and three afterwards, ending with a plague in Vienna in 1679. For none of these, however, does he uncover any pogrom or riots against Jews and certainly nothing akin to the mass incineration of entire communities seen in 1348–9.

So what was Tractenberg's harvest? In 1357 when plague struck Franconia, 'it was laid to the Jews, whose poisons had caused it'. In 1382, the Jews of Halle suffered an attack on suspicion of having poisoned wells, thereby starting an epidemic; the charge was repeated in 1397 in the towns of Rappoltsweiler, Dürkheim, and Colmar. In 1401 the Jews of Freiburg im Breisgau were charged with 'planning to exterminate Christendom by poisoning air'. In 1475, 'during a brief outbreak of endemic disease', Jews in Germany were again accused of seeking 'to poison all the wells in the land'; the same recriminations 'cropped up' in 1448 and 1453 in

---

[1] See Delumeau, *Rassurer et protéger*, esp. 571–2.   [2] See Chapter 3, note 3.
[3] On the exception of parts of Poland around Kraków and Miechów in 1360–1, see Chapter 2.

Schweidnitz, in Regensburg in 1472, and 'early in the 1500s' again in Halle. For 1580, Tractenberg lists his only case beyond German-speaking regions: during an epidemic in Aix, the English physician Thomas Flud claimed that 'poison which the Jews rubbed' on door knockers caused the plague. His next example comes a century later. Vienna's pestilence of 1679 erupted first in the Jewish quarter of Leopoldstadt. The Augustinian monk and popular preacher Abraham a Santa Clara (Johann Ultich Megerle, 1644–1709) claimed the plague was 'likewise ascribed to the Jews'. But this was a different matter. The popular preacher was not accusing Jews of intentionally spreading plague; rather, sympathetically, he saw them suffering in great numbers because of the 'bad living conditions in the ghetto'.[4]

First, all of these references derive from secondary sources—histories of the late nineteenth and twentieth century, several published in the Nazi era by authors sympathetic to the regime. More importantly, these 'incidents' were matters of accusation; none reveals collective violence, even individual acts of assault on property or persons. Tractenberg uses the word 'attack' only with one incident—in Halle in 1382—but his source, the mid-nineteenth-century historian of Jews, Otto Stobbe (1831–87), mentions no pogroms in Halle or anywhere else in 1382.[5] Moreover, from Tractenberg's source, it is unclear if plague triggered any of accusations of well poisoning in 1382 or even if plague were present in Halle, Rappoltsweiler, Dürkheim, and Colmar.[6] All his examples may have been matters of intellectuals' opinions, not actions or beliefs of commoners. Yet he concludes: throughout Europe, the Black Death established 'the habit of blaming Jews for such calamities' and 'once formed, [it] continued to assert itself'.[7]

By contrast, Paolo Preto's focus was Italy and, as might be expected, his harvest of anti-Semitic actions spurred by plague is modest. Traces of anti-Semitism during plagues are found in Piedmont at Moncalieri in 1429 and Savigliano in 1450.[8] In Calabria in 1422, 'the people (*popolo*) accused Jews of spreading powders of various diseases',[9] but he does not specify whether plague or any other disease was present in Calabria or if the accusation spurred violence. Further, in 1511, he claims Jews were chased from Udine, after the cessation of plague, and in 1556 they were accused of bringing plague to Padua. But his evidence, carefully combed from archives and published primary sources, reveals no arrests or popular violence.[10] In fact, Preto's conclusions are the opposite of Tractenberg's: before the plague of 1576, 'no physicians or philosophers seemed to have imagined any possibility that plague might have been spread intentionally', whether by Jews or anyone else.[11]

No doubt, further research into chronicles and administrative records scattered through state and municipal archives will reveal further incidents of plague accusations and perhaps some that ignited violence. One case, yet to be spotted in the

---

[4] Tractenberg, *The Devil and the Jews*, 106–7.   [5] Stobbe, *Die Juden in Deutschland*, 285.
[6] Ibid. Stobbe's last chapter, 'Die Judenverfolgungen', describes numerous outbreaks of violence against Jews from before the Black Death to 1516: Halle, Rappoltsweiler, Dürkheim, and Colmar are not listed, and he does not connect any of these to plague.
[7] Tractenberg, *The Devil and the Jews*, 106.   [8] Preto, *Epidemia*, 9.
[9] Ibid., 10.   [10] Preto, *Peste e società*, 52–3.   [11] Ibid., 53.

plague literature, may have occurred at Cuneo, in north-west Italy in 1451, the year of a particularly severe plague in that region lasting two years. According to a local chronicler, it killed 3000, 'debilitating the people'. His next entry recounts an attack at Cuneo against Jews: women and boys 'mowed them down with stones', and 'afterwards, [the Jews] dared no longer to reside [there]'. But the chronicler does not pin the incident to the plague or claims of poisoning. Instead, he notes usury as the motive.[12] A second incident arises in northern Italy, this one during the plague of 1463. A local Mantuan chronicler charged Jews with carrying it there from Ferrara.[13] But no actions were taken against them, nor was the charge one of intentional plague spreading; rather it resulted from their trade in used clothes and supposed careless violations of quarantine.

More than a hundred years later, during Italy's pandemic of 1575–8, another incident arises from archival sources that more clearly connects plague with accusations, and in this case violence against Jews. A letter from the Mantuan ambassador in Milan to the Duke's secretary in Mantua reported 'certain circumcised Spanish (*alcuni spagnoli circoncisi*)', in other words, *conversos*, had been arrested in Milan. The authorities surmised that the Turks had sent these religious renegades to inflict plague on Christians.[14] I have found no chronicler in Milan or Mantua to refer to the supposed plot and know no evidence corroborating it from judicial records. However, a similar episode occurred at Mortara, south-west of Milan, during the same month. Two sailors—'circumcised Spaniards' and 'renegade conversos'—were arrested. Moreover, in Milan a crowd seized four dressed as noblemen with concealed weapons and 'furiously beat them', after they had supposedly greased several door knockers.[15] In a plague tract of 1577, the physician Giuseppe Mugino may have been telling the same story: the Gran Cane had sent certain Spaniards, denounced as converts, 'to destroy poor Italy'.[16]

With this pan-Italian plague, Preto finds a significant shift in attitudes: 'something began to change around the time of this first great pandemic of the modern era'.[17] He is referring specifically to physicians and their suspicion of intentional plague spreaders or *untori*. The same might be said about attitudes seen in plague tracts at this time, accusing Jews of spreading plague, willfully or not. The doctor employed by the Comune of Udine, Gioseffo Daciano (whose tract was published in 1576) claimed the region's previous plague of 1555–6 had originated from 'perfidious and damned Jews', who brought their infected goods from Capodistra (now Koper in Slovenia) to Udine on their Passover. The Milanese nobleman and government official, Asciano Centorio Degli Ortensi, traced the plague's spread in 1574–5 from Trent to Venice's ghetto and then to Mantua, maintaining Jews had carried it by trading second-hand clothes. And the Genoese physician Andrea Gabrielli in his tract of 1577 called for 'stiff-necked Jews' to be

[12] *Cronache... di Cuneo*, 282.
[13] Schivenoglia, *Cronaca di Mantova*, 32. I thank Marie-Louise Leonard for this reference.
[14] Archivio di Stato di Mantova, busta 1693, c. 230. I thank Dr Leonard for this reference.
[15] Preto, *Epidemia*, 28.   [16] Ibid.   [17] Ibid., 11.

segregated from Christians in plague time because of their filth and sin.[18] Still, none of the accusations provoked new decrees, collective violence, or even reported individual attacks on Jews.

Can the same be said of places beyond Italy? An incident of far greater violence to a minority during a plague was the Lisbon massacre of 'New Christians' in 1506, when citzens slaughtered between two and three thousand former Jews over a two-day period. But was this massacre sparked by plague? The plague had been spreading through Lisbon and great swathes of the Iberian peninsula for at least six months before the massacre, and no source reports accusations of 'New Christians' creating it through their filth, sins, or by diabolical means. Nonetheless, historians have assumed the plague was the massacre's cause. To illustrate his conclusion that 'news of some disaster' such as the 'beginnings of an epidemic... trigger[ed] popular revenge', Yves-Marie Bercé focused on this massacre alone that supposedly occurred 'just as the city was threatened with plague',[19] which is incorrect. Yet others closer to the sources, such as Yosef Hayim Yerushalmi, have made similar claims: 'To anyone familiar with the dynamics of anti-Jewish massacres in the Middle Ages, the immediate background of the pogrom of 1506 betrays almost classic features.' He then pointed to 'the horrors of plague', a 'new plague' (although admitting it had been spreading through Lisbon since October 1505).[20]

More recently, Ami Isseroff has gone further, asserting that the plague 'aroused suspicion that it was "punishment" for secret Judaizing of conversos'.[21] However, none of the seven sixteenth-century sources describing the massacre identifies plague as the trigger. Instead, it resulted from a 'New Christian' questioning a miracle that supposedly appeared in Lisbon's Dominican church. By the chronicler Gaspar Correia's eyewitness account, a German merchant, whose daughter had been cured by the miracle, instigated the massacre because a 'New Christian' claimed the Dominicans had staged it.[22] Plague does not even appear in Solomon Ibn Verga's contemporaneous Hebrew account,[23] and in other sixteenth-century accounts, plague is mentioned only in the background to explain King Manuel's absence from the city. The humanist Damião de Gois, writing a half-century afterwards, mentions plague only to explain why Lisbon's 'most honourable' citizens were not around to protect the 'New Christians'.[24] Samuel Usque, who was six at the time of the massacre and escaped immediately to Ferrara, claimed almost fifty years later, that 'preachers in the pulpits, nobles in public places, and city-folk and rustics in the squares began saying that any famine, pestilence, or earthquakes that came

[18] Cohn, *Cultures of Plague*, 254, 251, 110, respectively. By contrast, in 1533, Francesco II Sforza protected Jews from claims that their goods were contaminated and assured them they would not be expelled from their houses and, if outside the Duchy, would be allowed to return; *The Jews in the Duchy of Milan*, II, 1045–51. I thank Monica Azzolini for this reference.

[19] Bercé, *Revolt and Revolution*, 119.   [20] Yerushalmi, *The Lisbon Massacre*, 7–8.

[21] Isseroff, 'Lisbon Massacre'.   [22] Soyer, 'The Massacre of the New Christians'.

[23] See Yerushalmi's translation in *The Lisbon Massacre*, 1–3.

[24] De Gois, *Chronica*: 'Nestes dia perecerão... mais de mil almas sem aver na cidadequem ousasse de resistir, pola pouca gente de sorte que nella avia por estarem os mais dos honrados fora, por caso da peste', 142.

to the land struck because these converts were not good Christians and practiced Judaism in secret.' But this general reference to calamities paid no attention to the specific plague that had engulfed the city half a year earlier. Like the others, Usque attributed the massacre to the New Christian's questioning the Dominicans' phoney light-show.[25]

PLAGUE SPREADING

Searching through a wide variety of sources—chronicles, physicians' plague tracts, and archival documents such as the vast records of the Sanità of Milan, of Venice, and of other northern Italian cities—Paolo Preto finds that 'theories of plague manufactory' do not appear until the late sixteenth century.[26] Yet, he has uncovered reports of these supposed acts ahead of the theory. His first 'true' example of 'greasing' (*unzioni*) appears at Casale Monferrato, Piedmont, in 1530; functionaries of the Health Board were accused of sprinkling poisonous dust and greasing places over the past seven years; twenty were 'spontaneously' arrested.[27] Six years later in the same town, the physician-scientist Gerolamo Cardano claimed that forty 'among men and women' were accused of attempting to murder fellow citizens with pestilential ointments rubbed on doorknobs and powders sprayed on clothing.[28] But no contemporary documents survive for this incident, and Preto suggests that Cardano, relying on oral testimony, may have confused his dates.[29] In 1545, the Health Board in Milan offered a 100-*scudi* reward for the arrest of 'two wicked men who had been spreading plague through the city'.[30] In 1554 at Saint-Albain (Savoy), a foreign pilgrim was arrested as a plague greaser ('ung semeur de peste') and lynched. Further trials against plague spreaders arose at Chambéry in the following two years.[31] With the plague of 1556 in Venice, several plague cleaners ('piccgamorti') were accused of throwing infected clothes into the canals to 'prolong the plague'.[32] In 1559, Genoa's Health Board alerted communes along the Riviera to be on guard against 'people dressed as pilgrims', who were instead *untori*.[33] The following year, Mantua's Health Board warned against four active in Brescia and Cremona, and Pavia notified Milan that *untori* from Venice were in the region. The same month Pavia posted notices that 'sad and evil people' were greasing doors and knockers. Finally, in May 1560, Milanese officials arrested the first victims of an official hunt for plague spreaders and hanged then quartered the body of Antonio da Treviso.[34]

Despite this collection of incidents, none appears south of a northern diagonal from Venice to Genoa, and Preto concludes that the real hunt for *untori* did not

---

[25] From Usque's *Consolação*, translated in Baron, *A Social and Religious History*, 46–7.
[26] Preto, *Epidemia*, 5 and 10.   [27] Ibid., 25.
[28] Cantù, *Sulla storia Lombarda* (1853 edition), np.
[29] Fiochetto, *Trattato della Peste*, 75, relates the same story.
[30] Preto, *Epidemia*, 26.   [31] Ibid., 27.   [32] Ibid., 26–7.
[33] Ibid., 27.   [34] Ibid.

begin until the plague of 1574–8.[35] A tradition of plague spreaders, however, had begun flourishing north of the Alps. Prosecutions, trials, torture, and executions of them occurred in Toulouse and Geneva in 1530, Montpellier, Nîmes, Aiguesmortes, and other Huguenot towns in 1563,[36] and Lyon by 1567.[37] For Geneva, William Naphy traces an earlier trajectory than seen for Italy. The first appearance of plague spreaders occurred in 1530 but accounted for only a handful of cases. By 1545 they increased to sixty-five prosecutions (nearly two-and-a-half-times those recorded in Milan's surviving court transcripts for its far more famous plague spreading of 1630).[38] The Genevan prosecutions then peaked with the plague of 1570–1: 115 criminal cases and forty-four executions.[39] Yet for this plague, cases of witchcraft and plague spreading were combined, with the plague spreaders accounting for only thirteen cases.[40] Thus, cases of plague spreading alone peaked in 1545 and after 1571 had disappeared in Geneva, well before they had begun in earnest in Italy.[41]

THE CASE OF MILAN

Even before Alessandro Manzoni's *Promessi sposi* (first written in Milanese in 1827, then in Tuscan in 1840) and *Storia delle colonna infame* (published in 1840, but written in 1823), plague spreading during Milan's diastrous epidemic of 1630 had commanded greater attention than for any other episode of it, the Black Death included. Already in the aftermath of this plague, it had stimulated at least ten chronicle accounts composed by those living through it and had appeared in chronicles outside Milan. It even gave rise to one contemporaneous work of imaginary literature.[42] The longest and most incisive of these accounts was by the canon Giuseppe Ripamonti (1573–1643).[43] His views on *untori* are also the most far-reaching and

---

[35] Ibid., 28. References to *untori* incidents cited by Preto during the 1574–8 plague are far less than those he cites between the plagues of 1530 and 1555–6. However, physicians in their plague tracts, 1576–9, paid greater attention to diabolic plague spreading than ever before. With Sicily's Ingrassia, *Parte quinta*, 6 and 12, physicians' preoccupations with purposeful plague poisoning extended beyond northern Italy; see Cohn, *Cultures of Plague*, 272.

[36] Littré, 'Les semeurs', 498.   [37] Rubys, *Discours sur la contagion*, 29–38.

[38] Naphy, *Plagues, Poisons and Potions*, 68.   [39] Ibid., 120.

[40] Ibid., 138–42, tables 10 and 11.

[41] Such trials certainly were not ubiquitous; for England, see Slack, *The Impact of Plague*, 293–4; and idem, 'Responses to Plague', 117. Moreover, for Italy, the late Cinquecento only anticipated what would become more widespread in the 1630s. On these anticipations, see Cohn, *Cultures of Plague*, 3, 101, 119, 271–2, and 277.

[42] Ripamonti, *De Peste*; Tadino, *Raguaglio*; Borromeo, *De Pestilentia*; Marioni, *Peste in Milano*; Lattuada, 'Cronaca'; Visconti, *Commentarius de peste*; Lampugnano, *La Pestilenza*; Somaglia, *Alleggiamento*; and Giulini, 'Un diario', although this last one concerns only Milan's liberation from the plague in 1632. Lupi, *Storia della peste* should also be included. It paid close attention to events in Milan, especially regarding *untori*. Finally, I include the play *La peste di Milano* by the Milanese Franciscan Observant at Santa Maria della Pace—Cinquanta, who was an eyewitness to the plague. In addition, chroniclers in other cities reflected on these events such as the Roman Gigli and the Modense Spaccini.

[43] For Ripamonti, see Repossi, 'Cronologia'; and Nicolini, *Peste e untori*, 47. Ripamonti had been imprisoned in 1617 for four years for his ideas and for another five in 1622; his term was, however, commuted to house arrest at Cardinal Borromeo's country palace.

critical before that of the Modenese erudite of the early Enlightenment, Ludovico Muratori (1672–1750), who, however, only briefly and vaguely touched this 'stravolgimento di fantasmi'.[44] The watershed in condemnations of these judicial procedures and torture that led to gruesome executions had to await Pietro Verri (1728–97) at the end of the eighteenth century.[45] Yet with the executions of Mora, Piazza, and Baruello, Ripamonti already attacked the ghoulish displays of corporeal punishment and the mechanisms through which Milan's governors churned rumours to abet mass hysteria.[46]

Ripamonti certainly did not go as far as Verri or Manzoni.[47] Instead, throughout his text, he condemned *untori* as 'true monsters of nature (*mostra naturae*)'.[48] With the supposed spree of plague spreading on 22 April 1630, he alleged 'everyone could absolutely see clearly with their own eyes' the greased marks left by the diabolical ones.[49] Further, he praised authorities such as Alessandro Tadino, head of the Sanità's tribunal, responsible for the punishment of *untori*, who, unlike Ripamonti, held few doubts or qualms about the torture and executions.[50] In addition, Ripamonti backed his patron, Cardinal Archbishop Federigo Borromeo, who not only decried the *untori*'s supposed crimes of killing an 'unlimited number' during the plague,[51] but also arrested and tortured the plague spreaders in his ecclesiastic tribunal.[52] Further, Ripamonti cited other places such as Volpedo in Piedmont, where he justified authorities hunting and executing plague spreaders.[53] He believed that *untori* had earlier threatened Milan in the plague of 1576[54] and more so in Palermo in 1624, when 'demonic forces mixed with the crowds and the treachery of mortals' and 'unscrupulous humans conspired with our eternal and implacable enemy'.[55]

In contrast to his contemporaries, however, Ripamonti charged that authorities from the king of Spain, Phillip IV[56] to the officers of Milan's municipal tribunals had fanned the rumours of *untori*, which led to wrongful arrests, torture, and

---

[44] Muratori, *Del Governo della peste*, 127. On Muratori's view, see Preto, *Epidemia*, 104; and Cottignoli, 'Il Trattato', 66–7. By the end of the eighteenth century, others began to have grave doubts about plague spreading as with the abbot-historian, Papon (*De la peste*, 180).

[45] Verri, *Osservazioni sulla tortura*, written in 1777, published posthumously in 1804. For this historiography, see Manzoni, *Storia della colonna infame*, 853–64.

[46] Ripamonti, *De Peste*, 114–27.

[47] Manzoni, *I promessi sposi*, 584, 599, 606; and *Storia della colonna infame*, 853–5.

[48] Ripamonti, *De Peste*, 146–7.   [49] Ibid., 107.

[50] On Borromeo, see Ripamonti, *De Peste*, book III, 192–249 and for Tadino, *Raguaglio*, 149–53.

[51] Borromeo, *De Pestilentia*, 78–9 (for citation) and especially 'capitolo V: De artibus spargendae pestis origineque artium earum', 40–51, his longest chapter.

[52] Marioni, *Peste in Milano*, 65. Curiously, Muratori, *Del Governo della peste*, 127–8, claimed that Federigo doubted the existence of *untori* in Milan in 1630 but supplies no references. Only at one point in his tract, does Federigo even say that the rabble ('vulgus') 'as was their custom' might have exaggerated the extent of the plague spreading, 'believing that the city was besieged by the devil' and that *untori* 'were everywhere' (34–5). On the other hand, he berated commoners ('plebe') who thought that *untori* were being falsely punished (46–7). In stark contrast to Ripamonti, the cardinal never admitted that some had been falsely accused. He even believed in cases of diabolic plague spreading where others questioned them, as when healthy young men recruited to join the sentinel of the palace of the Governatorato, died within four days of plague (84–5). In addition, between 1599 and 1621, he had approved the torture and burning alive of seven witches; Nicolini, 'Parte III', 519.

[53] Ripamonti, *De Peste*, 165.   [54] Ibid., 161.   [55] Ibid., 159.   [56] Ibid., 153.

executions.[57] The rumours plagued Milan with 'internecine hatred',[58] dividing the city to its familial core—'the matrimonial bed and the dining table'—turning husbands, wives, children, brothers, and neighbours, 'previously held with affection', against one another. According to Ripamonti, the erosion of these bonds further fuelled the plague's natural spread.[59] Many accusations were ridiculous ('ludibria'), so much so that people believed the Devil had rented an apartment in Milan to carry out his nefarious deeds.[60] To illustrate his point, he told stories such as one about a nobleman he refused to name, who at the beginning of the plague left Milan to visit churches in Rome. His sudden departure sparked 'the wildest rumours' that he must be the captain of the plague spreaders. The pope arrested him and locked him in an underground prison, doubled the guards, and sealed shut the doors. The terror was so great that no one, not even the nobleman's closest friends or relatives, 'dared open their mouths' in protest.[61]

Ripamonti railed 'against the gullibility of commoners along with the arrogance of the nobles', who defended rumours of omnipresent *untori* as though they were matters of 'religion and family': when he questioned reports of plague spreaders, immediately he was attacked for 'impiety'.[62] Surprisingly, few others questioned the frenzy and fantasies of 1630. Filippo Visconti, a friar at Milan's San Marco, mentioned that many of the clergy were forced to suffer false allegations, but unlike Ripamonti, he supplied no cases and treated the theme only in passing.[63] Not only in Milan but across Europe, until the eighteenth century, few comments have surfaced from chroniclers, churchmen, or intellectuals, condemning beliefs in supposed armies of *untori*. Instead, key figures at the forefront of seventeenth-century philosophy, science, and medicine—Fortunato Fedeli, Alessio Giarrusso, M. A. Alaymo, Jean Bodin, Paracelsus, Athanasius Kircher, and others[64]—argued that only demonic forces of manufactured plague could explain the increased plague mortalities of the late sixteenth and seventeenth centuries.

William Naphy has returned to the pre-Enlightenment view that the accused were not necessarily innocent; in fact, he believes most were guilty, engaged in spreading plague for the same reasons early modern observers often alleged—profit—and that the lowest echelons of plague workers—the *monatti*—were the ones to blame. To maintain their employment they struggled to prolong the plague.[65] Although his primary research centred on Geneva (and then Lausanne,[66] Milan, and Lyon), he held that across Europe patterns of plague spreading were much the same, especially in Geneva and Milan.[67] For both, those employed by

---

[57] Ibid., 109 and 127–37.   [58] Ibid., 13–15.
[59] Ibid., 113–15.   [60] Ibid., 108–9.
[61] Ibid., 141–3. The nobleman was Don Carlo Bossi, identified by Marioni; see note 162.
[62] Ibid., 147–9.
[63] Visconti, *Commentarius*, 506. The Milanese Observant friar and playwright Cinquanta may have held views similar to Ripamonti's. Cinquanta's characters certainly believed that diabolic *untori* had contributed to Milan's devastating mortality in 1630 (see *La peste di Milano del 1630*, 539, 661, 669, 671). However, the play turns on the hunt for Casimorio by two dimwitted soldiers, who without evidence falsely accused him as an *untore*.
[64] See Dollo, *Peste e untori*, 21, 25, 37–8, 45, 64, 79; and Preto, *Epidemia*, 11–17.
[65] Naphy, *Plagues, Poisons and Potions*, 5–6, 33, 77, 172, 182.
[66] Ibid., 159–61.   [67] Ibid., 182.

health boards in menial positions were in fact to blame: 'Destitute and desperate people placed in horrific and desensitising circumstances are capable of extremely bizarre and even evil behaviour.'

But if the *untori* were the low-paid *monatti*, worried over employment, why did the reported crimes of plague spreading decline and then disappear altogether when plague mortalities in Milan in September 1630 suddenly began to fall, at the moment when the *monatti*'s employment would have been threatened? In mid-July, plague deaths reached a high of 1800 a day[68] and continuing near that level until mid-August.[69] Then, by 11 September, they had fallen to seventy or eighty a day (in the city and its lazaretti combined),[70] and by 5 October had disappeared entirely.[71] On the other hand, from the near day-to-day correspondence of the *avvisi* from Milan to offices in Venice and Rome, which survive intact from 1630 to 1631, the last report of intentional plague spreading in Milan occurred on 31 August 1630.[72] And suspicions of plague spreading did not rise again with renewed plague cases on 7 December 1630 or with their decline soon afterwards.[73] The last execution for plague spreading, appearing either in the surviving trial transcripts of the Tribunal of Milan's Health Board (Sanità) or the execution list from the confraternity of San Giovanni Decollato, which accompanied the executed for all crimes to the scaffolds, was on 9 September 1630.[74] After that date, few fresh cases came before the tribunals, although plague lingered on until 7 February 1632.[75] As Milan's chief physician and head of the Sanità tribunal commented, by September, plague was on the wane and with it 'the diabolical evilness'.[76] The Observant friar and contemporary playwright also saw both trends 'going up in smoke' at the same moment.[77] One reason for the decline in the accusations or the authorities' reluctance to act on them may have been that they were coming too close to Milan's centres of power by mid-August, when rumours spread of two first cousins of Marcantonio Monti, President of the Health Board, being *untori*.[78] This may also explain why governments in Genoa and Naples, for example, were less inclined to act on rumours of plague spreading in Italy's next pandemic, 1656–7.[79]

Finally, if plague cleaners' desires to keep their posts can explain the plague-spreading spree, why did their attempts not blossom earlier in the fifteenth century, especially in Italy? After all, the corps of gravediggers, carters, and plague cleaners were then in place with the formation of new health boards in Italy before other

---

[68] BAV, *Avvisi*, Urb. Lat., 1100, pt 2, f. 437v. Delumeau, *Vie économique*, I, 25–36, remains an excellent introduction to the *Avvisi*.

[69] Somaglia, *Alleggiamento*, 482 and 485.   [70] *Avvisi*, Urb. Lat., 1100, pt 2, f. 580v.

[71] Ibid., f. 609v.   [72] Ibid., f. 520v.

[73] Also, explanations now turned to natural causes. From informants on Milan's Health Board, the *avvisi* reported that new cases resulted from families returning to Milan from localities still harbouring plague; ibid., f. 749r.

[74] *Elenco cronologico*, 37v.

[75] Moreover, in Novara and Bobbio, plague continued well into 1632; Paccagnini, 'Cronaca di un contagio', 94–5.

[76] Tadino, *Raguaglio*, 134: ch. 57: 'Cessa la Peste & frenò le diaboliche malie'.

[77] Cinquanta, *La peste di Milano del 1630*, 671.   [78] Tadino, *Raguaglio*, 78.

[79] For the few cases that continued after 1630 in Italy, see Preto, *Epidemia*, chs 3–4. For the plague of 1656–7 in Naples and rumours of plague spreading, Nicolini, *Peste e untori*, 191–3.

areas of Europe. But the first trials and executions arose and peaked beyond Italy's borders. More fundamentally, were *monatti*, other marginal 'outsiders', or more generally, 'the destitute and the desperate' the ones tried as *untori*?

THE ACCUSED: MILAN, 1630–1

We begin with the best-known, most-studied and documented case—Milan's. The transcripts of the Milanese trial cases (hereafter called 'the transcripts') are the only ones on plague spreading to have been published, first in 1839 and in 1988 as a critical edition, with a vast commentary and further discoveries of trial records.[80] Yet, despite the detailed attention given to these records over almost two centuries, no one has evaluated the completeness or representativeness of the surviving interrogations. These records derive from the tribunal of Milan's Sanità under the thumb of Milan's senate, as signalled by their occasional interventions into judicial procedures, recalling witnesses and even deciding if the accused should be executed.[81]

Two lengthy manuscripts—one of 499 folios; the other, 476—have been integrated into the modern edition. Both were copies prepared by the court for the lawyers of the highest-profile defendant for plague spreading, its organization, or financing, the Spanish aristocrat and soldier Don Giovanni de Padilla, son of one of Milan's highest-ranking officials, the Castellan of Milan. It is uncertain whether these records begin with the earliest cases. The transcripts' first case on 22 June—the soon-to-be tortured then executed Matteo del Furno—began before the two most notorious defendants had been summoned—the barber Giovanni Giacomo Mora and plague commissioner Guglielmo Piazza—and more than a month before Padilla's arrest on 30 July. Del Furno's case is not mentioned in any narrative source, not by Marioni, stationed in Milan to deliver daily dispatches to Venice, nor by later commentators or historians, including Verri and Manzoni. Marioni's first report on the Sanità's interrogations does not appear until 3 July, after plague mortalities had rapidly climbed to 500 a day and rumours of plague spreaders (*untioni et empiastri pestiferi*), smearing their poisonous concoctions 'within churches on doors and walls' had occurred 'daily'. By then, Marioni reported that 'several suspected men' had been imprisoned.[82] On the other hand, Ripamonti describes Milan's plague spreading as early as 22 April;[83] and by 19 May, the government was awarding fees to any witnesses coming forward with accusations.[84] Yet Ripamonti along with another eyewitness chronicler, Pietro Antonio Lattuada, reports no criminal interrogations of greasers until the infamous ones against health commissioner Piazza, after which the floodgates to prosecution opened.[85]

---

[80] *Processo agli untori.*
[81] Ibid., 404, 423, 429, 528. Also, see Cantù, *Ragionamenti*, parte X: Gli Untori.
[82] Marioni, *Peste in Milano*, 51; On the same day, he reported three *untori* arrested at Pavia; ibid., 52.
[83] Ripamonti, *De Peste*, 107.   [84] See notes 208–10.
[85] Ripamonti, *De Peste*, 115; Lattuada, 'Cronaca', 285.

San Marco's friar Visconti charts another chronology, seeing the first major suspicions of *untori* arising on 18 May ('commota est universa Civitas Mediolani ea suspicione'), 'when during the night men greased walls and other places people were accustomed to touch'. For these crimes, four men were arrested in the Porta Ticinese neighbourhood, soon to become the hotspot of this supposed criminal activity.[86] However, as the editor of Visconti's short chronicle speculates, Visconti was not in Milan from the famine of 1628 to the plague in 1630,[87] and his chronicle is filled with errors, as with mistaken names of the accused bankers and garbled stories, such as Senator Caccia's supposed poisoning.[88]

It is difficult to know the number of arrests of supposed *untori* made by the Sanità or other Milanese courts before its 'grida' of 19 May 'against those who went about greasing doors, doorknobs, and walls of this city'[89] or between that date and the first surviving interrogations more than a month later. But at least four had been apprehended on 19 May by the city's *podestà* and handed over to Gaspare Alfieri, head of the Sanità's tribunal, for questioning.[90] In addition, arrests must have mounted sharply after the great disillusion following the second procession of San Carlo's body on 11 June, when mortality rates soared and did not fall as expected because of the spiritual antidote.[91] Chroniclers concluded that such unexpected results could only have had diabolical causes and reported 'armies of *untori*' greasing the cathedral steps the night afterwards, murdering 4000 women.[92] According to Tadino, the cathedral's outside benches, where merchants and shopkeepers heard mass, were also greased, signalling 'the beginning of the "Untioni"'.[93]

While the transcripts record only twenty-seven arrested and jailed, the chroniclers suggest many more. First, those diabolically murdering the Milanese and considered *untori* were not restricted to smearing walls and other objects. Chroniclers reported fires that spread through certain neighbourhoods on 22, 23, and 29 July, burning a number of houses and killing individuals. According to ambassador-spy Marioni, the fires were the deeds of evil ones (*scellerati*), in other words, *untori*. By the 29th, he reported 'already more than fifty men' had been charged and imprisoned because

---

[86] Visconti, *Commentarius*, 501.   [87] Polidori, 'Avvertimento', 489–90.

[88] He lists the bankers as 'Turconius, Stracius [instead of Cinquevie], et Sanquinettus', and mistakenly records their arrests on 9 June, before those of Mora and Piazza (Visconti, *Commentarius*, 505). Further, the editor believed 'Stracius' was a mishearing of Lucinus, the scribe in Turconi's bank, who was not a banker. In addition, Visconti misconstrues the story of the servant Giambattista Ferletta, who supposedly murdered his master, Senator Caccia, describing Ferletta, helped by his wife, murdering 20,000 in Milan's lazaretto, mixing poisons in the sauces fed to patients (509).

[89] Paccagnini, 'Cronaca di un contagio', 54–5, printed in full, 55.   [90] Ibid., 54.

[91] Among others, see Somaglia, *Alleggiamento*, 481–2, on the procession and precautions. According to Manzoni, *I promessi sposi*, ch. 32, 608, the Cardinal resisted 'for some time' the government's pleas to carry out this procession, but Manzoni does not cite his source. Somaglia, *Alleggiamento*, 481–2, instead lauds Federigo as the 'difensore di questa patria' and for organizing the procession, assembling not only Milan's 'popolo' but those from towns and villages throughout the Duchy, 'che degnasse liberarla dal velenoso male'.

[92] Paccagnini, 'Cronaca di un contagio', 62–3.

[93] Tadino, *Raguaglio*, 101. Also, see Somaglia, *Alleggiamento*, 482, when 'people crueller than tigers attacked the city and state of Milan'.

of this '*unto*' alone. Yet none of these charges appears in the transcripts, nor do any interrogations allude to them. More significantly, on 11 September, 'around 200 men' imprisoned for plague spreading (*carcertai per le untori*) killed their guards and escaped with most soon recaptured. Yet nothing near that number enters the two-year history of the transcripts.[94] According to Marioni, a week earlier eleven of the escapees had confessed to having murdered fifty-four clergymen (*tra canonici et altri mansionarii*) and those captured were carted from Monza to Milan, where they awaited execution. None enters the transcripts.

Moreover, the transcripts concern only two neighbourhoods of Milan, one around the castle that focused on Padilla and a larger one, comprised principally of artisans of Porta Ticinese with its dives and taverns, such as the hosteria dei Sei Ladri, as the *untori*'s points of contact. The tribunal strenuously believed that the two were interconnected. However, from the defendants' testimonies, even after torture, few pointed to any signs of socializing between the two neighbourhoods, except for the notorious fencing master Carlo Vedano, who frequented numerous inns, scrounging food and drink, and whose contacts spanned noblemen, soldiers, artisans, and prostitutes. By contrast, the chronicles evince a citywide network of suspected *untori* with key nodes at the cathedral, Sant'Ambrogio, and churches in other parts of the city. It would be surprising if authorities had not investigated and made arrests in these supposed cells. Certainly, the court cast its nets widely as shown by interrogating witnesses at Ossona and gathering evidence as far afield as Naples and Rome concerning the case of the elusive Spanish soldier Pietro Verdeno di Saragozza.[95] Furthermore, the chroniclers mentioned cases of *untori* arrested, tortured, and executed not found in the transcripts. Ripamonti claims that 'every day saw bands of coarse peasants, armed with old weapons' dragging their suspects in chains to the city's prisons.[96] An episode related by the chronicle of Busto Arsizio supplies an example. In July a little boy at Cuggione reported to his father seeing a friar spreading the deadly grease. Church bells were rung; the villagers assembled, apprehended the friar, and marched him to Milan's prison, where he later died.[97]

A manuscript listing executions in Milan from 1471 to 1783, compiled by the religious confraternity of San Giovanni Decollato, now held at the Biblioteca Ambrosiana, may supply some sense of the transcripts' incompleteness. Instead of the transcripts' five executions, the confraternity lists ten executed in Milan between 30 June and 19 October 1630, charged as *untori*.[98] Those without a trace in the transcripts include Giacinto, called a friar of the Servites, executed on 14 August.[99] Perhaps he had been interrogated in an ecclesiastic tribunal. Another was Pietro Paolo Bigotto, a native of Milan, hanged first by a foot for six hours, then burnt to death, his ashes left to blow in the wind on 14 September. On 21 August

---

[94]   Marioni, *Peste in Milano*, 54 and 63.
[95]   *Processo agli untori*, 522. Manzoni, *Storia della colonna infame*, 837, claimed the soldier was a fantasy of the tortured barber Mora.
[96]   For instance, Ripamonti, *De Peste*, 127.   [97]   Lupi, *Storia della peste*, 138–9.
[98]   *Elenco cronologico*, 37r–v.
[99]   Also, Lattuada, 'Cronaca', 288–9, refers to the friar and his prison confession.

two men were executed for plague spreading ('che aver onto'): Gerolamo Migliavacca called 'il forese' or 'il Foresaro' well covered by the transcripts, but the second, Giovanni Battista Bianco, fails to appear.[100] A fourth without trace in the transcripts was Giovanni Battista Ferletta, burnt at the stake on 9 September for pestilential smearing under the guise of giving charity to the poor. According to chroniclers, he had poisoned his master, Senator Caccia, with a fragrant flower presented to him.[101] On the following day another unmentioned in the transcripts was Francisco Bermascin di Vegin, first broken on the wheel in Piazza alla Vetra ('arrotato alla Vetra') then flayed alive ('e poi scannato'). Finally, on 19 October, the painter Martino Recalcato, the last *untore* accompanied to scaffold, ended in the same brutal manner.[102]

These executions double those recorded in the transcripts. In addition, the Milanese nobleman and government official, Carlo Girolamo Cavatio della Somaglia, 'representing' the Spanish king, Philip IV, listed two other *untori* executed in Milan, Francesco Manzone called Bonazzo and Giovanni Andrea Barbero, not mentioned in the transcripts.[103] Still further executions of *untori* may have occurred in Milan. On 10 August, an *avviso* sent to Venice stated that two unnamed *untori* were to be ripped apart by iron thongs then broken on the wheel, but their executions were temporarily suspended.[104] On 14 August the Milan correspondent reported that two *untori* were tortured, broken on the wheel, strangled to death and their corpses burnt.[105] Whether they were the earlier suspended cases is not specified. On that date, the confraternity records only one execution—that of Giacinto called the Servite.[106] Finally, another *avviso* dated 11 January 1631 from Milan 'via Venice' cited letters dated 28 December, reported that 'three persons' having violated unspecified ordinances of Milan's Sanità were executed on the wheel,[107] and added that three plague spreaders had been burnt, but as usual these records did not specify their names or dates of execution.[108] However, no other source, narrative or administrative, corroborates the report. The last execution of an *untore* recorded by the confraternity had occurred almost three months earlier, and that of the transcripts, almost five months before, on 21 August, although the transcripts continue into 1632.

No corresponding document exists for comparing the transcripts with those arrested, questioned, and possibly tortured but who were either fined or acquitted and not executed. If the ratio of executed *untori* in the transcripts to those in the

---

[100] *Elenco cronologico*, 37v. Paccagnini, 'Cronaca di un contagio'; allegedly, Bianco murdered his own parents by greasing them ('l'unizione'), 80.

[101] Tadino, *Raguaglio*, 121; and Ripamonti *De Peste*, 163–5. Also, Preto, *Epidemia*, 41; and Paccagnini, 'Cronaca di un contagio', 77.

[102] For these cases, see *Elenco cronologico*, 37r–v.   [103] Somaglia, *Alleggiamento*, 498.

[104] *Avvisi*, Urb. Lat., 1100, pt 2, f. 481v.   [105] Ibid., ff. 487r–v.

[106] *Elenco cronologico*, 37v.

[107] *Avvisi*, fondo Vaticani Latini, no. 12948, ff. 9v–10r: 'Da Milano con lettere delle 28 passato havutesi per via di Venetia scrivere essere ivi state appiccate 3. persone sospette di contagio, perché praticare per quella città contro gl'ordini del tribunale della sanità, che anco erano state fatte morire su la Ruota'.

[108] Ibid., ff. 9v–10r.

confraternity list is applied to those arrested in the transcripts, the prosecuted doubles those of the transcripts (twenty-seven), so we would estimate that fifty-four had been arrested. With those from the *avvisi* added, the number of arrested climbs threefold to eighty-one. But from impressions given in the chroniclers, *avvisi*, and by the spy Marioni, these figures still appear to underestimate drastically the numbers actually arrested. Already by 17 July, Marioni had reported 1500 *untori* arrested in Milan but he seems to have taken the figure with a grain of salt, saying it came from a 'third-hand' source.[109] Moreover, this number surfaces in an *avviso* of 10 August[110] and still later in Giovan Battista Spaccini's chronicle on 18 September.[111] The Modenese's report might also be doubted further: on 28 August, he reported that 44,000 in Milan had been murdered by manufactured pestilential pastes,[112] and afterwards, the *avvisi* were still reporting arrests of plague spreaders.[113] How do we square these numbers with the twenty-seven 'imputati' found in the transcripts?[114]

One group not found in the transcripts were the clergy. The ecclesiastic courts may well have been more lenient with their colleagues than the secular ones and thus would have produced a smaller ratio of the executed to prosecuted. While in the confraternity's list only one *untore* from the clergy was executed (and given his naming, possibly he was a defrocked cleric), the narrative sources point to several notorious clerics accused of these crimes—some even accused as leaders. During his torture on 12 September 1630, Giovanni Stefano Baruello related a story about a French priest, who with incantations of 'Gola Gibla' and 'other Hebrew words', Baruello maintained, enlisted him along with two other Frenchmen and the aristocrat Padilla to take a phial ('ampolino') of greased poison to commit the diabolic slaughter. Yet, despite the story's abundant detail and its implication of a key defendant, the court never even asked the priest's name.[115]

Chronicles and letters also report the clergy heavily involved. On 16 August 1630 in a Milanese district ('contrada') within the city of Novara, the murderous greasing had occurred and the following morning a priest was charged.[116] At the same time, another priest was arrested in Milan, accused of greasing a nobleman in a public market.[117] Later that month, after the plague spreaders' prison break, one of the recaptured (and presumably tried) was a 'servitore' of Milan's cardinal-archbishop, Federigo Borromeo.[118] That he has no trace in the transcripts may

---

[109] Ibid., 52.

[110] *Avvisi*, Urb. Lat., 1100, pt 2, f. 481v, also reports 45,000 plague deaths over the past five months.

[111] Spaccini, *Cronaca di Modena*, 142.

[112] Ibid., 111. In Cinquanta's *La peste di Milano*, 578, a soldier pursuing *untori* claimed that 800 had been seized (which may have pertained to the entire Duchy): 'many had died in gaol without having been taken to Milan'.

[113] See, for instance, *Avvisi*, Urb. Lat., 1100, pt 2, f. 520v (31 August 1630).

[114] Recent scholars seem to have believed the figure of 1500 without considering its clash with the twenty-seven in the transcripts. See Nicolini, 'Parte III', 517; and Bertolli and Colombo, 'Capitoli introduttivi', 60; neither work cites the sources for 'over a 1000' or 'over 1500' arrested.

[115] *Processo agli untori*, 371–8, esp. 375–6. In a later interrogation, Padilla mentioned this priest again but without naming him; the court appears not to have chased the lead, 476–81, esp. 480. Also, see Ripamonti, *De Peste*, 127; and Somaglia, *Alleggiamento*, 497.

[116] Nicolini, 'Parte III', 529.   [117] Preto, *Epidemia*, 39.   [118] Ibid., 40.

suggest that he possessed clerical status. Another known to the archbishop and arrested at the time of Servite Giacinto was an unamed friar of Sant'Ambrogio ad Nemus.[119]

In October, Marioni reported that a priest from Abbiategrasso, a wealthy town ('terra grassa e piena') 25 km south-west of Milan, was apprehended and taken to Milan. Reputedly, he had murdered 'with his own hands more than 600 persons' and planned similar assaults throughout the Duchy.[120] At Busto, an itinerant friar, thirsty while working the vineyards around Castano, asked for water. A woman compassionately gave him bottles and gourds, which he surreptitiously poisoned 'leading to many deaths'.[121] In the vicinity of Legnano, boys herding cattle ran into town screaming that a lay friar had greased a shrub ('pianta').[122] Busto's chronicler reported another Servite friar arrested at Magnago on 12 July, who confessed to paying large sums through a certain 'scrittore' in Milan (perhaps the charged Benedetto Luchini of Turcone's bank) to spread the plague in eight towns and villages around Gallarate. When arrested, 60 gold coins ('cechini') were found in his pockets.[123] At Pavia, a Carmelite friar was gaoled for various greasings ('diversos untos').[124] The chronicler Lattuada maintained that 'many' among 'the innumerable' arrested were friars, but he lists only four, the Servite, the above-mentioned from Sant'Ambrogio, one from Milan's parish of San Giovanni in Conca, and another from San Vittore. Furthermore, he alleged that other friars committed their malicious crimes in the countryside,[125] and named another clerical greaser higher up the religious and social hierarchy. Before becoming an ambassador of the Duke of Parma, Messer Carlo Basso Teatino had been in religious orders and later continued to be a knight of Malta 'with priestly robes'. According to Lattuada, for 400,000 *scudi* he employed *untori* to commit the nefarious deeds, but escaped to Rome and was not apprehended.[126] Finally, as mentioned above, the Dominican chronicler Visconti maintained that 'many innocent clergymen' were arrested on false charges. Some were soon freed but others suffered the tribunal's atrocities and died as a result.[127] Among the innocent, several clerics were arrested, questioned, and tortured in Cardinal Borromeo's tribunal shortly after 4 December, but 'because nothing of importance was confessed', they were absolved.[128] Although clergymen tried in ecclesiastical tribunals may account for several not mentioned in the transcripts, given the few names of clerics noted in the narrative sources, they probably did not approach in number anything close to the supposed 1500.

---

[119] Tadino, *Raguaglio*, 115; Paccagnini, 'Cronaca di un contagio', 70.

[120] Marioni, *Peste in Milano*, 64, cited in *Processo agli untori*, 86. The Venetian ambassador also reported this case; see Preto, *Epidemia*, 40.

[121] Lupi, *Storia della peste*, 138.

[122] The case appears in a note by Cusani in Ripamonti, *La Peste* (1841), 83 (not reproduced in the 2009 edition). Cusani says he found numerous inquisitions and arrests of *untori* in public and private archives but notes none of them.

[123] Lupi, *Storia della peste*, 137.   [124] Preto, *Epidemia*, 66.

[125] Lattuada, 'Cronaca', 285.   [126] Ibid., 292.

[127] Visconti, *Commentarius*, 506.   [128] Marioni, *Peste in Milano*, 65.

COMPOSITION OF THE *UNTORI*

As these cases suggest, the accused were hardly restricted to 'the destitute'. On the other hand, did they cluster among the lowest echelons of the Health Board's employees—plague cleaners, carters, and gravediggers—motivated by economic interest to keep the plague alive as Naphy and others have claimed? Milan's transcripts, instead, show a wide array of indigenous artisans, shopkeepers, and skilled professionals: barber-surgeons, scissor-makers, tailors, dyers, and specialized soldiers,[129] along with wealthy bankers[130] with young scribes in their studios. Other sources reveal further skilled artisans and proprietors, such as a miller accused of grinding plague victims' bones and sprinkling the powder through streets and churches.[131] The confraternity executions add a native Milanese painter. But strikingly, not a single person accused of these deeds in Milan named in any of the sources was a *monatto* or even anyone working for the Health Board other than the 'commissioner' Guglielmo Piazza (to whom we shall return). Instead, people as high up the social register as the aristocrat Don Giovanni de Padilla were accused,[132] along with the Milanese nobleman Carlo Crivelli, charged as Padilla's accomplice and forced to pay a considerable fine of 6000 gold coins (*zecchini*) for surety.[133] The rich and powerful along with the artisans, moreover, were in the main 'insiders', geographically, socially, and economically.[134]

Milanese plague tracts, chronicles, and ecclesiastical sources bring to light others suspected as *untori*; and these too were not the destitute. Ripamonti recounts the story of a respectable eighty-year-old Milanese man, who entered his parish church, Sant'Antonio dei padri Teatini, to pray. When dusting a bench to sit, he set off women to attack him as a plague spreader. The swelling mob grabbed him by the hair, and kicked and punched him to death.[135] Another incident concerned young French students interested in Milanese art. Admiring the bas-reliefs on the Duomo's façade, they rubbed the figures, drawing a crowd, which attacked them for greasing the walls. Had the police not apprehended them, Ripamonti maintained, they would have been lynched.[136] Ripamonti relates other crowds taking justice into their own hands, surrounding suspicious-looking characters 'with shouts and a storm of stones and beatings' so that they 'yearned to be taken to prison as a safe haven'.[137] He believed such crowds were more common in the countryside and tells a story of feared plague-spreading at Senago, where Borromeo had his summer palace and Ripamonti was in residence for much of the plague.[138] The villagers

---

[129] Along with the Spanish castle guard, Pietro di Saragozza, there was Il Fontana, the *bombardiero*.

[130] In addition to the three, another banker, Ambrogio Melzo, was accused of paying *untori* (*Il processo degli untori*, 352) but was not charged in the transcripts.

[131] Lattuada, 'Cronaca', 288; Visconti, *Commentarius*, 508.

[132] *Processo agli untori*, 76, 150, 480.

[133] Ibid., 172, 175, 321, 354, 430, 495; Paccagnini, 'Cronaca di un contagio', 99; Nicolini, 'Parte III', 546; Preto, *Epidemia*, 49.

[134] Three were identified as born outside Milan: the two Spanish soldiers and Carlo Vedano from Ossona, 25 km from Milan, but he also resided in Milan.

[135] Ripamonti, *De Peste*, 126–9.   [136] Ibid., 129–31.   [137] Ibid., 127.

[138] Repossi, 'Chronologia', xciv.

established their own quarantine, not against the disease, but its 'demonic ministers'. Armed with muskets and pruning knives, they surrounded two young clerics dressed in black. Had one of the cardinal's servants not intervened, the peasants would have executed them. According to Ripamonti, their crimes were minding their own business and enjoying good literature and poetry—again not your usual riff-raff.[139]

The one targeted group totally missing from the accused in the transcripts was, in fact, the utterly impoverished—old widows, foreign beggars, the crippled and blind—along with those most often pictured as the prime suspects, the lowest rungs of plague cleaners and carters—*monatti*—supposedly reduced to diabolical straits to keep their jobs. The only accused employee of the Health Board was Guglielmo Piazza, one of the two infamous *untori* of the 'colonna infame'. Piazza, however, was not a *monatto*, said to be exclusively foreigners to Milan.[140] From interrogations and extensive testimony, no one ever referred to him as a 'monattum'. Consistently, he was called commissioner (*commissario della sanità*), and he announced proudly that he was head of the carters in his district.[141]

Moreover, less than a handful can easily be categorized as belonging to a criminal underworld, despite the name of one of the taverns regularly patronized by some of the accused—l'hosteria dei Sei Ladri.[142] Of the transcripts' twenty-seven 'imputed', only three were noted with previous criminal records—Gerolamo Migliavacca and Carlo Vedano, to be discussed, and the Spanish soldier Pietro Verdeno, employed at Milan's castle, earlier found guilty of attempted robbery.[143] In addition, the *mestatore* or trickster, Giovanni Stefano Baruello, suffered from 'mal francese', and was known as 'a big blasphemer'.[144] With his co-defendants, Gerolamo Migliavacca[145] and Pietro Gerolamo Bertone, Baruello's cousin, Ripamonti calls them, 'people of dives and whorehouses (*ex ganea, et popina homines*)'.[146] Of the three, Migliavacca's crimes were the worst: he had served time for murdering his brother and had come before the Holy Office on charges of witchcraft.[147] But even these accused were skilled craftsmen and property owners with fixed residences, who in their opening court statements proudly declared themselves 'Milanesi'.[148]

Baruello was a practising barber as well as a master knife-maker, owned his own shop and home, and employed his son, cousins, at least one apprentice, and a domestic

[139] Ripamonti, *De Peste*, 133–7.   [140] Ibid., 323.

[141] Ibid., 158, 242. Differences in status between a commissioner and a 'monattum' were sharp. For instance, Cinquanta's characters refer to *monatti* as 'a pack of thieves worthy of execution or at least the whip (*un branco di ladri | Degni di forca o della frusta almeno*)', 620 and 686, while commissioner Polimede is treated with respect and called 'Ser' or 'signore' (603, 604, 683).

[142] The transcripts mention numerous taverns—l'Osteria della Rosa, del Gambaro, della Brugnoni, della Rosa, della Stella, S. Paolo, del Gallo, di Cesere Pezzano (or Pisano), di Bremo, di Sisto.

[143] *Processo agli untori*, 556.

[144] Ibid., 249, 255, 257, 259. Nicolini, 'Parte III', 551, maintains that 'he was constantly in and out of prison for every sort of crime' and was convicted of fraticide and witchcraft, but Nicolini was here confusing Baruello with Magliavacca.

[145] Preto, *Epidemia*, 47; and Codero, *La Fabbrica della peste*, 82.

[146] Ripamonti, *De Peste*, 122–3.   [147] *Processo degli untori*, 246.

[148] Ibid. 249, and 76 (Giacinto Maganza detto il Romano); 204 (the barber Mora); his son Paolo (207), and Vedano, even though from Ossona, 371.

servant, Margherita Ciechetti, who was interrogated about his character.[149] In addition, he was the owner ('padrone') of a tavern, l'hosteria di San Paolo in Compita, just outside the Porta Ticinese. Migliavacca was also a master knife- and scissor-maker, owned his own shop, and employed at least one worker.[150] Both were artisans of the upper echelons, regulars at their local taverns, and well known within the neighbourhood. Less is mentioned about Bertino, but his son Melchione also owned a tavern, L'hosteria della Rosa, described as a spacious inn with several rooms and a large garden, which came under scrutiny because of allegations that worms, toads ('zatti'), lizards ('ghezzi'), and other animals were harvested there to be mixed into their deadly paste ('canepa').[151]

Another candidate for Milanese low life was Carlo Vedano, from Ossona. Before being accused of plague spreading, he had been charged with assaulting his parents and had been gaoled 'two or three times'.[152] Witnesses described him as universally disliked, one who beat his wife, his parents, even his sister-in-law. But he was a fencing master, owned his own school of fencing, and had tutored Don Carlo, the younger son of Milan's castellan. Moreover, he was a hanger-on at the castle, mixing with soldiers and aristocrats, and occasionally had sparred with Don Padilla.[153] As with most of the accused, Vedano was literate as shown by having followed court instructions, reading other defendants' interrogations.[154] In addition, he appears to have been a regular diner at the home of the chef of Prince Zandi.[155] One witness from Vedano's home town called him a vagabond.[156] He was not. Instead, he possessed two residences: one in Milan, the other in his native village, where he returned frequently and where his wife and child stayed.[157] There, he owned half of 'a large house (*una casa grande*)', which he purchased two years earlier for 4000 *lire*, along with 25 *pertiche* of arable land, some of which he leased out, and a dovecote.[158] Marioni refers to Vedano as 'a rich farmer (*massaro*)'[159]— again, hardly riff-raff.[160]

Nor do the transcripts picture the three accused Milanese bankers—Gerolamo Turconi, Giovanni Battista Sanguinetti, and Giovanni Battista Cinquevie, or their two scribes, Benedetto Lucini of Turconi's bank or Gerolamo Insula of Sanguinetti's— as 'destitute and desperate', possibly bankrupt by the harsh commercial climate that had engulfed the Duchy since the late 1620s. On the contrary, they were pictured as wealthy with large sums to spare for financing the colossal plot to kill Milan's population. Ultimately, for their release, they had to raise large sums for surety, which they paid immediately.[161] In addition, other sources mention those of high status, accused of financing or organizing plague spreading but who do not

---

[149] *Processo agli untori*, 249.   [150] Ibid., 80, 159, 168, 350, 358.   [151] Ibid., 249.
[152] Ibid., 405.   [153] Ibid., 386–9.   [154] Ibid., 388.   [155] Ibid., 388–9.
[156] Ibid., 415: testimony of Antonio Leva di Ossona, who then added that Vedano owned land.
[157] Ibid., 387.   [158] Ibid., 445.   [159] Marioni, *Peste in Milano*, 62.
[160] Preto, *Epidemia*, 50, lists Vedano as unemployed, but I find no indication of it, even if some claimed he no longer possessed his school. Witnesses from Ossona who called him 'un povero huomo' admitted he owned property. For Vedano's character, profession, and property holdings, see 168, 169, 173, 174–5, 386, 405, 406, 407, 441, 410, 411, 413, 414, 415, 419, 441, 442, 445, 482.
[161] Paccagnini, 'Cronaca di un contagio', 99.

appear in the transcripts. Marioni maintained that the Milanese count, Carlo Marliano, and Monsignor Carlo Bossi Teatino were arrested.[162] Lattuardo claimed that 'various important notables (*diversi principali signori*)' organized those committing the evil greasing; one of whom was the brother of the Marques of Memies [sic].[163] An *avviso* of Venice, dispatched from Milan on 10 August 1630, reported the illegitimate son ('figliuolo naturale') of Marchese Dogliani detained in Milan, charged along with Padilla for distributing money to the *untori*.[164] At Pavia, one of the first *untori* arrested was dressed as a knight of Malta.[165] The Servite friar mentioned earlier was denounced as operating factories of poison ('come fabbricatori di veleno'), employing forty workers, in which four knights from Brescia ('cavalieri bresciani') assisted.[166] Spaccini even singles out the nobility 'for being particularly involved in these despicable actions', and maintains that a reprehensible nephew of Cardinal Borromeo was also involved.[167]

The sole marginal character in this wide mix of artisans, bankers, and aristocrats may have been Giacinto Maganza, called the Roman, son of a friar, and labelled as a 'vagabond'. The transcripts reveal little else about him but leave no impression that he was a *monatto* or in any way dependent on plague for his livelihood. Nor was he an outsider; he also proudly declared in his opening interrogation: 'I am Milanese and well known in my neighbourhood of Porta Ticinese'.[168] He had been an apprentice ('ragazzo') of Signor Fabritio Landriano in the company ('compagnia') of Signor Verceillino Visconte. Whether it was a merchant or military company is not specified.[169] Later, he became an apprentice of the accused, Il Fontana, a master-builder ('mastro da muro') and 'bombardiero' at Milan's castle.[170] The slur 'vagabond' may have been just that: at the time of his arrest, Giacinto had a fixed residence in the parish of San Giovanni in Conca.[171]

To be sure, chroniclers had little good to say about *monatti*. Busto's chronicler complained that here and in the surrounding towns they were almost entirely foreigners who 'disgracefully' overcharged for their labour.[172] Luttuada censured them for their 'negligence and cowardliness'.[173] Ripamonti complained of their insolence, thievery, and unceasing desire to extort money. He called them a different race of men, 'desperate ministers of plague', who occasionally were 'driven to crazy sprees of ecstasy by the stacks of dead cadavers... the ultimate excess of the libido'. They did not cease robbing from the dead and extorting money from the dying.[174] He later added one accusation that might support present claims about these workers: fearing their salaries of six gold coins a day might end, they resolved to help those with 'infernal aims' to keep the plague alive.[175] Yet he supplied no cases and never called them *untori*. At most, they were helpers only. The physician Tadino poured on greater scorn, calling them 'a wretched people (*la meschina gente*)'

[162] Ibid., 76 and Marioni, *Peste in Milano*, 58.   [163] Lattuada, 'Cronaca', 287.
[164] *Avvisi*, Urb. Lat., 1100, pt 2, f. 481v; and repeated in Spaccini, *Cronaca di Modena*, 135.
[165] Lattuada, 'Cronaca', 289.   [166] Paccagnini, 'Cronaca di un contagio', 78.
[167] Spaccini, *Cronaca di Modena*, 142.   [168] *Processo agli untori*, 249.
[169] Ibid., 255.   [170] Ibid., 393.   [171] Ibid., 249.
[172] Lupi, *Storia della peste*, 147.   [173] Ibid., 293.
[174] Ripamonti, *De Peste*, 97–9.   [175] Ibid., 158–9.

and 'a wicked crowd (*questa canaglia de Monatti & Apparitori*)'.[176] He accused them of spreading the plague, however, not by intentional greasing but by greed, their reckless stealing from infected homes.[177] He also never referred to them as *untori*, at least not in Milan or Lombardy.[178] As for spreading plague through selling the goods of the plague-afflicted, he cited only one case and that one referred to Milan's previous plague in 1576.[179] Somaglia, who twenty years after the plague continued fervently to believe that only diabolical acts could have accounted for Milan's disastrous mortalities, also complained about *monatti*—their robberies from plague victims as well as from the healthy. He described them as outsiders from foreign places, housed separately from the Milanese but also never considered them *untori*.[180]

Finally, Manzoni, deeply absorbed in these seventeenth-century sources and their attitudes about *monatti*, reflected on them in chapters 33 and 34. With plague-stricken Don Rodrigo reaping his just desserts, his supposed trusted servant Griso returned not with the physician his master requested but with two *monatti*. They broke open his chests, taking all they could carry, thus reflecting contemporaries' image of them as low-life thieves, spreading plague unwittingly through greed.[181] In the next chapter, Renzo's return to Milan, dressed in his 'foreign' country fashion, immediately provoked suspicion and he was hounded as an 'untore', only to be saved by the carts of drunken *monatti*, who egged him on in his supposed zeal to annihilate Milan. In contrast to the previous chapter, this one diverges from the contemporary sources. In the city of Milan, none of those accused as *untori* had just wandered into town from foreign places, either from Italy or abroad, or were unknown in their neighbourhoods. The one contemporary source to back Manzoni's impression also derives from imaginary literature. Padre Cinquanta's Bolognese protagonist, Casimorio, rarely mentioned by modern scholars but known to Manzoni,[182] was a 'forastiere' freshly arrived in Milan, and may have inspired his chapter 34. Yet despite his liberties, Manzoni remained true to his sources in one essential respect: none of his *monatti* was an *untore*.

More to the point, in the transcripts not a single *monatto* was arrested or even questioned. In fact, they are hardly mentioned in hundreds of interrogations, even though a central figure in the trials, health commissioner Piazza, was their commander at the Porta Ticinese. On his interrogation of 1 July 1630, he confessed under torture to have received the froth ('spuma') of the pestilential dead from a *monatto* for 2 *scudi*, but he claimed never to have paid him and could not recall his name, only that he was 'a big foreigner with an ugly face (*chiera brutta*) and a black beard'.[183] On 26 July, the court cross-examined Piazza on the origins of his substance; again, he mentioned the big *monatto*, still could not remember his

---

[176] *Apparitori* walked in front of the carts transporting plague victims, dead or alive, ringing bells to warn the public; Manzoni, *I promessi sposi*, 612.

[177] Tadino, *Raguaglio*, 102.

[178] Tadino claims that in Sicily some *monatti* were *untori*; ibid., 119.   [179] Ibid., 118.

[180] Somaglia, *Alleggiamento*, 500; on their tasks and residences, 484.

[181] Manzoni, *I promessi sposi*, 625–32.   [182] Nicolini, *Peste e untori*, 37–8.

[183] *Processo agli untori*, 241–2.

name, but now thought he had worked for a commissioner named Beniamino.[184] The transcripts, however, show no signs of bothering to pursue this *monatto* or interrogate his boss. Nor from the hundreds of witnesses do any further suspicions arise of other *monatti*.[185] Instead, they themselves could be the victims of greasing: on 7 September, Pietro Paolo Rigotto was charged with having 'greased (*aver unto*)' a *monatto*, who worked at Milan's lazaretto.[186]

Given present assumptions that plague cleaners were the principal plague spreaders and that many, if not most, plague cleaners were women, the Milanese transcripts reveal another surprise—the total absence of women arrested, tortured, or accused of plague spreading in these records. Here, the transcripts appear roughly in line with impressions gained from the chronicles. In these (along with five published letters, the *avvisi*, and other sources), only one woman greaser is named: Caterina Rossana (or Rozzana). She boasted of having killed 4000,[187] but as stated earlier she does not appear in the transcripts. Borromeo adds a story of another unnamed *untorice*. In the quarter of Porta Vercellina, a mother denounced her own daughter as an accomplice to the poisonings,[188] but no such case is found in any other source.

Women's absence is especially surprising given charges of demonic activity and the association between plague spreading and witchcraft in the historiography, at least north of the Alps.[189] In late sixteenth- and seventeenth-century Venice, 70 per cent of accused witches were women,[190] which was below the European average.[191] One reason for their absence in Milan may have hinged on the pattern of this plague's mortality. Overwhelmingly, plague victims here were women. Before the procession of San Carlo's corpse on 5 June, when daily death tolls hovered around a hundred, Marioni claimed that of every hundred plague deaths, 90 were women. When the daily counts soared to 500, the gap closed somewhat, but by 3 July, with 14,000 plague deaths, 10,000 were women.[192] To explain the lopsided mortality, certain *untori* were imagined as killing women exclusively, as with the scissor-maker, Migliavacca detto il forbesaro, whom Marioni claimed murdered a hundred women by greasing their scissors.[193] According to Lattuada, *untori* targeted the whole of the College of Noble Widows near the hospital of the

---

[184] Ibid., 323.

[185] Nicolini, *Peste e untori*, 294, asserts that according 'to popular opinion, plague spreading would have been impossible without *monatti*' (294), but supplies no evidence for it.

[186] Paccagnini, 'Cronaca di un contagio', 83.

[187] Marioni, *Peste in Milano*, 60; Nicolini, 'Parte III', 529; Preto, *Epidemia*, 39. Borromeo, *La Pestilencia*, 1, also points to a lower-class woman ('muliercula'), who boasted of killing 4000 with her own hands, and another who killed 3000. Neither is named, and perhaps he was confusing rumours about the same Caterina. Although Paccagnini, 'Cronaca di un contagio', 89, mentions her condemnation, she does not appear in the transcripts and the editors do not explain her absence or that of others such as Bianco and Ferletta.

[188] Borromeo, *La Pestilentia*, 44–5. [189] Monter, 'Witchcraft in Geneva'.

[190] McGough, *Gender, Sexuality, and Syphilis*, 89. [191] Levack, *The Witch-Hunt*, 141–2.

[192] Marioni, *Peste in Milano*, 49–50, 51. Lupi, *Storia della peste*, 136, gives a higher figure, but his ratio for early July was roughly the same: of 17,000 plague deaths, 13,000 were women.

[193] Marioni, *Peste in Milano*, 62. The witness Caterina Baretta of Porta Ticinese said much the same; *Il processo degli untori*, 490.

male Fatebenefratelli (which was not touched): the widows' porters supplied them bread greased with pestilential paste.[194] Moreover, he alleged that the only named *untorice*, the woman who bragged about killing 4000, also specialized in women.[195] Other areas such as Piedmont may have differed, although no one has yet to assemble the names or sex ratios of the accused there. Nonetheless, a copy of a letter from a friar at Casale Monferrato in 1630 reported that the Devil gave orders to a branch of the imperial army then sweeping through northern Italy 'to spread powders and pestilential ointments'. From information received 'directly' from the Podestà of Nizza in Monferrato, the friar claimed this army of plague spreaders was comprised 'equally (*indifferentemente*) of men and women and mostly from the upper classes (*la più parte de migliori*). Over seventy were imprisoned and awaited execution.'[196]

With these exceptions, women appear not to have been accused, at least in Lombardy. Instead, they stood on the opposite side, as the prime accusers, testifying against the victims, especially in the earliest cases, leading to the condemnations of Mora and Piazza. These women, moreover, were the poor—widows, a midwife, washerwomen ('lavandarie'), and others identified only by name and parish.[197] As Ripamonti observed, women peering from their windows spotted the *untori* greasing walls and eagerly denounced them in courtroom examinations.[198] Perhaps these Milanese blame spreaders anticipated the poor in nineteenth-century cholera riots, who attacked doctors and high-ranking state officials thought to have instigated epidemics to cut costs by killing the poor. In the longest and most detailed account of the Milanese plague—Ripamonti's—plebeians and particularly porters and women ('apud plebem; baiulorum, atque mulierum') early on greeted Milan's most prominent doctor, the *protomedico* Lodovico Settala, with 'hostile screams' while he visited his plague patients.[199] Later, crowds attacked another leading physician of the Health Board, Alessandro Tadino.[200] Further popular insurrections erupted against Milanese Health Board officials in the countryside at Lecco,[201] and on 23 April 1630 a riot spread through several city neighbourhoods. With sticks and stones, the populace attacked plague cleaners and grave-carters (*i monatti*), as well as higher-ranking health authorities.[202] But except for one surgeon, to be discussed, doctors and other health workers rarely the targets of riots and were not accused or brought before the tribunals charged with the deadly greasing. In contrast to later cholera riots, a final group absent from the

---

[194] Lattuada, 'Cronaca', 290.   [195] Ibid., 291.

[196] Transcribed in Bollea, 'Untori piemontesi', 17. For the plague of 1599, the *Protomedico* of Savoy, Fiochetto (*Trattato della Peste*, 77), reported that 'men and women alike' were discovered greasing the city. While carted to the Piazza Castello, they were tortured with tongs ('tenagliati'), their legs, hips, arms, and ribs then broken, and, while still alive, put on the wheel; finally their throats were slit. For 1630, however, he names only one woman, a half-witted girl ('semi fatua'), who accused many innocents, including her mother, of greasing. Also, see Fiochetto, *Peste a Torino*, 68–9.

[197] *Processo agli untori*, 174–5, 212, 213, 460–1,489, 490, 491. On these 'donnicciuole', see Polidori, 'Avvertimento', 491; Manzoni, *Storia della colonna infame*, 757 and 758–9.

[198] Ripamonti, *De Peste*, 114–15; and Tadino, *Raguaglio*, 113.

[199] Ripamonti, *De Peste*, 80–3; and Manzoni, *I promessi sposi*, 590.

[200] Tadino, *Raguaglio*, 83–4.   [201] Nicolini, 'Parte III', 504.   [202] Ibid., 518.

surviving court registers as accusers or victims were children, even though Tadino maintained that the Podestà of Milan brought ten street urchins ('furbi') aged between twelve and fourteen before the Sanità. Enticed by food and drink and supposedly paid 40 *soldi* daily, they greased people in the Verzaro neighbourhood. When caught, they were publicly whipped and banished from the Milanese state.[203]

In contrast to the mass of later cholera riots, no straightforward class conflict emerges in Milan, provincial towns, or the countryside from the fantasies of 1630. Instead, the transcripts portray plague-crazed judges and the highest state officials loosely allied with the indigenous poor (usually women) against targets who were neither foreigners nor the marginal but instead native-born Milanese property owners. The chroniclers, however, suggest that other fears and animosities also were at play and perhaps more so in small towns and rural districts. According to Ripamonti, early on in the plague, 'crowds surrounded, hit with sticks, and stoned many innocent ones just because of worried faces and torn clothing'. The victims were then taken in chains to Milan's gaols. Ripamonti, however, does not name any of them or report any standing trial.[204] Later, during a popular revolt for which the chroniclers could not discern the motives, cries against the French rang through the city.[205] But no class or intellectual divide separated those who believed or disbelieved the stories of manufactured plague. Individuals from Milan's political and intellectual elites, such as Tadino, Borromeo, and Somaglia, members of the Health Board, judges, lawyers, Milan's titular ruler, Philip IV, king of Spain (1621–65),[206] and his leading minister, the count-duke of Olivares (1587–1645) were certain that demonic forces channelled by human plague spreaders explained Milan's soaring mortalities.[207] Milan's governors unwittingly encouraged the accusations, first by awarding 200 lire on 19 May for every supposed *untore* denounced—on 2 June, 'the reward (*il premio*)' was raised to 500 lire[208]—and then on 11 July, to 1000

---

[203] Tadino, *Raguaglio*, 115. Borromeo, *La Pestilencia*, 42–3, claimed that some parents 'lured their own sweet sons and daughters' into the practice 'with candies and delicacies'.

[204] Ripamonti, *De Peste*, 127.

[205] Ibid., 167–71. Suspicions of the French spreading plague emerge in 1629, when two men dressed as friars were arrested; Preto, *Epidemia*, 43; Tadino, *Raguaglio*, 102–3; and Nicolini, 'Parte III', 542–3.

[206] Nicolini, 'Parte III', 542–3; Preto, *Epidemia*, 43; and Paccagnini, 'Cronaca di un contagio', 86. Even if Nicolini, *Peste e untori*, 173, is correct that Philip's letter sent to the Milanese governor, Ambrogio Spinola, in 1629, reporting four French plague spreaders in Madrid escaping to Milan never existed, other evidence shows the Spanish king believed in artificial manufacturing of plague, and he acted on it at Madrid and Milan. See note 207 and *Bando di Filippo IV*; also the Spanish crown authorized payments to those in Milan who testified against *untori*; see Somaglia, *Alleggiamento*, 490–3.

[207] On 28 September 1630, Philip IV affixed placards across Madrid warning that 'algunos enemigos del genero humano' had joined forces, ready to spread 'los polvos, que con tan gran rigor han causado le peste en el Estado de Milan y en ostros Estados de aliados y amigos'. He offered 20,000 *scudi* for the capture of 'the diabolical enemies'. Olivares requested periodic inspections of Venetian and French embassies to search for *untori*; see Nicolini, 'Parte III', 542–3. In a letter of November 1630 to the Venetian ambassador at Madrid, Philip expressed fears that plague spreaders had entered Spain; idem, *Peste e untori*, 292. Not all, however, were convinced: a pamphlet by Seville's physician Don Fernando Solá expressed doubts; Villalba, *Epidemiologia española*, I, 4th Parte, 30–1.

[208] Nicolini, 'Parte III', 527.

scudi.[209] An *avviso* describes one instance of such an award being implemented: on 2 August, three unnamed 'accomplices' not only were freed but awarded the 'premio' to gather further accusations.[210] As Corrado Dollo has argued, those at the forefront of these new fantasies were among Europe's leading intellectuals.[211] To his cast of intellectuals, we need to add prominent heads of state and leaders of health boards. The horrific events of the seventeenth century did not depend on primitive fantasies and folkloric magic nestled in isolated alpine hamlets that suddenly escaped their rocky niches to ease down slopes to nearby cities, as Bercé has argued.[212]

A VARIETY OF MANIA

As clearly seen, the Milanese transcripts regarding accusations, arrests, and executions of *untori* are incomplete. Not only are cases enumerated in chronicles absent; entire constituencies are missing. The absence of clerics is understandable given the separation of secular and ecclesiastical jurisdictions, even if Cardinal Borromeo, according to the diary of Giacinto Gigli, obtained a special licence from the pope to have clerics accused of spreading plague tried in secular tribunals.[213] Another absence is more difficult to comprehend. The transcripts give little sense that popular and governmental fears of foreigners may have contributed to plague-spreading sprees. Not a single Frenchman or German was imprisoned or interrogated in the transcripts. Nonetheless, chatter heard from witnesses, spies (*delatores*), and occasionally the accused points to suspicions of the French as prime suppliers of the poisonous concoctions. As already seen, an unnamed French priest appeared as one of the conspiracy's leaders according to the forced confessions of Baruello and Padilla. Others cast similar aspersions on the French. As early as 25 June, Alvaro de Toledo, captain of the castle's gate, testified that the French were the true 'authors' of the plague spreading (*unizioni*).[214] In the 15 July interrogation of Piazza, he responded: 'along with the plague, the French were the ones supplying the poisonous substance (*di quell'onto*)'.[215] Half a year later, the court questioned Don Alvaro further. Now, he was more emphatic about what he alleged the Milanesi believed: the poisonous substances spread through the city derived from the French: 'no one talks of anything else'.[216] One of the baristi at the Sei Ladri corroborated this background noise. Under questioning, he claimed 'it was said' that plague spreading 'came from the French: they wished to destroy Italy'. But he cautioned: 'one person

---

[209] *Processo agli untori*, 69.   [210] *Avvisi*, Urb. Lat., 1100, pt 2, f. 464r.

[211] Dollo, *Peste e untori*, 4, 21, 25, 37–8, 45 51, 64, 79; also Tadino, *Raguaglio*, 119; Preto, *Epidemia*, 11–17, 33, who names other physicians and notable intellectuals. For physicians in Milan, beginning with Settala and Tadino, see Nicolini, *Peste e untori*, 107.

[212] Bercé, 'Les semeurs', 92.

[213] According to Gigli, *Diario Romano*, 117, 'some' were tried by these means, but I know no source to confirm it.

[214] Farinelli, 'Atti del processo', 174.   [215] *Processo agli untori*, 298.

[216] Ibid., 473, on 27 January 1631.

said one thing, and another, something else'.[217] Finally, the tribunal accused the banker Turconi of financing the French and Venetian governments for the paste and hiring the *untori*.[218] Yet the judges had little appetite to follow up these leads.

Chroniclers related more about the anti-French sentiment. Even with his story of French students admiring the Duomo's bas-reliefs, Ripamonti hinted that the attack was not random; 'the crowd recognized the students as French'.[219] Conspiracies of the French 'enemies' as the ones spreading plague peaked on 22 July, after fears of *untori* were on the wane. Suddenly, fires broke out in the neighbourhood of Porta Tosa, with several butcher shops burnt to the ground. Women led the revolt ('tumultus'), screaming: 'To arms! The enemy has entered the city!'. According to Ripamonti, commoners ('vulgus') believed that French troops on the city's outskirts had infiltrated *untori* into the city to kill the Milanese by disease and arson, even if, as Ripamonti noted, the notions were without substance.[220] Again, Piedmont may have differed, as seen in the one letter cited above: here, German soldiers organized by the Devil were the instigators.[221] The Roman chronicler Giacinto Gigli also pointed to Germans: during their siege of Mantua, the captain of the imperial army, aided by a 'heretic' named Guastaino, supposedly used pestilential liquids, which proved 'more deadly than their muskets' in killing the city's defenders. A dispatch from the Florentine ambassador in Milan, Domenico Pandolfini, supports Gigli's conjectures: the German soldiers sent to occupy Mantua were 'all Lutherans and among other things broke altars and sacred ornaments into a thousand pieces, poisoned Holy water with pestilential substances, and publicly rubbed their boots with the substance at Cremona'.[222] Gigli further claimed the Duke of Savoy before dying on 5 August 1630 had been implicated in plague spreading in Milan.[223]

However, as the beliefs of Milan's chief physician Tadino illustrate, fears of the French as plague spreaders were more prominent than those of other foreigners, and these beliefs were not restricted to commoners. He reported as fact that 'a number of French soldiers were in hiding just beyond the city walls, had started fires, and were wilfully infecting great numbers of people, out to annihilate the people (even if cautious ones called it a lie)'.[224] With his June report on the greasing of the cathedral's benches, he said some pointed to the plebeians because of their lack of respect for Milan's governor; others thought it was a joke played by students from Pavia. But the most plausible hypothesis, he claimed, implicated the French: already they had rubbed great quantities of their pastes on benches and walls.[225]

The canon Giovanni Battista Lupi, now thought to be Busto's chronicler, also believed the Milanese fires were the diabolic work of the French, but he added, 'with the cooperation of big shots (*molti principali*) in the city'. The French strategy was first to weaken the city with disease, then to conquer it by force.[226] He reported that a surgeon in Milan's lazaretto was manufacturing the poisonous paste and

[217] Ibid., 449.   [218] Nicolini, 'Parte III', 543.   [219] Ripamonti, *De Peste*, 128–31.
[220] Ibid., 166–71.   [221] See note 196.   [222] Cited in Nicolini, *Peste e untori*, 81.
[223] Gigli, *Diario Romano*, 116–17, entry for 5 August.   [224] Tadino, *Raguaglio*, 128–9.
[225] Ibid., 101.   [226] Lupi, *Storia della peste*, 135.

confessed that the French had paid him 15 *scudi* a day to kill his patients.[227] A letter from another canon, Francesco Maria Borri, of Milan's Collegiate Church, San Lorenzo Maggiore, to a priest serving on the Health Board, again suggests widespread belief in a French plot: their greasing of doors and walls had caused maximum confusion. Even the seat of the Milanese cardinal had been pestilentially smeared. One of the *untori* caught in the archbishop's palace and another three at Turin were thought to have been of a group of seventy sent by the French king to smear Milan's walls and doors: all three were 'dressed in the French fashion'.[228]

Not only did those in Milan and its environs blame the French, such prejudices crossed Lombardy and northern Italy. From archival sources, Paolo Preto has unearthed similar accusations at Pinerolo (Piedmont), where French doctors allegedly attempted to exterminate the local population, and at Cremona, Novara, Brescia, Mantua, and even Venice (despite being allied with the French).[229] Moreover, rumours accused other foreign enemies and allies alike. Lattuada claimed plague spreaders were afflicting other cities even more than Milan—in particular, Cremona. In Pavia, Brescia, Venice, and Bologna, many were apprehended, confessed, and executed for the crimes.[230] 'Among the arrested' he pointed to 'every sort, Italians, Spanish, Germans, French, Neapolitans, and others'.[231] Similarly, an official of Porta Romana held that 'some said the poisoning came from the Germans; others, from the French; others, the Spanish; and others that heretics were responsible, particularly ones from Geneva'.[232]

However, I have not found a single German, heretic, Genevan, or Neapolitan brought to trial or named as a plague spreader in Milan. Nor have I found stories of German *untori* in Milanese or other Lombard chronicles, even though these chroniclers saw German mercenaries as combattants in the siege of Mantua in August 1629 with troops billeted in Italian cities and the countryside during the autumn and saw their trade and troop movements from German cities into the Swiss territory of the Grisons and then into Lombardy as the conduit of the disastrous plague of 1630–2.[233] In addition, Tadino, Ripamonti, and Somaglia linked the first plague case in Milan to a Milanese soldier, Pietro Antonio Lovato, who became infected on 22 October 1629 from buying or stealing clothes from German soldiers.[234] But the Milanese did not blame these outsiders, despite tracking them as the ones carrying plague from German cities. Instead, Italians were convinced that of the foreigners, the French instigated the malicious acts and, after them, the

---

[227] Ibid., 136. The only complaint against Milanese doctors, however, concerned their stingy treatment of the poor, which 'scandalized the Health Board'; see Tadino, *Raguaglio*, ch. 56, 133.

[228] Legnani, 'Cinque lettere', Letter I, 400–1.

[229] Preto, *Epidemia*, 66, 67, 68, 70.

[230] Lattuada, 'Cronaca', 287. Despite these claims, Brighetti, *Bologna e la peste*, 43, finds in Bologna's archives only one decree (10 September 1630) against 'those who go about greasing doors, door-knobs, and other places in the city' but no executions of *untori*.

[231] Lattuada, 'Cronaca', 288, 27–8.   [232] *Processo agli untori*, 441; see also note 196.

[233] Visconti, *Commentarius*, 498; *Processo agli untori*, 509; Tadino, *Raguaglio*, 14–15; 20, 25, 26, 27–8, 50; Lampugnano, *La Pestilenza*, 22.

[234] Tadino, *Raguaglio*, 50–1. Ripamonti tells the same story but dates it a month later and calls the soldier Pier Paolo Locati; see Manzoni, *I promessi sposi*, ch. 31, 589. Somaglia, *Alleggiamento*, 479, names the soldier Pietro Paolo Locato and dates his infection to early February 1630.

Milanese's own allies and rulers, the Spanish. Spaccini maintained plague spreading was 'a Spanish invention' in alliance with the Milanesi.[235]

The last letter sent by the canon of San Lorenzo to his superior on 4 July reported that 'they [the antecedent is vague] have now discovered that the Castellan and his son [Padilla] had accomplices in their wish to annihilate all of Italy'. But it was not just a Spanish conspiracy. Among them were the Abbot of Torre, the ambassador of Savoy, his brother the Marquise of Gonzaga, and many others, amounting to more than 3000.[236] Other rumours turned to further international conspiracies pointing to various leaders of *untori*: the prince of Condé, the duke of Savoy, the pope, Cardinal Richelieu, the Genevan heretics, Albrecht von Wallenstein (supreme commander of the Austrian Habsburg armies), the Gonzaga of Mantua, the ex-governor of Milan, Don Gonzalo of Cordoba, and the king of Spain.[237] Yet despite rumours on the streets, within churches, and among the nobility, the only foreigners Milan's Sanità arrested were two Spaniards, the son of the Castellan and Don Pietro Verdeno di Saragozza, a former soldier at Milan's castle. Neither was an outsider or marginal; both belonged to the city's defences and establishment. Whether Milan was exceptional in Italy or in 1630 will need further research. In Mantua during this plague, the government made a list of 'foreign' *untori*, all eight of whom were from Genoa.[238] Moreover, the protagonist of Padre Cinquanta's drama, Casimorio, falsely hounded by Milan's soldiers as an *untore*, was (like Manzoni's Renzo) pursued because of his out-of-place dress, marking him as a foreigner: he was from Bologna.[239]

Finally, during the previous plague across Lombardy and other regions of Italy in 1574–8, Jews were mentioned as spreading it, but, as we have seen, through carelessness, not by diabolic arts. By contrast, from the records of 1630, it is as though Jews no longer inhabited Milan or Lombardy, but they did.[240] The only mention I have found of them in plague chroniclers comes from the physician Tadino, who was convinced of diabolical greasing by thousands. Yet, with the first

---

[235] Spaccini, *Cronaca di Modena*, 142.   [236] Legnani, 'Cinque lettere', Lettere V, 408.

[237] Paccagnini, 'Cronaca di un contagio', 68. These are taken from a number of sources. For Richelieu and Wallenstein, see, Nicolini, *Peste e untori*, 248 and 286.

[238] Preto, *Epidemia*, 66; Lattuada, 'Cronaca', 288. On 20 July a Genovese was found guilty and hanged for allegedly giving poisonous powders to prisoners to throw on the ground. By 26 June, in villages outside Genoa and along the Ligurian coast, walls and doors had already been reported as 'unti' with several arrests, including three Frenchmen; Nicolini, *Peste e untori*, 280. On occasion, 'foreigners' are mentioned in the transcripts as involved in plague spreading but not identified by nationality. Probably, they were from other Italian cities like the 'grande forastiero' in Piazza's trial; *Processo agli untori*, 242.

[239] Cinquanta, *La peste di Milano*; the soldiers call him 'that foreigner' (560, 562, 571, 578). Casimorio also referred to himself as a foreigner, and believed it was why he was taken as an 'untore' (613).

[240] Anti-Semitic violence occurred during this period in northern Italy but came from German Lutheran soldiers during their siege of Mantua. After stripping Mantua's Jews of their possessions, they sacked the ghetto on 25 July 1630 and chased 1200 Jewish 'men, women, and children' from the city. A German cavalry of 800 then pursued them, despoiling them of the little they had left 'down to their shirts'. The Jews arrived naked on the border with Ferrara (*Avvisi*, Urb. Lat., 1100, pt 2, f. 451v from Mantua to Venice, 457r to Rome, and 481v–2r to Venice). Around 10 August, the Jewish community ('Questa università d'Hebrei') sent 10,000 ducats to aid the 'banished Jews' on Ferrara's border (ibid., Supplemento, f. 482r). Before banishing the Jews, the German soldiers demanded 200,000 *scudi* from the Jewish ghetto. Also, see Spaccini, *Cronaca di Modena*, 106, 107, 116, 117.

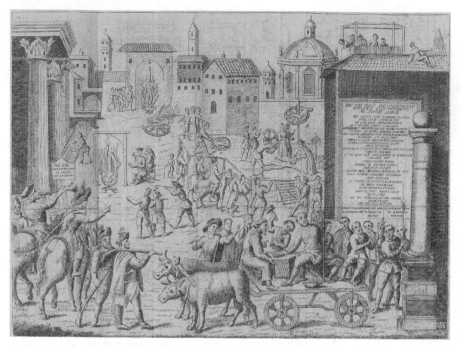

Figure 6.1. Plague in Milan, 1630, Colonna infame.

cases in late October, he advised his colleagues, physicians of Santa Corona, on how to treat cases of Jews in the neighbourhood of the borgo de Hortolani Catterina, suffering from malignant fever with pestilential symptoms. He added that these cases had arisen because of 'our sins'. He did not mention any sins of the Jews.[241]

ENGRAISSEURS IN FRENCH CITIES

Beyond Milan's, I know of no analysis of plague spreading from judicial transcripts, except for Monter's and Naphy's of Switzerland. Thus, for now, I rely on scattered court records and narrative sources for France. With the Reformation and religious wars in sixteenth-century France, the physiognomy of plague spreading emerges as differing radically from Milan's or Lombardy's. More blatant and graphic than in Italy, the Devil enters medical discourse as a causative agent of plague: operating through his 'instruments', magicians wilfully spread the disease in a new culture of blame.[242] The Reformation in France heightened attitudes

---

[241] Tadino, *Raguaglio*, 53. Given the means of transmitting plague through second-hand clothing (as contemporaries thought), Jews specializing in this trade could have easily been accused and persecuted. But they were not. For Italy, see Preto, 'Le grandi pesti', 125–6; idem, *Peste e società*, ch. 2; idem, *Epidemia*; Pastore, *Crimine e giustizia*; and *Processo agli untori*.

[242] See, for instance, Suau, *Traitez*, lib. I, 38r, 103r; lib II, 9r.

about the forces of good and bad within Europe, creating new medical writing that was political and patriotic, addressed to mayors, judges, presidents of regional parlements, and royal advisors. At the same time, staunch Catholic and royalist medical tracts saw evil machinations and threats to citizens' health coming from the 'Pretend Reformers', as in a tract by Bordeaux's physician Guillaume Briet and a similar one by an anonymous writer from Nîmes.[243] Plague became a battle hammering out Church positions. The Catholic Briet stressed sin as plague's principal cause, more so than in any previous plague tract I know by a physician or surgeon. After establishing plague's first cause as divine punishment, he rejected the standard Galenic-cosmological framework that had layered epidemic causation since the Black Death. For Briet, neither stars nor planets had great effect on disease, and impurity of air and corruption of foodstuffs and water were less important. Rather, his second cause also returned to God; plagues were His means for repressing our pride and fallen state ('nostre orgueil & le rabat'). Only with Briet's third cause—contagion—did plague enter the human realm, at least initially with contagion presented metaphorically as the military enemy, in this case, the forces of the Reformation.

In 1577, the Lyonnais historian and town councillor, Claude Rubys,[244] published a forty-four-page-long paragraph that again coupled sentiments of a religious and patriotic zealot in support of the French crown and Catholicism. More than Briet, Rubys left no doubt about who was performing the diabolical acts brought by God's wrath upon Lyon. Rubys too began with three causes of pestilence, showing similarities and differences with Briet. The first was the same as in all plague tracts that bothered mentioning it: God's scourge and will ('fleau & volonté') to punish mankind for its sin.[245] For the second, the lawyer-politician Rubys was more Galenic than the physician Briet: it was the air ('de l'infection ou mauvaise temperature de l'air').[246] As with Briet, Rubys's third cause was contagion, and it consumed most of his text. His definition began in the spirit of Fracastoro's second notion of contagion, *ad fomites*, in Rubys's words, contagion by bringing or touching infected things ('apport & atouchment de choses infectes').[247]

His notion then turned sharply from Fracastoro. This contagion was overwhelmingly caused by wilful spreading of plague by an outside population. To illustrate his point, Rubys took two cases from antiquity. The first was the supposed pestilence of Emperor Commodus' time, narrated by the late second-century CE Dio Cassius. But Rubys rewrote it, claiming Commodus created the pestilence that killed 2000 a day. By bribing certain wicked ones to go through Rome greasing ('engressees de venin') things people normally touched, the disease spread violently; Commodus became our first grand *engraisseur*.[248] Rubys then connected this disease to acts Dio considered separate and unexplained, criminals' pricking of people at random with poisoned needles. For Rubys, the prickers were *engraisseurs,* and the same had happened in Domitan's reign (despite Dio not mentioning

---

[243] Briet, *Explication*; idem, *Discours sur les causes*; and *Remede tres salutaire.*
[244] *Biographie universelle*, vol. 37, 22.   [245] Rubys, *Discours sur la contagion*, 5.
[246] Ibid., 6.   [247] Ibid., 7.   [248] Ibid.

any epidemic at that time). In describing the Black Death, Rubys's language also hinted at wilful plague spreading from foreign places: it was 'brought' from the Levant 'where the disease had reigned for a long time' to Genoa and thereafter 'inseminated through all of Italy *(& de puis de peu à fut semee par toute l'Italie)*'.[249]

But on plague greasers Rubys became more strident when he came to contemporary history: 'in our time experience has shown in many places evidence of these plague spreaders *(engresseurs)*'. He pointed first to Chambéry ('Chambrey'), where those accused of greasing objects confessed their crimes. He then reflected on his school days at Padua, when a Spanish doctor and several charged with cleaning houses of plague victims were found guilty, hanged, and strangled, for producing 'certain plasters composed of plague prepared by the Spanish doctor'.[250] No contemporary or subsequent secondary Italian source mentions the incident.[251] With his hometown of Lyon, Rubys's story comes into clearer focus and is given a motive. He first praised Lyon's officials for their well-organized policing of the city and charitable provisioning to the ill and poor. Their care 'was so well governed that two-thirds', he claims, 'recovered'.[252] Yet the plague still spread because of diabolic forces. In villages along the Rhone near Lyon, 'engresseurs' at night infected the gravelly beaches ('le gravier') along the Rhone to 'entrap' poor washermen and women, arriving the following morning. 'Miraculously' God intervened, allowing the 'bonnes gardes' of Lyon to discover the plot.[253] It had been a political conspiracy engineered by Calvinists, comparable to the Catiline conspiracy in ancient Rome. The Calvinists attempted to topple the French crown, taking by surprise one of its most important cities. He argued that previously the contagion in 1567 came from Protestant strongholds in Germany, especially Basel, where Calvinists put poisonous 'pastes' in bales of merchandise sent to Lyon. Again, thanks to God, the city's patriotic order, and threat of the 'gibet', the danger from 'Les Calvinistes predestinez' was averted.[254]

Finally, in the year of his pamphlet's publication (1577), 'when plague raged in Venice, Milan, and other Lombard towns', Rubys claimed 'engresseurs' from the Protestant mountain stronghold of Grison had manufactured the plague with 'the same ends' as the Calvinist heretics. Under the pretext of trading at fairs with the privileges of 'supposed Grisons', the Calvinists infiltrated Italy and from there carried the contagion to Lyon. But because the Lyonnais were loyal, loving servants of the crown, they carefully cleaned their city, and their guards zealously policed its gates. As a result, the plague's toll at the time of his writing was in decline.[255] Nonetheless, despite differences with Italy, Rubys's stories of purposeful plague

---

[249] Ibid.

[250] Ibid., 9. It was not clear that he had been a 'ieusne escolier' at Padua; instead, he is reported to have studied only at Paris and Toulouse; see 'Rubys' in *Biographie universelle*, vol. 37, 22.

[251] None of the plague tracts on Padua or Italy refers to this case. Nor does Preto, *Epidemia*, mention it or similar accusations in Padua. Only in Venice were there accusations at that time against 'some plague cleaners *(picegamorti)*' attempting to prolong the illness by spreading infected clothing along Venice's canals (26–7). Tadino, *Raguaglio*, 120, comes closest, listing 'quella di Padova dell'anno 1555' as an incident of plague spreading but says no more about it.

[252] Rubys, *Discours sur la contagion*, 26.   [253] Ibid., 29.

[254] Ibid., 30–3.   [255] Ibid., 33–8.

spreading also did not implicate the destitute. Instead, its myths turned on political and religious causes steeped in fantasies of Counter-Reformation hatred.

Although Rubys blamed regions within the Protestant Swiss Alps for sourcing the plague's manufactured poisons, his tales fail to support notions of these regions as primitive zones exporting their diabolic fantasies to big cities down the slopes.[256] Besides, Geneva, Lyon, and Milan were not the only cities infected by mythologies of plague spreading. In other regions far from the Alps—Cahors, Albigeois, Quercy, Toulouse, Paris, and Rouen—such accusations sprang forth, some antedating those at Lyon and Milan. The Parlementaire arrêts of Toulouse reveal elite and popular beliefs in plague spreading followed by the State's vicious measures of cere-monial torture and execution. These records also report cases beyond Toulouse's borders. In 1559, within Albigeois and Quercy, 'many' were discovered 'inseminat-ing plague artificially' and condemned to death. The court reported it because, at the same time, such people had been discovered in Toulouse, sentenced to death, and burnt alive. In the same year, one disguised as a poor man, was found greasing in the town of Espère,[257] north of Cahors in south-west France, and stoned to death. The same arrêt alluded to Jewish thieves 'in other times' punished for the same crime, one of whom was identified, but the dates and places were left vague.[258]

More tellingly, in Toulouse 'certain Italians' were tried in the royal courts for 'having promised to kill all the Huguenots' with plague. The proof against them rested on the supposed allegations that plague had hit Montpellier, Nîmes, Aigue-Mortes and 'other Huguenot towns', but 'not a single Catholic town was afflicted'. Several Italians were burnt alive, with notices posted assuring 'that execution would be promised to other of the said Italians'.[259] A lawyer of Nîmes, who edited a second edition of these sixteenth-century arrêts, reached further back in the century, finding the hunt and execution of plague spreaders at Toulouse as early as any in Geneva or elsewhere since the Black Death. This parlement noted prosecutions against two notorious ('si fameux') plague spreaders: one called Caddoz was tortured by pincers, decapitated, and quartered during the plague of 1530, and a second, called Lentille, met a similar end in 1545. Unfortunately, no more is noted about them, except that they infused scraps of clothing with their poisonous powders and scattered them in the streets and peoples' homes.[260]

M. G. de la Faille's early eighteenth-century chronicle of Toulouse comments that the city's rulers (capitouls) nipped plague in the bud in April 1542 by arresting two *semeurs*.[261] Further executions of plague spreaders, not mentioned in the published arrêts or by la Faille, can be found. In 1543 the annalist Louvet[262] reported 'two ministers of the devil' who made plasters from the bodies of plague

---

[256] Bercé, 'Les semeurs'.   [257] About 130 km north of Toulouse.

[258] *Arrests... de Tolose*, Arrest II, 202–3.   [259] Ibid., 202.

[260] *Arrests... de Tolose*, nouvelle edition, 237. Astruc, *Dissertation sur la contagion*, 88; and Chicoyneau, *Traité des causes*, 133, copied Graverol's note verbatim. These two Enlightenment intel-lectuals, the second the king's physician, added that 'the famous villains (*fameux scelerats*) were justly punished by the Parlement de Toulouse'.

[261] La Faille, *Annales*, 126. These were not recorded in La Roche-Flavin's summary of Toulouse's arrêts.

[262] An archival source, which Roucaud does not identify by name or date.

victims to grease the city ('pour semer par la ville') but were caught and condemned to death by fire.[263] In the following year 'other ministers of the devil' sought to poison Toulouse's wells and fountains but were also caught and burnt. In 1560, the only named woman in these arrêts, Jeanne de Saint-Pé, was convicted of plague spreading and hanged outside the gate of l'Isle, with her body afterwards burnt. [264] Finally, Joseph Roucaud from Toulouse's archives départementales reports the only case of plague spreading in seventeenth-century France that I have found, during what he called Toulouse's 'most memorable' plague, that of 1628–32.[265] It was also the only case from Toulouse to prosecute plague workers. In October 1629, two 'désinfecteurs' were discovered at night greasing the streets with infected wool. They were also charged with theft, then hanged, and their corpses burnt.[266]

These charges against plague spreaders affected not only southern France, as seen from Toulouse's arrêts. During a plague of 1581, Parisians noted plague deaths rising and believed the increase was caused by 'the wickedness of such people, who spread (*semoient*) it by certain gangrenous swabs (*pourritures*), plasters, and other infectious materials'. As a result, the king authorized citizens to kill without liability or future judicial scrutiny anyone found committing these acts. The Toulouse arrêts suggest that by the late sixteenth century such suspicions had become rife throughout France. To discover and seize plague spreaders, the crown recommended that guards be posted, night and day, in 'all towns and villages, and along the roads and byways of the great cities'.[267] Anticipatory of attacks against cholera spreaders in nineteenth-century Europe, the Toulouse arrêts signalled that doctors might be among the 'Maistres de cet art', using their knowledge of remedies not only to cure but to kill patients, treating 'ulcers on the chest with caustic herbs that give vent to the poison (*venin*), driving it straight to the heart'.[268] But only with this hint (and the previously mentioned conviction of two 'désinfecteurs') do these records point to the medical profession or to anyone else employed by a Health Board, and none indicted any from the lower echelons of 'destitute' plague cleaners.

As in Lyon, but in stark contrast to Milan, the major tensions exacerbated by early modern plagues in and around Toulouse concerned religious faith and the political conflict between Catholics and Protestants. Investigation of Toulouse's archives would surely uncover further charges of plague spreading. For the present, however, the published arrêts constitute almost the entire set of known cases of *engraisseurs* for early modern France outside of Lyon and indicate that Lyon was hardly alone in being riveted by these divisive accusations. Their timing was not the same as in Italy, where the accusations increased notably with the plagues of the last two years of the sixteenth century in Piedmont and more sharply during seventeenth century in Sicily, Lombardy, Piedmont, and the Veneto,[269] while in France they clustered between 1530 and 1582. Thus far, our sources point to no executions or even arrests in seventeenth-century France beyond one case in

[263] Roucaud, *La peste à Toulouse*, 464–5.

[264] Ibid., 445. Although Roucard comments at length on the arrêts published by La Roche-Flavin, he cites none of the documents on plague spreaders.

[265] Ibid., 112.   [266] Ibid., 446, from 'Déliberations capitulaires', 10 December 1629.

[267] *Arrests … de Tolose*, 202.   [268] Ibid.   [269] See Preto, *Epidemia*, chs 2–5.

Toulouse. As with Geneva, the hunt for plague spreaders was by then in deep decline or had disappeared entirely.[270]

On the other hand, even at their height in mid-sixteenth-century Toulouse, these trials and executions by burning alive cannot compete with the concurrent hysteria and brutality of witchcraft trials or with later waves of European cholera riots. Toulouse's la Faille records seventeen plague years between 1515 and 1610 and four other major epidemics—three of a disease called Coquelache in 1515, 1557, and 1580, the last of which resulted in the city closing schools, judicial courts, and prohibiting any public assembly,[271] and one of dysentery ('dissenterie') in 1545, infecting a third of the city and for which doctors could find no remedy.[272] But for only one of these—the plague of 1542—does he mention any hunt or execution of *semeurs de la peste*.[273]

Moreover, none of these incidents could be called a plague riot. The only such riots occurred far from France towards the end of the 'Second Pandemic' with the disastrous plague of Moscow in 1771. At the height of that plague on 15 September with 920 dying a day,[274] 'thousands' of rioters, composed mostly of domestic serfs, poured into the streets, ransacked monasteries and places of quarantine, freed the inmates and attacked soldiers and government officials, anticipating the cholera riots of the 1830s. Moreover, popular antipathies towards the medical profession had been provoked earlier in this plague by measures preventing the populace from touching the dead or performing traditional religious and funerary ceremonies. Yet this riot differed from the bulk of cholera riots sixty years later. The Moscow riot of 1771 was essentially a religious revolt, sparked by troops preventing crowds from assembling in front of an icon of 'the Mother of God', which commoners believed protected them from plague.[275] The chief victim of the riot was the city's archbishop, Amvrosii, who betrayed them by agreeing to the government's quarantines. Once the 'mob' found him, they tortured then murdered him, mutilating his body by piercing his eyes, pulling out his beard, and breaking his bones turning his body into 'a single wound'.[276] Although the house of the physician Mertens was pillaged and several other doctors were pursued, none appears to have been injured,[277] and rumours did not spread of physicians spreading the disease to kill off the poor.

---

[270] For the plague in Lyon in 1628–9, Papon, *De la peste*, I, 180, reports that there were claims of evil ones ('des scélérats') purposely spreading plague but reports no arrests, trials, or executions. Nor does he report any at Montpellier, Digne, Aix, and Marseille (185–93, 194–206, and 206). Monter, *Witchcraft in France*, 45, mentions plague spreading at Vevey in the canton of Vaud but no arrests or executions. However, Savoy had a different pattern: trials against *engraisseurs* appear as early as 1564 and continue until 1703; Greslou, *La Peste en Savoie*, 129–33.

[271] La Faille, *Annales de la ville de Toulouse*, 367–8.   [272] Ibid., 137.

[273] Ibid., 1515 (2), 1520 (22), 1521 (24), 1527, 1528, 1529 (65), 1542 (126), 1548 (151), 1556 (185), 1557 (188), 1559 (200), 1561 (247), 1585 (391), 1586 (395), 1587 (399–400), 1593 (469), and 1608 (542). His first volume is far less attentive to plague; the Black Death is not even mentioned (90–1).

[274] Alexander, *Bubonic Plague*, 186. This was the official figure; the resident physician at Moscow's Founding Hospital put it at 1200; Mertens, *An Account*, 23.

[275] Alexander, *Bubonic Plague*, ch. 7, esp. 186–95; and Mertens, *An Account*, 22–3.

[276] Alexander, *Bubonic Plague*, 194–5.   [277] Ibid., 193–4.

In summary, as far as disease-fuelled hatred and persecution of others goes, the Black Death did not cast a centuries-long shadow over Europe. Accusations of plague spreading did not resurface until the 1530s and were short-lived. In early modern Italy it turned inward against established insiders, even elites, and not the 'destitute and the poor' or marginalized minorities, while in France and Switzerland, it was aroused by religious enmity and turned against 'others'—Protestants in Catholic towns and Catholics in Protestant ones. Nonetheless, the poor, religious minorities, and the lowest orders of plague workers were never the principal victims. Finally, nowhere did it unleash mass violence as plague had in 1348 or as was to ensue with certain diseases in the nineteenth century. As Part III will illustrate, the hate–disease nexus blossomed instead with modernity.

PART III

MODERNITY:
EPIDEMICS OF HATE

7

Cholera's First European Tour
The Story in the British Isles

While early modernity gave rise to the blaming and persecution of plague spreaders, this violence was limited compared to the Black Death massacres, religious persecution of the sixteenth and seventeenth centuries, or witchcraft trials from Scotland to central Italy. The persecution and blame of supposed plague spreaders concerned individuals, rarely groups. Nor were those persecuted on the margins, such as plague cleaners as is supposed. Instead, those targeted were mainly insiders—male artisans and indigenous elites—clergymen, bankers, and military officers. Moreover, plague was the only disease to incite such violent blame in early modernity. The Great Pox aroused no riots against any group before the late nineteenth century, nor did it lead to persecution of any definable group, including women, before the late sixteenth century.

With the spread of cholera from the Ganges in India into Europe and Asia in the nineteenth century, matters changed: modernity, instead of decoupling the disease–hate nexus, intensified its lethality.[1] Under strikingly different political regimes and social contexts, cholera ignited waves of social violence against the rich, government officials, hospital workers, and especially doctors during its first pan-European outbreaks, 1830–7. Scholars have thus far studied much more intensively the social violence provoked by this wave than the subsequent six bouts combined that continue to the present. Before concentrating on the curious pro-longation of cholera's social violence, I shall examine cholera riots in the British Isles during the first wave, relying partially on the secondary literature[2] but, as with other chapters, more on primary sources, especially recent online newspaper archives.[3] These reveal seventy-two cholera riots from the disease's first landing in

---

[1] Historians have not found cholera riots in India, even when looking for them, as with Ian Catanach's 'Fatalism?', 184–5, when the agrarian Deccan Riots (1875) coincided with a cholera epidemic. I have found one Indian cholera riot. Its size, timing, character, and mythologies contrast sharply with Europe's. In August 1930, villagers at Gujal (Adilabad) performed ceremonies to propitiate the cholera goddess. A woman speaking as the goddess blamed another woman of the village for bringing it. Men beat the accused to death; *Singapore Free Press*, 11 August 1930, 18; and *Malaya Tribune*, 26 August 1930, 14. Also, see chapter 9, note 152, for possibly another Indian cholera riot in 1943.

[2] Morris, *Cholera 1832*; Durey, *The Return of the Plague*; and *Cholera & Conflict*.

[3] These include 'The Nineteenth Century British Newspapers', *The Times Digital Archive, Guardian and Observer, Scotsman*, and the BNA, accessed 22 July 2015. 'The Nineteenth Century British Newspapers' do not always show page numbers.

Britain in November 1831 to January 1833.[4] Rumours and myths of elites and especially of physicians employing the disease or inventing it to murder the poor galvanized communities to assemble in crowds in the thousands to attack hospitals and 'liberate' neighbours and kin from what the rioters perceived as death chambers.

Newspaper articles suggest that more cholera riots occurred than the ones I have been able to identify by place or date from thousands of newspaper pages and other sources. For instance, a paper claimed that in 'numerous instances in London and elsewhere... the misguided rabble have risen against... their only friends... the medical men'. It then listed three instances without specifying dates, places, or if the perpetrators were crowds or individuals, in which doctors were threatened 'and even assaulted': one narrowly escaped being thrown from a two-storey window; a ferocious dog was set upon a surgeon; and an Irishman, armed with a knife, attempted to stab a medical attendant.[5] Were these acts of collective violence? Another article, entitled 'Cholera Battles' reported 'several skirmishes with the doctors', concluding that they arose because 'the people' believe the sick 'are taken away to be dissected'.[6] It failed to report, however, the number of skirmishes, where they occurred, or if they constituted collective action. In Liverpool, eighty of the city's 'medical gentlemen' issued a circular, decrying the 'disgraceful outrages' to which they had been subjected, 'despite their offer of free treatment'. As with those above the places, dates, and character of the 'outrage' were unreported.[7]

Some riots may appear in local papers yet to be included in newspaper collections and others should be recoverable from police archives. For instance, in commenting on cholera's arrival in Belfast, *The Belfast News-Letter* expressed the hope that 'all classes will imitate the exemplary and noble conduct of the inhabitants of Edinburgh, and avoid such disgraceful acts as have occurred in Glasgow and Paisley.[8] This report appeared a week before Paisley's famous riot after boys discovered shovels and a hook in the town cemetery,[9] the only disturbance thus far found for Paisley. In other cases, the riots may have been too inconsequential or controversial for coverage. A short obituary of Thomas Rumley, a president of the Irish Royal College of Surgeons, reported a cholera riot even before the disease became epidemic there. At Kingstown, a seaport outside Dublin, a man with stomach disorders died in a back alley, and medical attendants diagnosed the cause of death as cholera. Kingstown's inhabitants called two doctors from Dublin, Rumley and William Stoker, for confirmation. According to the obituary, Kingstown's inhabitants rioted and attacked Stokes [sic] and Rumley because they pronounced the case as cholera. They 'narrowly escaped with their lives'. In the rapidly growing BNA, only one article has appeared concerning the incident, but it did not mention a riot.[10] Instead, by its

---

[4] For definitions of riots, revolts, and rebellions, see Cohn, *Lust for Liberty*, 3–9. In short, riots were collective actions consisting of groups larger than families or small gangs that used or threatened violence. In later chapters, I also distinguish riots from peaceful demonstrations.

[5] *Lancaster Gazette*, 14 April 1832 (from *London Medical Gazette*) sought to justify the decision of Paisley's surgeons to cease attending the poor afflicted with cholera, after the Paisley riots.

[6] *Corbett's Weekly*, 7 April 1832.   [7] *Liverpool Mercury*, 8 June 1832.

[8] *Belfast News-Letter*, 20 March 1832.

[9] *Morning Chronicle*, 30 March 1832; also see notes 64–6.

[10] Accessed 20 July 2015.

account Rumley and Stoker found 'the symptoms' insufficient to point to cholera.[11] However, as Ruth Newman has argued for cholera in Salisbury during the next wave of 1849, newspaper coverage by local papers could be problematic. For the commercial well-being of a town, a news blackout could ensue.[12] These problems, as we shall see, became more pronounced with later cholera waves at the end of the nineteenth and early twentieth century, when national governments in Russia and Italy and to some extent in Spain and other countries censored reports of cholera, and more so, any violence it might have spawned, to protect commerce, tourism, and national prestige. Often with the telegram and telephone, correspondents leaked the news to foreign papers. For these later events, small-town US or Australian papers could reveal more than local ones where the riots occurred.[13]

In addition, present technological problems of online searches lead to incidents being missed. First, unclear print and deficiency in the optical capacity in recognizing scans (OCR) affect keyword identification. 'Riot', for instance, is often read as 'not' and vice versa, and for other reasons words such as 'cholera', which appear clearly printed, can pass without digital recognition. More time consuming is the opposite problem of abundant false-positives. Searches for single words such as 'cholera' can generate thousands of pages of results, 99 per cent of which have nothing to do with any socio-psychological reactions to cholera. To make searches more economical, I employed double-word searches as with 'cholera' and 'riot' or 'cholera' and 'mob'. However, the vast majority of these searches produce pages without association between the words. The unit of analysis for these dual keyword searches is rarely the individual article but instead the page or multiple columns. With large formats and small print, these pages can contain 30,000 words and twenty or more articles on a wide variety of topics with one, for instance, reporting cholera mortalities, while another, Reform Act riots.

Moreover, cholera riots may have arisen with neither 'mob' nor 'riot' used. One riot I did not find in contemporary newspapers occurred in Exeter which resisted newly imposed burial regulations preventing cholera victims from being interred within consecrated grounds.[14] Moreover, the cholera doctor Thomas Shapter reported a second one at Exeter, sparked by the same myth of doctors poisoning cholera patients or giving them drugs to put them to sleep so they could be buried alive.[15] My keyword searches did not uncover it; nor has the secondary literature mentioned it. On the other hand, these searches have spotted cholera riots yet to be reported in the literature, even large ones such as at Wick, near mainland Scotland's furthest north-eastern point: an estimated crowd of 1500[16] ranks it the fourth largest cholera riot in British history.[17]

---

[11] *Saunders's News-Letter*, 21 April 1832, 2.   [12] Newman, 'Salisbury in the Age of Cholera'.
[13] See Chapters 8–10 on cholera, as well as the chapters on plague and influenza.
[14] Morris, *Cholera 1832*, 106, 127, says it was a resistance to burial regulation but does not date it, and cites Shapter, *Exeter*, as does Evesley, 'L'Angleterre', 175.
[15] Shapter, *Exeter*, 235–6, for the first riot, and 237 for the second.
[16] *Morning Post*, 1 August 1832, from *Edinburgh Evening Courant*.
[17] *Aberdeen Journal*, 4 August 1932, 6, revisited the event on its centenary.

Despite excellent analyses of British cholera violence in 1832, few comparisons have been drawn with riots on the Continent or elsewhere during the 1830s, for later cholera outbreaks, or between regions within the British Isles. First, of seventy-two cholera riots in the British Isles, thirty-two (44 per cent) occurred in England, twenty-two in Ireland, and eighteen in Scotland. From my survey none appeared in Wales, and I know of none reported in the secondary literature.[18] Perhaps cholera was less socially violent in Wales because it was less virulent there. However, with the next wave in 1849, when mortality and lethality figures become available, cholera proved as serious in Wales as anywhere else in the British Isles.[19] No one has asked: why no cholera riots in Wales?

As far as per capita ratios go, the number of riots in England and Wales, Ireland and Scotland is the reverse of that seen from the aggregate figures: based on their 1831 population (13,897,187), 2.30 cholera revolts per million inhabitants appeared for England and Wales in 1831–2; 2.83 per million for Ireland (7,784,539); and 7.61 for Scotland (2,365,114). Given these figures, the ratio of those dying from cholera was also higher in Ireland (20,070 cholera deaths or 3.76 per thousand) than in England and Wales (21,882 cholera deaths or 0.63 per thousand), and was considerably higher in Scotland than elsewhere in the British Isles (9592 cholera deaths or 4.06 per thousand).[20] In England, these riots erupted principally in the largest cities, led by London (13), Bristol (5), Liverpool (3), Birmingham (2), and Manchester (1), comprising all but seven disturbances (78 per cent). Moreover, the remaining ones also erupted in substantial towns—Exeter (2), Sunderland, Worcester, York, Durham, Wigan—and none in market towns or villages. Here, the Irish and Scottish riots differed from the English. Three flared up in Scotland's then largest city, Edinburgh; seven in its city on the rise, Glasgow; two in Greenock; and one in Aberdeen. The remainder arose in small industrial market towns, or villages— Paisley, Wick, and Leith (then a fishing village, separate from Edinburgh), Invergordon, a fishing village in Easter Ross, and the small village of Pathhead in Kirkcaldy (Fife). In Ireland, the provincial town and village context was more pronounced: five occurred in Dublin and one in Belfast, while the majority were in county towns or villages: Sligo (3), Boyle (2), Londonderry (1), Drogheda (1), Donegal (1), Kingstown (1); and then the villages of Claremorris (2), Ardee (1), Kilkenny (1), Killineer (1), Ballina near Killalal (1), and Blackrock (1).

Although cholera riots broke out in impoverished districts, whether rural or big-city slums, it would be difficult to argue that a strong correlation linked the severity of the disease in a place to the likelihood of a cholera riot. To be sure, there were towns badly hit, where rioting was prevalent. Ireland's Sligo, in the province of Connacht, was per capita the worst hit of any place in the British Isles. At least two-thirds of its population fled that year and of those remaining, the disease killed

---

[18] None appears in the online Scottish, English, or Irish papers. I have also searched 'Welsh Newspapers Online', containing all newspapers available at the National Library of Wales 1804–1910—1.1 million pages; accessed 23 July 2015.

[19] Michael and Thompson, *Public Health in Wales*, 16.

[20] These figures derive from Creighton, II, 816.

one in four.[21] According to Edinburgh's *The Caledonian Mercury*, the statistics were even bleaker: by 1 September only 2860 persons remained; 14,000 had left or died.[22] Nine days later, the paper revised its figures, claiming only 1000 stayed of a population that numbered 15,000 at the beginning of the year.[23] The paper painted a picture of children deserted by their parents, 'with the distress of the widows and orphans left in the town…frightful'.[24] Local papers argued that the people's 'most violent' resistance to medical services fuelled the virulence of the disease, resulting in medical attendants not being appointed. Further, 'the infatuated people crowding into the very rooms of the dying, and holding wakes' further fuelled 'the pestilence'.[25] By contrast, the most devastated town in England was Bilston in the West Midlands.[26] With a population of 14,500 before the epidemic, 2250 cases or 16 per cent of the population was infected and 693 died. Yet no source mentions a cholera riot here or even rumours of blame.[27]

Despite wide discrepancies in the places where cholera riots occurred, their targets of blame and violence, composition of crowds, prevailing conspiracies, and myths show a close resemblance across the British Isles. None pointed to the larger politics then swirling, the movements that led to the various reform acts of 1832. As elsewhere across Europe, the chief targets of the British and Irish riots were those in the medical profession, especially doctors and surgeons, along with hospitals and their equipment—cots, litters, and hearses (palanquins) used to carry victims to hospital or their graves. As the reports often make clear, these vehicles were expensive and, as revealed by their ritualistic destruction, possessed heightened symbolic value for the rioters. When the surgeon's assistant and his party came with an 'accommodation chair' to carry off an afflicted shoemaker of Lisson Grove to the Mary-la-bonne Cholera Hospital, Camden Town, a 'mob' of around 600 blocked his removal. On reaching its destination at Church Street, the crowd chanted 'they were going to Burke the man'. The chair was seized and 'the poor fellow in a state of nudity' pulled out 'in a lifeless state', placed on a rioter's back, and taken home. At Earl Street, 'the mob' tore the chair 'to atoms' and with its fragments 'furiously' pelted the doctor and his party.[28] In Manchester's riot of early September, 'several thousands of people, principally of the lower class', seized one of the new spring vehicles for transporting cholera patients, smashed it to pieces,

---

[21] See Henry, *Sligo*, 83: In the census before the cholera outbreak, Sligo's population was between 15,000 and 16,000; at the end of 1832, less than 4000 remained: 1230 cases with 641 cholera deaths. Because of concealment of cholera cases and deaths, both figures would have been higher here, where denial of the disease and disruption to medical services were severe.

[22] *Caledonian Mercury*, 1 September 1832.   [23] Ibid., 10 September 1832.

[24] Ibid., 1 September 1832. *The Belfast News-Letter*, 28 August 1832, reported 'many' inhabitants had taken shelter in the woods: 'Every house is closed'.

[25] *Freeman's Journal*, 31 August 1832, relying on *Sligo Journal* and *Mayo Constitution*. Papers also claimed that resistance to health officers fuelled cholera at Pathhead, Kirkcaldy; *The Times*, 22 August 1832, 3.

[26] Morris, *Cholera 1832*, 132.

[27] Durey, *The Return of the Plague*, 186. Greater attention has been paid to Bilston's high rate, but Sligo's was five times that of Bilston.

[28] *Morning Chronicle*, 31 March 1832.

then 'carefully burnt its fragments'. A police posse saved a second vehicle in the nick of time. These chairs cost the Board of Health 'a considerable sum of money'.[29]

Crowd anger in several cholera riots in Dublin focused totemistically on these vehicles. A litter transporting a cholera patient along Ormond Quay to the hospital mobilized 'a mob of ruffians'. The patient was 'forcibly' taken from the litter and 'carried off in triumph' with the litter flung into the river. Several then jumped in to break it 'into pieces'. That morning, two further riots produced similar occurrences with cots or litters demolished and burnt in the streets.[30] The same week, riots broke out in other parts of Dublin, again hijacking cholera vehicles and destroying cots, preventing patients from being taken to hospitals.[31] One 'mob', estimated at 200, injured officers with stones and yelled 'Sack' em up!', 'Burn the cot!' A tailor seized it and began leaping on top of it.[32] In Edinburgh a van carrying a cholera patient to the hospital at Castle Hill[33] met a similar fate. The crowd assailed the van and its driver with stones then ripped the van's top off. The driver escaped to the Fountainbridge quarantine but before he reached it, they seized his cart, drove it to Canal Basin, and threw it in.[34] More than half of the riots (37) turned on cholera vehicles with frenzied destruction by smashing, drowning, or burning these precious objects of the medical corps. On occasion, the assaults extended beyond their neighbourhoods, the hospital, or cemetery, as in Ballina in Ireland, where 'peasants' destroyed the vehicles between Ballina and Sligo and wrecked roads and bridges to prevent future cholera sufferers being removed to hospitals.[35]

BODY SNATCHING

While some of the reporting was matter-of-fact, without indicating the rioters' chants or speculating on causes or on what they believed, journalists in thirty-four of these incidents described rumours circulating among the rioters and speculated on motives. Overwhelmingly, the crowds believed doctors and hospitals were scheming to exterminate their patients. In this regard, cholera myths were uncannily similar, from Asiatic Russia to New York City, but the British ones had a particular twist and urgency stemming from events in the recent past. Surgeons such as John Hunter[36] had urged the medical profession to train a new generation of surgeons with demonstrations on human cadavers. As a result, new anatomy colleges spread across Britain in the 1820s, creating a soaring demand for cadavers. Three years before cholera's first appearance in Sunderland (November 1831),

---

[29] *Morning Post*, 3 September 1832; *The Times*, 5 September 1832, 3; and ibid., 6 September 1832, 4.
[30] *Morning Chronicle*, 27 April 1832, from *Courier*.
[31] *Saunder's News-Letter*, 25 April 1832, front page.   [32] Ibid., 27 April 1832, front page.
[33] It was one of the city's largest cholera hospitals, with 318 cases, with 187 dying, a lethality rate of 59 per cent; see Creighton, II, 812.
[34] *Scotsman*, 17 March 1832, 2.
[35] *Lancaster Gazette*, 6 October 1832, from *Literary Gazette* (Sligo), 9 September 1832.
[36] Morris, *Cholera 1832*, 101.

efforts to satisfy the new educational creed ignited a national scandal that quickly translated into a nightmare for the poor and labouring classes. In Edinburgh in 1828, to supply Dr Robert Knox with bodies for his anatomy lectures, William Burke and William Hare murdered sixteen people in ten months. The trial filled British newspapers, and remained alive in the minds of the poor when cholera reached Britain. These scandals were not restricted to Edinburgh. Two years earlier in Liverpool, three casks containing eleven salted bodies mysteriously appeared for anatomical dissection.[37] In January 1828, discovery of such a body sparked rioting in Dublin's streets resulting in a porter at Dublin's College of Surgeons being killed. According to the nineteenth-century chronicler of Ireland's Royal College of Surgeons, exporting corpses from Dublin had gone unchallenged before this discovery. Earlier, a company of purveyors made the Royal College's school a warehouse 'for their ghastly goods' destined for lecturers at other institutions in Dublin, London, and Edinburgh.[38] Still earlier, in 1822, mobs at Dublin wrecked and burnt down the house of Robert Adams, where he instructed apprentices in dissection.[39] As far as the politics of dissection and passage of the Anatomy Act go, the most significant scandal after Burke and Hare was a similar case of murder for cadavers by Bishop and Williams in 1831.[40] As chants and slurs recorded in newspapers during British cholera riots in Sunderland,[41] Liverpool,[42] Glasgow,[43] Bristol,[44] the East End of London,[45] Camden Town,[46] and Dublin[47] make clear, 'to burke', 'burking', and 'Burker' had entered working-class slang, reflecting new fears and obsessions.[48]

In one of the British Isles' earliest cholera riots,[49] the crowd went beyond chants to destroy an anatomy school. Curiously, this major riot—by newspapers' estimates,

---

[37] See McDuff, 'The 1832 Liverpool Cholera Riots', 95.

[38] Cameron, *History of the Royal College of Surgeons*, 183–4.

[39] Ibid., 520. Similar incidents occurred at Carlisle, Greenwich, Deptford, and Great Yarmouth; Richardson, *Death*, 75–6, 78, 87, 89.

[40] Richardson, *Death*, 132 and 143.   [41] See note 49.

[42] Durey, *The Return of the Plague*, 162 and 178, for four riots in early June; and *Preston Chronicle*, 9 June 1832, 3.

[43] It arose with Glasgow's first cholera riot in February 1832 and was repeated in March and April; see Durey, *The Return of the Plague*, 178.

[44] *Bristol Mercury*, 11 August 1832.

[45] *Scotsman*, 7 April 1832, 2; *Caledonian Mercury*, 5 April 1832; *Westmorland Gazette* 9 June 1832, 3.

[46] *Morning Chronicle*, 31 March 1832.   [47] Burrell, 'The Irish Cholera Epidemic', 230.

[48] More generally, see Durey, *The Return of the Plague*, 176–7; Gill, Burrell, and Brown, 'Fear and Frustration', 237.

[49] On 12 November 1831, a mob formed outside a meeting of the Health Board in Sunderland when cholera first entered Britain, chanting, 'Down with Clanning! Down with Clanning!' (the Health Board's chairman); *Morning Post*, 18 November 1831. A week before, Clanning had signed a letter published in the London papers, mentioning 'the undeniable fact' of cholera in Sunderland. *The Hull Packet*, 29 November 1831, reported that the mob would attack Dr Clanny's [sic] house. But no damage to property occurred. This 'mob' appears unusual for cholera. It must have been a newspaper-reading crowd who read the London papers, not local ones; it did not produce the usual myths of doctors murdering patients but protested restrictions on shipping that resulted from the Medical Board's communiqué (see *Morning Post*, 18 November 1831).

by far the largest in the British Isles[50]—has received little attention,[51] but contemporary papers described it in detail. In Aberdeen on the morning of 26 December 1831, a dog dug up the remains of a dead body, gathering 'a mob' which increased in number 'to nearly 20,000':

> A cry was raised of 'Burn the house; down with the burking shop'. Shavings, fir, tar, barrels and staves, were quickly procured and lighted, and within five minutes the back wall fell down with a tremendous crash. The building was completely destroyed, and had not the mob been kept in check by the sight of the military… other acts of violence would, no doubt, have been committed.[52]

Certainly, the estimation of the crowd size was exaggerated; it would have amounted to almost two-thirds of Aberdeen's old city population—men, women, children, and infants included.[53] All the same, this early cholera riot was one of the most significant in the British Isles by the damage it caused alone. It was the only one to have destroyed an anatomy college. Unlike on the Continent, where *carabinieri*, soldiers, *gendarmerie*, Russian troops, and Cossacks were regularly summoned to smash large crowds, this was the only one in Scotland to have summoned the military and one of four in the British Isles (two in Ireland and one in England).[54] Nonetheless, it did not result in mass arrests or executions: only three were brought to trial, and the judge expressed sympathy for the men: the three were sentenced to twelve months in the Aberdeen gaol and blame was partially placed on the medical profession for its gross negligence.[55]

Other riots across Britain expose similar fears and vocabulary. Less than week after the Lisson Grove riot, 'an infuriated mob' attacked a cholera hospital in another London neighbourhood, St George's Hospital in the East End, and threatened to kill its surgeons. The crowd's motives were clear: the surgeons were 'Burking the poor wretches who were admitted [to the hospital]'.[56] At the beginning of June, two further cholera riots in London raised suspicions of hospitals and hatred of 'medical gentlemen', invoking the new slang. Near Vauxhall Road, a child whose father just died and whose mother was afflicted called a surgeon. 'Imbib[ing] a strange prejudice against the doctors', 'the whole neighbourhood' of 'low Irish' assailed him, crying out that 'the doctors merely wanted to get the poor into their

---

[50] By the paper's estimate of 20,000 this would have been the largest cholera riot in Europe. Given that the population of Aberdeen's six parishes was 32,912 and the city and its vicinity numbered 58,019 (*The Statistical Accounts*, vol. XV, 143, and *City of Aberdeen*, iii), the figure is dubious. It would have been ten times larger than cholera crowds in the much larger cities of London and Manchester.

[51] Neither Morris, *Cholera 1832*, Durey, *The Return of the Plague*, nor recent essays in *Cholera & Conflict* refer to it. Gill and Holland briefly describe it ('Conclusion', 334–5), but do not question the estimate.

[52] *Manchester Times*, 31 December 1831, based on *Aberdeen Journal*.

[53] See note 50.

[54] The Irish ones were at Claremorris (*Morning Post*, 27 August 1832) and Londonderry (*Freeman's Journal*, 3 September 1832); for Manchester, see *Morning Post*, 6 September 1832. This was the only cholera riot Creighton, II, 828, noted; news of it, however, reached as far as Singapore; *Singapore Chronicle*, 7 March 1833, 2.

[55] Richardson, *Death*, 91.

[56] *Caledonian Mercury*, 5 April 1832; and *Scotsman*, 4 April 1832.

clutches to Burke them!'[57] The same day another incident occurred in another neighbourhood. At the Lime Street cholera hospital, the object of suspicion was not a doctor but a rare case in which a cholera sufferer became the victim of crowd anger. A crowd threw mud at a 'poor woman', calling her a 'Burker!' and chasing her as far as Islington.[58] Spurred by accusations of 'burking', a cholera riot the same week flared up in Liverpool, when bearers came to remove a sufferer to the hospital. The neighbourhood 'mob' assaulted the bearers and accused the 'medical gentlemen' of 'burking and poisoning'.[59] Four rioters were arrested—two men, two women; one was English, the others Irish.[60]

Without citations of the new vocabulary, other riots revealed similar anxieties, which the demand for corpses may in part have provoked. In August large crowds assembled around Bristol's cholera hospital of St Peter's, charging that 'the gentlemen' suffocate the poor to get them off their hands or poison them 'for the purposes of dissection'. The following Tuesday, 'a tumultuous assemblage' entered St Philip's churchyard, Bristol, after the burial service, just as coffins bearing several cholera victims were being interred. 'With many curses', they forced the gravedigger to disinter the coffins, snatched the spade from him, and forced off the lids, exposing 'the ghastly dead...to the gaze of hundreds of spectators'.[61] The following day a third Bristol riot centred on interment. A 'mob' at the Temple churchyard broke into the grounds and demanded two coffins be pried open to prove the bodies were dead. That Thursday yet a fourth cholera riot erupted with a 'mob' forming outside the gates of Bristol's cholera hospital: 'a sailor, in a straw hat and smock frock, intoxicated and flourishing a stick in the faces of the constables', declared he had been inside the hospital and witnessed the doctors 'burking the poor people'. He yelled for the hospital to be pulled down.[62]

At the beginning of March, cholera riots in Glasgow at Woodside, Springburn, and Bridgegate threatened surgeons and attacked gravediggers appointed to bury cholera victims, chanting that 'doctors are killing people for the sake of their bodies'.[63] Regarding the cholera riot in Paisley at the end of March, anxieties over body snatching were proven not to have been matters of popular superstition. Some boys discovered two small shovels and a hook and brought the evidence to town. A crowd assembled, marched to the cemetery, and began digging up graves. In one of the first, they discovered an empty coffin. The news spread rapidly, increasing 'the numbers collected round the scene of exhumation'. Armed 'with stobs broken from the cemetery gates, and bearing an empty coffin', the crowd processed through the town, breaking the windows of all the surgeons' houses, shops, and the hospital. They demolished a cholera hearse and 'everything connected with the [hospital] so far as possible'. Consisting 'almost entirely of half-grown lads and Irishmen', they marched on the hospital, forcing up its gate. A patient accidently

---

[57] *Westmorland Gazette*, 9 June 1832, 3.   [58] Ibid., 9 June 1832, 3.
[59] *Preston Chronicle*, 9 June 1832, 3, based on *Liverpool Courier*.   [60] Ibid.
[61] *Bristol Mercury*, 11 August 1832; also Hardiman, *The 1832 Cholera Epidemic*, 15.
[62] *Bristol Mercury*, 11 August 1832.   [63] *Manchester Times*, 3 March 1832.

struck by a rock died shortly afterwards.[64] 'Cholera battles' ensued between doctors and police on one side and 'the enraged people' on the other, who believed the sick were being 'carried away to be dissected'.[65] In this riot, neither local authorities nor newspapers condemned the mob outright. The evidence had supported the crowd. As they marched into town, Paisley's magistrates assembled to preserve the peace, offering a £50 reward to discover the body snatchers, 'in detestation of the resurrection system'.[66]

At the end of March, rioting erupted at Dublin's cholera hospital in Grangegorman Lane. Rumours spread of patients being culled 'to supply the schools with subjects for dissection'.[67] Several days later, crowds attacked drivers and carts transporting cholera patients to the hospital.[68] The papers maintained 'the poor people' believed 'their bodies' were being sacrificed 'to serve the dissecting table'.[69] As rioters in Glasgow's 'poorest' streets of Highland Close, Goose Dubbs, and Briggate[70] professed, the Health Board's strategy was to suppress the disease by weeding out the poor.[71]

At the beginning of September, 'a most serious disturbance' broke out near Manchester's cholera hospital with the streets 'thronged by several thousands', 'principally of the lower class', carrying a coffin, containing the body of a little boy, whose head had been severed from his trunk. Periodically, 'the mob' stopped to exhibit the headless body, and to exclaim that a doctor in the cholera hospital had murdered the boy for his head. As the aggrieved crowd passed through Manchester's principal streets, the numbers increased 'at every step' with 'cries against the doctors and an almost unanimous shout, "To the hospital, pull it to the ground" '.

The description, one of the longest for any British cholera revolt, details the crowd's progression, their demands and attack on the cholera hospital, the evacuation of patients, the patients' exhausted state with some dying in the streets, the breaking of the hospital's windows, destruction of beds, tables, every other piece of furniture, and the hospital's new spring vehicles. It was England's only cholera riot that required military intervention—four troops of the Fifteenth Hussars—and the only time the Riot Act was threatened for a cholera riot in the British Isles. Nine ringleaders were taken as prisoners—'chiefly Irishmen'—escorted by dragoons to the New Bailey.[72] Three days later, several newspapers published an addendum,

---

[64] *Morning Chronicle*, 30 March 1832; *Scotsman*, 9 May 1832, 3; and other papers based on *Glasgow Chronicle* of 27 March 1832. Nine ringleaders were charged. In addition to the violence described above, they attacked a corporal of police and a spirit dealer. News of these events spread to Australia, see *Sydney Gazette*, 11 September 1832, 3. Two police officers were seriously wounded. The mob spared the windows of 'anti-contagionists', while they 'utterly destroyed' those of Health Board.

[65] *Corbett's Weekly*, 7 April 1832.   [66] *Scotsman*, 28 March 1832, 3.

[67] *Morning Chronicle*, 27 April 1832; *Morning Post*, 27 April 1832; and *The Times*, 30 April 1832, front page.

[68] It was Dublin's largest cholera hospital with a capacity of 700 patients; Creighton, II, 821.

[69] *Morning Chronicle*, 28 April 1832: 'the people' claimed that 'if they were allowed to bury the bodies, so as to be sure they were not dissected', they would not object to patients going there.

[70] Neighbourhoods north of the Clyde, opposite Gorbals Bridge.

[71] *Aberdeen Journal*, 22 February 1832. *Caledonian Mercury*, 18 February 1832 and *Manchester Times*, 18 February 1832.

[72] *Morning Post*, 3 September 1832.

taking seriously the accusation against the surgeon charged with decapitation. He had bribed an Irish nurse to remain silent, but she informed her countrywomen and the boy's grandfather of the decapitation. The Hospital Board expressed its regrets and issued a warrant for the surgeon's arrest.[73] To regain public confidence, the hospital's chairman issued an apology to the people of Manchester, inviting any relative or friend of a patient taken to the hospital 'to visit him daily', and, if the patient died, to witness the body placed in the coffin and to be permitted to attend the funeral.[74]

Finally, an article in the *Medical Gazette*, copied by several newspapers, exposed the sale of cholera bodies for medical training, claiming it was not an episodic affair of a body snatched here or there; rather, it was occurring on an industrial scale with the tides of the Thames serving as a conveyor belt in the movement of cadavers. Engineers at Woolwich, instructed to dig large mass graves along the Thames discovered that:

> bodies of deceased cholera patients go down the river with one tide, and are brought up again to town with the next. They are, of course, intended for the dissecting-rooms; and we could mention some at which they have made their appearance, being easily recognised by the quantity of pitch with which they are covered.[75]

BURIED ALIVE

These 'resurrectionist' fears may have been behind other cholera riots presented with less detail than Paisley's or Manchester's. At least fifteen riots in my sample turned on questions of burial, and, as seen in Bristol, the scenes of the protests and confrontations with police occurred not only outside hospitals but in cemeteries. These appear, however, to have focused on a more traditional question going back to antiquity—that of being granted a decent burial. At Greenock on the Clyde estuary, a fourteen-year-old boy died shortly after being taken to the cholera hospital. 'It circulated' that the boy's treatment had killed him and rumours spread of his supposed secret burial atop a hill at nightfall. 'An immense crowd' of women and boys pursued his doctor, hooting and pelting him. With increased numbers, the crowd returned to the hospital to give the boy a Christian burial. To avert conflict, the magistrates agreed to bury the boy.[76]

Concerns over burial also dominated the second-largest cholera riot crowd, which gathered in Commercial Road in London's East End. Here, the papers said nothing about dissection. This cholera riot was unusual in that neither a hospital nor surgeon was attacked; rather, the crowd's animosity was directed against the parish curate and sexton conducting the victim's funeral. A woman who sold fish and oysters died at the Commercial Road cholera hospital and was buried in

---

[73] *Morning Post*, 6 September 1832; and *Freeman's Journal*, 7 September 1832. According to Richardson, *Death*, 228, the boy's head was later found in an apothecary; a warrant for the proprietor's arrest was issued, but he was never found.

[74] *Morning Post*, 7 September 1832.

[75] *Morning Chronicle*, 24 March 1832, from *Medical Gazette*.   [76] Ibid., 5 March 1832.

Stepney churchyard. A crowd assembled at the hospital and followed her procession to the church, alleging she was still alive. When the gravedigger filled in the dirt, the curate allegedly answered the crowd, saying 'he did not care' if she were alive, which drove the crowd to charge the grave and remove the earth. A police officer 'prudently' allowed the people to proceed to prove the woman was indeed dead. Still, the 'multitude', amounting to 'at least 2000', threatened to pull down the houses of the curate and sexton.[77] Two cholera riots in Birmingham in mid- and late August also revolved around fears of patients buried alive, without reference to the dissection table.[78] These fears fit wider anxieties then swelling in places as distant as Asiatic Russia: it seems that the horrific lethality of the disease, combined with the need to bury the dead rapidly and the insistence that cholera bodies be buried in separate cemeteries without relatives in attendance, persuaded the poor to believe elites were weeding out excess populations.

THE CHRONOLOGY OF RIOTS

Historians have held that the passage of the Anatomy Bill successfully allayed these anxieties of the poor and animosity towards the medical profession.[79] The chronology of the riots calls into question the centrality of the legislation at least for 1832.

Chronology of Cholera Riots

Months	Incidents
November 1831	1
December 1831	1
January 1832	0
February 1832	2
March 1832	15
April 1832	12
May 1832	3
June 1832	9
July 1832	2
August 1832	17
September 1832	3
October 1832	4
November 1832	0
December 1832	0
January 1833	1
Uncertain date	2
Total	72

[77] *Morning Post*, 25 August 1832; and *Scotsman*, 29 August 1832, 2.
[78] *Morning Chronicle*, 14 August 1832; *Scotsman*, 29 August 1832, 2; and *Chelmsford Chronicle*, 24 August 1832, 2.
[79] On the act, see Holland, 'Resurrectionists', 207; McDuff, 'The 1832 Liverpool Cholera Riots', 107, and Richardson, *Death*, part 2.

Across the British Isles, cholera riots peaked in March and April with twenty-seven (39 per cent) occurring in these two months alone. In May, June, and July, their decline had already taken place before the Anatomy Bill was promulgated by Parliament on 19 July 1832. Then, in August the riots rebounded, climbing to seventeen, the highest number for any month, and the riots persisted into January the following year. After the bill's passage, twenty-five further riots erupted—that is, over a third of them. Of course, not all riots are equal; some involved greater numbers, were more violent, and more thoroughly covered in the press. Yet, except for the Aberdeen riot, whose crowd figure is difficult to believe, the three largest riots occurred after the bill's passage: the one in Wick at the end of July, Stepney's at the end of August, and Britain's most publicized one in Manchester in mid-September. Of the five that had to turn to the military or police forces beyond a locality, all but the Aberdeen's arose after the act's passage.

As the table on previous page shows, fears that the poor were being slaughtered in hospitals, suffocated, or poisoned to supply corpses for anatomical training continued after the act was passed, with cries of 'burking' and dissection explicit. Another post-promulgation riot occurred in Wick at the end of July and is the only one I have found that traced lines of communication from one place to another. It was also the most detailed about fears of killing the poor to supply cadavers. According to newspapers, Wick's fishermen possessed no antipathy towards their physician Dr Allison, recently sent from Edinburgh to direct their local cholera hospital, until fishermen from Musselburgh, Fisherrow, and Dunbar east of Edinburgh arrived and spread stories that at Edinburgh, and now at Wick, he was profiting by killing the poor to supply cadavers for Edinburgh College: 'that all the patients whom Dr Allison had attended had died'. He had been sent, they maintained, to procure 'fifty subjects every week for Edinburgh College'. Twelve dozen coffins were ready for the operation and none would exit the hospital alive. The papers admitted that the 'rapidity' of the cholera deaths 'appeared to confirm these grossly unfounded stories'. As a result, crowds 'mostly composed of south country fishermen' assembled around the quarantine hospital and harangued Dr Allison 'with the most fearful imprecations and threatening language, horrid yells, and cries of "Murder him—off with the murderer" &c.' With these threats, Dr Allison left town.[80] As this narrative suggests, the ease with which rumours roused popular violence were due to the characteristics of the disease—its high lethality and the speed with which it advanced meant that few escaped surgeons' care or the hospital alive. The sale of cadavers constituted only one ingredient of this collective fear.

OTHER REASONS TO HATE DOCTORS AND TO REVOLT

Further myths bearing on doctors surfaced in other cholera riots. Instead of cries of 'burking', the poor of Glasgow's working-class wynds believed surgeons were

---

[80] *Morning Post*, 1 August 1832, from *Edinburgh Evening Courant*; and *Caledonian Mercury*, 2 August 1832, which repeats the story and adds details of the destruction wreaked by the crowd at the hospital. 'Two of the most violent rioters' were arrested but released the next day.

culling them with poison to slow the disease's spread.[81] The medical profession attacked these allegations without mentioning anatomy schools. In an editorial to the *Newcastle Courant*, Dr George Fox charged that no one knew how to manufacture or increase the disease, and besides, there was little chance of any payment coming from 'the class of patients' they treated, especially in the most heavily infected districts of Hetton in the Yorkshire Dales or Heworth outside York.[82]

Other cholera doctors described their threatened lives 'surrounded by a noisy mob', accused by 'the vulgar' of prescribing medicines 'calculated to produce the worst effects', and with cries of 'the mob to oppose every precautionary measure proposed by the Board of Heath'.[83] Similarly, a brief notice of a 'cholera riot' among the poor on Edinburgh's outskirts ('not many miles from the Cross') gave few hints of the crowds' motives other than suspicion and pure hatred of medical authorities. Removal of a cholera patient sparked the crowd's chant—'Kill the doctors, nae Board o' Health!'[84] A cholera doctor assigned to various places in Ireland since cholera began spreading there in April described the riots he had witnessed in Ballyshannon, Ballina, Claremorris, and Sligo. By his assessment, their prime reason 'was the old game played before my eyes for the fifteenth time since the arrival of pestilence at Sunderland. The doctors, it was stated, were to have 10 guineas a day: £5 of every one they killed; and to poison without mercy.'[85]

Was the medical profession generally despised by the lower classes in early nineteenth-century Britain or was the hatred triggered by cholera and largely confined to it? After all, cholera was not the only epidemic to produce mass mortalities in the early to mid-nineteenth century. In 1826, a typhus epidemic raged through the British Isles claiming 70,000 lives in Ireland and 20,000 in London alone.[86] Yet British and Irish newspapers do not report a single typhus riot; nor do the papers reflect on popular suspicions of poisoning, hospitals as death chambers, or hatred of physicians. With the Great Famine in Ireland of the 1840s, typhus again became a bigger killer, especially in the winter of 1847/8, and its venom concentrated on the poor.[87] While food riots spread through the country, I know of no typhus riots or cries against 'medical gentlemen', accused of plotting government culls of the poor. Also, a pandemic of influenza swept through Europe in the 1830s with no such cries, but these were slower killers with lower rates of lethality.

Although cholera mob anger almost invariably targeted hospitals, their litters, surgeons, or Health Board members, other concerns could spur popular outrage. The village riot of mid-August at Pathhead, Kirkcaldy, began similarly to other British cholera disturbances with a man or a woman suddenly dying of cholera. At Pathhead, however, none of the usual anxieties were voiced about the selling of

---

[81] *Aberdeen Journal*, 22 February 1832.   [82] *Newcastle Courant*, 4 February 1832.
[83] *Belfast News-Letter*, 24 April 1832.
[84] *Examiner*, 6 May 1832; also *Dublin Observer*, 29 April 1832, 17, from *Scotsman*; and *Morning Register*, 2 May 1832, 4.
[85] *Lancaster Gazette*, 6 October 1832, from *Literary Gazette*.
[86] *Morning Chronicle*, 27 April 1832; Newton, 'New Introduction', v.
[87] Hamonet, *Les épidémies de typhus*; Hardy, 'Urban Famine'; *The Great Irish Famine*; Crawford, 'Typhus in Nineteenth-Century Ireland', 121–37; *The Hungry Stream*; Kinealy, *The Great Irish Famine*; Henry, *Sligo*; Ó Gráda, *Ireland's Great Famine*.

cadavers, live burials, violations of traditional wakes, or improper burials. Instead, the crowd wished to conceal that 'cholera existed in the place at all'. Resistance began with women and children but after the head of the local Board of Health called out a constabulary of twenty to ensure the body's burial, men joined the ranks. Together, they barricaded the house and successfully defended the corpse against the officers.[88] Were anxieties over employment and economic prospects at play, or were other emotions at stake, the purity and prestige of their village, or evidence of God's judgement?

Cholera riots not roused by imagined plots of surgeons, hospital poisoning of the poor, or murder for cadavers were, however, rare. These turned on communities' efforts to guard themselves from outsiders whom they feared carried the infection, and fit patterns of fear and hate, which, as we shall see, lay behind violence connected with other infectious diseases, especially smallpox in late nineteenth- and early twentieth-century America and England. In the British Isles, these anxieties played a part in only six cholera riots. Moreover, they did not show the sharp class differences of contenders seen with other cholera riots: the poor and marginal against the medical elite and the state. In the Castle Hill district of Edinburgh, locals reacted angrily to the Board of Medicine's decision to erect a quarantine station at Fountainbridge to receive cholera cases from Leith.[89] Such concerns were slightly more common in Ireland. A letter sent to a Dublin paper on 8 May reported cholera raging in the village of Ardee. A cholera corpse was sent to the country to be interred. Believing that it would spread the disease, the country people stopped the corpse and demanded its return to Ardee. The corpse lay in the street for most of the day, until someone buried it in the Protestant churchyard.[90] Another exception occurred in Londonderry. As at Castle Hill, the 'tumult' began with the customary spark of a patient 'suspected' of cholera being removed to a cholera hospital, but in this case, popular opinion soon turned against the disease victim. Recently arrived en route to America, she was seen as a contaminating outsider. 'A concourse of persons, principally women...with a retinue of disorderly boys', took the patient back in the direction she came. To get the woman to hospital the Mayor had to call on the 331st Regiment, and when she arrived, she was dead.[91]

Two further incidents derived from anxieties over passengers entering communities from 'contaminated' districts concern the market town of Boyle in Connacht between Longford and Sligo. 'Several hundreds' of townsmen in one incident, and 200 in the other, assembled beyond the town's boundaries and made their way to a spot near Ruskey to block the coach approaching Boyle with a cholera victim.[92] At the end of August, Boyle's citizens again marched from town to defend against a feared cholera invasion this time from Sligo. The coachman from Sligo disobeyed their orders and continued towards Boyle. The townsmen destroyed a

---

[88] *The Times*, 22 August 1832, 3, from *Edinburgh Evening Post*; also in *Baltimore Gazette*, 15 October 1832, 2.

[89] *Scotsman*, 17 March 1832, 8.   [90] *Freeman's Journal*, 15 May 1832.

[91] Ibid., 6 September 1832, from *Derry Journal*.

[92] *Saunders's News-Letter*, 24 June 1832, 2, from *Boyle Gazette*.

bridge, preventing the coach's entry. Unlike other cholera riots explored in this chapter, the sympathies of a local press sided with the rebels.[93]

A sixth case from Blackrock outside Dublin fits what we will see as the quintessential smallpox pattern of class conflict with perpetuators of blame and hate and their victims switching sides: here, the aggressors were the wealthy, who broke the law and organized violence against the diseased victims, while the outsiders and the poor were the butts of their betters' hysteria and irrationality. In an about-face in cholera violence, the populace now defended the Board of Health, the hospital, and measures to protect the town from cholera. I paraphrase the lengthy proceedings presented in several newspapers.

Blackrock's Board of Health endeavoured to procure a house for a cholera hospital, but their applications were refused. So they built a wooden one, but because of protests by landed proprietors, the board could secure no site for it. Threatened by 'contagion and death', they placed the structure on a road adjoining Mr Saurin's demesne, setting this lord to begin plotting to remove it. First, he petitioned Lord Anglesey to intervene but instead of sending a cavalry 'to level the hospital to the dust', he donated £10 to the hospital. On 19 July, Saurin took to direct action by organizing his employees ('a mob of ruffians') to set the hospital ablaze. Several days later, his men armed with sledgehammers and led by his steward smashed the hospital to pieces and afterwards took refuge in Saurin's demesne. 'The people of the neighbourhood' pursued them, forced open Saurin's gate, and 'would in all probability have shed blood', had 'gentlemen' not intervened.[94] Immediately, the community charged Saurin and his servants with the crime, '*but the Government refused to prosecute* [italics in text]'.[95] As we will see, such alignments of elite mobs targeting the diseased victims became commonplace with smallpox, but with cholera Saurin's organized aggression is the only such instance I have found.

Finally, newspapers often identified the cholera crowds in vague, gender-free terms—the 'assembling of multitudes of people' at Fitzroy Market in London;[96] the 'mob' in Sunderland, London's East End St George's Hospital, and in the Gorbals;[97] 'ruffians' in Dublin and Blackrock;[98] 'drunks' in Killineer;[99] 'neighbours' in Kilkenny;[100] and 'the lower classes' in Aberdeen.[101] Yet when journalists delved further, women and children figure predominantly as the participants, and if

---

[93] Ibid., 28 August 1832, 3, from *Roscommon Gazette*.

[94] One of the accused confessed to have been in Saurin's pay.

[95] *Morning Chronicle*, 4 August 1832, from *Dublin Morning Register*; *The Newcastle Courant*, 4 August 1832. *Freeman's Journal*, 3 August 1832, copied the Kilmainham Quarter Sessions' report: 'riotous assembly and trespassing' on his land against five men, including a physician.

[96] *Morning Chronicle*, 23 March 1832.

[97] *Morning Post*, 18 November 1832; *Caledonian Mercury*, 5 April 1832; and *Scotsman*, 28 March 1832.

[98] *Morning Chronicle*, 27 April 1832; and ibid., 4 August 1832.

[99] Ibid., 20 August 1832.   [100] *Freeman's Journal*, 20 August 1832.

[101] Occasionally, rioters in English and Scottish towns were identified as 'mostly Irish'. For London: *Corbett's Weekly*, 7 April 1832; *Morning Chronicle*, 26 March 1832; ibid., 28 March 1832; ibid., 31 March 1832; Manchester: *Morning Chronicle*, 6 September 1832; Paisley: *Morning Chronicle*, 29 March 1832.

leaders were named, women and even adolescents emerge.[102] At the Castle Hill riot, 'blackguard boys' had been its mainstay, and 'had the diabolical suggestions of a number of females been attended to', the hospital would have been captured.[103] As we will see, women and children also filled the ranks of Continental cholera riots that endured into the twentieth century, but this was not the case with smallpox riots.

In conclusion, historians of cholera violence have concentrated on a particular context for the British Isles: fears of murder or body snatching to provide cadavers for new anatomy schools. The picture, I hypothesize, fits a larger one common across Europe from regions in Asiatic Russia to southern Italy, in which the poor and those on the margins were the aggressors, and elites and physicians, the victims. This violence depended heavily on characteristics of the disease—quick death and high rates of lethality—combined with the particular measures authorities took to resist it—rapid burial, separate cemeteries, and refusal to allow communities their traditional funerary practices. Cholera's social violence was a class struggle but one which few might now wish to celebrate, which may explain why Marx, Engels, and later New Left historians avoided mentioning the riots, despite their filling contemporary newspapers, and, in the case of Marx and Engels, swirling through their lives.[104] We now turn to investigate these patterns on the Continent.

---

[102] See the riots in Greenock, Paisley, Pathhead, and Edinburgh under Castle Hill.
[103] *Scotsman*, 17 March 1832.
[104] For a fuller discussion on Marx, Engels, the New Left, and cholera riots, see Cohn, 'Cholera Riots'.

8

Cholera on the Continent and in America

In Eastern European cities such as Königsberg (Prussia),[1] Posen (in Prussia before 1848), and Dessau (Eastern Germany), and in Russia, St Petersburg, Tambov, Toula, Novgorod, Kharkov, and others, the scale and violence of cholera riots were often greater than in places in the West.[2] Yet across strikingly different cultures, economies, and regimes—East, West, and South in Europe and on the east coast of the US—the content and character of conspiracies, divisions by social class, and the targets of rioters' wrath were similar.[3] Without obvious communication among rioters from New York to Asiatic Russia or evidence that the protesters (often illiterate) were aware of these riots occurring simultaneously across long distances,[4] the cholera conspiracies repeated stories of elites masterminding a Malthusian cull of the poor, with health boards, doctors, pharmacists, nurses, and government officials as the agents of the planned class mass murder. As we shall discover, these same myths could recur with cholera into the twentieth century, igniting widespread, deadly rioting, and the stories appeared as far east as Japan. Cholera's high lethality rates often meant that few patients returned alive from hospitals, triggering suspicions about doctors and authorities which led to collective violence.[5]

---

[1] Briese, *Angst in den Zeiten der Cholera*, I, 169–77; and Ross, *Contagion in Prussia*, ch. 8: 263 were arrested and 559 'implicated' (141). Smaller riots occurred at Memel and Stettin in 1831 with no lives lost and 'minimal' damage (139).

[2] Netchkina, et al., 'La Russie'; McGrew, *Russia and the Cholera*; and Baldwin, *Contagion*, ch. 2. Without estimates of those involved, numbers wounded or killed, the extent of the destruction during the first wave of rioting is difficult to compare over place and time. Although often mentioned in the secondary literature, the Stettin riot does not appear to have been extraordinarily violent: a letter from Stettin in *Freeman's Journal*, 15 September 1831, mentions only windows of a few houses broken; no one was reported killed or wounded. By contrast, 3639 were sentenced after the St Petersburg's riot in 1831 (Netchkina et al., 'La Russie', 154), making it possibly more extensive than Tashkent's in 1892. Some reported St Petersburg's crowds comprising a third of the city; ibid., 151. However, McGrew, *Russia and the Cholera*, 110, reports that on 22 June 1831 little more than a hundred were arrested with only one killed during St Petersburg's major cholera riot in the Haymarket.

[3] From my searches through various newspaper databases, no evidence of cholera riots has emerged for Latin America; however, the same cholera myths and violence appear to have been widespread. In the biography of her husband, Lady Burton, *The Life of Sir Richard F. Burton*, 30, recounts a cholera epidemic in Montevideo and Buenos Aires in 1869, when 'mobs' gathered in market squares, murdered doctors, and accused the government of poisoning.

[4] Although some among these marginal groups might have been literate, reformers believed the only way to counteract their beliefs was with placards and leaflets; articles written even 'in simple language' proved useless because 'the poor' do not 'generally read the public papers' (*Lancaster Gazette*, 23 June 1832, 3). In Ireland, June 1832, country folk spread news of protective tokens over 300 miles in a week (see Connolly, 'The 'Blessed Turf''), but natural and cultural barriers blocked the path of news, and it failed to penetrate Dublin.

[5] In 1897, when cholera hit Tokyo with few returning from hospitals, rumours spread of doctors draining blood from patients, plucking out their eyes, and sending them alive to the incinerator. As in

Certainly, myths of poisoning streams, wells, and other water supplies reached back to antiquity and were repeated in the Middle Ages and early modern period. But unlike the slaughter of lepers and Jews in 1319–21 or primarily Jews in 1348–51, the targets of the nineteenth- and twentieth-century cholera riots were rarely Jews or other marginal groups (and never lepers). Rather than attacking any 'other', popular rage turned in the opposite direction—against the dominant classes, especially the medical profession and forces of repression from local police to Cossacks and national armies. Only occasionally were groups such as Jesuits,[6] Jews,[7] or foreigners— Armenians, Persians, and Westerners (in China)—attacked.

Roderick McCrew interpreted the cholera riots in St Petersburg from 21 to 26 June 1831 within the context of Russia's war with Poland: 'hatred for Russia's enemies helped to identify physicians with Polish agents'.[8] He saw these riots as anti-foreign, targeting Poles. But as in other regions during the cholera wave of the 1830s, St Petersburg's crowds attacked cholera lazaretti and hospitals, ambulances and physicians, local guards and police. The only casualties mentioned in the inter-national press during these riots were physicians, and the only one killed was a German, not a Pole. Eight further physicians were severely beaten; two narrowly escaping death but were not identified as Polish or foreigners.[9] Instead, these riots reflect a general pattern: the rebels saw themselves as the patients' liberators against diabolic poisoning by the state and physicians.[10]

Except for one case to be investigated, when Jews were targeted, matters of reli-gion or race rarely sparked these riots. And this near-absence occurred against a backdrop of widespread anti-Semitic pogroms throughout the nineteenth and early twentieth centuries, especially in Eastern Europe and Russia. West of the Elbe, where anti-Semitic violence also flared,[11] Jews were never the targets of cholera violence. Despite similarities across vast terrains with strikingly different historical regimes and circumstances, historians have sought to explain cholera riots by turning non-comparatively to specific political events or national contexts. Peter Baldwin explained these Russian riots as arising from brutal repression by the

---

Europe, such stories sparked 'violent riots' against local authorities, requiring military intervention; see Rogaski, *Hygenic Modernity*, 152. In 1909–10, two cholera-related revolts erupted in Java. The first at Batavia (Jakarta) resulted from rumours of the government killing the 'people' with cholera to place their heads in the foundation stones of bridges. Cholera mobs attacked disinfectant parties, injuring several and killing two; *The Straits Times*, 4 October 1909, 7. For the second at Bandung (West Java), 'the populace' brutally attacked supposed poisoners, beating two to death; troops were summoned; 'many were arrested'; *The Straits Times*, 6 January 1910, 6.

[6] Vincent, 'Le cholera en Espagne', 54; and Chapter 10 in this volume.

[7] According to Baldwin, *Contagion*, 63–4, and others, Jewish physicians were among those singled out in St Petersburg and Königsberg. However, Ross's more detailed analysis, *Contagion in Prussia*, 135–53, lists no Jewish physicians killed; although gangs roamed streets, 'mistreat[ing]' Jews and physicians, 139. On St Petersburg, Baldwin, *Contagion*, 64, follows McGrew: foreign physicians were accused of an international plot to eliminate the poor.

[8] McGrew, *Russia and the Cholera*, 106 and 110.

[9] *Great Britain Privy Council*, 28; however, it concluded that 'the people' held 'all foreigners' accountable.

[10] McGrew, *Russia and the Cholera*, 110 and 116.

[11] On anti-Semitism before the Nazis, see Wasserstein, *Barbarism and Civilization*.

Cossacks and Czarist troops and harsh and rigid quarantine measures.[12] For Sir Richard Evans, such repressive measures were not peculiar to Russia or Eastern Europe, but provoked cholera riots across Europe. Yet, as seen in Chapter 7, troops were rarely marshalled to repress cholera riots in the British Isles, and the arrested generally counted less than a handful, not the hundreds as in Russia. Furthermore, the sentences in the British Isles were fines or short prison terms, not deadly lashes by the knout or execution. Nonetheless, in less than fourteen months, at least seventy-two cholera riots erupted in the British Isles, with several assembling crowds in the thousands.

Further explanations pinned on local or national contexts persist for other places in the 1830s. In France and especially Paris, Catherine Kudlick has argued that the revolutionary political climate created by the rise of the progressive July Monarchy that two years earlier had tossed out Charles X was the cause of cholera riots in Paris in 1832.[13] In England and Scotland, it was tensions over the Reform Act of 1832 or the scandals of Burke and Hare. In Sicily in 1837, the riots coincided with liberal and revolutionary fervour, resulting in widespread political threats to Bourbon rule and rebellion at Messina, Catania, and Siracusa.[14] But similar cholera riots arose in 1832 in places such as New York City in the climate of Jacksonian democracy and reason, when social and political calm prevailed.[15] And in places such as Sicily, the famous nineteenth-century historian and fervent supporter of the revolution against the Bourbons, Michele Amari, argued that the two revolts—one aroused by cholera; the other, a political one, against the Bourbon government—travelled along different tracks that hardly intersected. Instead of one movement reinforcing the other, 'cholera blocked every revolutionary tendency'; the cholera riots 'possessed no political character'.[16] Later, from his prodigious research into Sicilian archives, Alfonso Sansone concluded much the same: 'the horrible disease, cholera', had 'interrupted and broken the movement of *la Giovine Italia* and the message of Mazzini'.[17] More recently, Franco della Perutta maintained that the cholera chaos weakened the Bourbon state, providing opportunities for the anti-Bourbon forces. But still, cholera rebels had difficulty organizing their movements and achieved little success.[18] In addition, as argued in Chapter 7, no connection between cholera riots and the larger political struggles to enact the reform acts in England, Scotland, or Ireland appears from rioters' actions, chants, ideology, or commentary in newspapers that decried cholera rebels' 'ignorance and bestiality'.

[12] Baldwin, *Contagion*, ch. 2. Based on McGrew, Hays, *The Burdens of Disease*, 137, argues much the same: 'heavy police presence' and 'enforced isolation' caused the Russian riots. Henze, *Disease*, follows Evans, 'Epidemics and Revolutions', but documents that quarantine was not as stringent as is often assumed. Medical authorities had yet to define what constituted effective quarantine, and it varied radically from place to place (17). For the central riot of her analysis—Saratov on 28 June 1892—the medical institutions and organizational structures to combat cholera came into play only after the violence. Instead, of quarantine and repression, the riot rested on the opposite: failure by local government to act (74–5).

[13] Kudlick, *Cholera*. Also, Salomé, 'Le massacre', 105, 118, 123, fails to place these Parisian reactions comparatively, framing them instead within the political context of the July Monarchy.

[14] Sansone, *Gli Avvenimenti*; Preto, *Epidemia*, 121–66; and *I moti del 1837*.

[15] Rosenberg, *The Cholera Years*.   [16] Preto, *Epidemia*, 140, from archival sources on Amari.

[17] Sansone, *Gli avvenimenti*, 204.   [18] Della Perutta, *Mazzini*, 274.

In summary, Europe presents a kaleidoscope of contrasting political events and regimes on the eve of cholera's first European tour of the 1830s, but across regions and regimes cholera riots prevailed with much the same fantasies. Fernand Braudel's lesson for comparative history must be taken to heart: local events cannot explain pan-regional phenomena.[19]

The absence of interplay between cholera riots and the general milieu of political activism is equally telling with the next cholera wave in 1848–9. Cholera cases and mortality reached their highest levels for any cholera wave in European history. These years, moreover, coincided with the worst famines and economic crises of the nineteenth century, and provoked the century's most threatening class conflict and national revolutions. Yet, neither cholera's mortalities nor this background of revolutionary fervour and state repression produced a repeat of the first wave of cholera riots. The revolutionary years instead diverted cholera's social violence, creating a pause in its power to provoke blame and hatred. Evans explained this absence of cholera riots by referring to 'the almost universal relaxation of the very strict police controls'.[20] But was this the case in Ireland, for instance, where police tensions and repression of famine riots increased?

Back to 1831–3: as seen earlier, epidemics of typhus spread through the British Isles within the same social-political milieu as cholera and scored as high and, in places, higher rates of mortalities. The same was true of a typhus epidemic in Paris in 1831, which continued to be a benchmark for a terrible epidemic in 1842, when the city was dealt another serious blow by this disease.[21] Yet no riots arose from these outbreaks. In addition, Paris was stuck by a disastrous influenza pandemic in 1831, outstripping cholera's mortalities a year later.[22] Although chronologically closer to the political and ideological upheavals of the July Monarchy, the influenza epidemic failed to provoke any recorded social violence, hatred, or blame. Moreover, in cities such as Marseille,[23] Lille,[24] Bordeaux,[25] and Rouen, equally affected by the political changes and tensions of the July Monarchy and with a crippling European-wide depression in commerce and textiles worsening workers' economic conditions,[26] nothing comparable to Paris's cholera riots emerged. In Lille, labourers and the poor produced myths of the government poisoning wells.[27] In Rouen, a rumour spread that the government desired to eliminate the poor by poisoning fish and water sources.[28] But unlike in Paris, these rumours did not spark riots.

*   *   *

With few exceptions, the social and psychological reactions to cholera have focused almost exclusively on the disease's first major European tour. Unlike the Black Death, cholera's dance with social loathing did not come to an abrupt halt

[19] Braudel and Spooner, 'Prices in Europe', 437.
[20] Evans, 'Epidemics and Revolutions', 169.   [21] *Scotsman*, 31 August 1842, 2.
[22] Quinn, *Flu*, 104–5.   [23] Guiral, 'Le choléra à Marseille'.
[24] Dineur and Engrand, 'Le choléra à Lille'.   [25] Fréour, 'Le choléra à Bordeaux'.
[26] Vidalenc, 'Les départements normands'.   [27] Dineur and Engrand, 'Le choléra à Lille'.
[28] Vidalenc, 'Les départements normands', 106 and 108.

after its first performance; rather, subsequent waves in the 1860s to its sixth in 1904–11 provoked hatred and collective violence—that is, after John Snow had mapped cholera's mode of transmission in 1854, after his ideas had been accepted by 1866,[29] after Robert Koch cultured the bacillus in 1884, and with effective modes of treatment in train.[30] To date, no one has compared these waves of cholera over the long term to evaluate changes in their social repercussions or production of fantasies and conspiracies. Where comparisons have been made, they have been limited to two cholera waves and mostly within the context of a single city, region, or country.[31] Cholera's social disruption is generally assumed to have declined dramatically after the 1830s and to have lingered on only in backward corners of Europe, as in Russia or southern Italy (Mezzogiorno). Although cholera social violence may have mostly ended after the 1830s in Britain and France, this was not the case in Russia, Italy, Spain, and other regions. As late as cholera's sixth wave in the early twentieth century, when the disease no longer possessed many mysteries, the old myths of poisoning to cull populations of the poor could still rage with violent force.

FRANCE

Yet to be recognized, the most dramatic decline of cholera's social violence after the 1830s occurred in France, the US, and the British Isles. Only for the British Isles have historians emphasized that cholera riots did not recur in subsequent waves after 1832 (which is not entirely correct).[32] In France and the US, the first cholera

[29] Hamlin, *Cholera*, 191, and Echenberg, *Africa in the Time of Cholera*, 64, appear to overstate the extent which Snow's ideas were ignored before James Farr rejuvenated them during the epidemic of 1866. See Acland, *Memoir on the Cholera at Oxford*: 'few persons will doubt the connection between some Cholera outbreaks and the condition of the Water—as . . . elaborately and meritoriously investigated by Dr. Snow' (77). The Broad Street pump was not the only water source closed during the 1854 epidemic. Based on similar suppositions, a pump handle was broken off at Oxford; ibid., 77. In 1854, Acland claimed 'it is generally supposed' that 'sewage, Foul Water, or the like' spread cholera (78). In the same year, citizens of St John, Quebec suspected foul water and sewage caused cholera; Bilson, *A Darkened House*, 173 and 138. Also see Zeheter, *Epidemics, Empire, and Environments*, chapters 3–5, on the importance of Edwin Chadwick and the sanitation movement.

[30] Riots against doctors accused of spreading cholera erupted in Le Var (Toulon), Arles, and Auriol in southern France in 1884 (Baehrel, 'Épidémie et terreur', 114–15, 128). Riots in Puerta del Sol in Madrid continued to 1885; Vincent, 'Le cholera en Espagne', 54–5; and major cholera revolts erupted in Sicily, Naples, Puglia, Calabria, around Rome and possibly as far north as Venice until 1911; see Chapter 9.

[31] Snowden, *Naples in the Time of Cholera*, for late nineteenth- and early twentieth-century southern Italy; Evans, *Death in Hamburg*, for late nineteenth-century Hamburg; Bourdelais and Raulot, *Une Peur Bleue*, comparing 1832 with 1854; Kudlick, *Cholera*, 1832 and 1849 in Paris; and Henze, *Disease*, 1892 and 1904–10 in Saratov.

[32] Durey, *The Return of the Plague*, 211; Gill and Holland, 'Conclusion', 340. From BNA, I have discovered four cholera riots during the epidemic in 1849—one in County Kerry, Ireland (*Leeds Intelligencer*, 16 June 1849, from *Kerry Evening Post*), another at Findhorn, northern Scotland (*Inverness Courier*, 20 September 1849; *Elgin Courier*, 14 September 1849), a third at the Scottish fishing village of Dubeath (*Scotsman*, 24 November 1849, 2), and a fourth at Totnes, South Devon (*Western Times*, 6 October 1849). Except possibly the one at Totnes, these were tiny riots without myths of poisoning, murders for cadavers, or beliefs in physicians culling populations of the poor. Only in Totnes were the targets similar to those in 1831–2. 'The mob' smashed the door and windows of a recently converted cholera hospital. The motive, however, was fear of cholera entering their neighbourhood.

wave of 1832 never produced the same levels of blame, social disruption, and rioting as in most other European countries. Given historians' attention to cholera and social violence in France from the pioneering research of René Baehrel in the early 1950s, Louis Chevalier's in the 1960s, and Patrice Bourdelais', Jean-Yves Raulot's, and Catherine Kudlick's in the 1980s and 1990s, such an assertion may sound far-fetched. The Parisian riots of 1832 are the most thoroughly studied for any city at any time. These were unusual for cholera disturbances during the 1830s as well as later in that they were seemingly integrated with national politics. Here, the cholera myths percolated to the top of society and may have even started there. The monarchist right used this explosive, quick-killing disease to challenge the newly minted progressive politics of the July Monarchy, blaming it for the spread of cholera to the capital. Royalists claimed that the government of French Premier Casimir Périer had disseminated the poison into public drinking fountains and barrels of wine, and had smeared it on the stalls of food markets.[33] The Parisian préfet of police rebutted the charges by issuing his own, accusing the new regime's enemies of being the riots' *agents provocateurs*.[34] Yet the religious right dominated cholera's politics, preaching that it was God's punishment against the new reformist government, and 'harangued the people' to overthrow the 'Government of assassins, which sheds the blood of the citizens, massacres prisoners, and leaves the poor to die of hunger'.[35]

The Parisian riots of 1832 were also unusual in galvanizing the economic interests of at least one sector of the middle classes, proprietors of garbage collection, along with the 1800 rag-and-bone men and vendors of water throughout the capital, threatened economically by new sanitary decrees.[36] In addition, Paris's anti-cholera measures targeted supposed dietary dangers of consuming fruit and vegetables, thereby threatening these vendors' livelihoods.[37] Yet, despite these differences, Parisian rioters produced much the same conspiracy theories and accusations seen elsewhere.[38] As in Russia, other places in continental Europe, and throughout the British Isles, Parisians targeted physicians and their assistants as the instigators of the poisoning. Along with setting wagons of garbage ablaze, cholera crowds in Paris drowned a medical assistant in the Seine in 1832[39] and attacked numerous other physicians.[40] An eyewitness account by a correspondent for a US medical journal explained the riots: 'the Paris mob' saw physicians in all the hospitals poisoning the people, 'because few patients came out alive'.[41] An English

[33] Bourdelais and Raulot, *Une Peur Bleue*, 224.   [34] Chevalier, 'Première partie: Paris', 19.

[35] *The Times*, 12 April 1832, 2. Salomé, 'Le massacre', argues that cholera violence in Paris lacked 'a clear and intelligible political dimension' (120).

[36] *Saratoga Sentinel*, 15 May 1832, 2.

[37] Delaporte, *Disease and Civilization*, 67; also Salomé, 'Le massacre', 114: those charged with committing deadly attacks ranged from apprentices to artisans of relatively comfortable means.

[38] For instance, Salomé, 'Le massacre', 107.

[39] Snowden, *Naples in the Time of Cholera*, 151, and Delaporte, *Disease and Civilization*, 66; Salomé, 'Le massacre', does not refer to this incident but cites others, when crowds blamed doctors for poisoning, 110 and 111.

[40] Salomé, 'Le massacre'. Also, *Le Figaro*, 10 April 1832, front page.

[41] *The Cholera Gazette* (Philadelphia), 1/1–16 (1832), 85.

medical account of the Parisian cholera fantasies maintained 'people were persuaded' of poisoning everywhere; at one moment it was the water, then 'the provisions', then 'the wine'.[42] A Parisian during the riots declared: 'There are too many of the poor, and they would rather poison than feed us'.[43]

Historians have claimed that the Parisian riots spilled into the provinces with near or equal force in 1832.[44] The evidence assembled by them, however, fails to show any city or province with reactions comparable to Paris. Moreover, beyond French borders, arrests, damages, death tolls, and executions from cholera riots could climb beyond anything seen even in Paris. In Siracusa, for instance, in a single riot, rumours of cholera poisoning drove crowds to lynch forty people.[45] By contrast, the most dramatic case presented by Bourdelais and Raulot of a cholera disturbance in the provinces in 1832 comes from Casteljaloux in the département of Lot-et-Garonne. The mayor received an anonymous letter alleging that four individuals had poisoned public fountains, and the préfet of the town claimed that 'enemies of the July Revolution had been the culprits in an effort to weaken the lower classes'.[46] But these were words, not acts of destruction or murder. Similarly, essays edited by Chevalier dedicated to cities and regions outside Paris in 1832 report panic, fear, mass religious processions, rumours, and occasionally accusations of poisoning against government agents, but no murders or riots. In Lille, the populace initially considered cholera as 'purely an invention of the police' and that government agents had poisoned public water supplies. But despite their fears, no rioting followed—not even peaceful demonstrations. Instead, in 1832, 'the Liloise working class remained entirely passive'.[47]

Throughout the départements of Normandy even less was reported: few myths of poisoning arose and no rumours accusing the government or physicians of attempting to murder the poor. In smaller Norman communes such as Pont-de-l'Arche, panic was not even manifested,[48] and for Normandy as a whole: '[T]he reactions of the population seemed in most respects to be normal'; the populace sympathized with the victims, and the local press 'exalted the generosity of the sovereign, who had donated large sums for public relief'.[49] Only at the beginning of the cholera outbreak did Rouen's newspapers allege that cholera was the work of poisoners, but such suspicions faded quickly without violence.[50] In Bordeaux, no hints of the cholera myths or panic are recorded.[51] On the other hand, in Marseille, where the spread of cholera followed the Mediterranean pattern of not striking until 1834–5, archival records claim that 'fear struck this city with greater force

[42] Shrimpton and Smith, *Cholera*, 71–2.
[43] Cited from Salomé, 'Le massacre': 'Il y a trop de pauvres, et on aime mieux nous empoisonner que de nous nourrir' (107).
[44] See Bourdelais and Raulot, *Une Peur Bleue*, 275, The provincial ones 'plus souvent restent proches des réactions parisiennes'.
[45] Preto, *Epidemia*, ch. 5 and 226, and also for Siracusa, Bercé, *Le chaudron*, 157.
[46] Bourdelais and Raulot, *Une Peur Bleue*, 225; and Rollet and Sauriac, 'Épidémies et mentalités, 962–5.
[47] Dineur and Engrand, 'Le choléra à Lille', 93–4.
[48] Vidalenc, 'Les départements normands', 103.   [49] Ibid., 107–8.
[50] Ibid.   [51] Fréour, 'Le choléra à Bordeaux'.

than anywhere in France',[52] but still no cholera riots or myths of doctors poisoning surfaced. Instead, Marseille's solution to fear was religious and passive: 30,000 people processed and prostrated themselves at the feet of their saints.[53] *Le Figaro* reported that 'the poisonings' troubled security in Lyon, Grenoble, the Vendée, and several towns in other provinces, and the army was put on guard, but mentioned no riots or violence.[54]

Finally, a study of cholera in 1832 through the region of Seine-et-Oise emphasizes panic, fear, and flight sparked by cholera's explosive spread and the rapid deaths of the afflicted. While the authors' demographic and epidemiological analysis pertains exclusively to this region, their descriptions of the socio-psychological reactions derive from secondary sources and are taken almost entirely from other places. The few accusations of poisoning that the authors uncover within Seine-et-Oise show no evidence of cholera rumours spurring violence or mass movements. Even mistrust of doctors here differed from that in Paris or other European countries: in Seine-et-Oise only doctors sent from Paris were feared; they trusted their own.[55]

NORTH AMERICA

Similarly, little has been found of cholera myths or violence in the US, and yet this difference with Europe has gone without comment, even in Charles Rosenberg's classic, centred on cholera in New York City, but which spans the continent across its three major cholera waves, 1832 to 1866. He found repeated bitter controversies between politicians, the clergy, and medical professions over the character of the disease, whether it was contagious, and the best means to combat it. But even these wars of words, mostly among intellectuals, brewed during cholera's successive waves in 1849 and 1866. As far as collective violence goes, he spotted only a handful of incidents, the first three of which can hardly be called riots.

1. In Chester, Pennsylvania, several persons suspected of carrying the pestilence were reportedly murdered, along with a man who had sheltered them.

2. Armed Rhode Islanders turned back New Yorkers fleeing across Long Island Sound.

3. At Ypsilanti, a local militia fired on a mail stage from cholera-infested Detroit.[56]

'Mob' first appears in a fourth incident in New York City, but its collective violence appears limited to the inmates of a single tenement: 'a miscellaneous mob of

---

[52] Guiral, 'Le choléra à Marseille', 121.   [53] Ibid., 138.

[54] *Le Figaro*, 10 April 1832, front page. Salomé, 'Le massacre', suggests that collective violence may have occurred at Meung-sur-Loire in le Loiret, but 'the documentation is insufficient' (104).

[55] A single case of scapegoating uncovered pertained not to persecution, murder, or attempted murder of a government official or doctor, but to a worker—a pulverizer of paints ('un ouvrier broyeur de couleurs')—who appeared with a yellow face, but it is unclear whether he suffered any physical abuse; Rollet and Sauriac, 'Épidémies et mentalités', 962–5.

[56] Rosenberg, *The Cholera Years*, 37.

men and women' blocked hallways of their building, forcing the authorities to lower a coffin out of a window. When it reached the ground, the women of the building 'stood upon it to prevent its being taken away'.[57] Other newspapers not used by Rosenberg, however, report it as more than a fracas within a tenement and more in line with disturbances occurring at the same time in the British Isles. A 'mob' of 300 assembled to prevent health officers entering a house to remove and bury a cholera victim. Five quarts of rum were carried into the house (no doubt, for the wake), which, according to the journalists, fuelled the mob's 'serious resistance'.[58]

A fifth incident also shows European characteristics. At Utica, New York, 'an infuriated mob of Irish workingmen stormed the cholera hospital'. But no injuries, arrests, or damages to the hospital were reported. Finally, Rosenberg adds that 'even in enlightened Philadelphia, physicians and attendants were vilified and abused'.[59] It is not clear, however, whether the 'abuse' amounted to collective violence. More recently, new historical and archaeological evidence has uncovered the remains of fifty-seven of the 120 Irish labourers hired to cut the difficult fifty-ninth mile of the Philadelphia and Columbia Railroad at Duffy's Cut, who became devastated by cholera in 1832. Four of the fifty-seven show catastrophic head injuries, one with a bullet hole. The archaeologists speculate that the burial site was an enforced quarantine from which the four may have escaped, were captured, executed, and thrown back in what became a mass grave of cholera victims. A near-contemporary unpublished history of the event reports the Irish workers tried to flee to local homes for assistance but were turned away. Eventually, four Sisters of Charity attended the dying Irishmen. The history, however, reports nothing about a quarantine or violence to victims.[60]

For the next two cholera waves, Rosenberg finds two further riots. The first erupted on 16 May 1849. New York City's Board of Health established a cholera hospital, a 'crude loft', which 'a mob' threatened to burn down, but the crowd was dispersed,[61] preventing the threats from going beyond words. Rosenberg's second case, on Staten Island in 1858,[62] was significant, in fact, one of the largest and most costly in lives and damage to property sparked by an epidemic in US history. Yet this riot, organized and staffed by elites against a quarantine centre with hospitals, isolation buildings, and sheds to house passengers coming into New York City's harbours who were suspected of carrying any infectious disease, did not occur during a cholera epidemic. Moreover, numerous newspapers pointed to the presence of smallpox and yellow fever but none to cholera or any anxieties about it.[63]

---

[57] Ibid., 33, from the _Commercial Advertiser_, 3 July and 13 August 1832.
[58] _Philadelphia Inquirer_, 4 July 1832, 2; _Baltimore Gazette_, 5 July 1832, 2, from _New York Commercial Gazette_; and _Portsmouth Journal of Literature and Politics_, 14 July 1832, front page.
[59] Rosenberg, _The Cholera Years_, 95.
[60] Watson, 'The Sisters of Charity', 14–16; and Dan Barry, 'With Shovels and Science', _New York Times_, 24 March 2013; also Shah, _Pandemic_, 126.
[61] Ibid., 107–8; from _The New-York Tribune_, 18 and 19 May 1849.
[62] Rosenberg, _The Cholera Years_, 203.   [63] Chapters 12 and 18 will explore this incident.

Such a meagre return does not result from any lack of diligence on Rosenberg's part. I know of no one to extend his list, and now, aided by online newspapers, I can only offer a few, which do not reshape his picture: compared with Europe, cholera riots in the US remain a rarity. When cholera reached Detroit via Canada in early July 1832,[64] three incidents occurred in surrounding small towns desperate to prevent what was perceived as a highly contagious disease from entering their communities. Rosenberg mentions the first of these, at Ypsilanti. Further details can be added: citizens sought to prohibit all intercourse with outsiders, fired on the mail stage, and killed its horse. In a second incident at Rochester, Oakland County, passengers from Detroit were chased from public houses with 'their baggage thrown after them'; bridges were destroyed, and 'other measures taken to prevent persons from Detroit entering the village'. In a third, at Pontiac, a body of armed men established sentinels along the highways leading to the village with orders to stop all from Detroit. These differed from the European riots fuelled by mythologies of hospitals as death chambers and physicians as poisoners. Moreover, not all communities in southern Michigan behaved alike. At Auburn, physicians and town leaders convinced their citizens that cholera was not a contagious disease. In a town meeting, they resolved not to follow in the footsteps of their neighbours and insisted it was 'every citizen's duty' to extend 'all the assistance in their power to the unfortunate sick'.[65]

During the second wave of 1849, rioters attacked a cholera hospital in Quebec City. It was more menacing and successful than the New York City protest of the same year [66] and was the only one in North America to approach European dimensions. 'About two thousand, riotously disposed, assembled in front of the Police Barracks' and demolished the city's cholera hospital. 'Yelling and hooting all the time', they destroyed 'everything that could be broken'.[67] The military had to be summoned. Yet even here, European mythologies of physicians or state agents poisoning the populace fail to appear. As with later attacks on smallpox pesthouses, none of the perpetrators of violence in Quebec was named.[68]

---

[64] More research is needed for Canada. Most recently, see Zeheter, *Epidemics, Empire and Environments*, which compares cholera in Quebec City and Madras but pays no attention to cholera riots and seems unaware even of the largest and most destructive cholera riot in North America having occurred in Quebec City in 1849. I have searched through one of the few online papers available for 1832, the *Kingston Chronicle*, producing 124 hits for 'cholera' and 'riot' and 84 for 'cholera' and 'mob'. None, however, reveals cholera disturbances in the region, even though Kingston imposed strict quarantine measures with patients removed to new cholera hospitals and the dead to a new cholera cemetery out of town (*Kingston Chronicle*, 23 June 1832, 3). The paper also refers to the cholera epidemic at Quebec, Montreal, and the enforced quarantining of arriving immigrants at Grosse Isle. On the long life of this quarantine centre, see Zeheter, *Epidemics, Empire and Environments*, 71–2, 82, 208, 230.

[65] *Democratic Free Press* (later *Detroit Free Press*), 19 July 1832, 2.

[66] Other papers in 'Chronicling America' report this incident: the *Evening Post*, 17 May 1849, 3; *Baltimore Sun*, 19 May 1849, front page; *Trenton State Gazette*, 19 May 1849, 4.

[67] *Trenton State Gazette*, 23 July 1849. The Australian press mentioned it briefly: for example, *The Maitland Mercury*, 21 November 1849, 3, which adds that the Customs House was 'completely gutted'. These papers estimated the crowd at 2000. Numerous British papers mentioned it, for instance, *Glasgow Herald*, 30 July 1849.

[68] Bilson, *A Darkened House*, 125–6. Also, during the epidemic of 1849, residents of Prince Edward Island burnt a cholera hospital for immigrants 'as a dangerous nuisance to the neighbourhood' (125).

In July 1854, a sixth cholera disturbance surfaced in New York City's Fifth Ward. A 'meeting of indignation' was called to oppose the Emigration Office's decision to open a cholera hospital in the neighbourhood. 'Earnest remonstrances' were 'uttered', but the citizens' protest did not become a riot. Instead, citizens proposed 'candid and plain-spoken resolutions' that questioned the board's decision to build the hospital in a densely crowded district. The *New York Times* supported the neighbours' protest.[69] In contrast to this paper's detailed reportage of European cholera riots into the twentieth century, this was the only cholera protest within the US of any sort that it mentioned since the paper's foundation in 1851.[70]

Two further cholera riots, however, erupted in 1866. A mob in St Louis torched the 'dead house', where bodies of cholera victims were stored,[71] and a similar incident occurred several days before in Philadelphia. But here the citizens' motives were clear: in line with US smallpox riots, the 'mob' was comprised of property owners, who would not accept a hospital for the infectious in their backyard. Again, the protesters voiced none of the conspiracies heard in Europe.[72] Finally, disorder occurred during the next European cholera pandemic in 1892, although that cholera wave failed to spread through America. Instead, the disturbance was a European import. Steerage passengers on a ship—the *Normannia*—who probably became infected while docked in Hamburg, were transferred to another ship ordered to dock at Long Island's Fire Island quarantine station. Three hundred oystermen greeted the ship 'armed with shotguns, oars, and other weapons' and prevented the passengers from landing. The crowd yelled obscenities and calls for the passengers to return to New York. The governor sent troops.[73] Only after several days, suffering from heat and overcrowding, were the passengers allowed ashore.[74] The oystermen's threats concerned fears of infection spreading to their community,[75] not Old World conspiracies that were continuing to affect parts of Europe. Beyond Rosenberg, few have studied the social characteristics and consequences of cholera in US history. One study to do so for New Orleans, St Louis,

---

A year and a half later, a cholera incident flared up among emigrants on a steamer approaching Mobile, Alabama, 20 miles north of Montgomery. When cholera broke out on board, passengers became belligerent; a militia was summoned to suppress the mob.

[69] *New York Times*, 15 July 1854.

[70] Cholera may have provoked another incident in 1866 in the Bronx. Newspapers reporting it, however, leave in doubt whether this bar-room brawl was connected to cholera.

[71] *Evening Public Ledger*, 20 August 1866, 2.

[72] From 'Chronicling America', only one newspaper reported the early-morning burning of the hall. The night before, citizens held a meeting to 'appeal to the mayor' to rescind the Health Board's decision to build a cholera hospital in such a densely built neighbourhood (*Evening Telegraph*, 3 August 1866, 3). The paper surmised collusion between the incendiaries and the fire department; ibid., 4 August 1866, 5.

[73] *Guardian*, 20 September 1892, 9, from the *New York Evening Post*'s editor aboard the *Cepheus*.

[74] *Guardian*, 14 September 1892, 8.

[75] The Australian press paid great attention to this cholera riot, supplying details not found in US papers, such as attempts to drown Dr Vought, director of the sanitary arrangements on Fire Island, and those illegally quarantining the *Normannia* included Long Island oystermen, clam diggers, merchants, and 'a so-called lawyer'; *The Argus*, 14 September 1892, 5; and *Kapunda Herald*, 17 January 1893, 3.

San Francisco, Sacramento, and smaller staging posts on its westward move across the continent, 1848 to 1855, reports not a single incident of mob violence or even accusations against physicians. As in Rosenberg's study, the antagonisms centred on medical debate: theories of transmission and controversies between contagionists and anti-contagionists.[76]

RUSSIA AND EASTERN EUROPE: THE LATER WAVES

While the 1848–9 outbreak may have marked the end or near disappearance of cholera's social violence in the British Isles and for major cities and regions in France, it proved only a pause in cholera's social violence in other European states. For Russia, the violence spread through the Volga basin and overland northward to Nizhnii-Novgorod, the lands of Russia's cholera vortex since its first wave in the 1820s. Here, cholera riots continued to strike cities such as Tsaritsyn, Saratov (Saratoff), Samara, and further east in Tashkent on the Uzbekistan–Kazakhstan border in Asiatic Sydiria, as revealed in foreign newspapers, relayed by correspondents, which undercut Czarist censorship of cholera riots that embarrassed the Empire's autocratic rule. Despite scholars' focus on cholera in 1831–2, cholera violence had not steadily declined over the century and may even have reached a crescendo during Russia's penultimate cholera wave in the summer of 1892. To date, no one has compared the number, range, or ferocity of these incidents, or detailed how their conspiracies and myths may have changed.

In 1892 the British physician, sanitary officer, and Russian correspondent for the *Lancet*, Frank Clemow, described 'the terrible riots in Astrakhan, Saratov, Khvalynsk and other places'. He maintained that the rioters' 'reign of terror' spread the disease not only directly by removing patients from hospitals, 'leaving them to die in the streets', but also 'by paralysing' authorities' efforts to check the epidemic. In Astrakhan, an administrative centre on the Volga, for five days 'panic was absolute', disrupting medical services: 'It will never be known how many people were attacked with cholera during that period'.[77] As early as 21 June, rumours declared the city's sanitary measures were unnecessary and that the sick were being brought to hospitals to be buried alive. After removing the patients, 'the infuriated populace' set the city's hospitals ablaze and attacked the Governor's house. A military detachment arrived, arrested the leaders, and dispersed the crowd, killing three.[78] Reuters news service held the municipality partially responsible because of its carelessness in transporting patients to cholera hospitals 'in wretched carts like packing cases'. It estimated the rioters' numbers at 10,000—the highest seen for any cholera riot, those of the 1830s included.[79] A US paper based on correspondence put it at

---

[76] Roth, 'The Western Cholera Trail'.

[77] Clemow, 'The Cholera Epidemic in Russia', 1059. Cholera had attacked the city and its region since the earliest cholera wave, reaching the Volga in 1823; Creighton, II, 794.

[78] *Pittsburgh Dispatch*, 12 July 1892, 12. Australian and British papers followed these Russian cholera disturbances. Henze, *Disease*, 62–3, adds that the crowd tore down tearooms and police stations.

[79] Except for the questionable estimate of Aberdeen's that nearly equalled the city's adult population.

20,000 to 30,000, in a city of 80,000. In addition to burning the hospital, leaving some patients 'horribly mutilated', and 'beating all the doctors severely', rioters attacked Persian merchants, believing the epidemic had originated in Persia, a rare instance when origins appear to have spelled blame.[80]

On 10 July, rumours spread through another administrative centre—Saratov—a major port on the Volga.[81] Alleging that cholera victims had been hospitalized without cause, the crowd dragged them from hospitals 'to save them' from what 'the mob' perceived as their fate—burial alive.[82] To counteract the doctors' supposed poisons, the 'liberators' carried the sick to the banks of the Volga to give them milk, believing it an antidote to the physicians' poison.[83] They attacked medical assistants, killing two and mutilating their bodies, smashed windows, burst into the dwellings of policemen and doctors, destroyed the residence of the Chief of Police, ransacked shops, and forced their way into the police station to burn documents. They destroyed the carts for transporting patients to hospitals, and 'invaded the sheds' where cholera victims were treated, 'ruthlessly massacring' all members of the hospital staff in spite of 'supplications for mercy'. The 'mob' then set the sheds on fire, looted the new Central Hospital, and was poised for 'fresh excesses', when troops arrived, killing several and wounding more. The following day, Saratov was reported as having 'the appearance of a military camp', its streets full of soldiers with canons positioned near the cathedral.[84] The mob threatened to take over the city and, according to a St Petersburg correspondent, would have succeeded, had troops not fired on them.[85] Another account blamed the riots on 'ignorant peasants, small tradesmen, and mechanics', asserting that they resented 'any attempt to improve the sanitary conditions'.[86] Another hinted that women were the leaders and were arrested 'for inciting the mob to violence'.[87]

Yet the *Scotsman* held the Saratov riot was well organized, despite 'the lower classes' holding the old beliefs about doctors poisoning cholera patients. By early July 1892, protesters held meetings, delivered speeches to large crowds in public squares, and were no longer confined to neighbourhoods. Now, an entire town was placed 'completely at the mercy of the rioters'.[88] In November, Paris's *Le Temps* summarized Saratov's revolts, describing two having occurred that summer—one on 28 June, another on 11 July. It stressed that the rioters' targets were planned, with the burning of the Demidov hospital, murder of police agents, invasion of the central police station, and sacking of the residences of Doctor Bonvitch and

---

[80] *Scotsman*, 19 July 1892, 5. On crowd estimates, see *Pittsburgh Dispatch*, 27 July 1892, 12.

[81] On Saratow before 1892, see Henze, *Disease*, 67–79.

[82] *Scotsman*, 19 July 1892, 5.

[83] *Morning Call*, 15 July 1892, front page; and *La Presse*, 20 July 1892.

[84] *Scotsman*, 20 July 1892, 8, from St Petersburg.

[85] *Evening World*, 14 July 1892; *Morning Call*, 15 July 1892, front page; and *Scotsman*, 15 July 1892, 5.

[86] *Morning Call*, 23 July 1892.

[87] *Pittsburgh Dispatch*, 24 July 1892. According to *Le Temps*, 12 November 1892, 2, only five of the 155 accused were women. Henze, *Disease*, 88–92, adds that the crowd 'began a systematic hunt for doctors and police', attacked the police office, and destroyed all its documents.

[88] *Scotsman*, 20 July 1892, 8.

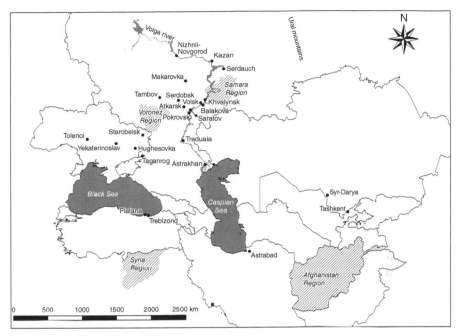

Map 8.1. Cholera riots, Russia, 1892. Shaded areas correspond to regions of cholera riots outside major towns.

of the musician Dostoevski. Unlike in most earlier cholera riots, key leaders appeared: a junk dealer ('marchand de bric-à-brac') directed the course of events and one named Martianov planned sorties against individual policemen and doctors. A third was Alexandre Papov, who covered himself with whitewash, claiming he had been thrown in a dog cage and coated in paint to be buried alive, but escaped 'by a miracle', and used his tale to rouse followers. A fourth leader called Chkadronov spread rumours among peasants and city dwellers that ambulance doctors forced patients to swallow a liquid that killed them after 'atrocious suffering'. The article recounted the complex movements of separate groups of rioters and coordinated attacks on specific targets ('Chacune de ces bandes, suivant un itinéraire évidemment fixé à l'avance'). Against general impressions of cholera riots in the past—that they sprang up more or less spontaneously without prior meetings or leaders—this article argued that these were well organized ('avoir été organisée d'assez longue main') and had been directed by 'intelligent and determined' leaders. The numbers arrested suggest their scale, filling 'no less than' twenty-seven columns of *La vie russe*, comprised mostly of 'peasants and townsmen' but also twenty military reservists and others off duty.[89]

In July, 'a serious riot of the same character' erupted at Pokrovsk, near Saratov, that followed in the provincial capital's footsteps: 'the mob' broke into the hospital,

---

[89] *Le Temps*, 12 November 1892, 2. According to Henze, *Disease*, 91, seventeen were from the military.

wrecked the resident physician's lodgings, and assaulted a medical assistant, who died the next day.[90] One hundred and sixty were arrested and tried.[91] Further riots spread to other towns in the province at Volsk[92] and Khvalynsk, where the 'mob' took over the town for more than three days.[93] Again, at Astrakhan, riots targeted doctors, killing a resident physician, sacking the hospital, and threatening the police. As a consequence, the Minister of the Interior posted notices in towns along the Volga, 'warning the public that all disorders and acts of violence' would be put down by armed force and tried by court martial.[94] Several days later, villagers at Balakova in the same province marched to a recently completed cholera hospital and dismantled it, 'plank by plank', 'methodically and in silence'.[95] Despite the perseverance of the old myths, these riots again appear well organized. In reaction, the authorities and foreign journalists now created their own myths, claiming outside agitators must have instigated them. As far as Nizhnii-Novgorod, the government posted inflammatory proclamations and Reuters reported that 'self-constituted leaders in the mobs' carried out 'preconcerted' plans, 'declaring that they had escaped from coffins'.[96]

During the same week, further disturbances arose in the province of Astrakhan (Figure 8.1). In the small town of Treduaia (Srednaia-Akhtouba), inhabitants united with recently arrived emigrants from other parts of Russia, rebelled against sanitary measures, pillaged commercial offices, killed a pharmacist and his assistant, attacked postal and telegraph offices, and assaulted the police. A priest attempting to pacify the crowd was seized and beaten. Disturbances spread to the surrounding villages of Tolenoi and Zamosc; disinfectants were seized and destroyed.[97] Although not reported in the foreign press until a month later because of the government's 'strictest censorship', the same week witnessed cholera riots by peasants, who attacked physicians along the Syr Darya river.[98]

In late July (though not reaching St Petersburg correspondents until 1 August), 'serious riots' erupted at Tashkent: tribal Sarts believed that cholera among their tribesmen came from Russian doctors poisoning them. Armed with revolvers and daggers, 5000, 'driven to madness over the reported cruelties to cholera patients', invaded the Russian quarter of the city, plundered shops, and stoned 'all citizens in their way'. They attacked and destroyed the residence of the Deputy Governor, Count Poutinstinoff, chased him through the streets, trampled, stoned, and beat him to death, 'mutilating his features beyond recognition'. Cossacks and the army momentarily quelled the revolt, but the Sarts regrouped in their mosques and

[90] *Guardian*, 20 July 1892, 8, from Reuters, and *Scotsman*, 20 July 1892, 8.
[91] *Reynold's Newsletter*, 11 September 1892, front page.
[92] *Scotsman*, 22 July 1892, 5, from St Petersburg.
[93] *Edinburgh Evening News*, 19 July 1892, 3. The crowd also later brutally murdered the physician A. M. Molchanov; Henze, *Disease*, 92.
[94] *Scotsman*, 20 July 1892; and *Nottingham Evening Post*, 19 July 1892, 3.
[95] *Scotsman*, 25 July 1892, 7. Also, Henze, *Disease*, 92.   [96] *Scotsman*, 22 July 1892.
[97] Ibid., 26 July 1892, 5, from St Petersburg; *Western Times*, 27 July 1892, 4.
[98] *Record-Union*, 2 August 1892, front page. On Russian cholera censorship, see *Manchester Evening News*, 2 August 1892, 4.

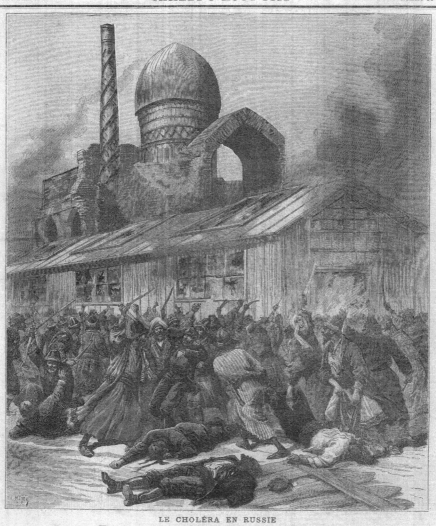

Figure 8.1. Cholera riot Astrakhan, 1892, *Le Petit Journal.*

battled against the army. Sixty Sarts by one account, seventy by another,[99] were killed and 'hundreds' wounded. The soldiers also suffered heavily with 'many' wounded and fifteen dead.[100]

Authorities and news correspondents no longer considered the outbreaks spontaneous. Like the examples cited here, they pointed to skilled leaders and prior organization. From its St Petersburg correspondent, the *Observer* claimed the 'recent disturbances were regularly organized some days before by Mahommedan malcontents'.[101] Almost a month later, conflict still smouldered,[102] with disturbances against sanitary precautions spreading into 'even the remote Ural districts', requiring military intervention. In Tambov and Atkarsk, inhabitants were 'so terrorised by the threatening mob that no individual dares to inform the police'.[103]

On 22 July, 'fearing cholera riots', the Russian government proclaimed 'a state of siege' at Nizhnii-Novgorod,[104] and at the end of the month the military had to defend a ship anchored in the Volga that served as a cholera hospital.[105] Riots spread eastward to Seradanach [Serdauch], Toubanound, Astrakhan, Tolenoi [Tal'ne], Zamosc, and Tashkent,[106] killing pharmacists, their assistants, doctors, and police.[107] Further disturbances arose in the central Russian province of Samara; its governor had to summon the 159th Regiment and establish tight security around physicians' residences. In the village of Balakova, peasants demolished a cholera ambulance. At Nizhnii-Novgorod and Kazan, local governments acted in ways that recall early modern plague-spreading trials but not seen elsewhere in the nineteenth and twentieth centuries: municipal governors joined the rioters, 'relentlessly' pursuing and indicting those charged with spreading the disease by poison.[108]

At the end of the month, a US paper concluded that cholera rioting in Russia during 1892 'scarcely finds a parallel in modern history since the plague riots of the Middle Ages...or only in Russian annals of the seventeenth-century uprisings of Stenka Razin and Pugacheff'.[109] Surely, it was an overstatement. The earlier Russian movements stretched over years, not hours or days, mobilizing peasant troops in the tens of thousands and with corresponding numbers killed.[110] It is striking, however, that the journalist did not recall earlier cholera riots such as those in St Petersburg in 1831. From their memories, the earlier riots certainly did not tower over the present ones. How many of the cholera riots in 1830–2 had

---

[99] *St Paul Daily Globe*, 29 December 1892.
[100] *Scotsman*, 2 August 1892, 6 and 30 August 1892.   [101] *The Observer*, 7 August 1892, 5.
[102] *The Record-Union*, 2 August 1892, front page. A number of US papers followed the story. On the harsh punishments meted out to rioters from August to the end of the year, see *St Paul Daily Globe*, 29 December 1892.
[103] *Morning Post*, 30 July 1892, 5. Papers from Gallica paid less attention to these riots; the 'Ashkend' *émeute* was an exception: *Le Figaro*, 28 August 1892.
[104] *Morning Call*, 23 July 1892.   [105] *Pittsburgh Dispatch*, 30 July 1892, 7.
[106] *Witchita Daily Eagle*, 26 July 1892. Serdauch is the province of Tatarstan. I could not find Toubanound. I thank Professor Evan Mawdsley for his help.
[107] Ibid., *Morning Call*, 30 July 1892; *Pittsburgh Dispatch*, 27 July 1892, 12; *Record-Union*, 30 July 1892, front page.
[108] *Le Temps*, 25 July 1892, 2. According to the *New York Times*, 24 July 1892, Balakhna's villagers demolished their cholera hospital, despite troops guarding it.
[109] *Pittsburgh Dispatch*, 27 July 1892, 12.
[110] Avrich, *Russian Rebels*, chs 1–2; and Parker, *Global Crisis*, 181ff.

occupied entire cities, even momentarily, or could count 5000–10,000 among their ranks?[111] Moreover, the cholera riots of 1892 were not confined to cities, even though few specific reports detailed ones in the countryside. San Francisco's *Morning Call* claimed they had spread all the way to Afghanistan and by early August had raced throughout Russia.[112]

Cholera rioting, however, had yet to end. In August, disturbances continued apace, and their territory expanded, no longer confined to central Russia. First, they recurred in Saratov with destruction of property and the murder of Dr Moltchanoff (or Moltehanoff), whose body the 'mob' beat 'into an unrecognizable form'.[113] Thirty were arrested; seven were women.[114] A hundred miles away in cholera-stricken Serdobsk, rioters burnt 300 houses, causing 'great distress' and homelessness. Serious riots began on 1 August at Hughes' steelworks and collieries in Hughesovka (also called Youzova, now Donetsk in the Ukraine), but because of Czarist censorship were unknown to the West until the end of the month. The alleged cause was 'the lower classes' opposing sanitary precautions. A 'mob' stoned the police while they were removing a woman to the hospital, and then attacked Cossacks dispatched to protect the police. The Cossacks drew their swords; 200 rioters and thirty soldiers were 'disabled'. The crowd next sacked the hospital, and, 'excited by drink', tried to set the town on fire. According to an Odessa correspondent, 10,000 rioters began the day by massacring several Jews, then succeeded in burning down the town, 'every house reduced to ashes, including even the church'. They invaded the factories, 'taking everything not nailed down'. Mr Hughes and his family had to run for their lives.[115] It took three days to restore order and only after the arrival of two regiments and a battery of artillery.[116] According to *Le Temps*, on the first day of fighting alone, the rioters killed or gravely injured twenty-five Cossacks, while 200 rioters were 'put out of combat'. Yet by the second day, 'the Cossacks still were unable to defend themselves against the thousands of workers and were mostly killed'.[117]

The August riots spread to other places in the region. The governor of Taganrog dispatched Cossack troops to stop riots at Yekaterinoslav (Dnepropetrovsk); many buildings were wrecked and set ablaze.[118] Rioting reached other regions such as Voronež Province (about 700 km south of Moscow) and the 'village' of Makarovka (now on the outskirts of Voronezh), then comprising a population of around 8000. 'As at Astrakan and elsewhere', the mob attacked the hospital along with its ambulance conveying medicine and disinfectants. The doctors fled, and order

---

[111] On estimates of riots in 1830–1, see note 1.

[112] *The Morning Call*, 9 August 1892. The paper took the Czarist line that Nihilists had incited them.

[113] *Evening Bulletin*, 19 August 1892.

[114] *London Daily News*, 9 August 1892, 5; and *New York Herald*, 10 August 1892, 6.

[115] *Scotsman*, 27 August 1892, 7. John Hughes (1814–89) was a Welsh engineer, inventor, and entrepreneur, invited by the Czar to build steelworks in 1868.

[116] *Wichita Daily Eagle*, 27 August 1892, front page.

[117] *Le Temps*, 28 August 1892, 2. A worker with an iron rail knocked the Cossacks' commander from his horse; *Scotsman*, 27 August 1892, 7.

[118] *Evening Bulletin*, 19 August 1892; and *Birmingham Daily Post*, 5 December 1892, 4.

was not restored until soldiers arrived. The 'instigators' were 'publicly knouted'.[119] A week later, north of the Black Sea, 'a mob' attacked a floating hospital at Starobelsk, 'completely demolishing it'. The assaulted doctors, 'would have been killed' had troops not intervened.[120] In other places, the rioting assumed a different face from cholera's usual conspiratorial fantasies. In Astrabad (Persia, then part of the Russia), priests (mollahs) sparked the violence, preaching that alcoholic beverages had brought on this 'Plague'. The religiously inspired mob raided the dram shops and destroyed the goods of Armenian traders (Russian subjects). The Czar sent twenty-five mounted Cossacks and a Russian gunboat to guard the consulate.[121]

Cholera riots spread into Syria,[122] and Platana (Akçaabat in present-day Turkey), 7 miles west of Trabzon (Trebizond) on the Black Sea. Townspeople escaping a lazaretto were shot; seven were killed with 'many more' wounded.[123] According to a Constantinople dispatch, the trouble arose from the sanitary regulations. Nearly 1500, detained at the lazaretto, attempted to break its sanitary cordon.[124] Two months later, a more menacing rebellion struck Trabzon, 'an open revolt' against the town's governor and the head of the Sanitary Department, accused by the rioters of poisoning the sick. The alleged reasons for it, however, were now different: local officials were rumoured to have poisoned townsmen so that the central authorities would believe cholera had spread to the region, and, as a result, the local officials would be decorated for their efforts to suppress it.[125] On 18 August, cholera conspiracies and riots spread to other parts of Russia with the places and motives left vague. Despite the brevity of the reports, the riots must have been large: military intervention was required to quell them.[126]

CHOLERA RIOTS IN EUROPE IN THE 1890s

By September, the disturbances had spread beyond Russia into Eastern Europe and from there into Europe's cultural heartland. On 2 September, peasants in Kiszacs, near Neusatz in Hungary, rioted when cholera patients were removed to hospitals.[127] The events and motivation differed from the Russian ones: the village assembled and insisted an autopsy of a cholera victim should not be performed. Such acts, the villagers believed, violated the body and would thereby bring hailstorms destroying their crops. Armed with scythes and pitchforks, the peasants appear to have succeeded: the victim was buried without a post-mortem examination.[128]

[119] *Scotsman*, 8 August 1892, 9; *Chicago Daily Tribune*, 7 August 1892, 2; and *Observer*, 7 August 1892, 5, from St Petersburg, 5 August. Knouting was a severe public flogging with a special whip called a knout or knut. *Western Champion*, 9 August 1892, 6, reported another disturbance in Voronež: a mob destroyed the hospital and the doctors fled.

[120] *Daily Inter Ocean*, 17 August 1892, 3; and *Freeman's Journal*, 17 August 1892, 6.

[121] *Evening World*, 8 August 1892.   [122] *Sedalia Weekly Bazoo*, 9 August 1892.

[123] *Daily Gazette for Middlesbrough*, 12 August 1892, 2.

[124] *Evening World*, 11 August 1892.   [125] *Sheffield Independent*, 5 October 1892, 5.

[126] *Sun*, 18 August 1892.   [127] Ibid., 3 September 1892.

[128] *Sheffield Daily Telegraph*, 5 September 1892, 5; and *Glasgow Herald*, 5 September 1892, 7; among others.

Three weeks later, villagers of Lyssobiki (Łysobyki) in the 'Congress of Poland' attacked officials investigating a cholera outbreak. Rumours spread of officials sent to poison cholera patients or bury them alive. A 'large and excited mob' stormed the hotel where the officials were staying, smashed windows and doors, and threatened their lives. Troops were dispatched.[129] The US paper did not comment on the composition of the crowd, but, as we will see, its leadership and rank and file were unusual. Further, cholera and anti-Christian riots broke out in Ostrovo (Ostrowo), Poland (then within Russia), north of Gdansk.[130] A single brief report fails to reveal whether the two riots were intertwined.[131]

By early October, cholera and its associated violence invaded Budapest, even if the riots were not as large or bloody as Russia's. According to a local correspondent, 'the ignorant classes' prevented sanitary authorities performing their tasks and attacked them while disinfecting houses. The first assailants were women, who poured kettles of boiling water on the sanitary officers. 'Finding the situation literally too hot for them', they fled.[132] Later, men joined, showering the sanitary workers with stones. When the police arrived, they were attacked, leaving some 'quite severely injured'.[133] Two years later, further cholera riots spread to Hungarian villages.[134] In November, at Huszt, protest erupted over a decree requiring the cholera dead to be buried in a separate cemetery. A peasant was killed, 'many wounded', and sixty arrested, including twenty women.[135] The same proclamation sparked another village riot, though less well reported by the Anglophone press, even though greater casualties ensued: at an unnamed village in Marmaros Comitat, troops killed four and wounded twenty.[136] Meanwhile, cholera riots spread to villages in Romania with attacks against doctors followed by deadly repression.[137]

From the summer of 1894 to 1895, sparked by burial decrees, Poland became a hotspot of cholera rioting. In July, 'serious disturbances' erupted at Sharnoff in the Russian-occupied Government of Radom. At the funeral of four victims, a 'mob' attempted to prevent their burial in a cemetery constructed solely for cholera victims. Crowds chased off the coffin bearers and stormed the huts housing patients, 'rescuing' twenty but injuring several. The ringleaders were arrested.[138] Two months later at Blasseki (Blaszki), the district of Kalish (Kalisz) in Russian Poland, a mob torched sixty houses with the inmates left inside 'consumed by fire', several too

---

[129] *St Paul Daily Globe*, 24 September 1892.   [130] *Pittsburgh Dispatch*, 14 October 1892, 9.

[131] 'Chronicling America' papers produce only one earlier cholera revolt in Polish regions or Lithuania and Estonia. Outside Vilnius in 1871, a reputed monk from Galicia, selling rosaries and other religious objects, spread the belief that the sanitary controls had no object but to poison the peasantry. Three hundred peasants attacked officials disinfecting. Thirteen were arrested; *Jackson Daily Citizen*, 3 October 1871, 2.

[132] According to *Scotsman*, 6 October 1892, 5, the mob arrived with pickaxes and brooms, preventing officials carrying out the operation'.

[133] *The Evening Bulletin*, 10 October 1892; also reported in less detail by the English press: for instance, *Birmingham Daily Post*, 10 October 1892, 8.

[134] *Evening World*, 19 September 1894; ibid., 7 November 1894.

[135] *Scotsman*, 7 November 1894, 9; and *London Standard* 7 November 1894, 5.

[136] *Worcester Journal*, 10 November 1894, 6.

[137] *Chicago Daily Tribune*, 30 September 1893, 5, for Brahilov.

[138] *Gloucester Citizen*, 26 July 1894, 3.

weak to move. The newspaper does not clarify whether the rioters intended to kill the cholera-afflicted; nor did it speculate on their motives.[139] In the same month, riots spread to other places in Poland, 'owing to the ignorance of the peasantry', but a paper described only one. As in Sharnoff, and Ottynia, the crowd 'forcibly removed' cholera patients from the hospital and set the Sanitary Officer's house on fire. The military was summoned.[140] The following year (1895) riots flared in northern parts of the Austro-Hungarian Empire, in the Kingdom of Galicia at Podolia, where inhabitants resisted the construction of temporary cholera hospitals. Troops were summoned.[141]

Cholera rioting also penetrated Western Europe. Reminiscent of German pogroms against Jews during the Black Death, it began before the disease appeared. Fear drove the populace in Munich to what 'almost amounts to a frenzy': 'An immense throng of butchers, clerks, mechanics, and others' gathered in front of the guardroom, demanding that all traffic by railway be stopped. The police charged the 'mob' but successfully resisted. A detachment of infantry arrived to assist the civil authorities, drove back the rioters, arresting 'those who were the more demonstrative'. In the struggle, protesters were wounded by sword thrusts; 'others had their heads broken'.[142]

The following year at the end of September and into October, possibly two cholera riots flared in Hamburg's working-class suburb of St Pauli. Both had similar causes and consequences, although the second appears to have stemmed from a mistaken copying of a previous news file. According to the *New-York Tribune*, both stemmed from 'the poor and ignorant classes, who seem to have a horror of being compelled to observe cleanliness and the ordinary sanitary regulations'.[143] Although the *New York Times* repeated the same phrase, it showed more sympathy towards the workers, attributing their reactions to the authorities' attempts to enforce sanitary ordinances, which the populace claimed interfered with 'their way of life'.[144] On 26 September, health officers, accompanied by police, entered St Pauli to impose ordinances of cleanliness. Exactly what these entailed is not described, but the community resisted by stoning the officials. A rioter was arrested. The 'mob' then turned on the police to rescue him, captured an officer 'and trampled him to death with their thick workers-class clogs': his body became 'a mass of bruises'; his face unrecognizable. The military was summoned; many were arrested; eight were charged with murder.[145] Two weeks later, a similar story appeared. Now, the captured policeman whose face was kicked beyond recognition received a further insult: the mob danced on his corpse.[146] Almost immediately, newspapers began questioning whether the second one had occurred, claiming it a 'fake',

[139] *St. Louis Republican*, 26 September 1894, 5.
[140] *London Standard*, 19 September 1894, 5.   [141] *New York Times*, 7 August 1895.
[142] *Sun*, 3 September 1892.   [143] *New-York Tribune*, 11 October 1893, from Hamburg.
[144] Ibid., 27 September 1893, from Hamburg; and ibid., 11 October 1893, from Hamburg.
[145] Ibid., 27 September 1893.
[146] Ibid., 11 October 1893; *Evening World*, 10 October 1893; *New-York Tribune*, 11 October 1893, 4; *Alexandria Gazette*, 11 October 1893, 2; and *Capital Journal* repeated the story almost verbatim. *The Shenandoah Herald*, 13 October 1893, 2, added: 'These are the kind of brutes that our government has been allowing for years to pour into this country by the hundreds of thousands'.

produced by a 'bogus news association'.[147] Hamburg's authorities demanded that Reuters retract the story.[148] The papers, however, never claimed the first riot had been a fake, and the *New York Times*, whose reports were sent from Hamburg correspondents, never retracted even the second story.[149] For the first one, papers claimed that more arrests were expected, the name of the freed rioter had been ascertained, and he would be found.[150] Cholera riots spread further west, in fact, into one country, where I have spotted no cholera riots during Europe's wave of the 1830s. In mid-October 1893, a 'mob' in an unspecified town in Belgium revolted against sanitary enforcements, attacked police and health officers, kicking and beating to death one officer and a policeman. Troops 'charged the mob'.[151]

During the 1892–5 wave, cholera riots also re-emerged in Italy. The most remarkable of these occurred not in the south but in Tuscany's port city, Livorno. First, the *Lancet* claimed that half the population of 110,000 abandoned the city from panic, 'leaving their poorer fellow-citizens to die of disease or hunger'. Then on 27 September 1893 a strange confrontation between 'the indigent' and police developed. Instead of the usual conspiracies, the prevailing myth reached back to supposed Hippocratic measures in antiquity to dispel epidemics—building fires to purify the air.[152] The violence and confrontation with the authorities was, nonetheless, as intense as several cholera riots in Russia with extensive loss of property and life. 'Energetically', the 'people' broke up doors and furniture of their houses, piled them in the main thoroughfares and set them on fire. The fire brigade, 'already taxed beyond its strength', tried to control the conflagration. Resenting the interference, the people 'indignantly and passionately' attacked the firemen and police sent to protect them. From their windows, people hurled 'missiles' 'onto the devoted vindicators of public order'. Hand-to-hand combat between the two ensued, 'until, in self-defence and against overwhelming numbers', the latter drew their revolvers.[153] Unknown to these journalists, such efforts by Livorno's populace to preserve their city from cholera was not new. In the epidemic of 1867, crowds had taken the same measures.[154]

While cholera riots had disappeared from parts of Western Europe before its fifth wave, 1892 to 1895, such actions still inflicted horror and terror in cities in Russia, Central Europe, and Italy, and not just in isolated backward villages. Moreover, many of the same mythologies rampant in the 1830s—fear of doctors,

---

[147] *New York Herald*, 11 October 1893; *St Paul Daily Globe*. The *Herald* seems to have denied the first but not the second riot.

[148] *Morning Post*, 14 October 1893, 5. According to the *San Francisco Chronicle*, 11 October 1893, 2, the Associated Press confirmed that the second riot had not occurred.

[149] In his authoritative *Death in Hamburg*, 366–8, Evans does not refute nor even mention either riot in St Pauli. Instead, he emphatically maintains that 'no unrest' broke out in this working-class quarter that bore the brunt of the cholera from 1890 to the city's last wave in 1906, 'not even any small incident of collective hostility to the authorities' (367). He then explains why Hamburg supposedly avoided violence.

[150] *Chicago Daily Tribune*, 27 September 1893, 5.　　[151] *Irish World*, 21 October 1893, 6.

[152] 'Cholera at Leghorn', *Lancet*, 14 October 1893, 948. On these measures, see Cohn, *Cultures of Plague*, 80, and their last catastrophic consequence at Honolulu; see Chapter 15.

[153] 'Cholera at Leghorn', *Lancet*, 14 October 1893, 948.

[154] *La Nazione*, 22 August 1867, 2, from Livorno.

hospitals, and of the state's supposed scheming to kill the poor—continued to propel cholera revolts. In Russian cities, these occurred in more backward regions but also surfaced elsewhere in cosmopolitan cities at the forefront of a central European Renaissance, as in late nineteenth-century Budapest and Munich, or cities experiencing unprecedented commercial and industrial success, like Hamburg and Livorno. To be sure, these were cities riven by class struggle, but the same was true of major cities in Britain, France, Germany, and the Austro-Hungarian Empire, where cholera riots no longer flared. Exactly why such violence should have persisted in some places and not in others will be discussed later. But it is clear that the spread of modernization, capitalism, mass education, and commerce had not eradicated cholera's power to inspire hatred and blame in fin-de-siècle Europe.

Europe and Asiatic Russia were not the only places to experience cholera riots in 1892. For one that struck much further afield, in Fanchew in China, the character of blame differed from Europe's. Approximating present expectations that epidemics spur the blaming of 'others', here 'haters of foreigners' spread rumours of Chinese in the pay of Europeans, poisoning wells. 'Consequently, all strangers are imprisoned and many have had their heads cut off and their entrails and hearts thrown into the river'.[155] Yet the Chinese conspiracy and ensuing witch-hunts were staged along class lines similar to European cholera violence: the rich (in this case, foreigners) bore the brunt of the terror. With the next cholera wave in 1902, a similar outburst occurred at Chenchou (Chin-chou) in Hunan Province. The populace erupted in a 'superstitious frenzy', convinced that newly arrived missionaries had caused the epidemic by poisoning the drinking water. The mob wrecked the mission and murdered the missionaries.[156] A cholera outbreak at Shanghai resulted in riots, in which 'a number of foreigners' were injured with natives killed. Marines from several foreign legations were posted and 'large bodies of Chinese troops' were stationed with Gatling guns at street corners. 'Sharp engagements' ensued between soldiers and 'mobs'. According to a US missionary in Shanghai, the 'trouble' arose because of quarantine measures coupled with the belief that the quarantine authorities stole babies to make medicine.[157] Cholera's propensity to blame westerners attached to religious foundations in China continued into the Communist era and may even have intensified. In 1951, 'the Communists' accused five Canadian nuns of murdering Chinese orphans. Earlier, the nunnery, along with other denominations 'in many parts of China', had been accused of spreading cholera at Canton in 1938.[158] As Chapter 9 will show, cholera's power to spread hate and violence endured in parts of the world well into the twentieth, even the twenty-first, century.

This chapter has shown cholera riots manifesting differences in different environments and historical contexts. Comparing cholera riots in the 1830s and in the

---

[155] *Daily Public Ledger*, 15 October 1892, front page; *Jasper Weekly Courier*, 21 October 1892, front page; *Fair Play*, 22 October 1892, front page; *Cape Grardeau Democrat*, 22 October 1892, front page.
[156] *Anaconda Standard*, 25 August 1902, 2. At least fifty Australian papers reported it (for instance, *Register*, 2 September 1902, 5): one of the 'martyred' missionaries was Australian.
[157] *Detroit Free Press*, 18 December 1910, 8.   [158] *The Argus*, 5 April 1951, 6.

1890s shows changes in leadership, organization, and mythologies. Yet from the start, cholera established a discernible pattern that was more or less unique to this disease and that emerged nearly universally across wide areas of Europe into the Americas and Asia. In the main, these were not attacks on outsiders—Jews, foreigners, or the poor. Nor were the victims of disease doubly victims of blame and social violence. Instead, cholera rioters pictured themselves 'liberating' the cholera-afflicted from the clutches of evil doctors, hospitals, and the state. Underlying the rioters' brutal attacks that often reached ritualistic frenzies of murder, mutilation, and destruction of key objects were abiding myths that the medical community, armed by sanitary officers and agents of the state, sought to cull populations of the poor. These myths emerged in widely diverse social, economic, and political contexts. Imitation and direct communication might explain the repeat performance of some of these rituals of violence and belief, as seen with fishermen near Edinburgh spreading rumours to mainland Scotland's far north. But for the bulk of these incidents, which appeared almost simultaneously over vast distances, crossing linguistic divides, nations, empires, and even oceans, such communication is difficult to imagine. These myths, moreover, did not disappear with cholera's first European wave. Instead, they continued after the disease's mechanisms of transmission were understood and the bacillus had been cultured.

Something about the disease, and not just particular social and political contexts, contributed to these enigmatic reoccurrences in places into the twentieth century. Contemporaneously with the cholera riots of 1892 in regions such as the Volga basin, epidemics of typhus and plague scored death counts equal to cholera's but did not spawn accusations against physicians or violence. Peculiarities of cholera, its rapid infliction of death and high fatality rates combined with demands that cholera corpses be buried immediately in separate grounds, appear to be the factors that spawned people's deep suspicions of diabolic happenings. Despite the discovery of cholera's aetiology, scientific knowledge that it was primarily waterborne, and could be prevented by systems of sewage disposal, cholera's lethality rates remained high in places into the twentieth century. The market town of Verbicaro, Calabria, in 1911, is a case in point. In one day, its population of between 5000–6000 experienced eighty-two fresh cholera cases; forty-eight resulted in a quick death—a fatality rate just under 60 per cent. The next day, extensive violence erupted.[159] In one place after another, independently of one another, it was easy to think that with so few returning from cholera hospitals something was awry. The fact that the majority of those afflicted and hospitalized were the poor further fuelled suspicions.

[159] For instance, when cholera broke out among Turkish troops at Habdenkeim in 1901, of seventy-nine cases, forty died; *La Stampa*, 1 November 1910, 2. For Verbicaro, see Chapter 9.

9

Cholera Violence
An Italian Story in Comparative Perspective

As shown in Chapter 8, cholera riots did not decline everywhere after the disease's debut. On the contrary, in the Russian Empire, cholera's social violence may have reached its apogee with its fifth wave in 1892, expanding geographically beyond the better-studied ones of the 1830s. From their vortex north of the Black Sea, they spread in 1892 east into Asiatic Russia and West beyond the traditional borders of Russia into Persia, Syria, and Poland and into Hungary, Germany, and Italy. The chapter may have left, however, a false impression that Western Europe was fundamentally different from places further east: that after the 1830s, Europe west of the Elbe experienced few cholera protests and the ones to occur happened in out-of-the-way places, like fishing villages in Scotland's far north. As we argued, for France and the British Isles, cholera disturbances declined sharply after 1832. However, it would be wrong to assume that the disease had lost its power to ignite hate and violence or regenerate myths of doctors poisoning the poor through prominent zones of Western Europe.

THE IBERIAN PENINSULA

During the 1880s (the first decade of cholera's fifth pandemic wave), cholera's social violence was instead concentrated in Western Europe. Moreover, the beliefs underlying many of these disturbances cut along class lines similar to those of the 1830s and repeated the old phobias of doctors and the state inventing cholera to poison commoners. As far as international attention goes (in part because of the development of organizations and technologies of communication such as Reuters and the telegram[1]), cholera outbreaks in Spain in 1885 sparked as much, if not greater, notoriety for the capital, Madrid, than any previous wave of any infectious disease in Spain. In June, with the rise in cholera cases, tensions mounted over the city's water supply in the poorer neighbourhoods. When inspectors arrived in the working-class quarter of La Latina, the populace greeted them with stones. Soon the riot became more serious at la Puerta del Sol,[2] a focal point of the troubles in

---

[1] On the telegraph and news agencies from the mid-nineteenth century, see Wenzlhuemer, *Connecting the Nineteenth-Century World*, 88–92.

[2] In the seventeenth century, it became Madrid's central square, a meeting place for news.

1832. In this and surrounding neighbourhoods, 'the people' prevented health authorities from performing their tasks.[3] The crowd captured the queen; three rioters were killed, and dozens wounded.[4] Through its Spanish correspondents, US papers questioned the official statistics, claiming that seven, not three, were killed[5]—more recorded deaths than in any single cholera riot during the first wave of cholera rioting in France, the British Isles, or the US. Similar movements spread into various Catalan towns from Valencia to Murcia.[6] Entire villages were deserted with the sick abandoned and the dead left unburied. As with earlier cholera waves, suspicion of doctors in Granada grew among the populace: doctors were forced to swallow medicines before administering them to others. In other villages, rioters attacked government officials, and in Logroño (La Rioja, in northern Spain) small riots arose against sanitary regulations.[7] Yet at the same time and in some of the same places, a new wrinkle appeared in cholera riots that ran in a contrary direction: several doctors were 'brutally assaulted', because they declined to grant their patients what the public judged as adequate attention.[8]

At the end of August, a riot in Almeria, Andalusia, added another dimension to cholera's class cleavages. 'Labouring people' were incensed that wealthy residents had deserted their city, leaving them without employment. With the wealthy as the targets, and not hospitals, doctors, or government officials, 'the mob' wrecked their homes, and the military had to be summoned. Here, the death tallies and those seriously wounded (eight and twelve, respectively) exceeded the better-reported Madrid casualties a month earlier.[9] Moreover, Spain's cholera troubles were not limited to the mainland. At Santa Cruz de Santiago, capital of the Canary Islands, the entry of a Captain-General and Civil Governor from Cadiz violated the island's quarantine regulations, mobilizing the local population into street fighting: bombs exploded; the local authorities resigned en masse and hundreds fled into the island's interior.[10] A decade later, the recalcitrance of the Portuguese followed a similar pattern. Central government in Lisbon insisted that Portuguese ships coming from cholera-infested ports should be allowed to dock at the island of Madeira, violating the island's quarantine regulations. Riots erupted. As in the Canary Islands, participants included more than the rabble. After negotiations with Lisbon failed, mass meetings ensued. Crowds pelted officers with stones; a new governor sent to Santa Cruz threatened the crowds, aiming big guns at them; and officers stabbed to death a grocer's boy, who attacked the new Chief of Police.[11] Another new wrinkle had

---

[3] *The Hickman Courier*, 3 July 1885. [4] Vincent, 'Le cholera en Espagne', 54–5.

[5] *Springfield Globe-Republic*, 22 June 1885; and *Scotsman*, 22 June 1885, 5.

[6] Vincent, 'Le cholera en Espagne', 54–5.

[7] *McCook Tribune*, 27 August 1885; and *San Francisco Chronicle*, 18 August 1885, 8.

[8] *Middlebury Register*, 14 August 1885.

[9] *Sun*, 31 August 1885; *San Francisco Chronicle*, 31 August 1885, 3, and *New York Times*, 31 August 1885, plus at least nine papers in 'Chronicling America', *New York Times*, 22 June 1885 and 18 August 1885, and numerous ones in BNA.

[10] *Sacramento Daily Record-Union*, 22 August 1885, front page.

[11] *Scotsman*, 2 June 1894, 11, from a Scottish correspondent aboard the *Funchal*, which broke the quarantine. No notice of this cholera revolt is seen in 'Chronicling America' or 'Nineteenth-Century British Library Newspapers'. Another cholera riot occurred in Madeira during the next cholera wave in 1910. Brief notices of it in the *San Francisco Chronicle*, 16 December 1910, 5, and the *Western Star*,

appeared, no doubt implicit earlier, when health officers, doctors, and police from capital cities imposed their medicines and sanitary regulations on the periphery. Now, however, a capital's arrogance and abrogation of the rights of an incorporated region triggered violence that cut across classes and possessed a political base.

This politicization of the cholera riot and inclusion of the middle classes, even the elites, is best seen in Madrid and Seville in 1885. The events, however, did not unite communities but divided the country along other axes. The issues were political and concerned King Alfonso XII's movements and his perceived political loyalties to Madrid, splitting those who supported the municipal government from those behind the monarchy. Instead of myths of poisoning and hospitals as death chambers, the causes galvanizing Madrid's citizenry possessed trappings of bourgeois respectability. On 20 June with 'every shop closed, even the cafés', 'an orderly crowd' occupied the streets. They debated the king's responsibilities and his allegiances regarding whether he should visit the cholera-afflicted in Murcia as announced. Those of Madrid were aggrieved that he would channel 'his energies and compassion' away from the capital and risk his life, when he had yet to sire an heir to the throne. If he made the visit, Madrid's municipal government threatened to resign.[12] Later that day, the politics and constituency of the crowds changed. Protest turned against the municipal government for declaring Madrid infected. In the late afternoon another 'immense crowd assembled', cheering the king and queen, and demonstrated against Madrid's civil authorities. That evening the king tried to form a new Ministry for Madrid with the Liberal Party but failed. He then decided to forgo his visit; the Conservatives returned to office 'without modification'.[13]

Madrid's events did not end the political turmoil exacerbated by the epidemic. In September, further cholera riots touched other municipalities, demonstrating the same bourgeois respectability as in the capital. In Seville, the protest spread to ladies, members of gentlemen's clubs, and theatre-goers. A government official arrived to inspect the city's lazaretto but refused to enter it. Immediately, crowds demonstrated in front of Government House against his cowardice and health officers' irresponsibility. Stones were thrown, windows broken. The civil guard was summoned and charged 'the mob', wounding three boys and an old man. The municipal council resigned, and when the governor or his supporters entered a club, the members got up and left. 'Even ladies' left theatres when he entered.[14]

Yet in other towns and regions of Spain cholera's old patterns persisted. At the end of July 'the populace' of Tudela, Navarre, made 'hostile demonstrations' against the doctors, who declared the presence of cholera, and a 'mob' wrecked a train.[15]

17 December 1910, 2, reported the rioters were the 'uneducated'; twenty were arrested resisting sanitary measures.

[12] *Scotsman*, 22 June 1885, 5.

[13] Ibid., from telegrams from Central News and Reuters; and *South Australian Weekly Chronicle*, 15 August 1885, 8.

[14] *Scotsman*, 5 September 1885.

[15] Ibid., 31 July 1885, 5, telegram from Madrid. It is unreported in papers from 'Chronicling America', *The Times*, *Guardian*, and *Observer*.

With the disease 'raging throughout Spain' another 'mob' murdered three doctors, influenced by popular beliefs of doctors poisoning cholera patients,[16] and in Valencia, a 'mob' destroyed a hospital van carrying cholera medicines.[17]

THE 1904–11 WAVE: RUSSIA

Spain was not alone in Western Europe to experience a revival of cholera riots that sprung from the old mythologies, while developing new twists. Well after Koch had cultured the bacillus and great strides in treatment and sanitary measures had ended most of cholera's mysteries, a sixth cholera wave spread into Russia in 1904, reaching Italy a year later and lasting until 1912. It continued to stir panic, fear, and violence, stemming from the same class mythologies. Hospitals were torched; physicians and governmental officials were attacked. Some were killed and others gruesomely mutilated. These flared up first in Russia with local governments braced for the large-scale cholera revolts suffered eighteen years earlier.[18] Local authorities decreed 'severe pains and penalties for concealment of cases' or for resisting sanitary detachments: 'the lives of the doctors and nurses [were] in constant peril . . . the benighted peasants are persuaded that they sow the germs of the disease'.[19]

In August 1909, a cholera riot at Pskow (Pskov) resulted in forty-one peasants being arrested.[20] Later that month, villagers refused to hand over cholera patients for treatment, attacked cholera barracks, and endangered the lives of nurses. The police were summoned, and gendarmes had to escort doctors making their rounds.[21] The following year, cholera riots against sanitary measures spread throughout southwestern Russia;[22] the old patterns stretching back to the 1830s persisted. In September 1910, a peasant mob killed a doctor in Yekaterinoslav Province with 'medical men' throughout the region, 'constantly' being beaten and needing police escorts to visit patients. New elements, moreover, entered these plots. The correspondent claimed that 'reactionary demagogues' incited peasants to attack medical attendants, and Jews were accused of being 'agents of the plague'. The 'right-wing press' was behind the propaganda, and the editor of the *Black Hundred Newspaper* was fined $100 for circulating the stories.[23]

As in the past, Russian correspondents to foreign newspapers had no qualms in exposing their own upper-class bias: 'Wherever the authorities make the slightest effort to enforce sanitary measures, a clash with the ignorant populace is almost sure to follow'. But now they reported a new element: religious fatalism. In south-western Russia, townsmen not only objected to officials invading their

---

[16] *Northern Territory Times*, 5 September 1890, 3. The paper did not specify where the incident occurred.
[17] *Chicago Daily Tribune*, 14 January 1885, 5.
[18] *Times and Democrat*, 6 September 1910, citing *Bovoe Vremya*.
[19] Ibid.   [20] *Gainsville Daily Sun*, 27 August 1909.
[21] *New-York Tribune*, 29 August 1909; and *New York Times*, 29 August 1909.
[22] *Washington Times*, 29 June 1910.   [23] *New York Times*, 10 September 1910.

homes; 'they also have a vague idea that heaven has willed the pestilence and [that] the authorities have no right to attempt to check its ravages'.[24] Yet because of the Czarist regime's preparedness, improved medical services, and developments in social welfare and philanthropy,[25] the extensive rioting of previous cholera waves had finally subsided. Now, the protests were limited to villages or small towns. Widespread riots in cities such as Astrakhan, Tashkent, Saratoff, and Nizhnii-Novgorod, with crowds in the thousands, hundreds killed, and more injured, had become a thing of the past.[26] Yet the violence had not ended. With famine and outbreaks of typhus, and 'a severe cholera epidemic' in Soviet Russia in 1921, cholera riots erupted 'in many cities and villages, and [were] raging on a vast scale'. 'Red troops' were dispatched 'in a desperate effort to restore order'.[27] Another occurred a year later at a hub of cholera and violence since the 1830s, Astrakhan.[28]

ITALY, 1910

Such was not the trajectory with a more urbanized and market-orientated Western European society, Italy.[29] Nor were these outbursts wholly confined to supposed backward regions of the South. The prime stage for cholera panic and widespread violence during Italy's first cholera wave—Sicily—appears to have been exempt from major riots during this sixth wave, even if beliefs in *untori* and governmental poisoning persisted there. The largest of the riots and the ones to receive widespread reportage occurred on the mainland. In Naples towards the end of February 1911, cholera tensions became intertwined with national politics to an extent never before seen in Italy, even in 1837. No longer confined to the local rabble, the political classes entered the protests with organization and leadership from the top—the Mayor, City Council, and Chamber of Commerce galvanizing popular support against Italy's Prime Minister, Luigi Luzzati, and national impositions restricting Neapolitan commerce, transforming cholera protest into a political revolt on a national scale. However, because of the background of violent cholera riots then brewing in Puglia and threats that a cholera revolt organized by municipal elites might prove efficacious, Rome backed down, repealing its sanitary strictures on Neapolitan trade and leaving Luzzati humiliated.[30]

Frank Snowden attributes Naples' success in part to the background of violent cholera uprisings already afoot in other southern regions.[31] He mentions, however, only three—in Barletta, Molfetta, and Taranto—and describes only one in any

---

[24] *Washington Times*, 29 June 1910.   [25] Henze, *Disease*, 107–9, 119, 155–6.

[26] Nonetheless, cholera violence continued in towns such as Iuzovka in 1910; physicians in villages in the Volga basin were beaten, even by Cossacks assigned to protect them; ibid., 130, 142–5.

[27] *New-York Tribune* 24 July 1921. I have found only one other paper (*Evening Telegraph*, 25 July 1921, 4) to corroborate the report.

[28] To be discussed in Chapter 10.

[29] Evans, 'Epidemics and Revolutions', 151, claims this sixth wave 'had virtually no impact on western Europe'.

[30] Snowden, *Naples in the Time of Cholera*, 292–5.   [31] Ibid., 293–4.

detail, that of Taranto from 30 December 1910 to 1 January 1911. It began as an economic uprising against health measures prohibiting cultivation and sale of shellfish, principally oysters,[32] causing unemployment and hardship to the local economy.[33] The composition of the crowds was probably similar to previous ones dominated by impoverished women ('donnicciuole'). Those who rampaged through Taranto's densely populated streets, breaking windows and streetlamps were 'fishing folk and children' ('gente di mare e di ragazzi'). The class character of this riot, however, may have differed: the demonstrators were predominantly from the large commercial class of vendors of oysters and fish.[34] The first night's rioting left only one person, hit by a vase of flowers thrown from a window, seriously injured.[35] The following morning, however, causalities mounted, when 'thousands' congregated along the streets. Here, new knowledge of *vibrio cholerae* reservoirs in shellfish beds[36] gave rise to new economic forms of protest. Yet the riots also harked back to older cholera mythologies. When health officials sought to remove a cholera victim against his family's wishes, 'thousands' poured into the streets and attacked the barracks of the *carabinieri*, charged with enforcing the city's sanitary regulations. They hit the traditional sites of suspicion, completely destroying a pharmacy and wounding the pharmacist,[37] and showed their contempt for local authorities by storming the office of the urban police, triumphantly destroying its coat of arms.[38] Three rioters were killed and many wounded. Only with the army's arrival was order restored. But now another wrinkle appeared: instead of mass arrests and serious punishments, Taranto's mayor opened soup kitchens ('le cucine economiche') to feed the unemployed, and the Italian government negotiated with the president of the oystermen to revoke the redundancies of twenty-eight fishermen and granted the company a subsidy of 5000 lire, 3000 to be distributed to unemployed fishermen and 2000 to soup kitchens.[39]

In the Naples' hinterland and across the southern mainland more riotous consequences stirred than Snowden may have imagined. At least three major outbreaks erupted during the autumn and winter of 1910, before Taranto's riot. All three, moreover, equalled its numbers or exceeded them. Surprisingly, the earliest is not found in keyword searches through US and British online newspapers, especially since it occurred in a major city—Bari. On 5 September, 'a mob of 2,000' attacked the city's sanitary office and 'maltreated' employees. Twenty-three were wounded. The reason given for the uproar was the promulgation of an ordinance soon to wreak havoc in other towns in the province—prohibition of eating figs, seen as spreading cholera. The measure threatened the region's fig-growing economy and was seen as 'worse than the disease'.[40]

A second riot was also of considerable size and importance. Unlike Bari's, this one at Bisceglie, 40 km to the north, was well reported in the US and Italian

---

[32] *Corriere della Sera*, 1 January 1911, 5. [33] Snowden, *Naples in the Time of Cholera*, 293.
[34] *Corriere della Sera*, 1 January 1911, 5. [35] Ibid.
[36] See note 159. [37] *Corriere della Sera*, 1 January 1911, 5. [38] Ibid.
[39] Snowden, *Naples in the Time of Cholera*, 293–4; *The Times*, 2 January 1911, 7; *La Stampa*, 2 January 1911, 4.
[40] *Daily Herald*, 5 September 1910, 5.

presses. It sprang from concerns over restricting shellfish fishing but also rested on ancient beliefs. When the Red Cross attempted to fumigate the city's cathedral, a 'mob' of men and women attacked the officers; the municipal guard had to be summoned. A man was shot dead, a woman health worker seriously injured from stoning, and scores were wounded in hand-to-hand combat. The rioters, however, prevailed until extra troops arrived. A correspondent from Bari along with Milan's *Corriere della Sera* saw the underlying cause as economic: the restrictions on the sale of fish, the region's 'chief food supply', enraged the populace, just beginning to recover from commercial depression.[41] Still, traditional concerns were as pivotal: the municipality had fanned discontent by prohibiting a religious procession, and the cathedral became the riot's central battlefield.[42] Health workers' fumigation at the cathedral blackened its sacred figures, sending women against the Red Cross workers, 'trampling them under foot' and destroying their disinfection pumps. Three hundred local fishermen with revolvers came to the women's defence and forcibly expelled the 'doctors' engaged in disinfection.[43]

> Some ascended the belfry and set all the bells ringing violently. In a few minutes practically the whole of the population assembled, eager for the opportunity of attacking the local authorities for their vexatious cholera measures.[44]

According to *Corriere della Sera*, women began the struggle and formed its leading edge: 'many hundreds of them poured into the cathedral as though a swollen river and ran to the high altar, screaming and yelling'.[45]

A third cholera revolt of 1910 in Ostuni, in the province of Brindisi, escaped the notice of the British and US press but at least fifty Australian papers covered it along with *La Stampa* and *Corriere della Sera*. If crowd estimates are trusted, oversight of this riot in the secondary literature is all the more remarkable. By one paper's count the 'mob' reached 8000,[46] making it as large as any in Europe or Asiatic Russia and perhaps Italy's largest, even including the Sicilian riots of 1837 (for which crowd estimates were never given). More realistically, other papers put it at 3000.[47] Nonetheless, Ostuni's would have been among Italy's largest. As in Bisceglie, offences to religious practice set it off.[48]

'Ten days or so' before the riots, a crowd went to the mayor requesting permission to hold a procession with a statue from a country sanctuary to end the epidemic. Because of the supposed danger of crowding during a procession, the mayor tried to prevent it, saying the cathedral already possessed a statue of the martyr, but citizens believed that only the village one possessed the needed powers. The uprising also

---

[41] *Washington Times*, 24 October 1910; *Los Angeles Herald*, 28 September 1910, from a Milanese correspondent.
[42] *Corriere della Sera*, 23 September 1910, front page.
[43] *Alliance Herald*, 27 October 1910; *Los Angeles Herald*, 28 September 1910.
[44] *Los Angeles Herald*, 28 September 1910.
[45] *Corriere della Sera*, 23 September 1910, front page.
[46] *Barrier Miner*, 17 November 1910, 2.
[47] *The Advertiser*, 17 November 1910, 9. The Italian papers put it vaguely at 'over a thousand'. Ostuni's population in 1910 was only 18,500.
[48] Ibid. According to Australian papers, the clergy initiated the riot.

rested on other traditional phantasms: the 'popolino' believed *untori* among the health authorities had 'imported the disease'[49] and were also engaged in live burials. The riot erupted not at the beginning of a cholera outbreak or when mortalities soared, but at its end, after most of the patients had died or recovered. Suspicions over burial were the spark. Summons from the health authorities to build two coffins—one for a wife, the other for her husband, still alive—aroused rumours of intentional killing. When the wife's coffin passed through town, a crowd demanded that the coffin be inspected.[50] Rapidly, the crowd grew to a thousand, charged the lazaretto, and 'reduced its furnishings to rubble'. 'Rebels' seized the remaining patients and carried them to their homes, shouting 'Death to the doctors and to the sanitary officers'. In ensuing battles with *carabinieri* and attacks on the town hall, which they set ablaze,[51] a peasant boy of nineteen was shot dead. The crowd took possession of the square, attacked doctors' residences, and cut telegraph and telephone lines.[52] With the boy's cadaver, they processed through the streets, behaving like a 'foreign army of invaders', badly injuring health workers and eight *carabinieri*. Reinforcements of *carabinieri* arrived from other districts; eighty rioters were arrested.[53] As usual, the papers blamed the protesters as testimony of 'the recent and saddest proof of the profound ignorance of the people'.[54]

A fourth cholera riot erupted in the winter of 1910. This one, however, was in the north, at the seaside resort of Terracina, near Rome. No crowd estimates appear, but *La Stampa* reported it as comprised of 'large popular demonstrations and riots (*grandi manifestazioni popolari e tumulti*)'[55] and *Corriere della Sera* as 'numerosa e tumultuosa'. A Sydney paper called it reminiscent of 'medieval savagery' for its ritualistic destruction of cholera litters and suspicions over intentional killings by hospitals and doctors. When health officers came to remove a stricken shopkeeper, 'a hostile throng' seized the litter, smashing it to fragments. The mayor hurried to the scene with 'a bodyguard of *carabinieri*', but they were beaten back by heavy sticks. Women ripped the uniforms off the soldiers and 'bit them so savagely that they were provoked to lash the rioters with drawn swords'.[56] According to *La Stampa*, Terracina's cholera patients had been taken to Rome's lazaretto, causing its residents to complain, not because the patients never returned alive, but because they returned too soon, sparking fears of a contagious threat. The populace persuaded Rome to keep the patients for longer.[57] However, for unexplained reasons, the protest changed from fear of contagion to cholera's traditional objective, liberating the diseased victims from the clutches of the state. Similar to other cholera riots that year and earlier, the crowd was composed primarily of women, with one woman 'more violent than the rest' probably the group's leader.[58]

---

[49] *La Stampa*, 15 November 1910, front page. I have taken the story from two long articles in *Il Corriere della Sera*, 15 November 1910, 2; and 16 November 1910, 2.
[50] *La Stampa*, 15 November 1910, front page.   [51] Ibid.
[52] *Il Corriere della Sera*, 15 November 1910, 2.
[53] Ibid., 16 November 1910, 2. *La Stampa*, 15 November 1910, front page, said it was seventy.
[54] *La Stampa*, 15 November 1910, front page.   [55] Ibid., 18 October 1910, 2.
[56] *World's News*, 26 November 1910, 18.
[57] *Corriere della Sera*, 18 October 1910, 2.   [58] Ibid.

At the same time, cholera riots were said to be happening in Naples. Negotiations between the city's political elites and Rome had not ended its troubles. However, even before Prime Minister Giovanni Giolitti's official census of cholera in July 1911, Italian press censorship was 'working overtime'. US papers insisted that further riots were occurring in Naples, even if they were unable to ferret out the details.[59] Further information gained from their Italian correspondents, however, allowed the press to reveal a fifth cholera riot in 1910, this one in Barletta in the province of Bari. Although in a provincial farming town, the riot was on the same scale as Taranto's.[60] Conforming to earlier cholera patterns, it pitched a desperate, impoverished population against hospitals and doctors. But now it was the government's irrationality and fears—not the poor's—that triggered the rioting: a belief that figs caused cholera. An ordinance from Rome prohibited eating them, cutting deeply into the region's economy, already penalized by economic recession.[61] Further, Barletta had been placed under 'virtual martial law' before the rioting began to enforce a *cordon sanitaire* that further depressed its failing economy. As a result, 'several thousand starving and unemployed people' (by another account, 2000) clashed with the militia, broke the cordons, stormed the town hall, invaded the hospitals, and 'chased all the doctors out of the city'. They sacked soup kitchens, besieged the principal pharmacy, and assassinated the head chemist. Thirty officers and troops were wounded 'before charging the miserable wretches with fixed bayonets'; fifty rioters were arrested, comprised of 'men, women, and children'.[62] The *popolo* were convinced: 'the medical profession had no aim other than to create the epidemic'.[63]

The one Italian paper I have found to report the riot, Milan's *Corriere della Sera*, emphasized the role of 'many hundreds of shrivelled and emaciated women', who orchestrated the riot's first movements, demanding that all Barletta's doctors leave town immediately. To quell the fighting on the second day, a special train of 500 soldiers from three regiments arrived. On the following day, calm was restored. The paper then shows another facet of the Italian state's solution to cholera unrest in 1910 not revealed by foreign newspapers. The peace was also restored by free meals distributed through soup kitchens to Barletta's starving. A day later, health authorities eased travel restrictions and modified restrictions on selling foodstuffs, now sequestering only rotten fruit and vegetables.[64]

---

[59] *Democratic Banner*, 25 October 1910. On Italian censorship of cholera and its riots, see the *Colorado Springs Gazette*, 8 October 1911, 22. On the enactment of Giolitti's censorship, Snowden, *Naples in the Time of Cholera*, 445. On Italian censorship of cholera in 1893 and the mechanisms by which correspondents leaked the information across borders, *Chicago Daily Tribune*, 13 August 1893, 9.

[60] In addition, *New York Times*, 4 September 1910, reported the riot but treated it in less detail than smaller provincial papers.

[61] *Wenatchee Daily World*, 3 September 1910, front page.

[62] Ibid.; *Los Angeles Herald*, 4 September 1910, 4; other papers in 'Chronicling America', and *Guardian*, 5 September 1910, 12.

[63] Ibid. Several long articles in *Corriere della Sera*, 3 September 1910, 2: 'Tumultuosa dimostrazione a Barletta contro i medici e gli agenti municipali', 4 September 1911, 2 'I tumulti di Barletta per i provvedimenti contro il colera. La caccia ai medici'; and 5 September 1911, 2.

[64] Ibid., 6 September 1910.

From the international press, I have found no further cholera riots from early September 1910 to 27 August 1911, but Italian papers reported at least eight other disturbances in and around Naples, Bari, and Sicily. The first of these erupted in Naples' most impoverished neighbourhoods on 10 September, where food was often indigestible with 'cases of gastro-enteritis'[65] rife. After only two cases of suspected cholera, 'a large crowd' pursued an automobile of sanitary officials arriving to disinfect a suspected house. With the agents' entry blocked, 'immediately' a violent struggle erupted between the 'popolani' on one side, and nurses and agents on the other. Several 'wretched women (*donnicciuole*)' joined by bricklayers facilitated the escape of the suspected cholera victim.[66] Less than a week later, a similar riot struck Castellammare di Stabia, also provoked by disinfecting an impoverished neighbourhood. Again, 'wretched women' formed the front line. 'As though possessed by the devil', 'gossip-mongering women' surrounded health workers, accusing them of spreading poison in the air to ignite cholera with their disinfectant guns. Men with hoes and spades joined in and tried to lynch the sanitary workers. Even after the police arrived, crowds of women continued threatening health workers.[67]

At the end of the month, 'savage scenes', if not riots, broke out at opposite ends of the Mezzogiorno. In Bagheria, east of Palermo, 'the people' nailed a black cross to the town hall with a letter threatening that if cholera arrived, the mayor and counsellors would be killed. During the night peasants suspecting *untori* patrolled their neighbourhoods armed with guns, and an effigy of the mayor, portrayed as shot, appeared. In Molfetta on the Adriatic north of Bari, 'occurrences of clamorous disorder... ran up and down the city with crowds chanting "Down with the Red Cross"', and ended with a disinfectant car thrown into the sea. Although the target of their anger may have been the car, the economies of the health sanctions provoked it, in this case, prohibition on sales of small fish.[68]

About the same time, according to *Corriere della Sera*, despite the absence of epidemic cholera in Sicily, villagers 'possessed by the fear of cholera viewed everyone involved in public affairs or who did not belong to the lowest classes as enemies'. As a result, 'they engaged in the most unbelievable actions we have seen'. The paper, however, mentioned only two incidents. In Burgio and Villafranca Sicula, peasants shot off thousands of shotgun shells at night to intimidate local authorities, who supposedly 'came to spread the cholera among the poor'. If cholera became epidemic, they threatened to direct the shells at the powers that be.[69] In Lucca Sicula, 'it was worse': the *popolo* affixed placards publicizing the names of supposed *untori*, threatening them with summary justice if cholera became epidemic.[70]

A week later a cholera demonstration of a different sort erupted. It was one of the few to occur in Sicily's capital, Palermo. Unlike the riot in Naples in the autumn, confined to the city's poorest neighbourhoods, Palermo's was city-wide

---

[65] With Giolitti's censorship the following year, it became the coded term for cholera.
[66] *Corriere della Sera*, 11 September 1910, 4.
[67] Ibid., 16 September 1910, 4.   [68] Ibid., 30 September 1910, 2.
[69] Ibid., 1 October 1910, front page.   [70] Ibid.

and its participants were the propertied. 'About a thousand merchants, shopkeepers (*commercianti*) and citizens of every class' protested on 4 October against the government because it had declared the city 'infected'. No violence or attacks on hospitals, medical corps, disinfectant wagons, or pharmacies ensued. Instead, with protest turning to economics, shop closures were the form of protest.[71]

Finally, in November an incident flared up at Torre del Greco, 12.5 km south of Naples. 'An enormous crowd of the lower classes (*popolani*)' gathered outside the town hall, protesting an anti-cholera ordinance shutting off the town's water supplies. They screamed 'Down with the authorities!', and their numbers swelled. Some tried setting the town hall on fire; 'in the confusion' the rioters' leader was wounded. A column of the rioters attacked the mayor's house but a platoon of foot soldiers stopped them, and the town hall was placed under military guard.[72] Again, myths of poisoning or *untori* did not circulate. The *popolani*'s revolt appears economic and humanitarian: how could they survive without fresh drinking water? However, as we have seen from the other examples, these new protests were not the norm. By the end of November 1910, the *Lancet* described the unsanitary conditions and destitution prevailing in Puglia: communes 'at the end of their resources' with 'many places so demoralised' that the 'terror-stricken people' took to flight, concealed suspected cases, and relived 'all the old mediaeval traditions of poisoning and wilful spread of disease by doctors'.[73]

ITALY, 1911

Cholera returned the following summer and, despite government efforts to censor reporting of the disease, and especially of the associated riots, the consequences of violence and accusation can be seen to have widened. On the night of 10 July 1911, the population of the small town of Belmondo Mezzagno, near Palermo, assembled before the town hall,[74] where the mayor, town council, and the district's public physician ('medico condotto') were planning a location for a quarantine camp ('un locale di isolamento'). In compliance with the Giolitti censorship, which had just gone into effect, Italian papers no longer mentioned the word 'cholera'.[75] 'Hooting and hostile cries' brought the prefectoral commissioner to the balcony, but 'a volley of invectives' drowned out his words, followed by a shower of stones that 'made havoc of the windows'. The mayor and councillors escaped by the back door. The assailants drew revolvers, while others used logs to break down the door, all shouting 'Morte al medico! Morte al commissario!' They marched on the physician's home, sacked it, flung his splintered furniture into the street, set the house on fire, then returned to the town hall and burnt it, destroying all its documents.[76] Order was not restored until the next day. Sixty were arrested.[77]

---

[71] Ibid., 5 October 1910, front page.   [72] *La Stampa*, 18 November 1910, 2.
[73] *Lancet*, 12 November 1910, 1453–4.   [74] Ibid., 22 July 1911: 274.
[75] *La Stampa*, 12 July 1911, 2. *Il Corriere della Sera* did not report it.
[76] *La Stampa*, 12 July 1911, 2; and *Lancet*, 22 July 1911: 274.
[77] *La Stampa*, 12 July 1911, 2.

Cholera riots spread across southern mainland Italy, several on a scale equal to those in Russia in 1892 or Sicily in 1837. The first of these erupted on 9 September 1911 in Gioia del Colle, south of Bari. Like the contagion itself, cholera rioting spread to the agricultural town of Massafra in the Province of Lecce, then to Mola di Bari, on the Adriatic, south of Bari, then further north to Carpinone, in the province of Campobasso, and finally across the peninsula to Cosenza in Calabria.[78] These were well reported in US papers, often as front-page stories with glaring headlines—'Cholera at Large in Italian Towns on Dreadful Rumor'; 'Fanatical Inhabitants Empty Hospital';[79] 'Cholera Patients Carried through Streets in Ghastly Processions'.[80] Reflecting the state censorship, the dispatches derived mostly from Chiasso on the Swiss border.

The cholera epidemic at Gioia del Colle gave rise to 'savage excitement'. Health officials issued orders separating those showing signs of the disease from the suspected and confining them in separate hospitals. Rumours spread that the authorities intended to kill the victims. Crowds rushed through the streets to attack hospitals. A small corps of *carabinieri*, trying to resist the crowd, was overwhelmed. The protesters then rescued cholera patients from the hospital and 'carried them in a ghastly procession through town', shouting 'imprecations against the government'.[81] 'The scene was gruesome in the extreme.'[82] Troops were sent in. At least one Italian newspaper, *La Stampa*, reported the riot under the noses of the censors, simply by avoiding the word 'colera'. According to its account, the riot arose in a curious context: 'the condition of the patients had greatly improved'; 'for several days no new cases or deaths were reported'.[83] By 1910–11 even in southern Italy medicine and care of cholera patients had improved: not all cholera hospitals could be described as places from where few returned alive. Yet the old cholera myths died hard.

About the same time, scenes similar to Gioia's occurred at Massafra. 'Thousands men and women',[84] 'armed with spades, sticks and other farm implements',[85] congregated in front of the city hall, chanting 'Death!' 'Death!', while the council of Lecce discussed sanitary measures. The 'mob' chased the mayor and councillors from the building, attacked the cholera hospital, battled against police, and succeeded in carrying away patients, then smashed the furniture and set the building ablaze:

> The patients, some in a dying condition, were carried triumphantly through the streets. The general belief of the people is that the doctors inoculate cholera-stricken persons with poison.

In addition to mass destruction and the death of several cholera patients, prominent government officials and doctors were seriously wounded.[86] Two days later, martial law was declared: soldiers patrolled the streets; sentinels guarded cholera

---

[78] *The Sun*, 12 September 1911, 2.   [79] *Bisbee Daily Review*, 10 September 1911, front page.
[80] *Salt Lake Tribune*, 10 September 1911, front page.
[81] *Times Dispatch*, 10 September 1911, front page.
[82] *Bisbee Daily Review*, 10 September 1911, front page.
[83] *La Stampa*, 9 September 1911, front page.
[84] Simonetti and Sangiorgi, *Il colera*, 189. Some papers estimated 3000.   [85] Ibid.
[86] Ibid. For earlier ones, also see Snowden, *Naples in the Time of Cholera*, 292–6.

patients; and those who had stormed the hospitals were arrested.[87] Yet a second assault on the lazaretto occurred within two days.[88] A patient left behind died the following morning and the doctors, followed by nurses, escaped only by the lazaretto's windows.[89]

According to the *New-York Tribune*, the 'excesses' arose from 'preventive measures to combat the plague', and similar protest arose in 'a number of other Italian towns', where doctors were accused of poisoning and attacked while treating their patients.[90] Other papers were more specific: cholera hospitals in Mola di Bari were raided. At Carpinone, a street vendor was accused of poisoning wells and narrowly escaped lynching, and sanitary cordons placed around villages near Cosenza caused riots, followed by forty-six arrests.[91] Here, the epicentre of cholera violence was close at hand—Verbicaro. Two weeks before, its inhabitants, incensed by cholera measures, travelled to the provincial capital, Cosenza, where they rioted, killing two members of the Red Cross, and burnt down the city hall.[92] No doubt, the Giolitti censorship blocked information on other cholera uprisings that research into judicial archives might bring to light. But despite the censorship, Italian papers reported further disturbances not found in the foreign press and which historians have yet to mention. For one in Salerno in the second week of July, sanitary ordinances (as in Taranto, Massafra, and Mola di Bari) threatened the livelihoods of labourers in a region suffering from economic recession, even famine.[93] These prohibited the sale of shellfish ('dei molluschi e dei crostacci') and vegetables customarily eaten uncooked. The city's fishermen closed their shops and attacked the city hall. *Carabinieri* were summoned; 'violent scuffles' ensued: 'bats and stones went flying'. Eventually, the 23rd Infantry arrived. 'Many' of the demonstrators were wounded along with three *carabinieri*, including their captain.[94]

The most notable case, however, was the revolt of Verbicaro at the end of August 1911. Despite the censorship, it made front-page headlines and filled columns for several days. Even the hush-word 'colera' appeared at least once. This revolt was too extraordinary for either the press or government to ignore. *Corriere della Sera* even blamed 'Onorevole Giolitti' for underestimating the strength of 'the myth of the choleric powder rampant throughout the South, especially among the illiterate

[87] *New-York Tribune*, 12 September 1911, 5.

[88] *Washington Herald*, 12 September 1911, 7; and *Sun*, 12 September 1911, 2; and *The Times*, 11 September 1911, 7.

[89] *La Stampa*, 9 September 1911, 6. The article did not use the word 'colera' but referred to the 'colerosi'. It supplied fewer details than found in the foreign press; see *San Francisco Chronicle*, 5 March 1903, 8.

[90] *New-York Tribune*, 12 September 1911, 5, claimed the physicians would have been killed had soldiers not intervened, but failed to mention the places or numbers involved. *Sun*, 12 September 1911, 2, and *El Paso Herald*, 11 September 1911, 3, printed similarly vague reports.

[91] *Sun*, 12 September 1911, 2.

[92] *Mahoning Dispatch*, 1 September 1911, 2.

[93] Among other places, see the headline stories on these economic conditions in southern Italy that created famines and rebellion in 1910 and 1911: *Aberdeen Journal*, 18 August 1910, 5; *Evening Telegraph*, 18 August 1910, 2.

[94] *Corriere della Sera*, 22 July 11, 2, not reported in *La Stampa*.

peasantry'.[95] This isolated town of 6000 in Calabria's mountains did not even possess a road passable by automobile or horse-drawn coach to its nearest railway station at Paola, 18 km away. Moreover, Verbicaro had a long pedigree of cholera violence. The present riots appear as a repeat of the accusations of 'plague spreading' made against the mayor and agents of the state in 1857. In fact, the mayor then was the grandfather of the present mayor. The 'leggenda' lived on. According to interviews collected by a *Corriere della Sera* reporter, who travelled by train to Paola, then trekked through the mountain passes to Verbicaro, the revolt was vengeance against cholera poisoners, past and present.[96]

While the mayor was holding a meeting, rebels ('i rivoltosi') numbering 1200 attacked the town hall. At first, women 'animated by the desire to do violence against the mayor, Signor Guaragna' comprised the rebels, but soon men and boys armed with axes, scythes, and knives and chanting 'Death to the Mayor!' joined in.[97] An employee, late for the meeting, was discovered to have been recently involved with the town's census. A woman struck his head with a knotty stick. Another shot him with a revolver, and while on the ground, a third slashed his head off with a pruning knife.[98] The horrific scene had not happened at random. The employee's role in the census was viewed with contempt. Harking back to a basic plot recurring in cholera conspiracies across time and space, the peasants believed it to have been the means for choosing who to eliminate to resolve overpopulation: 'Certain ones' had been selected in advance 'for the sacrifice'.[99] One of the town's priests was charged with instigating the riots by stoking such fears that ignited peasant memories.[100] Yet, while neither *Corriere della Sera* nor any other paper described similar scenes then erupting in the immediate vicinity, the Milanese paper claimed that stories of the same terror were circulating in Scalea, Falconara, Belvedere Marittimo, and the provincial seat, Paola. In Grisola Cipollina, news spread that 'the people' stopped a fugitive from Verbicaro 'with a suspicious smile and the accustomed face of death (*con una boccetta di sublimato, con il solito teschietto da morto*)', said to be a plague spreader (*untore*), and massacred him. Authorities at Paola denied the story. But the *Corriere* claimed similar ones were spreading 'everywhere'.[101]

Reports on Verbicaro filled over four long front-page columns of *Corriere della Sera* on 30 August along with others in *La Stampa*,[102] and front-page retrospectives continued into the second half of September. Yet the foreign press supplied more details about the riots themselves, though paid little attention to underlying causes: for them, Verbicaro's protest had arisen simply because of 'popular superstition'. A 'mob of 500' (or 1200 depending on the account), armed with spades, knives, sticks, and agricultural implements, paraded through town, shouting 'Long live

[95] *Corriere della Sera*, 30 August 1911, front page.
[96] Ibid., 31 August 1911, 2: 'La folla paura degli "untori": Una visita a Verbicaro. La popolazione in fuga'.
[97] Ibid, 31 August 1911, 2.   [98] Ibid.   [99] Ibid.
[100] Ibid., 4 September 1911, 1–2: 'Una terra italiana da redimere', 2.
[101] Ibid., 31 August 1911, 2.
[102] *La Stampa*, 30 August 1911, front page; 29 August 1911, front page; 1 September 1911, 2; 2 September 1911, 3: 'Dolorose constatazioni dopo i gravissimi fatti di Verbicaro'; 4 September 1911, 2: 'Profughi verbicaresi che, spinti dalla fame, assaltano a fucilate la stazione'.

the king!' and 'Death to the Mayor!' They knocked down telegraph poles and cut the wires to isolate Verbicaro further, preventing the authorities from summoning troops. The rebels besieged the town hall, wrecked the furniture, burnt the archives, then the building, along with the praetorial court, the telegraph office, and the mayor's house, and released prisoners from the local gaol. The mayor, town clerk, and judge fled. A group of eleven, including three women, caught the clerk and 'hacked [him] to pieces'; the judge 'died of fright' as he reached the train station. The police wounded several and killed a woman. Troops did not arrive until the following day and arrested eleven ringleaders. Corpses were left unburied; half the population fled to the mountains, and cholera lethality rates rose to higher percentages, reflecting the chaos and destruction of quarantine and medical facilities. In close to 60 per cent of the cases, the patient died, while official figures for Italy stood at 659 deaths out of 1687 cases:[103] 39 per cent. Verbicaro's mayor escaped, but not for long: two days later, when the provincial prefect threatened to dismiss him, he returned and was murdered, tragically, repeating his grandfather's fate fifty-five years later.[104]

Verbicaro's revolt transfixed the Italian press to an extent not seen with any other cholera disturbance for this or any previous cholera wave. After the riots ended, articles continued through September, but instead of dwelling on the events, they attempted to explain the violence and 'irrationality of the rabble'. *La Stampa* and *Corriere della Sera* saw the problem as peculiar to the South (Mezzogiorno) and its isolated places known for historic backwardness. According to *Corriere*, hundreds of 'paesi' in the South were exactly like Verbicaro.[105] In a special editorial, its renowned journalist, Luigi Barzini (Sr.), asked the insightful question: 'why had such irrational violence erupted from cholera?' But his argument had nothing to do with cholera; instead, it focused exclusively on the 'southern problem', which in his eyes was more specifically a Calabrese problem, resting on its peasants' conception of the state and the relationship between government and the people ('popolo'). According to Barzini, it was a 'feudal' relationship. The 'popolo' considered the government a 'foreign power', 'an occupying army'. Taxes were a tribute of war that failed to benefit the peasant. The state's only interest was to squeeze the peasant as much as it could, and this explains their great distrust of the government. 'He felt abandoned, disarmed, and betrayed'. To these long-term sentiments, Barzini added contemporary facts: over the past half century, the government had built no new roads in Calabria, and its population had declined 20 per cent in the last decade, with 60 per cent of its men emigrating to America, leaving an adult population mainly of impoverished women.[106] In these retrospective articles, neither Barzini nor other journalists or intellectuals returned to his first question: why cholera? Why had this disease and not others of epidemic force during the nineteenth and early twentieth century created such antipathy, violence, and myths of poisoning? Against

---

[103] *The Sun*, 29 August 1911, front page, from Naples.
[104] Papers such as the *Sun* mistakenly said it was his father. See *Corriere della Sera*, 31 August 1918, 2. Seventeen were tried for slaying the judge and town clerk; *Sun*, 14 October 1911.
[105] *Corriere della Sera*, 30 August 1911, front page.   [106] Ibid., 4 September 1911, 1–2.

the backdrop of depopulation, why had peasants believed the government wished to cull their numbers? Why had they turned with such rage against the medical profession? And why had such violence arisen with cholera in other regions of Italy beyond Verbicaro and Calabria, places in central Italy, even cosmopolitan cities such as Naples and later that year (as we shall see) in northern Italy?

An even longer editorial on Verbicaro's tragedy led *Corriere*'s front page on Sunday 17 September.[107] Among discussions of 'the southern question', prejudices, fantasies, and oppression under Bourbon rule, and Calabria's failure to become culturally incorporated into the new national state, this article described a consequence of the riots unmentioned by the foreign press. As many as four thousand, two-thirds of Verbicaro's population, had fled, 'disappearing into the gorges and ravines between the bramble and vineyards'. Dispersed in the mountains, they scavenged to survive, chased away by those within the surrounding villages 'as though lepers'. According to Barzini, the reason for the mass exodus was the belief that the government planned to poison them.[108]

Against these explanations, cholera riots were not exclusive to the South, even in this, Italy's last major cholera wave, as Barzini and others assumed. After reporting that Italy had been the worst hit in Europe by the 1910–11 epidemic and that the southern provinces of Naples, Palermo, Caserta, and Salerno suffered the highest caseloads and casualties, a *Lancet* correspondent condemned the mob violence 'against municipal authorities, doctors, and nurses'. He made his point from one case, not a southern town but an unnamed one near Rome, and followed conspiracies reaching back to the 1830s. Believing that 'cholera patients were purposely poisoned in the hospital, rioters overpowered the military guard and stormed the cholera hospital, shouting, "Death to the doctors and nurses!"' After parading the sick to their homes, 'the mob' wrecked the town hall and threatened to kill the mayor and his staff.[109] Another *Lancet* correspondent recorded mob violence in the province of Rome, now naming the seashore towns, Anzio and Nettuno. Similar to those in the South, crowds prevented doctors and their assistants from visiting cholera patients and accused them of purposefully spreading the disease. On one occasion, the crowd attempted 'to lynch' them.

Despite Giolitti's censorship, at least two Italian newspapers, Rome's *Il Messaggero* and *Corriere della Sera* described multiple incidents of cholera violence at Nettuno (without mentioning 'colera', 'quarantina', or 'lazaretto'). Instead, cholera was called acute enteritis ('casi di enterite acuta'), the quarantined, 'le persone contumaci', and the lazareto, 'la casa contumaciale'. Otherwise, the Italian papers were more specific than the *Lancet*'s correspondent. Economic causes had conditioned Nettuno's anger and resort to violence. For some days, measures taken by sanitary authorities and the commune damaged tourism during the summer bathing season. Yet signs of the old traditions surfaced: with 'noisy demonstrations (*dimostrazioni chiassose*)' in front of the lazaretto, crowds sought to liberate the quarantine. Another incident

---

[107] Ibid., 'Perchè non è scomparsa la credenza nel veleno di Stato'.
[108] Ibid., 4 September 1911, front page. On Verbicaro in 1911, see Lorenzo, *Colera sovversive*.
[109] 'Cholera in Europe', *Lancet*, 30 December 1911: 1856.

at Nettuno resembled aspects of recent events at Ostuni, used earlier by papers to illustrate southern Italians' 'ignorance and superstition': about 500, 'mostly women and peasants', had gone to a little sanctuary ('tempietto') dedicated to Saint Roch, a kilometre from town. They woke up the friars and demanded that their patron's statue be handed over to them for a procession. The brothers tried to persuade the 'popolani' that presently such action was unwise but failed to convince them. The crowd then processed with the statue through Nettuno's streets.[110]

A third incident at Nettuno, grounded in cholera's old conspiracies, proved more violent. Mounting numbers of patients transported to the lazaretto 'exasperated ever more the most ignorant of the people'. On 4 July, the head of the sanitary office, a doctor from the Red Cross, went to a peasant's house to take his child 'suffering with serious conditions' (e.g. cholera) to the lazaretto. Large numbers of 'the lower classes' gathered to prevent the child's removal, attacking the litter and freeing the patient. That evening the crowds reassembled in front of the boy's house with women screaming 'they want to kill that poor child'. *Carabinieri* tried to calm the crowd and free the doctor. After striking a deal to free the doctor, the *popolani* instead 'hysterically rushed on him with fists, batons and pieces of iron, beating him atrociously'. An officer fired into the air, killing a seventeen-year-old boy. 'A veritable bloodbath (*carneficina*)' ensued with commoners charging the outnumbered *carabinieri* with sticks, knives, and stones. From around 300, the crowd grew to 500. 'Women and peasants' ran through the streets, ringing bells into the night. The town's well-respected archpriest intervened but to no avail. Later that night, 200 riflemen ('bersaglieri') restored order.[111] The *Lancet*'s correspondent claimed 'a similar uprising, equally inspired by superstitious dread of hygienic precautions and the institution of a lazaretto', occurred in Venice, 'doubtless to be followed by others'.[112] Although this article circulated widely in the US press, I have not spotted another independent source for it. But the Giolitti censorship was especially concerned with suppressing such news in northern centres of lucrative tourism.[113]

The most significant cholera riot in the north during this epidemic was not reported by the *Lancet* or any US paper in the vast 'Chronicling America' archive; nor does it appear in Snowden's coverage of cholera in Italy,[114] or any secondary source I know.[115] Instead, the *Scotsman* picked up the report through a circuitous route. A Milanese correspondent sent it by post to the frontier, where it was probably received by Reuters. Nonetheless, this was no small incident. The crowd at Segni (Lazio), then, only an hour's train ride to Rome, was put at 3000, making

---

[110] *Corriere della Sera*, 5 July 1911, 4.
[111] *Corriere della Sera*, 5 July 1911, 4. *La Stampa* mentions none of these events.
[112] *Lancet*, 22 July 1911: 274.
[113] *The Democratic Banner*, 25 October 1910; Rütten, 'Cholera'; and Snowden, *Naples in the Time of Cholera*, 307–11.
[114] Snowden, *Naples in the Time of Cholera*.
[115] Simonetti and Sangiorgi, *Il colera*, mentions riots outside Puglia but none in central or northern Italy.

it one of Italy's largest cholera riots. As with those in the South, myths of government and physicians out to massacre the innocent underlay it:

> Segni has just been the scene of grave cholera riots, the origin of which was the same as that of the recent troubles in Calabria. The municipality took steps to prevent the spread of cholera. A hospital was formed, in which there are five cholera patients, and a quarantine establishment.... The idea spread among ignorant people that the municipal authorities, the Government, and the Carabineers were in league to poison them, and had organized a slaughter of the innocents. A mob of three thousand marched on the Town Hall, shouting for the release from the hospital of their relations and friends. Soon the whole military force of the town, consisting of only five Carabineers, was overwhelmed.... The Carabineers were pelted with stones and injured, and...retired, and the rioters, by this time numbering several thousand, battered down the Town Hall's door, intending to sack and destroy it and murder any they imagined responsible for the cholera.
>
> The chief objects of their anger were the Mayor and hospital clerks, who, however, escaped by the roofs.... The women were particularly ferocious, and one of them seized a Carabineer by his tunic and threw him to the ground. He was disarmed, trampled upon, and wounded...the mob broke into the Town Hall, and threw all they could lay their hands upon out of the windows. A woman seized the municipal flag and shouted, 'To the hospital'. Her cry was taken up immediately, and the mob surged through the town, crying 'Death to the doctors and nurses.'...
>
> On reaching the lazaretto the rioters removed three patients suffering from cholera, as well as ones in quarantine, and carried them in their arms in a procession to their homes. The scene was ghastly in the extreme.... Troops from Rome have now occupied the town. Many arrests have been made.[116]

Despite the censorship, at least one Italian newspaper recorded the events at Segni, adding elements suggesting why its women were so incensed. As with others during the 1910–11 wave, this riot coupled new economic reasons with the old mythologies of protest. On the eve of the riots, the municipality had imposed a sanitary decree of dubious merit for combating cholera, prohibiting hens roaming freely through town. Tending chickens was women's 'industry'. Now, forbidden to leave them in their courtyards, they had to keep them penned in the house, which destroyed their household goods. In addition, these women suffered from damages caused by disinfection, which the state refused to reimburse.[117]

Despite new elements of economic rationale and a clearer sense of organization, planning, and leadership, myths present at the outset in the 1830s persisted— intentional poisoning and planned massacres of the poor, with hospitals, doctors, and governments as the agents. They were present not only in isolated and neglected districts such as Verbicaro but also within Rome's metropolitan ambit and possibly in Venice. No doubt, this wave of cholera produced further incidents of social violence that state censorship successfully concealed. *Corriere della Sera*'s long editorial of 17 September maintained that 'the echo of Verbicaro's atrocious event

---

[116] *Scotsman*, 17 October 1911, 8: from Reuters; *The Times*, 17 October 1911, 5. Also, Australian papers reported them; see, for instance, *The Maitland Daily Mercury*, 17 October 1911, 5.

[117] *La Stampa*, 17 October 1911, 4: 'Una ripetizione dei fatti di Verbicaro'.

had not yet run its course . . . beliefs in the intentional origins of the disease persisted at Massafra, Sant'Angelo in Grotte, Cetara and several other rural communes of the South'. Except for Massafra, my searches have turned up none of the others. This same editorial, moreover, alleged that belief in the state using cholera to poison the people became stronger in 1910–11 than in the previous cholera waves of 1866–7 or 1884–5.[118]

COMPARISONS OF CHOLERA VIOLENCE WITHIN ITALY

Because of improvements in communication with the telegraph, telephone, and international networks of newspaper correspondents, a comparison over time of the diffusion of cholera riots and beliefs in its intentional spread is problematic. Certainly, the cholera revolts in the summer of 1837 in the four principal regions of Sicily—Palermo, Messina, Catania, and Siracusa—might compare in numbers of participants and levels of violence with cholera riots in Russia and Eastern Europe. From prodigious archival research, Alfonso Sansone unearthed violent cholera rioting, especially in villages and small towns, with sharp class divisions between peasants and workers ('la plebe') on one side against large property holders ('dei più cospicui possidenti') on the other.[119] He listed at least twenty-nine places in Sicily that rose up in arms against supposed disseminators of cholera and made clear that there were more, as in a list of sixteen small towns and villages in the valley of Siracusa, which ends: 'and in other communes of the Valley'. As for violence, riots even in villages and small towns such as Villagrazia, Villabate, Misilmeri, Marineo, Prizzi, and Termini-Imerese were bloodier than any in the British Isles. In Marineo in the Val di Palermo, for instance, crowds destroyed communal archives, devastated homes, and killed thirty-three, including the town's mayor, chief justice, and head priest ('l'arciprete').[120] Between July and October in the same valley of Misilmeri, 156 were charged with rioting, with eight put before the firing squad.[121] For villages and towns of La Valle Minore di Palermo, 650 were sentenced and the crowds killed at least eighty, in addition to 'innumerable burnings of houses, devastations and sackings'. One hundred and forty were condemned to death, ninety of whom were executed.[122] Sansone mentions no incidents within Palermo, yet a House of Commons report on quarantine referred to one there in June: three 'vaguely suspected' of poisoning public fountains were 'torn to pieces'.[123]

---

[118] *Corriere della Sera*, 17 September 1911, front page.
[119] Sansone, *Gli avvenimenti*, 71, 72, 74, 75, 142, 204; della Perutta, *Mazzini*, 273–7; and idem, *Società e classi popolari*, 211, taken largely from Sansone.
[120] Sansone, *Gli avvenimenti*, 76.   [121] Ibid., 82–3.
[122] Ibid., 93. For the four regions, the plebeians killed 130 'innocents'. In addition to those condemned to death, 'many hundreds' were sentenced to life in prison; others, put in irons; others in solitary confinement; and an 'inestimable number' killed in personal vendettas; ibid., 204–5.
[123] Bowring, *Abstracts*, 52.

The geographical patterns of cholera uprisings differed in Sicily from most places in Europe during this first cholera wave as well as in many afterwards. In Sicily, they concentrated in small towns and villages with the capital Palermo mostly spared, despite deadly riots swirling through the adjacent valley to the east. And when cholera struck cities, the violence became interlaced with general uprisings against the Bourbon monarchy, as at Messina with cries of 'Messinesi! Gridate vendetta contro gli oppressori della vostra patria' (People of Messina! Cry out against the oppressors of your country). Here, the violence was politically organized; its targets mostly government buildings and symbols of power rather than persons. The crowds broke into the offices of the maritime police and health commissioners, destroying the latter. They ripped down the maritime police's coats of arms and threw the furniture and registers of the health commissioner into the sea, tore apart the royal flag and 'attacked' paintings on the walls. At the customs house, they disarmed the collector. But despite the scale of these demonstrations, Sansone records only one attack that led to serious personal injuries—an assault on an inspector of the maritime police. Unlike uprisings in the Valle di Palermo, no brutal repression with numerous capital punishments followed.[124]

In Siracusa and Catania, the cholera revolts were more clearly entwined with the liberal and nationalist rebellion against the Bourbon monarchy, and some of their leaders came from the intelligentsia and professional classes. Yet their attacks relied on accusations of intentional cholera spreading. In Siracusa it took the form of legal inquisitions and trials against supposed poisoners and spreaders of cholera, reminiscent of Milan's prosecution of *untori* in 1630. More so than with any other cholera wave in Italy or elsewhere, the accusations derived from the educated classes, with the liberal lawyer, Mario Adorno, at the commission's helm, blaming cholera's spread on 'a devilish sect bent on poisoning the people'.[125] Here, such rumours were not restricted to the immigrant poor, as in Dublin or Astrakhan, but 'freely circulated in cafés, judicial tribunals, piazze, and before magistrates'.[126] Taking their lead from legal elites, those in small towns such as Floridia, Modica, and Solarino fanned the accusations of poisoning through the Val di Siracusa, inciting uprisings against the suspected, who included large landholders and government officials.[127] In Catania, on the other hand, the protesters' targets resembled Spain's in the 1830s: crowds attacked monastic communities, in this case, Benedictines, and assaulted the town's cholera hospital, smashing it asunder. The class nature of the violence, however, differed from patterns in the rest of Europe: instead of the instigators being the rabble, the organizers and their ideology came from the 'Piazza dell'Università', where Sicily's flag of Independence was unfurled, and its leader was the Prior of the municipal government, 'an old liberal Catanese'.[128]

Moreover, perhaps because of cholera's intertwining with political uprisings in Sicily, attacks against hospitals and the medical core were rare. In Sicily, the reaction focused instead sharply on agents of the state. Despite numerous attacks on

[124] Sansone, *Gli avvenimenti*, 96–101.   [125] Ibid., 106.
[126] Ibid.   [127] Ibid., 130 and 142.   [128] Ibid., 156.

individuals suspected of poisoning with at least 180 ending in murder or execution in the summer of 1837, not a single nurse or pharmacist was suspected. Only in Messina did crowds attack sanitary officials, and only in Siracusa was a doctor targeted, and here it amounted to 'whispers' against the town's protomedico.[129] Finally, of the hundreds of houses and government offices attacked and burnt, the 'popolo' rose against only two cholera hospitals (as far as Sansone's descriptions go), and in Siracusa it was limited to broken windows.[130] Only in Catania, did crowd action against a hospital spiral to ritualistic levels of frenzy seen across the Alps (or in later cholera waves in Italy): the Catanesi charged the hospital, destroyed everything they could lay their hands on, and gathered the broken pieces in the streets with 'cries of exalted glee'. Even here, however, these actions differed: they were directed against the pro-Bourbon municipal government, which they succeeded in overthrowing.[131] In 1985 Carmello Vetro took Sansone to task for underestimating attacks against doctors during this first Italian cholera wave, citing instances at Palermo, Caltanissetta, and Siracusa of doctors stigmatized in derisive verse and accused of poisoning.[132] His qualifications, however, corroborate Sansone's earlier conclusions: major attacks on hospitals and massacres of the medical profession fail to surface.

No other region of Italy has been so thoroughly studied for cholera during its first wave, especially concerning socio-political ramifications. Nor has anyone drawn comparisons between these events and other places in Italy to speculate on differences in political alliances, political consequences, levels of violence, or rioters' targets. In 1836–7 cholera disturbances spread much less decisively into the mainland South. The few to do so, as in Sicily, broke out in small towns and villages. Franco della Perutta briefly described protests in the Cilento, south of Salerno. In August 1837, in Marina di Camerota villagers demanded care and spiritual assistance from their mayor and archpriest, but these did not possess the slightest 'tint of a political reaction'.[133] Nor did the usual myths of the cholera revolts—accusations of mass poisoning or conspiracies by the rich to annihilate the poor—emerge. By contrast, at Atena Lucana, 'the alarm of the *popolo*'s warning of poisoners' was heard. Their protest, sparked by a mixture of religious and social concerns, however, differed from those in Sicily. While privileged families continued to be buried within parish churchyards, health commissioners forced the 'popolo' into new grounds designated for cholera victims alone. From this, anger and 'more seditious voices' arose against the landowning classes.[134] Yet, even here, destruction of property and attacks on cholera hospitals, health officers, doctors, mayors, or other agents of the state failed to arise. Della Perutta maintained that 'analogous episodes' occurred in other villages in the Cilento, listing five that reopened private vendettas and turned against the 'galantuomini'. At Padula, peasants murdered three presumed poisoners.[135] He held that attacks 'with similar characteristics' spread through 'many other localities in the Mezzogiorno'—in the Abruzzo, Calabria,

---

[129] Ibid., 105. The trials against accused spreaders targeted mostly the police ('i rondieri'), 115–47.
[130] Ibid., 156.   [131] Ibid.   [132] Vetro, 'Società, medici e terapie'.
[133] Della Perutta, *Mazzini*, 265.   [134] Ibid.   [135] Ibid.

and especially Puglia—where 'the riots were particularly intensive'. But beyond the Cilento, he named only six places. One was Ostuni, where cholera riots, as we have seen, reached a high pitch in 1910 during the peninsula's last major cholera wave. As in 1910, those in 1837 were directed against burial inequalities: the *popolo* would not tolerate 'being thrown into ditches'. Little else, however, is reported: nothing about targets, destruction, arrests, or the usual cholera mythologies. Della Perutta maintained that no evidence points to organized popular movements but, given the general 'discontent of the popular classes', an anti-Bourbon political dimension cannot be ruled out.[136] For him, cholera riots of the peninsula's first wave were confined to the South. Nor do other sources—primary or secondary—reveal any beyond the Mezzogiorno.[137] Still, some historians have suggested that the epidemic led to a collapse of order, fears of the medical profession, and myths of poisoning erupting in northern cities. But when specific incidents are described, they appear meek by comparison with Sicily's brutality in 1837. In Brescia in 1836, Anna Forti Messina recorded that the cholera-stricken were left to die of thirst and were prevented from swallowing any medicines prescribed by municipal doctors. She maintained that similar incidents were occurring elsewhere in the Veneto, in Naples, Genoa, Massa Carrara, Sardinia, and in villages and towns in Tuscany (though she produced no examples). She claimed that 'Veleno!' was a cry of the people during the first cholera outbreak in northern Italy but provided only one example: at Livorno doctors were accused of poisoning, not, however, because of the usual story, wishing to exterminate the poor, but rather to alleviate human suffering. She further suggested that 'the supposed poisoners were not only doctors but the wealthy (*i signori*) in general, at times foreigners, those in authority, the king, the government'. While in Sicily in 1837, it was the Bourbons, in Turin in 1835 it was the king and the nobility, and in Genoa, the present government of Republicans.[138] But she describes no northern cholera riots or collective violence of any sort. Moreover, the closest suggestion of collective violence north of Naples, 1835–7, that I have found comes from a doctor's description of a fellow doctor's experience in the region of Cesena (Romagna): 'the plebes rose up tumultuously against' a dottor Cassani, accusing him of poisoning. But no physical violence ensued. Instead, 'honest citizens . . . convinced them otherwise', and the doctor did not 'find himself in serious trouble'.[139] The only mass movements cholera sparked in the north in the 1830s were religious and peaceful. In Genoa, where cholera 'raged with particular vehemence', a great assemblage of the people arose' in religious processions, 'characterized by incomprehensible manifestations of

---

[136] Ibid., 265–6.

[137] A recollection by a patient of Brierre de Boismont, (*Hallucinations*, Case LX, 146), refers to 'a near relative', massacred at Rome by 'an ignorant and furious mob' accused of poisoning children during a cholera epidemic. The author does not date the incident, and I know no northern Italian cholera riots reported before the book's publication.

[138] Messina, 'L'Italia dell'Ottocento', 481.

[139] From Barbacciani, *Storia sul Cholera-Morbus*, 79, cited in Pieri, *Lo Zingaro*, 54.

fanaticism and credulity'. And in Rome the pope led 'an immense crowd' in a solemn procession.[140]

Medical articles written by cholera doctors, serving their communities during the 1835–7 pandemic,[141] provide further observations and insights into attitudes and actions of various classes during this first cholera wave. At Brescia in 1836, a cholera doctor in an article devoted principally to cures and procedures described lower-class 'preoccupations':

> First and foremost, they deny that cholera exists. Instead, it is as if the governors and the doctors wished to frighten the people so that they would flee their homes and the city. Similarly, the plebes put the blame on doctors, that the disease was created by our terrible craft or that we wished to reduce their numbers by poisoning them without any pity.

He concretized his generalizations with incidents of cholera patients accusing him of spreading the disease, and concluded that their opinions 'sadly were simply signs of the time'. Yet, despite his low opinion of the 'vulgo', the doctor did not report any collective violence or suggest that his life was ever endangered.[142] A thirty-eight page summary of Pietro Betti's three-volume study of Tuscany's first cholera wave (1926 pages) cites his condemnation of the Tuscan 'plebi', blaming them for their 'docility', 'resistance', 'stupid fatalism', 'cowardice', and 'indifference', which he argued accentuated the spread of cholera. He contrasted their attitudes with the 'efficacious vigilance' and 'informed actions' of those in government, who strove to meet 'the needs of all'.[143] But despite his contempt for commoners, no violence or resistance to sanitary measures or accusations against doctors or anyone else purposely spreading the disease is reported. Moreover, detailed reports on cholera statistics and popular reactions during the 1830s in individual cities from Sardinia to Lombardy[144] make no mention even of rumours of intentional cholera spreading outside the South. Instead, several praised their local populations for their charity, diligence, and self-sacrifice in combating the disease.[145] A report on several cities in the state of Sardinia singled out twelve doctors from Genoa as 'martyrs', who fell victim to the epidemic caring for fellow citizens.[146] And a report on cholera in Bergamo praised all its citizens: despite every danger, they 'competed to offer charity and help' to shelter the needy.[147]

In cholera waves after 1837, reactions of local populations beyond Sicily, however, did not continued to be so positive. One of Italy's major medical journals of the nineteenth century, *AUM*, unlike the *Lancet*, did not commission articles to investigate the social consequences of epidemics. Nevertheless, in analyzing

---

[140] Simonetti and Sangiorgi, *Il colera*, 23.

[141] These derive from Emeroteca online, Braidense Library, Milan.

[142] Fornasini, 'Intorno al cholera di Brescia'. In her long introduction to Amari's account of cholera in Sicily in 1837 (*Descrizione del cholera di Sicilia*), Castiglione cites Dottore Menis on mistrust of doctors in Brescia (1836) but reports no incidents against them (62).

[143] Morelli, 'Pietro Betti', 608.

[144] The AUM from 1817 to 1874 and as *Annali universali di medicina e chirurgia* to 1888.

[145] Morelli, 'Pietro Betti', 616.   [146] Calderini, 'Cenno istorico', 443.

[147] Borsani and Freschi, 'Osservazioni…Bergamo', 115.

mortality and lethality and debates on transmission, its authors occasionally provided glimpses into these reactions. Here, too, the popular mentality north of Sicily changed from the 1830s, and its direction was the opposite of that seen with the decline in cholera violence in the British Isles and France or what we might have expected from steady advances in the understanding of the disease. During the epidemic at Milan in 1855, a physician reported that some in the city resisted any medical intervention; they were convinced that the medical profession was out to poison them.[148] At this time, such beliefs had become diffused in the Romagna. A letter of 14 April 1855 on Cesena's sanitary conditions claimed that, 'part of the population believed that the government had secretly ordered doctors to adminster poison to the afflicted under their care to kill them'.[149] No praise of citizens' charity appears in these pages.

Furthermore, attacks and minor riots can be collected from these reports. In the next cholera epidemic of 1865, a Neapolitan doctor interrupted his clinical statistics to narrate an incident at San Giovanni Teduccio, a village on the coast south-east of Naples. The disease began in a single household and continued to strike only those in that household. A crowd formed and burnt the 'maladetta' house to the ground.[150] With the next cholera wave in 1884, a doctor reported two incidents from the district of La Spezia (Liguria). At Lerici, the army had to be sent to clear a *cordon sanitaire* illegally imposed on the town by its citizens. The heads of the *popolo* were arrested, but as soon as the *carabinieri* left, 'as if by magic', citizens reconstructed the blockades. Similar cordons formed along provincial highways near Buonviaggio with 'serious disturbances' erupting and many arrests.[151]

In contrast to the heavy concentration of social violence in Sicily during the peninsula's first cholera wave, riots of the 1850s, 1860s, 1880s, and especially in 1910–11 focused on the mainland South and ran north to towns and villages in Lazio, Tuscany, Liguria, Piedmont, Lombardy, and the Veneto. In 1910–11 these occurred in at least twenty-six cities, towns, and villages from Bari to Rome's hinterland and in Venice. In Italy, cholera conspiracies, mythologies, and social violence paved no straightforward progressive history. Over time, they may have become more bound with economic causes but spanned a wider expanse of the nation, repeating fears and accusations that exploded into collective violence against the state, hospitals, and physicians.

CHOLERA VIOLENCE AFTER 1911

To be sure, cholera's break with social violence after 1911 in Europe and across the globe resulted from the disease's decline. But as we have seen, large-scale cholera riots erupted in Italian cities such as Ostuni, Gioia del Colle, and Segni in 1910–11,

---

[148] Sacchi, 'Relazione della commissione sanitaria'.
[149] Pieri, *Lo Zingaro*, 36.
[150] Pepere, 'Rapporto...S. Giovanni a Teduccio'.
[151] Oldoini, 'Storia delle epidemie', 344.

when almost all the patients had been cured. Furthermore, cholera riots continued later in the twentieth century, often recalling the old mythologies of intentional poisoning. They erupted in Soviet Russia as late as 1922, and in Kolkata (Calcutta) and surrounding towns and villages in 1943.[152] During World War I, in German-occupied France, the old cholera myths resurfaced, when the German general staff notified its embassy in occupied France that a French doctor and his two assistants were trying to poison wells near Metz with cholera microbes. They were court-martialled and shot.[153] These experiences of cholera terror and blame may have been more widespread with deeper roots in the German populace than suggested by German war propaganda. Four months later, an Australian living in Berlin reported rumours of doctors, now Russian, poisoning city fountains with cholera and of other Russians feeding German children sweets laced with the bacilli. Such reports, the Australian held, had become everyday occurrences of Berlin life.[154]

Even the seventh cholera wave of El Tor isolates, previously dated to 1937 and now to 1905 but which struck with epidemic force first in Indonesia in 1961,[155] and is present today[156] continues to provoke prejudice, blaming, and rioting, despite few mysteries remaining with this disease and case fatalities usually below 1 per cent.[157] As with cholera in the past, the conspiracies and blaming continue to divide communities along class lines. When cholera reached Peru in 1991, government ministries attacked the poor as 'pigs', accusing them of spreading the disease by their 'pig-like' habits. The poor retaliated with mass demonstrations against state officials.[158] A year later the Venezuelan government blamed cholera on the poor's dirty, uncivilized habits, especially their diet of crabs, while the poor

---

[152] *New York Times Magazine*, 2 October 1943: 'India's Starvation Toll Soars'. This one appears to have been triggered, however, more by an accompanying famine than cholera. Mobs attacked 'rice-loaded boats', not hospitals or doctors, and rumours spread of rice disappearing from markets.

[153] *Clarence and Richmond Examiner*, 6 August 1914, 4. Similar stories spread further afield, and in Berlin became a problem for the German army command; *Bendigo Advertiser*, 3 October 1914, 3.

[154] *Clarence and Richmond Examiner*, 11 February 1915, 2.

[155] Cases appeared in 1937, see Shah, *Pandemic*, 169.

[156] See examples of such cholera violence in Zimbabwe and Haiti: A. Mutreja, et al. 'Evidence for Several Waves'; 'Global Epidemics'; Echenberg, 'Cholera'; and idem, *Africa in the Time of Cholera*, part II. On cholera riots in Haiti, see Farmer, *Haiti after the Earthquake*; and 'Haiti: Protesters Stone U.N. Patrol', *New York Times*, 18 November 2010: 'Several hundred protesters stoned a United Nations patrol and yelled anti-United Nations slogans in the capital, Port-au-Prince…The protest followed several days of riots against the peacekeepers at Cap Haitien, where at least two people were killed…' Also, Shah, *Pandemics*, 122–3. Unlike in Venezuela in 1992, I have not seen here conspiracy theories of elites purposely killing off the poor. For cholera riots in Harare, Zimbabwe, *The New York Times*, 4 December 2008 and 13 December 2008: doctors and nurses protested against government inattention, denial, blaming the West, and closing, understaffing, and ill-equipping hospitals. Mugabe's officials invented conspiracy theories of British 'biological chemical warfare' and 'a genocidal onslaught'; see Echenberg, *Africa in the Time of Cholera*, 168. Cholera continues to kill an estimated 100,000 annually; see Clemens et al., 'Cholera'.

[157] Cueto, 'Stigma and Blame', 269. From 1998 to 2009, Zimbabwe case fatalities averaged 4 per cent soaring to 7.7 per cent in 2006; Echenberg, *Africa in the Time of Cholera*, 168.

[158] Cueto, 'Stigma and Blame', 281–3.

accused the government and multinationals of poisoning their food (especially crabs) to kill them off.[159]

Such reactions have not been limited to impoverished districts of developing countries. In August and September 1973, the El Tor strain afflicted Naples and surrounding communities, provoking mass demonstrations and strikes. These, however, differed radically from those of Italy's previous cholera waves. Instead of resisting vaccination, disinfection, or state intervention by health officials and physicians, protests from Naples' poor now attacked state incompetence in treatment and delivery of medicines and services. Because of black-market profiteering, prices of drugs and lemons—popularly believed to prevent, even cure cholera—skyrocketed, and vaccination kits became difficult to find. As a consequence, 200 in Torre del Greco, comprised principally of women with their infants and children in tow, marched against the municipal government and demonstrated in front of the health office, which locked its doors, but through which they soon entered. Instead of suspicion of doctors and their medicines, the demonstrators demanded information and immediate vaccination for themselves: 'Vaccinateli!'; 'Dammi qualche informazione'; 'Vogliamo il vaccino subito'. At the beginning of September, women of Naples' proletarian neighbourhood of Cavalleggeri Fuorigrotta and of the 'Legge 640' built barricades and blocked traffic. Instead of attacking health services, they demanded the municipality clean their streets and disinfect their homes.

Not all sanitary measures, however, were welcomed. On 3 September fishermen of Santa Lucia joined the women, protesting against the government's destruction of their mussel beds as a sanitary precaution. On 14 September, protest reached its peak when between 2000 and 3000 workers from the district of Massimo D'Azeglio marched on the city hall, mounted barricades, and staged a rent strike, demanding 'Free health assistance'. Incidents of violence followed. The unemployed destroyed the prefect's automobile and threw rocks at health officers and police. The police responded with tear gas and smoke bombs, and rammed their jeeps through the crowds.[160] But their repression failed: at the end of September the municipality's mishandling of the epidemic accompanied by fifteen days of protest brought down Naples' government.[161] Yet the resulting death toll, despite the corruption, chaos, and misadministration, amounted to nine in a two month-period over the vast population of Naples and its surrounding towns.[162]

Although the aims of this Neapolitan protest and popular understanding of the disease's transmission had changed sharply since the early twentieth century, cholera still could divide populations and continued to bring women and children onto barricades in violent clashes with the state, only joined later by male workers whose livelihoods were threatened by sanitary measures. The composition of the

---

[159] Briggs, 'Theorizing Modernity Conspiratorially', esp. 164–72. On crabs as an alternative host of *Vibrio cholera*, see Hamlin, *Cholera*, 275. In the Philippines from 1882 to 1902, similar patterns of accusations from regimes and elites, blaming the poor for 'pig-sty carabao barbarism' and 'stupidity and criminal carelessness' provoked resistance and violence; see Sullivan, 'Cholera and Colonialism', 289.

[160] *Anche il colera*, 11–12, 16, 21, 35, 41–2, 46, 95.   [161] Ibid., 95.

[162] Ibid., 46. The lethality rate was 1 in 92 reported cases.

crowds and their class alignments resembled cholera riots going back to the 1830s and especially those of the fig-growing and fishing towns of Puglia during the spate of cholera riots in 1910–11. A crucial difference, however, now was patent: cries of 'untori' and myths of physicians killing off the poor had finally disappeared. Yet despite this endpoint, Italy's socio-psychological history of cholera does not trace a progressive understanding or trust between *popolino* and the state. Chapter 10's cholera comparisons expose further deviations from any Whig history of disease and its socio-psychological consequences.

10

Cholera Protest over Time

In terms of hate and disease, cholera has been the most thoroughly studied. Yet historians rarely comment on the reasons for its explosive power to provoke prejudice, conspiracies, and class divisions across widely contrasting social and political contexts. From the previous three chapters, two factors have emerged—the clustering of victims among the impoverished and the high lethality rates. Another factor might be cholera's power to transform the body so suddenly and horrifically, from the onset of violent diarrhoea to the last gasps of rice-like vomit, reducing living bodies in hours to blue-hued shrivelled corpses. Cholera, however, was hardly the only epidemic to cluster among the lower classes, and with yellow fever in the Deep South, the clustering was greater. Yet yellow fever never produced anything approaching cholera's levels or frequency of social violence, or anything akin to its patterns of class suspicion, prejudice, or blame. Moreover, diseases such as plague, smallpox, yellow fever, and even influenza could rapidly and horrifically transform bodies, with black bile streaming from orifices with yellow fever; bodies rotting before death with 'black smallpox'; bursting buboes with plague; and lungs reduced to spongy mush and oxygen depletion (cyanosis) turning bodies blue with the Great Influenza's pneumonic complications.

Cholera remains enigmatic, especially in its first European *grande tour*. Its provocation of hate covered territories vaster than the Black Death's for Europe alone. Whereas the pogroms of 1347–51 were concentrated in German-speaking lands, spilling over to parts of France, Spain, and the Low Countries,[1] cholera riots of the 1830s spared few countries in Europe. Across diverse political regimes and cultures, from autocratic Czarist Russia to sophisticated Paris and liberal-democratic Edinburgh, the responses were similar. As seen repeatedly in their writings, physicians and journalists may have laid their prejudices bare, blaming the poor and 'ignorant' for spreading the disease. But the poor and marginal—the Irish in Liverpool and Glasgow; tribal Sarts in Tashkent; fig-growers in Puglia; peasants in Hungary—resorted to violence, accusing government officials and medical professionals of poisoning the poor with hospitals as chambers of mass execution.

As seen with the British Isles, different places produced different twists on these core plots. For instance, in one of the most murderous of the cholera riots in Madrid in 1834, the supposed culprits were not doctors or municipal rulers. Rumours, instead, spread of monks and friars poisoning wells and fountains. At the Convent of San Isidro, twenty, by some accounts, fifty by others, were massacred

---

[1] See Cohn, 'The Black Death'.

in their cells. 'Scarcely any religious house escaped a visit from the mob'.[2] An article in the *Madrid Gazette* (translated in the *Observer*) added further stories: a boy of ten was supposedly discovered with a small vessel in his hand at the fountain of Avapies; two cigar manufacturers were found with small cakes of *nux comica* and suspected as poisoners; and a young man was accused of poisoning the fountains at the Puerta del Sol. He died en route to the police station, beaten to a pulp by the quarter's residents. In another part of the town, another body of people scaled the walls of the College of Jesuits and killed six in their cells and another four behind a bolted gate. Later that night, others attacked the Convents of the Franciscans and La Merced, killing an unspecified number of friars, while others attacked the Convents of San Cayetano, the Trinity, the Carmen, and Los Basilios, but here 'mediators' quelled the crowds. Similar attacks against religious orders occurred at Zaragoza, Murcia, Reus, and Barcelona in 1834 and the following year.[3] Another difference regards the levels of violence and the severity of repression. In Italy, Spain, Eastern Europe, and Russia, the riots often led to the death of the targeted, followed by greater casualties for the rioters from armed retaliation or execution. By contrast, in the British Isles, despite at least seventy-two riots, and crowds climbing to 2000 or more, fewer than a handful of deaths have come to light, either from rioters' assaults or state repression.

In addition to the rarity of comparative analysis from one national context to the next, scholars have paid scant attention to how cholera protests may have changed from the 1830s to the present. Such differences pose new questions. As we have seen, the second European wave during the revolutionary years 1848–9 produced almost everywhere in Europe cholera's highest mortalities; yet neither the increase in diffusion nor cholera's virulence renewed its social violence.[4] Cholera, however, had not lost its power to inspire hate and violence. In Russia, Poland, Hungary, Spain, Portugal, Germany, Italy, the Middle East, and China, this second wave proved at best a momentary pause. To examine these changes over time, I concentrate on Italy with comparative forays into countries from Venezuela to Muslim North Africa.

ITALY, 1867

After the momentary pause in cholera riots in the late 1840s, they reappeared with a vengeance with the third wave in the late summer and autumn of 1867. Presently, however, hardly a trace of them is seen in the secondary literature. A Florentine

---

[2] *Observer*, 3 August 1834, 4.

[3] Rodríguez Ocaña, *El cólera*, 123 and 125. In Granada, however, 'open hostility towards the Church was not evident' (123).

[4] In 1848–9, cholera mortalities in the British Isles more than doubled those in 1831–3 (Morris, *Cholera 1832*, 11; for increases in France, see Kudlick, *Cholera in Post-Revolutionary Paris*, 213–19. Despite underestimates for both waves in Russia, reported cases soared almost fourfold from 466,457, 1830 to 1832, to 1,742,439, 1848–9, and cholera deaths by the same ratio, 197,069 to 690,150; Clemow, *The Cholera Epidemic*, 31; and Patterson, 'Cholera Diffusion in Russia', 1176 and 1179.

correspondent reported a number of them in Calabria in August; these followed cholera's earlier conspiracies. In the village of Porcilla, 'the populace, maddened as usual by the notion that poison had been disseminated amongst them', broke into the houses of a family, accusing them of being the authors of the evil, and butchered five of them. Forty were arrested.[5] According to an Australian paper, it was 'the worst instance of savage ignorance', and blame lay with the Church and State of Italy's 'defunct regime'.[6]

Perhaps reflecting the large numbers of Italian emigrants in Australia, the Australian papers paid great attention to this fourth cholera wave in Italy. They argued that these 'tumults and horrible atrocities' centred on Sicily, explained by its 'superstitious terror' and famine. But the papers failed to mention concrete cases,[7] and for Sicily none appears from my survey of foreign papers and only one from the Italian press. Instead of resisting quarantine or pretending the disease did not exist, Messina's populace protested because they saw their municipal government not doing enough. On 1 July 1865, the docking of a steamer bringing mail from plague-ridden Alexandria prodded them to engage in direct action, vowing not to allow any ship from countries in Europe or Africa to land.[8] Old cholera myths, however, re-emerged: the populace set fire to hospitals and quarantine buildings. The National Guard had to be called in to restore order,[9] and the civil militia patrolled the city 'for some time' thereafter.[10] Certainly, rigorous enforcement of quarantine and other sanitary restrictions were not always the key elements sparking cholera riots or other social violence connected with epidemics, as has been hypothesized.[11] In this case and others to follow, the reason for popular outrage was the opposite—governments' reluctance to impose quarantine.

On the other hand, the Italian papers give further hints of cholera protest in Sicily that did not lead to rioting. The first came early during the epidemic at Aderni (Adrano) in the Province of Catania: the population 'at first' was convinced that government troops had purposefully planted cholera, but quickly their complaints changed, requesting their government to do more for them. Instead of resorting to collective violence, they posted their demands in the town's café.[12] Another threat came from Palermo when the disease's 'dangers had almost completely passed'. The rabble ('popolaccio') 'became rowdy (*comincia a far baldoria*), giving everybody the usual trouble (*a darsi a tutti gli strazzi*)', but rioting did not ensue.[13]

Certainly, cholera had not spared Sicily in 1867; instead, newspapers portrayed it as more severely stricken than any region in Italy. Before cholera had risen to

[5] *Scotsman*, 29 August 1867, 4, from *Daily News*; *Fife Herald*, 12 September 1867, 2.
[6] *Fife Herald*, 12 September 1867, 2. *Il Giornale di Roma*, 21 August 1867, front page; and *La Riforma* (Florence), 13 September 1867, 4.
[7] *Argus*, 15 November 1867, Supplement, front page.
[8] *Public Ledger*, 18 July 1865, 2.
[9] Ibid., and *Scotsman*, 3 July 1865, 3. *Corriere di Roma*, 5 July 1867, front page, reported that the Maritime Health office was also burnt, and firemen extinguishing the fire were driven away.
[10] *Corriere di Roma*, 5 July 1867, front page.
[11] Evans, 'Epidemics and Revolutions', 167–9.
[12] *La Riforma* (Florence), 14 August 1867, 2.
[13] *La Nazione* (Florence), 14 September 1867, 2: from Palermo.

epidemic levels on the mainland, parts of Sicily had been decimated. Palermo was described as 'an immense hospital of the sick and dying, a camp of the dead'.[14] By the end of September, its death counts were in decline; yet families had fled to the countryside and were too frightened to return. The *Giornale di Napoli* asserted that commerce was 'totally ruined'; 'misery cast a lugubrious veil over the entire island' with 'new and terrible difficulties looming'.[15] Messina had been reduced 'to a state of desperation; panic was everywhere and the local government feared unrest'.[16] In Catania, the general panic was so great that it had become impossible to draw up a will: all thirty of its notaries had fled.[17]

In turn, these conditions led Sicily's municipal governments to pass stringent anti-cholera controls, more so than on the mainland and of the sort that would produce violent reactions with future cholera waves. Already by mid-August, Messina had established 'a rigorous *cordone sanitario*' that prohibited goods or persons entering from any infected country.[18] In the second week of September, even with cholera in steep decline, Palermo issued a decree 'strictly prohibiting' the return of those who had left the city during the epidemic until everything could be carefully disinfected.[19] Yet concrete cases of cholera disturbances during this fourth cholera wave centred on other regions.

In Percile (or Peroile), near Naples, a gruesome story resembles the cruelty inflicted on smallpox victims in nineteenth-century America. Here, it was not cholera's usual story of rioters seeing themselves as the victims' liberators. Hearing that a family was quarantined because they were suspected of carrying cholera, a 'mob' broke into the house at midnight and hacked them to death, except for a little girl, discovered ten hours later 'covered in wounds and half dying' amidst 'the dead bodies strewed about the floor'.[20] The press reported 'not a single neighbour' sounded an alarm or offered aid.[21] Further incidents flared in Calabria, stretching from its south-easternmost tip at Reggio to Avellino near Naples. The papers point to stories of poisoning wells that returned to early modern notions of *untori*. Most of these galvanized small crowds, but what they lacked in numbers, they possessed in savagery. Most important of these, reported widely in foreign and Italian papers, was a disturbance in early September in the market town of Ardore, 45 km east of Reggio. With the first case of cholera, the 'populace' (its crowd size not estimated) assembled outside the town's pharmacy, which they threatened to burn to the ground. On hearing of the riot, Signor Garzoni, commander of a nearby military company, came to calm the protesters. 'Having lost all respect for the authorities', the populace answered Garzoni's pleas for peace by trampling him to death. They then set the pharmacy ablaze, after 'butchering ruthlessly' the whole family within. Their 'thirst for blood not yet appeased', they killed another twenty of Garzoni's officials,[22] and fed Garzoni's body to their pigs.

[14] *Giornale di Roma*, 20 August 1867, front page.
[15] *La Nazione*, 28 September 1867, 2.   [16] *Giornale di Roma*, 31 August 1867, front page.
[17] *Giornale di Roma*, 21 August 1867, front page, from *L'Amico del Popolo* (Palermo).
[18] *La Riforma* (Florence), 21 August 1867, 3.
[19] *La Nazione*, 14 September 1867, 2.   [20] *Empire*, 22 November 1867, 6.
[21] *Fife Herald*, 12 September 1867, 2.   [22] *La Nazione*, 13 September 1867, 2.

Another trophy of the rioters' rage was Lo Schiavo, captain of Ardore's National Guard and a native of the town. The Italian papers indulged in the gory details. Before Garzoni was fed to the pigs, he and Lo Schiavo were stripped and roasted alive in flames.[23] The 'plebegia' 'drunken by the taste of blood' murdered 'many' of Lo Schiavo's relatives, burning them alive with another fourteen 'obscenely mutilated', killed by being dragged down city streets.[24] One of the first thrown in the flames was the local pharmacist also named Lo Schiavo.[25] In addition, the barracks of the *carabinieri* and the National Guard were torched.[26] The crowd searched not only for Captain Lo Schiavo's relatives but any 'liberals' in town, inflicting 'infinite and cruel suffering', sacking and setting on fire 'an immense number of their houses'. Local sources put the number of victims at forty-nine[27]—more deaths inflicted by rioters than in any single cholera disturbance in Sicily in 1837. *La Nazione* highlighted the violence with individual stories: four women were dragged almost to death, then tortured by burning off their feet and arms, then made to suffer 'unheard agonies, disfiguring them obscenely'. Another concerned a woman, whose only child, a baby nursing at her breast, was shot as the mother gave it her last kiss.[28]

According to Italian papers, the massacres stemmed from an incident a week earlier when an Ardorese butcher went to nearby San Nicola to buy oxen. Its *popolo* suspected him of poisoning and brought him to the municipal authorities. 'In an instant', the crowd dragged him through the streets and massacred him with axes.[29] Unlike the foreign press, the Italian papers emphasized the longer-term causes, lodged in national politics of the new nation, where southern remnants of the Bourbon regime and clerical reaction remained strong. According to Florence's *La Nazione*, the revolts were the fruits of the 'scheming clergy and Bourbons', who believed they could profit from the epidemic's 'sad circumstances to plant hate against the government'. At Ardore, the paper alleged priests had been working diligently with the people, 'where they found easy ground to sow superstition'.[30] The targets of the revolt—the National Guard, liberals, and residents from other regions ('forestieri')—along with the rebels' chants, 'Morte agli avvelenatori! Morte ai complici del governo! Viva la religione! Viva Francesco! [the king of Spain]' (Death to the poisoners! Death to the government's accomplices! Long live the Church! Long live Francesco!) lent credence to the paper's view.[31] Despite its anticlerical bent, the paper, nonetheless, praised the one hero of this sorry saga—a priest. The day after the revolt, a 'bravo sacerdote' ran through the district, assisting

---

[23] Ibid., 14 September 1867, 4.   [24] Ibid., 24 September 1867, 3.

[25] Ibid., 13 September 1867, 2.

[26] Ibid., 10 September 1867, 2; 14 September 1867, 4; 24 September 1867, 3.

[27] Ibid., 14 September 1867, 4.   [28] Ibid., 25 September 1867, 3.

[29] Ibid., 24 September 1867, 3.

[30] Ibid., 13 September 1867, 2 and 3. The town was infamous for its reactionary sentiments; in 1861, the Spanish general, José Borges, began his campaign here to reconquer the Kingdom of Two Sicilies (ibid., 14 September 1867, 4).

[31] Ibid., 14 September 1867, 4. Also, see the brief coverage in *La Riforma* (Rome), 13 September 1867, 4; and *Giornale di Roma*, 7 September 1867, front page; 9 September 1867, front page; 14 September 1867, front page; 21 September 1867, front page. At the BNCR and the BNCF—the two largest depositories for historical newspapers in Italy, no southern papers survive for 1867. A principal source for *La Nazione* was *L'Italia di Napoli* (see for instance *La Nazione*, 24 September 1867, 3).

wounded soldiers and arming *carabinieri*.[32] Because of the savagery, the state sent an extraordinary number of troops to the town—2000 from the National Guard—a number not witnessed for any other cholera outbreak.[33] Many fled, estimated as high as 3000 from this small town of '5000, subtracting the old, women, and children'.[34] The guardsmen scoured the mountains in pursuit of the rioters but did not report numbers arrested or killed.[35] Nonetheless, if accurate, this repressive force exceeded any ever sent by the czars to quell their cholera riots with crowds as large as 10,000.[36]

This Calabrese town was not the only place where conflict between the new state and old guard, especially the priesthood, fuelled cholera unrest. Less than a week later, the 'plebe' of the Amalfi region, armed with sticks and poles and 'infused with the fantasy that cholera was the product of intentional poisoning', attacked four or five young men in Positano, marked as poisoners. The 'good people' of the town, intimidated, stayed locked in their homes. The four ended 'covered in wounds', but were rescued by a small band of *carabinieri*.[37] A priest led 'the gang (*masnada*)' with shouts of 'Down with the heinous Government poisoning the people!' Scuffles ensued for three hours before troops from Salerno arrested thirty.[38]

Again spurred by rumours of supposed poisoners ('pretesi avvelenatori') further violence arose on 5 September. Armed residents of Tolvi (Tolve di Basilicata) entered the town's piazza, claiming poisoners were about town ('paese').[39] They surrounded the house of Antonio Sabellino, chanting that he was a cholera spreader. A party broke into the house in search of poison. A woman, 'one of the foremost among the savage crew', found a jar of a paste Sabellino kept to kill rats. A dog, forced to swallow it, died 'of course'. No sooner had the dog dropped dead than the 'plebe' went wild, mercilessly massacring 'the three unfortunate ones'. The rebels marched through town, chanting 'in eight days we will be rulers here'. The *carabinieri* stationed at Tolve were helpless and called Potenza for troops.[40]

The Italian press (north and south), emphasized the political background and causes of this cholera cruelty. According to *La Nazione*, based on reports from *Giornale di Napoli*, 'with the first cases' of cholera at Tolve, the Bourbon–clerical alliance began arousing the 'plebes', asserting there was no cholera, claiming instead that 'government agents used poison to murder the population'. At first, the people took no heed of the jabber ('ciarle'), but as the disease spread, large numbers lost trust, began refusing prescriptions, and blocked the municipality's attempts to disinfect houses. This led to the murder of Sabellino, a guardsman of

---

[32] *La Nazione*, 24 September 1867, 3.   [33] Ibid., 13 September 1867, 2.

[34] Ibid., 10 September 1867, 2; others estimated the population at just over 4000; ibid., 14 September 1867, 4.

[35] *The Sydney Morning Herald*, 18 November 1867, 2; *The Goulburn Herald*, 23 November 1867, 2; *Freeman's Journal*, 23 November 1867, 11; *Empire*, 26 November 1867, 2; *Kiama Independent*, 5 December 1867, 4; and others.

[36] *La Nazione*, 14 September 1867, 4. Only one or two cases had appeared when this revolt erupted.

[37] Ibid., 14 September 1867, 4.   [38] Ibid., 17 September 1867, 3, from *Giornale di Napoli*.

[39] *La Nazione*, 12 September 1867, 2, from Naples.

[40] *La Nazione*, 12 September 1867, 2; 13 September 1867, 4; and 14 September 1867, 4; and *Giornale di Roma*, 11 September 1867, front page; 14 September 1867, 4; 16 September 1867, front page.

the government,[41] and the two others in his house.[42] However, this political divide between the new liberal state and the old regime was anything but straightforward. Three weeks after the revolt, the Prefect of Basilicata dismissed Tolve's mayor. Not only had he failed to calm the crowd or call the National Guard, the National Guard had made common cause with the rebels![43] Three weeks later, people of Tolve's district resisted the *carabinieri* and the state.[44]

Further incidents in September 1867 suggest that recent scientific findings on cholera transmission by waterborne bacteria had filtered down to the populace but had become fused with the old myths of poisoning. In Lioni, in the province of Avellino, 'the people' assembled, 'riotously' shouting that public wells had been poisoned, and demanded a scientific analysis of the water.[45] They suspected the work of *untori* and pursued them. The government had to send troops to protect the innocent.[46] The 'popolo' continued patrolling their streets in search of *untori*, taking the law into their own hands 'with scuffles' and 'tumulti' erupting between the peasant patrols and the accused.[47] Similar hunts through Avellino were reported but only one by name.[48] At the estate ('tenimento') of Monticchio, peasants suspected three 'mysterious men'. Armed with clubs and scythes, they caught and handed them over to the authorities: two were French; the third, Algerian. It was an unusual case when foreigners were the suspects.[49]

Several hundred kilometres further south, parishioners of Corigliano (province of Cosenza) also adopted modern notions of disease to illuminate old fears, 'firmly believing poisoners went door to door blowing *germs* through keyholes'. According to the correspondents, the idea became so deeply rooted that many from the lower classes abandoned their homes and camped outdoors to avoid the poisonous fumes. Those who stayed constantly fired their muskets from their windows 'to paralyse' the poison's action.[50] Sharp-shooters and *carabinieri* were sent in, but it took time 'to calm the tumult and arrest the leaders'.[51]

An action in Rossano (Bocchigliero) appears more menacing, but as with the events in Corigliano, physical violence may have been averted. It illustrates the populace's deep distrust of the state and that peasants could have their own political agenda. Armed, a hundred of them paraded through the streets, demanding that the chief of the police and *carabinieri* 'leave the place at once' and that the peasants

---

[41] *La Nazione*, 17 September 1867, 3, from *Giornale di Napoli*.

[42] *Giornale di Roma*, 16 September 1867, front page.

[43] *La Riforma* (Rome), 21 September 1867, 4.

[44] *Giornale di Roma*, 21 September 1867, front page and 26 September 1867, front page. Riots also erupted at Cogliano; see *Chicago Daily Tribune*, 5 October 1867, 2.

[45] See the Australian papers cited in note 35; plus *La Nazione*, 12 September 1867, 2; and *La Riforma* (Florence), 16 September 1867, 4.

[46] *La Riforma* (Florence), 13 September 1867, 4.

[47] *Giornale di Roma*, 11 September 1867, front page; and *La Riforma* (Florence), 16 September 1867, 4.

[48] Another incident occurred at Paduli (Avellino), where peasants killed a public functionary; *Giornale di Roma*, 5 September 1867, front page.

[49] *La Riforma* (Florence), 16 September 1867, 4. Also, see note 58, with those from other Italian regions, called foreigners.

[50] See Australian papers, note 35; and *Giornale di Roma*, 5 September 1867, front page.

[51] *Giornale di Roma*, 5 September 1867, front page.

be allowed to elect a mayor, 'a peasant like ourselves'. But this was not simply a political protest; rather, the old cholera conspiracy of authorities seeking to murder the poor was the spark. When the National Guard's captain tried to persuade them to disband, the peasants responded: 'We are tired of seeing the poison brought into our houses', and threatened that if the captain did not do their bidding, 'his house would be first on their list'.[52] Further, two brothers in Rossano wounded a man they accused of poisoning their mother with cholera; others murdered the municipal assessor, whom they claimed had 600 *untori* in his pay.[53]

Further cholera disturbances sparked by accusations of poisoning spread through Calabria at Apricena, Civita, Longbucco, Tirolo, Minervino, Cutro, Savelli, and Frascineto.[54] Others surfaced in San Paolo Albanese and Albano, near Genzano, in Basilicata,[55] Pescarenico, near Lecce, and Nardi, a comune of Gallipoli (Puglia).[56] But unlike the detailed articles that filled papers for Ardore and Tolve, single-line notices described them as tumults against cholera measures. Others remain geographically unspecified, as with an entry of 28 August: 'riots continue in Calabria propelled by the intemperance of the plebes and the ferocity of their false beliefs about cholera'.[57] In villages along Calabria's southern shores, where 'large numbers of "foreigners" from northern provinces' worked, locals regarded them ('con occhio torvo') as poisoners. Municipal governments also clearly believed in the myths, ordering armed guards to be placed continuously around wells, inspected every thirty minutes to see if the eels and fish they placed there were alive.[58]

When papers specified the actions or motives of these rioters, they appear as attacks on supposed *untori*[59] or against health workers transporting patients to cholera hospitals.[60] Yet several of them resulted in more deaths than any cholera riot in the British Isles. In Frascineto in the provence of Cosenza, for instance, five members of the same family, suspected as poisoners, were butchered.[61] Not all these brief mentions pertained to small, even obscure villages, difficult to find on modern maps. Some occurred in neighbourhoods of Naples but were only vaguely indicated in the Italian papers.[62]

As in 1865, cholera violence arose not only from fears of doctors and others poisoning the poor; it also turned against the state because it refused to act. With news of cholera in Messina and Naples, residents of the seaside town, Pizzo, near Calabria's southernmost tip, prevented ships from landing. They chanted but refrained from acts of violence until a steamship ('piroscafo') arrived from Naples. When the

---

[52] Ibid.   [53] *Mercury*, 21 September 1867, 3.
[54] *Giornale di Roma*, 19 August 1867, front page; 21 August 1867, front page; 24 August 1867, front page; 27 August 1867, front page; 2 September 1867, front page; and *La Riforma* (Florence), 28 August 1867, 3.
[55] *Giornale di Roma*, 21 August 1867, front page; 5 September 1867, front page.
[56] *La Riforma* (Florence), 28 August 1867, 3; and *La Perseveranza* (Naples), 3 August 1867, 3.
[57] *La Riforma* (Florence), 28 August 1867, 3.   [58] Ibid., 20 September 1867, 4.
[59] Ibid., 28 August 1867, 3; 20 September 1867, 4.
[60] *Corriere di Roma*, 28 August 1867, 3.   [61] *La Riforma* (Florence), 28 August 1867, 3.
[62] See, for instance, ibid., 29 August 1867, 3: Naples' 'brutal' *plebaglie* 'repeatedly' attempted to prevent the municipality aiding the cholera-stricken.

passengers disembarked, the 'popolo' threw stones at them,[63] including at a military general, and marched them to an uninhabitable hut, where they locked them up, causing 'a poor pregnant woman' to abort her child. According to later sentencing, captains of the National Guard had coordinated the *plebaglia*'s actions.[64]

Furthermore, beliefs in *untori* were not exclusive to the South. A Florentine correspondent reporting 'a deplorable' riot in Crescenzano, near Milan, admitted that 'even' in northern Italy, 'evil' cholera myths could be found. With the substitution of a few words such as 'plague' for 'cholera' and 'barbiere' for 'chemist', his description might be mistaken for Manzoni's plague of 1630. Only now, the authorities neither fostered nor accepted the populace's myths.[65] Such beliefs also surfaced in cosmopolitan cities of Italy's rich city-state past. On 2 September the Patriarch of Venice ('cardinale patriarca') felt compelled to order his parish priests to preach against 'absurd rumours' and 'dangerous prejudices' of the 'weak and ignorant', that doctors were diagnosing cases as cholera when there was none, to gain profit or 'still worse, to spread the disease'.[66] A week later, Venice reported 'the most base superstition'. In its hospitals, 'those stricken with cholera strenuously refuse to take medicines prescribed by their doctors from fear of being poisoned!!! [sic]'.[67] In response, the Venetian municipality published a magazine entitled 'L'educazione popolare', distributed free of charge to combat the 'ignorance and superstitions of the people on their notions about cholera'. *La Riforma* lamented: 'Still today, in the midst of the nineteenth century, the press must record such enormously absurd deeds.'[68] In mid-September, when cholera invaded Genoa's quarter of the Comune della Foce,[69] rumours accused those entering the quarter of purposefully spreading cholera. Florence's *La Riforma* charged that three members of the government ('consiglieri comunali') supported the claims.[70] An editorial made clear that the beliefs were not limited to this quarter: regularly, *carabinieri* had to be called to protect health workers. As in Venice, to combat the 'pregiudizi popolari', the municipality distributed free copies of 'a little book', *Errori volgari intorno al colera*, written 'in simple and popular language'.[71]

Beliefs more ancient than early modern ones of *untori* could spark cholera disruption, arrests, and collective action in northern Italy. In Camin, on Padua's outskirts, the priest announced that because of the epidemic, the annual procession of the Madonna of the girdle would not be held. A group of 'madmen', however, assailed the church and forced the pastor to take the relics and hold the procession as usual. *Carabinieri* and national guardsmen stopped 'the wicked ones' by arresting two priests and a chaplain, despite pleas that 'fanatics' forced them to break the law.[72]

---

[63] Ibid., 30 August 1867, 3.

[64] Ibid., 31 August 1867, 3; *Giornale di Roma*, 27 September 1867, front page; and *Corriere di Roma*, 28 August 1867, 3. *Fife Herald*, 12 September 1867, 2. Pizzo's 'popolo' besieged the train station, preventing passengers from leaving.

[65] *Scotsman*, 29 August 1867, 4.   [66] Cited in *La Nazione*, 5 September 1867, 2.

[67] *La Riforma* (Florence), 10 September 1867, 4.   [68] Ibid., 18 September 1867, 4.

[69] Comune della Folce was autonomous from Genoa until 1873.

[70] *La Riforma* (Florence), 15 September 1867, 4.   [71] Ibid., 6 September 1867, 4.

[72] *La Perseveranza* (Naples), 6 September 1867, 3.

Such acts of small-scale cruelty aimed at suspected *untori* and health workers were not the only ones then stirring up cholera outbreaks. As we have seen, the new state could enter the fray with the National Guard on either side of the barricades. Glimpsed only dimly earlier, cholera could also unite the lower classes with journalists and the bourgeoisie. Journalists now raised new political questions that attacked the new state because of cholera ravages under their watch. Their reports reveal a groundswell of resentment from Neapolitan labourers informed by new knowledge of cholera's dissemination. Bad water and the state's neglect of urban hydraulic infrastructures were already perceived as the chief causes of cholera. In late November, a Tasmanian paper translated a Neapolitan editorial published three months earlier that linked Naples' foul conditions to its cholera disaster:

> There is not a street or lane from which putrid exhalations are not omitted from many openings, poisoning the air and rendering it almost compulsory to cleanse the mouth even at the expense of imitating the dirty customs of the Italians.

The anonymous Neapolitan journalist did not then proceed to blame the poor for their 'dirty' habits, as earlier had been the press's call. Instead, he sided with them, placing the blame squarely on government. First, a legacy of neglect from the previous 'bad government' of the Bourbons was to blame. The journalist, however, was not scoring political points by turning against a rival regime; his more trenchant criticisms targeted the present 'liberal institutions' of post-Garibaldi Italy. As far as the infrastructure of urban health was concerned, nothing had changed. For the past seven years, Neapolitans had demanded basic sanitary improvements but were met with 'criminal neglect'. As a result, residents 'are still without the most necessary element of existence—water'. He accused the authorities of poisoning the people. His notion of 'poisoning' pointed not to *untori* but to neglect and improper sewage systems that 'choked the city'. He held that these 'unsparing reproaches' against the authorities no longer derived from 'civilized foreigners' but from 'the inhabitants themselves'.[73] Yet conspiracy theories reminiscent of Sicily in 1837 remained in places, according to the press, due to the 'sanguinary excesses' of the peasantry and the work of Bourbon and clerical instigators.[74]

THE FIFTH CHOLERA WAVE: 1884

Cholera beliefs and protest in Italy fail to plot a straightforward history of progress and civilization. With the next wave of the disease, the old patterns and myths persisted, provoking small acts of cruelty along with larger movements. However, the cause now giving rise to the greatest number of protests concerned municipal governments' refusal to initiate strict quarantine. The reasons for the change had to do with government recognition of the scientific discovery that cholera's agent *vibrio cholera* was spread by excrement, water, poor plumbing, and squalid sanitation.

---

[73] *The Mercury*, 21 September 1867, 3.
[74] *Sydney Morning Herald*, 18 November 1867, 2.

Newspapers, mainly in the north—*La Libertà*, *La Capitale*, la *Gazzetta del Popolo*, *Corriere della Sera*—began speaking out against quarantine and *cordon sanitaire*, arguing that these inconveniences to passengers and commerce did not affect cholera's spread.[75] But citizens across much of Italy, especially in southern ports, remained sceptical, prompting changes in protest. Now, it was not governmental controls but their absence that brought citizens into the streets.

The arrival of steamships from infected countries sparked demonstrations, as seen with Messina's resistance to such ships docking in 1865 and 1867. What was new was the frequency and procedures of these protests: rarely did they torch hospitals or town halls. Instead, they were often peaceful, even democratic, as seen with one of the first cholera protests of 1884. On 20 August, a steamship from infected Gaeta landed its fifty passengers at Messina. Immediately, the *popolo* elected 'a commission' to express the citizens' wishes. Assembling at the prefect's office, they demanded the ship's departure. Given the 'votes of the Messinesi', the government prevented further dealings with the ship; the citizens returned home peacefully.[76] The following day, another vessel approach from a suspected region, triggering 'dimostranti' to assemble again beneath the Prefect's window, and again he met their demands.[77] Such demonstrations were not always successful. In Castellammare (29 km south of Naples) and Pozzuoli (13 km west of Naples), 'demonstrators' pleaded for quarantine measures to prevent passengers from Naples entering their towns. The municipal officers refused.[78] At Pozzuoli, the populace then turned to interrupting trains.[79] As we shall see, at Castellammare, conflict became more violent.

Demands for quarantine were not the only reasons citizens demonstrated. By the third week of September, the disastrous situation in Naples, which surpassed threefold the casualties of 1837,[80] had finally begun to improve, and many wished to return. Quickly, 'a peaceful demonstration' was organized to present criteria concerning who should be readmitted.[81] Before the disease had taken epidemic proportions in Sicily, a mass demonstration marched through streets of Messina and assembled at the Office of the Prefect, demanding measures be taken not only in Messina but throughout Sicily, to prevent cholera 'invading' the island.[82] Not all of these cholera protests were comprised of the better-off citizens or were non-violent. A year later, after cases of cholera had declined, concerns over quarantine continued to excite crowds 'throughout all Sicily's principal cities'. They prevented trains departing from cholera-afflicted districts from entering their towns. In 'several places', 'mobs threatened' and troops were dispatched.[83]

---

[75] *Il Messaggero*, 6 August 1884, front page; and *Giornale di Sicilia*, 9 August 1884, 3.
[76] *Giornale di Sicilia*, 21 August 1884, 2.   [77] Ibid., 22 August 1884, 2.
[78] Ibid., 5 September 1884, 2.   [79] *Scotsman*, 5 September 1884, 6.
[80] *Giornale di Sicilia*, 29 September 1884, 3.
[81] *La Riforma* (Florence), 27 September 1884, front page.
[82] *Giornale di Sicilia*, 20 August 1884, 2. They had followed Palermo's lead, after its 'distinguished citizens' met to discuss best policies for cholera prevention.
[83] *Scotsman*, 22 September 1885, 6.

However, the more menacing protests came principally from the mainland, not Sicily. As early as July, mobs in Naples protested against authorities' laxity in handling the cholera outbreak, chanting 'We will not have the cholera here'.[84] Towards the end of August, the demonstrations increased throughout the southern mainland. A mob in Calabria established their own quarantine regulations and threatened passengers arriving from cholera-afflicted Naples. A Neapolitan correspondent aboard a train that stopped at the station of 'Sile' (probably Sila in Calabria, east of Cosenza) was 'surrounded by a howling mob, armed with spades and pitchforks'.[85] At the same time, a demonstration staged in front of the offices of the Prefect of Cosenza demanded that trains be stopped from infected Buffaloria. The Prefect refused; the crowd fired on the train.[86] Throughout Calabria, 'violent scenes' against trains from Naples ensued until troops were sent.[87] In Catanzaro and Reggio Calabria, 'sparked by superstitions and fear of cholera', armed 'popolo' interrupted postal services by blocking trains.[88] In Morra, Starle, Stile,[89] and Riccella,[90] armed inhabitants shoved passengers back into their trains, forcing them to return to Naples. Certain train routes in Calabria temporarily ceased because of peasants firing into them and destroying tracks.[91]

At the end of August, the National Ministry declared similar acts would not be repeated.[92] But they were. After days of 'arduous travel', a hundred Italian immigrants returned to their homes in Cosenza from America. 'Dreaming of relatives' embraces and rest from their great fatigue', they instead met 'a furious crowd' who greeted them at the station with bats, stones, and muskets, screaming: 'We do not want you *colerosi*! Go back to Naples! You bring us the plague!' Without money or friends, the Cosentini were forced to return.[93] Were these victims the 'outsider', germs poised to invade a pristine country, or does an analogy with autoimmune diseases fit better— the body repulsing its own?[94] Not all these stories of lawless quarantine, however, were as inhumane as Cosenza's. On 6 September, when Messinesi lined their wharfs to prevent *l'Assiria*'s passengers entering the city, a northern newspaper praised them for providing the passengers with all their needs, allowing them to wash and disinfect their clothing and luggage: 'The Messinesi exhibited true and providential charity, attesting to their ancient spirit of kindliness'.[95]

Unlawful acts of community-imposed quarantine were not unique to Calabria or the South. A 'mob' in Marino, near Rome, insulted a priest arriving from Naples and hounded him out of town.[96] Further north in Orvieto in southern Tuscany,

[84] *The Times*, 29 July 1884, 4, from Naples.
[85] *New York Herald*, 1 September 1884, 5, from Naples.
[86] *La Nazione*, 1 September 1884, 2; and *La Riforma* (Florence), 1 September 1884, 2. See a similar incident at Reggio Calabria, *La Nazione*, 2 September 1884, 2; and *La Riforma* (Florence), 1 September 1884, 2.
[87] *Giornale di Sicilia*, 1 September 1884, 3.   [88] *La Nazione*, 1 September 1884, 2.
[89] Ibid., 1 September 1884, 2.   [90] *Giornale di Sicilia*, 31 August 1884, 3.
[91] *New York Times*, 7 September 1884.   [92] *Giornale di Sicilia*, 31 August 1884, 3.
[93] *La Nazione*, 2 September 1884, 2.
[94] For examples of violent and illegal quarantines in villages around Campobasso, see *New York Times*, 7 September 1884, from London.
[95] *La Nazione*, 9 September 1884, 2.   [96] *New York Times*, 7 September 1884.

townsmen refused admittance to travellers from Naples. Meanwhile in Turin, the Hygienic Society demanded the abolition of fumigation and internal quarantine regulations, calling them useless. But when municipal governments acknowledged cholera's latest findings and prohibited quarantine, as in the resort town of Santa Marinella north-west of Rome, or in Civitavecchia, 10 km to the north, local populations revolted. At Civitavecchia, they assembled, marched to the train station, and destroyed the rails, blocking all communication with Rome to prevent cholera-exposed emigrants from entering. The quarantine ended only after the 37th Regiment arrived and arrested the ringleaders.[97] During this fifth cholera wave, anger concerning quarantine could, however, rage in both directions within the same town. In Civitavecchia a week before the revolt to impose quarantine, a false report circulated that the city was poised to adopt the very same. 'Tourists and visitors of all classes' rioted against the violations to their freedom. Again, railways were targeted. A crowd of 1800 'besieged the stations and took a freight train by storm'.[98]

While questions of quarantine may have become a dominant theme of cholera unrest in 1884, the old mythologies fuelling cholera violence since 1837 continued. At the end of August about 300 of the 'popolo' 'invaded' the house of a Signore Barrese, believing him to be hiding a Doctor Ferro, whom commoners ('il volgo') accused of cholera spreading. Not finding him, they beat Barrese to a pulp with bats and dragged him by the feet through the streets, leaving his life in the balance. Moreover, the article referred vaguely to other 'grave injuries and rebellions', flaring at other places in the province.[99] In Resina (presently Ercolano) in the Bay of Naples and neighbouring Portici, schools closed after mothers ('le mamme') 'discovered' that municipal doctors were poisoning their children 'through special papers'. They 'stampeded' the schools and carried their children home.[100] In Candino in Calabria, two forest rangers knocked at a farmhouse ('una masseria') and jokingly told the farmer that the mayor was spreading cholera. Quickly the news spread; within the hour, 400 peasants assembled with bats and rifles to kill the mayor.[101] On 24 September, in the village of San Ferdinando Laureana (Reggio Calabria) 'many from the countryside' went to the house of a certain Larussa to destroy 'all her supplies of cholera poison'. Failing to enter, they continued to the house of a De Simone with the same intent.[102]

As in earlier cholera waves through Europe, removal of cholera victims to hospitals continued to spark terror in Italy. From the villages of Giffoni Sei Casali in the district of Salerno, 'many armed people' assailed the local lazaretto, broke down its door, 'liberated the quarantined', threw out the beds, and sounded the bells 'calling the locals to come out squawking (*il paese schiamazzando*)'.[103] Such

---

[97] *Scotsman*, 5 September 1884, 6; *Il Messaggero*, 5 September 1884, front page; and *La Lombardia*, 5 September 1884, 5. Similarly, near La Spezia, passengers were stopped, faced with shotguns; *New York Times*, 18 September 1884, 3.

[98] *New York Times*, 27 August 1884, from Rome.   [99] Ibid., 1 September 1884, 2.

[100] Ibid., 2 September 1884, 2.   [101] Ibid., 2 September 1884, 2.

[102] Ibid., 29 September 1884, front page.

[103] *La Riforma* (Florence), 18 September 1884, 4; *Il Pungolo* (Milan), 17–18 September 1884, 3; and *Bendigo Advertiser*, 29 October 1884, Supplement, front page.

fears of poisoning and, in this case, live burials, arose not only in villages and small towns. At the outset of cholera in Naples in 1884, a man was arrested 'for inciting a rebellion' among the *popolo*, claiming the municipal government had started the epidemic through injecting poison into tomatoes.[104] Around the same time, a riot erupted in the Neapolitan alleyway of Stufa San Giorgio. A patient recovering from another disease, mistakenly thought to have died from cholera, was dumped in a funeral cart containing cholera cadavers. When it became clear that he was alive, popular anger mounted. With 'their numbers continually growing', they chanted: 'See how they come and take the living'. 'Had the funeral carriage and its custodians not run away quickly', the paper asked, 'who knows what would have followed?'[105] In August, papers condemned the 'superstitions' of the lower classes in the most 'uncivilized quarters', reporting 'battles', 'uprisings', threats, and assaults against Naples' municipal doctors, considered *untori*, and chants of 'Ecco tutti i medici nostri! Assassini! Assassini!'[106] As cholera reached its peak in September, with its poorer streets 'silent with death', interrupted only by 'joiners hammering rough coffins together', a woman selling fruit on a corner fell over. Since the poor believed fruit to be a prophylactic against cholera and ate it in greater quantities when cholera struck, they feared foul play: a crowd gathered, made a bonfire of her chair, stand, and fruit, and left her to die. All refused to carry her to the hospital.[107] According to a Neapolitan correspondent, such disturbances 'on the part of the rabble' were now constantly occurring. The *New York Times* corroborated the story: 'the utmost panic' prevailed in the poorer districts; 'a number of riots had occurred in the market place'; 'and troops have been used to suppress them'. Even Cardinal San Felice, 'who visits the hospitals and slums all day long was hooted in the streets...as a poisoner'.[108] In October, another rumour circulating among 'the lower classes' repeated mythologies of the 1830s: the people believed doctors received 20 lire ($4) for every cholera patient dying under their care. When the number reached a thousand, the doctor could retire with a life pension.[109]

For Naples, however, the major reason for sending troops against the populace during this epidemic was because the religious processions they held violated cholera sanitary ordinances (especially on San Gennaro's feast day, 19 September).[110] Crowds, mostly women, assembled outside the Church of San Gennaro, because the Virgin Mary was reputed to have descended there. To witness her appearance they tried to break down the church doors.[111] Later, 'swarms of urchins' and women with candles filled the streets, singing litanies, and the authorities vowed no further 'barbaric spectacles' would occur.[112] Such faith in the power of religion

[104] *Il Messaggero*, 4 September 1884, front page.
[105] *La Riforma* (Florence), 6 September 1884, 2.
[106] *La Lombardia*, 29 August 1884, 2; and *Il Pungolo* (Milan), 28–9 August 1884, 2.
[107] *Bendigo Advertiser*, 29 October 1884, Supplement, front page. These scenes recall Matilde Serao's descriptions in 1884 (*Il Ventre di Napoli*).
[108] *New York Times*, 7 September 1884.   [109] *San Francisco Chronicle*, 12 October 1884, 4.
[110] *Giornale di Sicilia*, 17 September 1884, 3; and 20 September 1884, 3.
[111] *New York Times*, 7 September 1884.
[112] *La Riforma* (Florence), 6 September 1884, 2. In addition, municipal authorities stopped a religious procession in Palermo's port on 27 September; *Giornale di Sicilia*, 28 September 1884, 3.

to eradicate cholera was not particular to the South. In late August 1884, in cholera-stricken Busca (Piedmont), peasants repelled doctors and put their trust 'in charms and superstitious observations'. These included religious processions, which, as in Naples, secular authorities had banned because of fears of 'contagion'.[113] In Lucca on 26 August 1884, the violence over processions may have been worse than in Naples: 'a serious tumult' erupted, after the Prefect prohibited them. The military was summoned, which resulted in rioters being wounded.[114] This new intensity of state repression of religious processions went against the latest scientific findings regarding cholera. Unlike early modern plague, cholera was not a person-to-person disease likely to be spread by walking in procession. Clearly, with the evolution of cholera protest and violence into the nineteenth century, irrationality was not the sole preserve of the impoverished.

As with the fourth cholera wave, the disease's social violence focused predominantly not on Sicily, but on the mainland South with epicentres in Naples and Calabria. But as in 1867, the north was not immune from these 'pregiudizi'. In fact, in 1884, the earliest incidents of cholera's social violence occurred in the far north and were well-engrained in the old mythologies. In Borgo San Dalmazzo (Cuneo), the rabble ('la plebaglia') rose up against doctors and pharmacists, accusing them of poisoning a girl under the guise of cholera.[115] With early cases of cholera in Livignano (Garfagnana), rumours circulated that people were spreading the disease by scattering material composed from cholera victims' excrement on the streets.[116] A month and a half later in Camporazione (Garfagnana), fear turned to violence with peasants stoning soldiers charged with maintaining the 'cordone sanitario'.[117] Further west in Tuscany at Pietrasanta 'grave fears' arose that health workers were incapable of performing their tasks because of rage against doctors; troops were summoned.[118] In the mountain village of Corchia in the Parmese, 'all the inhabitants' gathered to demand the speedy departure of cholera doctors, claiming they were planning to cull victims to end the epidemic.[119]

THE FIFTH WAVE: 1887

With this epidemic, social violence in Sicily returned centre stage for the first time since cholera's Italian debut. The most serious of these occurred in Santa Maria di Licodia in the province of Caltagirone.[120] This 'turba di malfattori' ('uproar of the wicked')[121] did not flare up with the first cases. Unusually, the papers offer a glimpse of a small town suffering from cholera before any social violence developed.

[113] *New York Times*, 27 August 1884; and Snowden, *Naples in the Time of Cholera*, 164.
[114] *New York Times*, 27 August 1884.   [115] *Giornale di Sicilia*, 5 August 1884, 3.
[116] *Il Messaggero*, 3 August 1884, front page.   [117] *La Lombardia*, 18 September 1884, 3.
[118] Ibid., 4 September 1884, 2.
[119] *Il Pungolo* (Milan), 17–18–19 August 1884, front page. One doctor alleged superstitious priests were behind these notions. Similar threats against doctors were heard at Giareto.
[120] Ibid., 19 August 1887, 2–3. Its population in 1887 was 7000.
[121] *Giornale di Sicilia*, 18 August 1887, 2.

Already by the beginning of August, cholera had sent the 'maggiorenti'—that is, the town's authorities, who were wealthy and, as the article makes clear, responsible for sanitary conditions—fleeing. The poor who remained were uplifted by the arrival of outside volunteers, whom they greeted with cheers: 'Viva le squadre democratiche!'[122] At this point, the papers made no remarks about the ignorance or 'pregiudizi' of the rabble. With the town's 'misfatto', however, newspapers north and south changed their tune. Rome's *Il Messaggero* now reported that as soon as cholera 'exploded' in the town, peasants formed a sentinel carrying rifles ready to fire at any 'they thought were spreading cholera'.[123] For the *Giornale di Sicilia*, it happened when health authorities began isolating those with the disease or who had had contacts with them.[124] Along with Florence's *La Nazione*,[125] papers told much the same story: 'contadini' united with 'workers' ('operai') in town and became 'organized' in a military fashion, with 'blind allegiance' to their leaders. They distributed their platoons across the city; even the 'darkest corners (*cantuccio più buio*)' were guarded to show the supposed poisoners that they were being watched. Rebels fired their rifles all night so that no one could sleep or leave their homes before dawn.[126] As *Il Giornale di Sicilia* stressed, chief among the suspects were the government and *carabinieri*. At night on 13 August, armed conflict erupted, when a patrol of *carabinieri* encountered the paramilitary peasants and workers. A *carabiniere* was killed, the other four wounded. The next day, soldiers from Caltagirone, the regional capital, made arrests and restored order.

In the following weeks, the 'misfatto' became a cause célèbre. An editorial in Turin's *Gazzetta del Popolo* compared the town with 'the most inhospitable' regions of Africa ('dei Negua e di Ris-A-lula!'), and called on the new 'patriotic' nation to 'civilize this Abissiminia!' *Il Giornale di Sicilia* responded angrily: 'Ours is not a nation of cannibals, and such evil exists everywhere, even in Tuscany. The Bourbons' bad governance, their education of ignorance produced sightings of *untori* and accounts for their treatment of doctors. Why doesn't the paper report that the intelligent classes and honest workers are here united in assuring that the thugs (*i ceffi brutti*) of Licodia and Leonforte will be punished?'[127]

In 1887, beliefs in intentional poisoning spurred further localized cholera disturbances, but these did not provoke riots with participants mounting in the hundreds. In early August in Ricocca, Sicily, rumours of governors as poisoners mobilized peasants to arm and accost a municipal guard burying a cholera victim.[128] In mid-August, furnace workers railed against several carters transporting wine from Misterbianco, outside Catania, accusing them of carrying substances to spread cholera at night. A squabble ('battibecco') ensued leaving two carters badly wounded; seven were arrested.[129] At the same time, 'a drama of superstition, sad scenes, and general panic', unfolded in Sicily's interior. In Francaville, someone

---

[122] Ibid., 5 August 1887, 2; also see *Il Messaggero*, 4 August 1887, 2.
[123] *Il Messaggero*, 19 August 1887, 2–3.   [124] *Giornale di Sicilia*, 18 July 1887, 2.
[125] *La Nazione*, 15 August 1887, 3; and 21 August 1887, 2.
[126] Mainly from *Il Messaggero*, 19 August 1887, 2–3.
[127] *Il Giornale di Sicilia*, 28 August 1887, 2.
[128] *Il Messaggero*, 3 August 1887, 2.   [129] *La Nazione*, 21 August 1887, 2.

'whose name is not even known', pretending to be an *untore*, entered houses demanding money not to spread cholera. No arrests or injuries were reported.[130] On the same day, the rabble ('popolino') of Castellammare[131] called the mayor and town's doctors poisoners, but again no injuries, arrests, or mass movements were reported.[132] Towards the end of the month, in Maletto (north-west of Catania), a gang apprehended a peasant accused of spreading the disease and buried him up to his neck. One of the gang, however, sneaked back and freed him.[133] On 7 September in Troina (province of Enna), shots rang out against two *carabinieri* but only tore their uniforms. A journalist from Catania asked: 'What was the motivation?' The answer: 'The usual, belief that *carabinieri* sprinkle the poison.' The newspaper then defended the town, saying, 'it was an isolated case' without any sympathy from commoners ('popolani'), by virtue of the authorities, the middle classes, and an educated public.[134] The following day, shots rang out in Catania while gravediggers buried a cholera victim. The gravediggers ran, and *carabinieri* had to finish the job.[135]

Finally, the same week, another cholera uprising erupted at Naso. To restrict intermingling, authorities postponed the town's animal fair. To defend their livelihoods, herders and peasants assembled the night before the market's closing, broke down the fence and 'invaded' the fairground. While this cholera riot appears to have been centred on economic concerns, the paper characterized the general fear and cholera panic in the province of Messina as much the same as before: 'superstitions reigned supreme among the lower classes (*il popolino*)', who believed cholera inevitably ended in death and blamed the doctors for it. The paper picked one case to illustrate its point. On the previous Saturday night, a young physician registered a pregnant woman as having died of cholera and began disinfecting her apartment. A crowd gathered, hooted, and threw stones at the doctor, who escaped after the police arrived and had drawn their sabres. The paper added that most families refused to allow sufferers to take prescribed medicines and treated themselves instead with olive oil and crushed herbs.[136]

The international press reported none of these stories. However, it described five cases not found in the Italian papers I have read; all of them occurred in Sicily. In early September 1887, a mob shot a postman suspected of spreading cholera through distributing letters in Villabota (probably Villabate, near Palermo),[137] which had been the scene of one of Italy's earliest cholera riots in July 1837.[138] A second incident was grislier. A 'mob' captured three soldiers sent to Trapani to disinfect cholera-stricken neighbourhoods. Accused of poisoning, they were forced to drink the carbolic acid used to disinfect streets and houses. One obeyed and

---

[130] *Il Messaggero*, 17 August 1887, front page.
[131] This Stabia may have been the one near Naples or del Golfo, near Trapani.
[132] *Il Messaggero*, 17 September 1887.   [133] *La Nazione*, 1 September 1887, 2.
[134] *Giornale di Sicilia*, 12 September 1887, 3.   [135] *La Nazione*, 9–10 September 1887, 3.
[136] *Gazzetta Piemontese*, 2 September 1887, 2.
[137] *Worcester Daily Spy*, 23 September 1887, front page; *Barton County Democrat*, 29 September 1887, 2.
[138] Sansone, *Gli avvenimenti*, 71 and 73.

quickly 'died in horrible agony'; the other two refused and were executed.[139] A third was more chilling still. At Monreale, less than 10 km from Palermo, a mob met those fleeing from cholera rampant in Palermo, some returning to their native village. With guns, the mob forced the refugees to camp in the fields, and stabbed to death and cremated a nine-year-old boy, who approached the town for safety, 'driven by hunger'.[140]

Only a fourth incident, however, was a riot. Given the number of arrests, it was probably the largest and most destructive cholera incident of 1887. In Leonforte, in Sicily's interior, inhabitants accused the government of wilful cholera spreading. They attacked *carabinieri*, killing two, and over fifty peasants were arrested.[141] Ten days later, a letter from Palermo, published first by a Viennese paper, elaborated further, saying that the villagers had killed the brigadier of the gendarmes sent by the mayor to end the unrest. The rioters barricaded themselves in a local monastery; a state of siege ensued. The letter claimed the villagers believed cholera had originated from a victim transferred to their recently built hospital. A band of peasants, 'armed to the teeth' set the building ablaze and murdered the sick man, accusing him of being in the government's pay to spread cholera. It was one of the few cholera riots anywhere, at any time, to victimize a victim of the disease. The letter also claimed that another riot with 'similar events' erupted at Caltagirone[142] with seventy-eight peasants arrested. But the incident is not described, and I find no trace of it in Italian or foreign papers.[143] Certainly, the old mythologies continued in 1887 and not just in small Sicilian villages of the interior. At Messina, not marked for its cholera violence, even in 1837, and praised in 1884 for its 'ancient spirit and goodness', rumours of physicians and pharmacists poisoning the poor now reached panic proportions. As a result, these professionals fled the city, and because of urgent need for medical care, Messina's police pursued them to force them back to town.[144] A long editorial in the *New York Times*, comparing cholera violence in southern France and Italy, generalized: in contrast to France: 'Everywhere [in Italy] the belief is prevalent that doctors spread the poison, having received orders to kill the people, and hence the poor hide their sick and mob the doctors in the streets.'[145]

The comparison was overstated. Cholera social violence in the previous epicentres during 1867 and 1884—the southern mainland—were clearly on the decline by 1887. Here, only a few incidents appear, and none was on the scale of the previous two epidemics. The first was in mid-September: an incident spurred by popular beliefs that the government was killing the poor arose at Pozzuoli, the scene of a cholera riot only three years before. Now, however, the threatened violence failed to materialize. A woman from one of the most squalid quarters died of cholera. When the coffin was brought to remove her, a crowd gathered, invaded her room, and threatened the gravediggers. The commander of the municipal guard calmed the crowd, and the gravediggers made haste 'through the horrific screams of the

---

[139] *New York Herald*, 13 September 1887, 7.   [140] *Scotsman*, 23 September 1887, 3.
[141] *Derby Daily Telegraph*, 20 July 1887, 3.   [142] About 70 km south-west of Catania.
[143] *Gloucester Citizen*, 26 August 1887, 3; *Bury and Norwich Post*, 30 August 1887, 3.
[144] *Bunyip*, 11 November 1887, 2.   [145] *New York Times*, 7 September 1884.

crowd', but without injuries or arrests.[146] This was the only incident on the mainland, north or south, in 1887, mentioned in northern newspapers I have examined.

Curiously, a southern paper, Naples' *Il Pungolo*, found others, but these occurred mainly in northern Italy. Market towns ('comuni') near Turin were 'crazily' instituting cordon restrictions around their communities that even restricted doctors' movements. Given doctors' abnegation and courage in treating cholera cases, the paper called it an 'insult'.[147] In Genoa, fifty youngsters ('di giovanastro') protested against the city's cordon by acquiring 'as many copies as they could of a local newspaper, *Caffero* (which presumably supported the quarantine) and burnt them in front of the city's health office, chanting: 'Down with *Il Caffaro*! Down with the Cordon!' The protest appears successful: the following morning, the cordon was lifted.[148] Further down the coast at Portovenere, concerns over protecting a community grew more violent. The cause of this 'sommossa' was transporting cholera victims from Le Grazie to Portovenere's lazaretto. The 'population' barricaded the roads leading to the town. Armed forces arrived, destroyed the barricades, and made fourteen arrests. In the same region, 13 km to the north, 'disorder' erupted over quarantine at La Spezia, but here for the opposite reason. The municipal government stubbornly maintained its quarantine, which was 'suffocating' the city. Commercial groups organized a protest, closed their shops, and at the civic theatre held 'a tumultuous meeting'.[149] A week later La Spezia kept its military cordon, and the Neapolitan paper chided it for its backwardness, charging that the cordon was in flagrant ignorance of recent evidence about cholera now 'accepted in every other region of the Nation'. In addition to the Italian evidence, the paper pointed to Paris, which recently opened its doors to refugees fleeing cholera-ridden Toulon and Marseille, 'and the city has remained immune!'[150]

Except possibly for barricades built at Portovenere and the arrest of fourteen rebels, these examples north of Sicily reveal little, if any, collective violence and no signs of the old cholera myths of intentional poisoning. *Il Pungolo*, however, suggested that they had not disappeared from central or northern Italy. Based on Genoese sources, it claimed that 'the fatal superstitions of the rabble (*popolino*)' in La Spezia had led inhabitants to conceal early cases of cholera, hampering health authorities and fanning cholera's spread.[151] For Bergamo, it revealed that not only in tiny villages ('borgate') but also in the city, 'ignorance and superstition' reigned with 'crude, stupid, evil, or cruel individuals believing that doctors spread the cholera poison'.[152] Finally, in Parma, 'popolani' expressed the same suspicions. They assembled in the streets to scream obscenities at doctors and nurses when performing their duties. No physical injuries were inflicted, but afterwards several physicians declared they would not treat cholera patients in Parma unless accompanied by police escorts.[153]

---

[146] *Il Messaggero*, 20 September 1887, 2. [147] Ibid., 3–4 September 1887, front page.
[148] Ibid., 16–17 September 1887, 2. [149] Ibid., 18–19 September 1887, front page.
[150] Ibid., 24–5 September 1887, front page. [151] Ibid., 26–7 September 1887, front page.
[152] Ibid., 31 August–1 September 1887, 2. [153] Ibid., 1–2 September 1887, 2.

As in 1884, newspapers continued to chastise the religiously zealous for processions, prayers, and religious images to remedy epidemics. Again, San Gennaro's feast day was the flashpoint. Rome's *Il Messaggero* described Neapolitan streets in popular quarters 'filled with images of the Madonnas [sic] and saints, lit with candles' and berated their 'ignorance' and 'superstitions', 'fed by priests'.[154] The national government's position, however, had changed: instead of sending troops to arrest those in the procession, it joined the celebration, offering a twenty-one-cannon salute in Naples.[155] The paper most critical of the city's religious festivals was now Naples' own, *Il Pungolo*, which called this notion of salvation, with cholera cases on the rise, 'the shame of religious festivals (*la vergogna delle feste*)' and condemned the deputies and councillors, who 'forced the hand of the authorities to obtain permits and block ordinances…to provide cheap distractions for the poor'. As a result, the poor, it maintained, paid for this entertainment with their lives.[156]

Finally, only rarely had papers supported popular outrage against the behaviour of elites, as in 1884 during Naples' worst cholera epidemic, when opposing the city's maladroit sanitary practices, the 'popolino' ran through streets crying, 'Get out, get out of your houses if you don't want to be poisoned to death'. The papers had to admit that the sulphur used to fumigate the city was pouring into houses through the plumbing, threatening to asphyxiate the inhabitants of via Cavour.[157] In 1887, such condemnations increased. At the beginning of August, the mayor of Paternò was destitute because his chief minister fled the city when the epidemic erupted.[158] The following day, the inhabitants complained they lacked medicines and a lazaretto, and their doctors had fled town.[159] On 10 August, papers decried the flight of doctors, pharmacists, and elites from Catania.[160] Four days later, the doctors who had fled were invited to return but refused, and other doctors, along with municipal councillors, fled the district too.[161] The *Gazzetta Ufficiale* published a list of doctors and pharmacists who had deserted their posts, and were now put under arrest.[162] Naples' *Il Pungolo* pointed to the flight of elites ('la classe commoda') north of Rome. In Castelnuovo (Garfagnana), not only had they fled, but the mayor joined them, 'leaving everything in squalor, a sepulchral silence prevailed throughout, broken only by the sound of muskets and explosives'. The streets were deserted; the houses left empty; 'only occasionally might someone dart past rapidly with a Bengali torch'.[163] At La Spezia, trains were insufficient to carry off the fugitives ('i fuggiaschi'). 'All sorts of vehicles clogged country roads, transporting goods and the old from the city'.[164]

In 1887, cholera still possessed its power to trigger the old suspicions and myths of intentional poisoning with occasional violence against the medical profession, as often now in the north as in the south. But times had changed. The cholera violence that remained was confined to neighbourhood incidents and could hardly

---

[154] *Il Messaggero*, 20 August 1887, 2.   [155] Ibid., 21 August 1887, front page.
[156] *Il Pungolo* (Naples), 8–9 August 1887, 2.
[157] *La Riforma* (Florence), 30 September 1884, 2.   [158] *Il Messaggero*, 3 August 1887, 2.
[159] Ibid., 4 August 1887, 2.   [160] *La Nazione*, 10 August 1887, 2.
[161] Ibid., 14 August 1887, 2.   [162] *Il Pungolo*, 13–14 August 1887, 2.
[163] Ibid., 18–19 August 1887, 2.   [164] Ibid., 25–6 August 1887, 2.

be called riots. Large demonstrations and illegal quarantines imposed at major southern ports and railway stations had drastically declined in number, size, and violence, and alliances between newspapers and the 'popolino' had been created, attacking the abuses and self-interest of elites. For the next cholera epidemics of 1892 and 1893, despite the disease raging in cities such as Palermo and Livorno,[165] I have found only one serious riot in Italy, and it was in Tuscany.[166] Had we ended our analysis here, we might safely speculate that attitudes in Italy had finally moved on. Yet from Italy's next cholera wave, we know 1887 marked no endpoint in sedating cholera's social toxins.

ABANDONMENT AND CHARITY

As with the Black Death, stories of professionals fleeing their posts when their services were most needed appear with cholera. During the epidemics of 1867, 1884, and especially 1887, newspapers and official gazettes reported, shamed, and fined notaries, doctors, pharmacists, city councillors, mayors, and administrators for abandoning the cities of Messina, Catania, and Castelnuovo di Garfagnana. Further examples can be added. In 1884, administrators of religious charities ('opera pie') and one of the municipal deputies fled from Genoa.[167] Because of the exodus at La Spezia, the municipality lacked personnel to bury corpses and had to form a 'Committee of Eighty' to search for cholera cadavers house to house.[168] In 1887, doctors took flight from Regalbuto, then in the province of Catania, and when asked to return, refused.[169] A week later, in Scicli (in the province of Ragusa), all the municipal employees abandoned their posts.[170] By mid-September, elites ('i signori') and white-collar workers ('impiegati') had fled Messina, and shopkeepers shut their shops, 'leaving the city bereft of necessities and deprived of assistance with the afflicted left in the streets'.[171]

Mass abandonment during cholera epidemics was not unique to Italy, as earlier attested by Sligo's experience. Another side to Italy's cholera crises, however, seems exceptional. These were waves of charity, abnegation, and community volunteerism, especially beginning in 1867.[172] On occasion, abandonment itself led to charity, as in 1867 in Naples when doctors, pharmacists, and councillors fled. To fill the breach Monsignor Dusment with a few helpers 'made rounds night and day distributing charity and comforting the dying'.[173] In 1884, civil authorities escaped the Tuscan village of Sillicano, leaving cholera victims unburied; 'with great sacrifice', the army volunteered to bury them.[174] In 1887, after the elites fled Messina,

---

[165] *Le Petit Parisien*, 2 October 1893, 2; and *Gazzetta Piemontese*, 12 October 1893, 3.
[166] See Chapter 8.   [167] *Il Messaggero*, 29 September 1884, 2.
[168] *Giornale di Sicilia*, 30 August 1884, 2.   [169] *La Nazione*, 14 August 1887, 2.
[170] Ibid., 23 August 1887, front page.   [171] *Il Messaggero*, 18 September 1887, front page.
[172] As early as 1835 examples of martyred doctors were praised, such as the Genoese who went to Sardinia, dying of cholera as a consequence; see Chapter 9.
[173] *Corriere italiano*, 20 September 1867, 2; from *Gazzetta Piemontese*, 18 September 1867.
[174] Ibid., 4 September 1884, 2.

volunteers of the Golden Cross (Croce d'oro) intervened along with doctors from Naples.[175]

Praised in the press, these acts of compassion took various forms and developed in different ways. In the 1867 crisis, they relied on traditional structures of Italian charity: first of all the Church, exemplified by Dusment above. Palermo's and Catania's archbishops received equal praise: 'without resting, they went through streets, entering the smallest hovels to assist the afflicted'.[176] Second, the papers praised doctors, nurses, and pharmacists who refused to leave, 'sacrificing night and day' to attend the 'colerosi'.[177] Third, the military volunteered, as in Aosta, when eight soldiers from a local detachment 'with intelligence and zeal nursed cholera sufferers for over forty days in the town's lazaretto'. In gratitude, the municipality offered them 250 lire, but they insisted it should go to the poor devastated by the disease.[178] In 1867, new transregional assistance appeared. Florence's *La Riforma* organized a subscription for families stricken by cholera in Sicily, with monies sent to Palermo's worst-affected neighbourhoods.[179] The 'Assembly of Bolognese Workers' raised 100 lire for fellow workers in Palermo, crippled by cholera, to be distributed by its Lincoln brigade. Workers in Florence were organizing the same.[180] Milan's municipal government raised 2000 lire to benefit the neediest in the worst-hit provinces. Again, Palermo was the principal recipient and expressed its gratitude.[181]

With the next cholera wave in 1884, these organizations further changed the face of charity across Italy. Milan's *La Perseveranza* organized 'subscriptions' for 'all impoverished Italians hit by cholera'.[182] Northern municipalities—Verona's provincial government,[183] the giunta comunale of Livorno, and the Venetians—collected funds to buy sheets and covers for afflicted southerners.[184] Northern cities were not the only ones to make donations: Palermo contributed 202 crates of lemons to the hecatomb of this cholera crisis, Naples.[185] Homeopathic doctors offered their care to Naples free of charge.[186] Workers' groups such as Livorno's firemen[187] and Venice's gondoliers (la Società Bucintoro)[188] sent goods and money to Naples, and across Italy *carabinieri* pledged funds.[189] Banks, entrepreneurs, and political leaders led by charitable example: the Banco di Napoli gave the large sum of 31,000 lire to the city's poorest neighbourhoods;[190] and Milan's Bocconi brothers donated

[175] *Il Messaggero*, 18 September 1884, front page.

[176] *Corriere italiano*, 26 August 1867, front page. Also the cardinal patriarch of Milan was praised for visiting cholera victims.

[177] *La Nazione*, 5 September 1867, 2. In Turin, the community thanked the medical staff and nuns ('suore di carità') who cared for cholera victims in its military lazaretto; ibid., 9 September 1867, front page.

[178] *La Riforma* (Florence), 28 August 1867, 3; for other examples of military assistance, see ibid., 5 September 1867, 3; *La Nazione*, 5 September 1867, 2.

[179] *La Riforma* (Florence), 18 August 1867, 3.   [180] Ibid., 10 September 1867, 4.

[181] *La Perseveranza* (Milan) 23 August 1867, 3.   [182] Ibid., 12 September 1884, 2.

[183] *Giornale di Sicilia*, 15 September 1884, 3.

[184] *La Riforma* (Florence), 28 September 1884, front page.

[185] *Giornale di Sicilia*, 13 September 1884, 3.   [186] *La Lombardia*, 6 September 1884, 3.

[187] *La Riforma* (Florence), 28 September 1884, front page.

[188] *Giornale di Sicilia*, 15 September 1884, 3.   [189] *La Lombardia*, 26 September 1884, 2.

[190] *Giornale di Sicilia*, 13 September 1884, 3.

10,000 lire to purchase sheets for them.[191] Clubs, such as the rowers of Rome (La Società dei canottieri) raised money for Naples and organized a festival on the Tiber on their behalf.[192] Those in Florence, Piacenza, 'and other places' organized public walks ('passeggiati') to benefit the Neapolitans.[193] In Naples, a volunteer association to help bury the cholera dead was organized.[194] Committees of volunteers formed also to protect their communities in places yet to be stricken, as in Milan.[195] Agostino Depretis, President of the National Council of Ministers, visited cholera patients in Busca and donated an unstated large sum ('la generosa elargizione lasciata') to their families.[196] Soon-to-be president, Francesco Crispi, sent seventy-one crates of lemons to Naples;[197] and King Umberto visited the afflicted, donating a colossal sum, 300,000 lire, to Naples' poorest quarters.[198] Municipalities sent relief to other cities, as with the northern town of Sondrio, whose councillors voted unanimously to send funds to hard-hit La Spezia and Naples.[199] In addition, new charitable organizations, such as La Congregazione di Carità di Roma, sent 2000 sheets.[200]

Another charitable development of 1884 was notable. New 'squadre' instead of raising collections in northern cities, removed from cholera's dangers, took trains to worst-hit Naples, risking their lives to assist directly with problems of sanitation and care. These organizations were tied to the anti-clerical, democratic politics of the new republic: la Squadra dei garibaldini livornesi di soccorso,[201] la Croce Bianca,[202] le Squadre Toscana e Lombardia, organized by the radical deputies Felice Cavallotti, Antonio Maffi, and Ettore Ferrari, and Florence's Squadro di socialisti.[203] Another regional group to travel south with donations and services, some paying with their lives, was la Squadra dei romagnoli, and Naples' city council thanked them profusely in letters published in northern papers.[204] As with the Florentine workers of La Confederazione Operaia, who formed their own 'Comitato di soccorso' to care for Naples' *colerosi,* young men ('molti giovanotti') comprised these organizations.[205] Among other services,[206] they organized and staffed soup kitchens ('le cucine economiche'),[207] which would have a long future, blossoming during the Great Influenza of 1918–19, not just in Italy, but globally. In 1884, the new squads crossed the Alps to assist hard-hit villages in France's Basse

---

[191] Ibid., 19 September 1884, 3.   [192] *Il Pungolo* (Milan), 21–2 September 1884, 2.
[193] Ibid., 17–18 September 1884, 2; 22–3 September 1884, 2.
[194] *La Lombardia*, 6 September 1884, 3.   [195] Ibid., 26 September 1884, 2.
[196] *La Nazione*, 31 August 1884, 2.   [197] *Giornale di Sicilia*, 17 September 1884, 3.
[198] *La Perseveranza* (Naples), 22 August 1884, 3; 12 September 1884, 2; *La Nazione*, 16 September 1884, 2; *Giornale di Sicilia*, 13 September 1884, 3.
[199] *Il Pungolo*, 17–18 September 1884, 2.   [200] *Giornale di Sicilia*, 15 September 1884, 3.
[201] *La Riforma* (Florence), 28 September 1884, front page.   [202] Ibid.
[203] *Giornale di Sicilia*, 16 September 1884, 2; *La Riforma* (Florence), 20 September 1884, 2; 23 September 1884, 2; *La Lombardia*, 13 September 1884, 3; and *Il Pungolo* (Milan), 17–18 September 1884, 2.
[204] *La Riforma* (Florence), 30 September 1884, 2.   [205] Ibid., 27 September 1884, 2.
[206] In contrast to those of 1887, papers of 1884 rarely specified the volunteers' contributions; see *La Nazione*, 5 September 1887, 2.
[207] *Giornale di Sicilia*, 16 September 1884, 2; and *La Riforma* (Florence), 28 September 1884, front page.

Alpi; Milanese doctors went to Marseille,[208] and cities formed societies to send money and goods to 'our French brothers'.[209]

Three years later with the next epidemic, still more volunteer groups travelled north to south—the Croce d'oro and le Squadre democratiche—to join local associations in the worst-hit cities, now Messina and Catania.[210] The volunteer traffic also crossed Sicily as with Corleone's citizens joining Catania's volunteers to treat the afflicted at Catania.[211] Northerners not only travelled south but attended communities nearby as with the Genovesi sending beds, sheets, and covers to La Spezia.[212] During this epidemic, references to soup kitchens and the names of volunteer societies increased. But as with cholera's social violence, the history of cholera charity did not trace a steady progressive trajectory. For Italy's last major cholera wave, 1910–11, I have found soup kitchens established only in cholera-hit Taranto and Barletta. In both cases, moreover, regional governments—not volunteers—founded them to relieve populations but only after they had revolted. More significantly, the political and humanitarian zeal of young northern *squadristi*, rushing to succour their southern 'fratelli', disappeared. Northerners now viewed the desperately afflicted in towns such as Verbicaro and Bisceglie not as 'fratelli', but as the uneducated, superstitious, and exploited. Instead of beds, monies, and volunteers, their assistance now came in the form of words, explaining the roots of these communities' backwardness. Nonetheless, this mass volunteerism and self-sacrifice in Italy for the cholera-afflicted over two decades is striking in comparison with earlier waves of cholera in Italy as well as in other countries.[213]

THE MIDDLE EAST

It seems that major cholera riots began to erupt in the Middle East only at the end of the nineteenth century or else foreign newspapers only then began to report them.[214] However, the Western press had certainly addressed earlier disturbances in the Ottoman Empire. Six cholera revolts have surfaced from my research on Muslim countries. The first, found in a single Australian paper, resembled European ones in its underlying beliefs and conspiracies but possessed another element—anti-colonial sentiment and antipathy towards foreigners. The paper's description

---

[208] *La Perseveranza* (Naples) 22 August 1884, 3.

[209] *La Lombardia*, 11 August 1884, front page; and 20 August 1884, front page.

[210] *Giornale di Sicilia*, 18 September 1887, 3; 21 September 1887, 2; *La Nazione*, 23 September 1887, 2; *Il Pungolo*, 17–18 September 1887, 2; and *Il Messaggero*, 18 September 1887, front page.

[211] *La Nazione*, 11 August 1887, 2.   [212] *Il Pungolo*, 25–6 September 1887, 2.

[213] Ross, *Contagion in Prussia*, 249, explains Berlin's escape from mob violence in 1831. Learning lessons from the riot at Königsberg, the king modified strict quarantine regulations. But the middle classes also played a part by organizing soup kitchens for the unemployed and providing for orphans. During the cholera outbreak in Denmark in 1853, private charities distributed food to the afflicted; Bonderup, *Cholera-Morbo'er og Danmark*, ch. 3 and 401. But neither case shows the organized charity of volunteers criss-crossing a country or that endured over several epidemics.

[214] Echenberg, *Africa in the Time of Cholera*, 70, reports what appears to be a minor cholera riot in March 1850 at Bizerte, when a French physician was attacked.

is brief, no more than a notice taken from a London correspondent: 'The mob' accused English doctors sent to Egypt of poisoning their cholera patients. Rioting ensued and a government ambulance was destroyed before troops arrived and suppressed the disorder.[215]

A second incident is more fully reported yet more difficult to analyse. It derives from an interview with a British Consul colonel, one of the few to have survived a Bedouin attack on Russian, French, and British diplomats in Jeddah on 30 May 1895. The motivating fears and targets of attack, however, are reminiscent of European cholera disturbances. After describing his 'hairbreadth escape' and the murder of several diplomats, he speculated on the Bedouins' motives. The most probable one, he concluded, was a matter of mistaken identity: the Bedouins thought the diplomats were quarantine doctors because of the present cholera epidemic. 'Bedouins and Arabs' believed them to be 'willing instruments of the Turkish Government' spreading cholera to conquer the Bedouin. Simultaneously, a third outbreak of violence occurred in Mecca, where attackers looted and partially destroyed the cholera hospital, causing doctors to flee. The 'mob' dragged out the disinfecting machines, seen as the tools to kill Bedouins and smashed them to bits.[216]

During this decade and into the twentieth century, three further Muslim cholera revolts presented new elements. First, two riots, one in Turkey, the other in Cairo, were the first cholera protests that were student revolts. Both hinged on orthodox Muslim burial customs and violations of sacred ceremonies. In December 1893, the treatment of cholera patients in the hospital and neglect of Muslim burial rites 'agitated' the Softias, or religious students, to hold meetings:

> placards were secretly posted on the walls of the Mosque at Stamboul [Istanbul], urging the faithful to take notice of the scandalous manner in which the Mussulman dead were interred, of the bad treatment of the sick, and the wholesale squandering for personal profit of sums assigned for sanitary measures.[217]

Two and a half years later, sanitary measures enforced by secular authorities sparked another student uprising 'at the Great Muslim University Mosque of El Ashar [Cairo]'.[218] When the Governor and Sub-Governor entered the university to inspect a cholera case and enforce sanitary regulations, students showered them with stones, wounding the Governor and maltreating the Sub-Governor and other officials. Later that day, reinforcements arrived; the students resisted. Ultimately, the police restored order by firing on the crowd, killing one, critically wounding three, and arresting 120, 'mostly Syrian Turks'. The papers praised the Governor for his 'great judgement and promptitude' and the police for their exemplary behaviour.[219] *Le Temps* corroborated the scale of the resistance, elaborating further on the arrests: forty released, seventy-two imprisoned, fifteen sentenced without

---

[215] *Sydney Morning Herald*, 14 August 1883, 7.   [216] Ibid., 26 December 1895, 3.
[217] *Scotsman*, 19 December 1893, 7, from Vienna.
[218] *Le Temps*, 5 October 1896, 2, It was founded in 970 or 972 as a madrassa (centre of Islamic study).
[219] *Scotsman*, 2 June 1896, 6.

reporting their punishments (127 in total).[220] The *New York Times* claimed 200 were arrested,[221] with the police killing the leaders.[222]

Despite the underlying sentiments of the foreign press—assertions of 'Mohammedan fanaticism', praise of the police's 'exemplary behaviour'—the scripts above suggest another story, one that compares in brutality, numbers killed, and especially numbers arrested with Cossack repression in 1892. Yet the student protests point to none of the rioters' excesses described in Russia, such as the murder and mutilation of doctors, torching of hospitals, and the destruction even of an entire industrial town. Nor were they underpinned by conspiracies of poisoning and live burials. Instead, the students protested against intrusions into their religious customs, especially burial practices, and in the Turkish case, the protests were secular and economic—against scandalous treatment of the sick and the authorities' pilfering of monies apportioned for sanitary relief.

A fifth cholera riot, again in 'Turkey', in Monastir in Tunisia which lay in the African part of the Ottoman Empire, illustrates another Muslim response to cholera. In September 1911, rioters attacked the aggressive preventive measures and zeal of Monastir's health officer (praised by the Constantinople correspondent for his diligence) in isolating cholera contacts, closing off or diverting water supplies in infected neighbourhoods, and prohibiting the sale of melons and other fruit in the bazaar. Residents saw the measures differently and organized a protest that initially was peaceful. 'Several thousand persons, mostly of the poorer classes' held a public meeting outside the Club of the Monastir Committee of Union and Progress. Led by a religious leader (*hodja*), they accused sanitary authorities of violating Islamic law, and drafted resolutions to remove 'the obnoxious' sanitary inspector, abolish many of the 'prophylactic measures', and reopen supplies of fresh water. Led by Yahia and other *hodjas*, fruiterers, water-sellers, and sweepers, whose businesses had suffered from the regulations, damaged the windows of a club, marched to the Konak, 'where the Vali had capitulated without a murmur', annulled the regulations and dismissed the chief sanitary inspector.[223] Sale of fruit was resumed, water supplies reopened, and the faithful were permitted to wash cholera-inflicted corpses.[224] Two days later, supported by the military with orders from central government, the Vali reinstated the regulations and threatened any resistance with armed force. In the foreign press, nothing was reported about any retaliation, peaceful or violent. But, as with the other two Muslim protests, no myths or conspiracies are evident and, despite the community's *hodjas* having led the protest, their demands were secular (except for the washing of corpses), opposing the government's disruptive and deadly shutting off of water supplies. In proposing to boil water before using it, the protesters acknowledged recent science

---

[220] *Le Temps*, 5 October 1896, 2.   [221] *New York Times*, 2 June 1896.
[222] Ibid., 3 June 1896. Also, *Pall Mall Gazette*, 28 May 1896, 7–8; and *Coventry Evening Telegraph*, 2 June 1896, 3.
[223] *The Times*, 26 September 1911, 3.
[224] *Sun*, 17 September 1911, 2, from Vienna. The same day, the *Observer* published a similar report from Reuters; *Daily Herald*, 24 October 1911, 6; and *Derby Daily Telegraph*, 18 September 1911, 4.

that pinned cholera to contaminated water. More than the student protests, this revolt focused on economics.

An earlier cholera riot, curiously reported by only a few papers, erupted in the Labat (or Labor) quarter of Alexandria on 11 August 1883. By contrast, its outlines reproduced the fears behind European cholera disturbances: the rioters believed that English doctors were poisoning 'natives' and attempted to destroy the ambulances, crying 'Death to the Christians!' British troops easily quelled the uprising.[225] Yet an English paper referred to none of these myths nor to anti-British, anti-Christian violence. Instead, according to its version, the 'native quarter' opposed 'some measures of disinfection' and consequently the sanitary Commission decided that a guard of Egyptian soldiers would accompany its officials.[226]

Finally, in October 1947 a cholera epidemic erupted in Egypt. First, the UN's newly formed World Health Organization (WHO), in cooperation with the Egyptian government and international volunteers won praise for their measures controlling the epidemic. The outbreak was successfully contained to Egypt and ended in six weeks—a record time for a major cholera epidemic. Moreover, the mortalities were a seventh of Egypt's previous cholera epidemic deaths in 1902.[227] Yet, this one produced more riots and recrimination than any in the Middle East. At the same time, it engendered volunteer assistance across political parties, religious groups, and gender. Often the two—charity and protest—came from the same organizations and individuals. As Nancy Gallagher has shown from Egyptian newspapers and archival materials, indigenous political organizations rushed to help. Forty thousand from the Muslim Brotherhood alone volunteered, distributing leaflets on cholera prevention, helping to cordon off infected areas, and caring for patients through the Nile valley. Muslim students distributed leaflets in mosques and in the streets, promoting the latest research from British medicine, and volunteered to care for the afflicted in Cairo's poorer quarters.[228] As with the Great Influenza of 1918–20, women played a prominent role. After the Ministry of Health had burnt patients' clothing in isolation camps, women of the Red Crescent and the Mabarra Muhammad Ali distributed new clothes to the impoverished. Other women's groups visited the houses of Cairo's poor and advised on cholera prevention.[229] Again, reminiscent of the Great Influenza, the international community responded to this cholera crisis: organizations from Bombay, the Soviet Union, Iraq, Syria, Lebanon, Turkey, Italy, Switzerland, Holland, Sweden, France, and Denmark sent vaccine and medical missions to Egypt.[230]

The Egyptian government, however, refused donations from two groups—the Hebrew University of Jerusalem and the Women's Zionist Organization of America (Hadassah). And here began the repeated tale of suspicion, conspiracies, and violence that historically and geographically has comprised the predominant response to cholera. The Egyptian press portrayed the Jewish offerings as a plot under

---

[225] *New York Times*, 11 August 1883 from London; and *San Francisco Chronicle*, 11 August 1883, from Alexandria.
[226] *Exeter and Plymouth Gazette and Daily Telegraph*, 11 August 1883, 4.
[227] Gallagher, *Egypt's Other Wars*, 135.   [228] Ibid., 124–6.
[229] Ibid., 135.   [230] Ibid., 129.

humanitarian guises to destroy Egyptian cities.[231] The Muslim Brotherhood also spun conspiracy theories, alleging British vaccines were intended 'to poison the people'. Furthermore, they blamed British troops coming to Egypt from the Punjab, where cholera had erupted in September, a month before arriving in Egypt, claiming it was a plot to annex Sudan from Egypt.[232] The Brotherhood suggested a third plot that chimes with earlier European cholera conspiracies now placed in a larger geopolitical sphere: the British had introduced the pathogen to drain Egypt of its resources, thereby derailing its nationalist movement. The only way to eradicate cholera, the Brotherhood preached, was by holy war to expel the British from Egypt.[233]

Other Egyptians spun similar conspiracy theories. Radical students, who entered poor urban neighbourhoods to distribute purified water, gasoline, soap, and DDT, also visited mosques 'to explain' the role of British troops 'causing the epidemic'. Given the timing of the cholera outbreak in the Punjab and British troop movement into Egypt, the British probably had unwittingly carried the disease into Egypt. In fact, British physicians writing in the *Lancet* and P. M. Kaul, an expert at the WHO, refuted Britain's official line that pilgrims carried it from Mecca or Medina to Egypt, the route of previous transmissions. This time cholera had infected Egypt a month before appearing at Mecca or Medina.[234]

Only two weeks into this cholera epidemic, a new form of conflict arose with violence erupting within volunteer groups and between volunteers and the government. The Ministry of Health refused to work with the students, and police attacked charitable associations sponsored by the opposition party—the Haditu—arresting their participants, while the Haditu party claimed the 'secret police' had instigated violence to justify police intervention.[235] Student groups demonstrated against government negligence and publicized complaints against the Health Ministry.[236]

Anger and violence also stemmed from the communities of the victims—the poor—who resented the military's heavy-handed measures that forced suspected victims and their families into isolation camps and burnt their possessions.[237] Across Lower Egypt, the poor attacked guards at isolation camps; troops fired on canal boatmen trying to evade a cordon near Alexandria; the poor stoned an ambulance in al-Rashid (Rosetta), carrying suspected cholera cases to a hospital. The next day more than a thousand inmates of an isolation camp tried to escape by stoning their guards, and at Buhayra, the quarantined burnt their tents.[238] Yet, despite the violence, the old European mythologies of the invention of cholera to cull the poor fail to appear. Instead, the protests of the poor against government abuses resemble the more politicized protests of Indian plague riots at the end of the nineteenth century against the British army. In addition, as with Indian plague riots, the poor were not alone in opposing harsh and economically ruinous measures; opposition now cut across classes creating a clear political agenda.

---

[231] Ibid., 129. [232] Ibid., 145. [233] Ibid., 146. [234] Ibid., 150 and 157.
[235] Ibid., 126–7. [236] Ibid. [237] Ibid., 123.
[238] Ibid., 123–4; also Echenberg, *Africa in the Time of Cholera*, 70–82, relying on Gallagher.

EVOLUTION OF CHOLERA'S SOCIAL TOXINS

While old myths of poisoning the poor continued fuelling cholera protests into the twentieth century, they began in the 1860s to show new features, becoming more grounded in secular and economic grievances against disruptive sanitary measures and gaining middle-class support. Instead of criticisms against state actions, imagined or real, protesters attacked the state for abandoning its responsibilities in sanitation control and neglecting services for workers and the poor. In addition to examples discussed in this chapter, when quarantine severely restricted employment and the supply of food in Palermo during the 1884 epidemic, its 'workers' staged a mass demonstration, demanding that the state supply bread and work to the population: many were arrested and wounded.[239] These demands continued with the next epidemic in 1887 in Catania: 'crowds of the poor' demonstrated in front of the town hall, 'chanting and cursing' the government for suspending its distribution of bread and rice.[240] Ten days later, with the disease raging in parts of Sicily, marches of the poor on town halls occurred in Paternò and Riposto, west of Catania, demanding bread.[241] With these shifts, strategies changed from mass violence with ghoulish atrocities to largely peaceful demonstrations with petitions and resolutions voted on by democratic processes. Moreover, the economic character of cholera riots became more pronounced in Italy with the sixth cholera wave of 1910–11, in Barletta and other towns in Puglia when anti-cholera regulations banning consumption of figs and shellfish, crippled two mainstays of southern coastal economies. These prohibitions recurred with cholera's seventh wave, forcing fishermen to mount the barricades in Naples in 1973 and in eastern Venezuela during the 1990s.

Along with these economic concerns, a darker side crept into cholera riots during the 1880s and 1890s rarely seen earlier—attacks against minorities, even if they may not have been the principal targets.[242] In addition to attacking Cossacks, sacking the hospital, and setting a company town ablaze, rioters in Hughesovka also killed several Jews,[243] perhaps reflecting residual anti-Semitism.[244] At the same time, crowds in Astrakhan targeted another minority, Persian merchants, and alleged the disease originated in Persia.[245] Less than a month later, another cholera riot erupted in Astrakhan, attacking another ethnic minority, Armenians blamed for the disease.[246] In Italy, 1910–11, gypsies were the minority accused of spreading cholera. Here the government (led by a Jewish Prime Minister) expelled them from cities, thereby encouraging incidents of mob violence against them.[247]

---

[239] *Il Pungolo* (Milan), 17–18 September 1884, 2.

[240] *Il Messaggero*, 1 August 1887, 2, from *La Gazzetta del Popolo di Catania*.

[241] Ibid., 10 August 1887, front page.

[242] In Paris 1832, foreigners were targeted with several thrown into the Seine.

[243] *Wichita Daily Eagle*, 27 July 1892.

[244] 'Our Risk in Cholera'. *The Times*, 30 August 1892, 3, asserted that Jews were the principal targets but no other paper in my sample made such a claim.

[245] *Guardian*, 19 July 1892, 8.   [246] *Guardian*, 11 August 1892, 8, from Tehran.

[247] Snowden, *Naples in the Time of Cholera*, 238–9; Bewell, *Romanticism*, 260, claims that nineteenth-century British literature represented 'cholera as a companion of Gypsies'. In Italian '*lo zingaro*' (gypsy) could mean cholera; see *Il Messaggero*, 25 August 1884, 3: 'Lo spettro dello zingaro'.

Yet scapegoating minorities was the exception, especially outside German-speaking regions and Russia, despite the general milieu of anti-Semitic pogroms throughout the second half of the nineteenth and early twentieth century. Far from being cholera's usual targets, Jews could even become the instigators as in Lyssobiki (Łysobyki), in the district of Lukow, then in the 'Congress of Poland' in 1892.[248] According to a St Petersburg correspondent, a riot here exhibited cholera's old traits of 'ignorant prejudice'. But now a Jew, the coach-driver Abraham Migdal, propagated the myths of health officials poisoning and burying alive the indigenous poor. As a result, residents refused to host them, and when the officials went to an inn, a 'mob' assembled, threw stones at the windows, and tried to break down the doors, forcing the sanitary party to seek refuge.[249]

As we have seen, such myths remained the impetus behind significant and violent cholera riots in Russia and Italy until 1911, but largely disappeared afterwards. Nonetheless, incidents with doctors or local authorities bearing the brunt of cholera-related violence continued. One of the largest massacres caused by a cholera riot occurred during the Russian depression and famine of 1922. I have found only one notice of it, a brief one in the *Guardian* from a Parisian communiqué. It occurred at that hub of numerous earlier cholera disturbances, Astrakhan, and began by 'maltreating' doctors and attacking Communist Commissars. Two hundred were killed in the disturbances.[250]

With the present cholera wave of El Tor, cholera's force to produce myths and conspiracies remains alive, as seen in eastern Venezuela with theories held by indigenous Indians of authorities purposefully contaminating seabeds to cull the poor. In a globalized economy, these myths now penetrated beyond local or national boundaries to embrace multinational capitalism. The Venezuelans accused international vessels fishing in their waters and docking in their ports of purposely planting cholera-stricken crews in their midst and dumping products ridden with the bacillus in their waters. Others accused British Petroleum of inseminating cholera in Venezuelan rivers by oil exploration. Another invented further international causes: when Venezuelan dock workers refused to fill Trinidadian boats with crabs, the workers believed that the entrepreneurs retaliated by producing cholera. Most global of all, rumours spread among Venezuelan Indians during the Gulf War that US bombs exploding in Iraqi deserts on the other side of the globe created *vibrio cholerae* in eastern Venezuelan waters.[251]

During the seventh wave, cholera protests have also turned about-face, as in Torre del Greco and Naples in 1973. Instead of fear and hatred of medical intervention, disinfectants, and vaccinations, the poor have railed against state officials because of their corruption, lack of medical attention, and price gouging of medicines. Such reversals were anticipated in Egypt, 1947, and earlier still, in

[248] Poland became a dependency of Russia with the Congress of Paris in 1815 and was converted into a Russian province by the late nineteenth century. I thank Hamish Scott for the clarification.

[249] *Observer*, 25 September 1892, 5.

[250] *Guardian*, 23 July 1921, front page. For cholera riots against the Soviets a year before and in 1922, see Chapter 9.

[251] Briggs, 'Theorizing Modernity Conspiratorially', 169–70.

the small Sicilian town of Paternò in 1887. Our comparative study of cholera shows variations in reactions and riots from central Russia to the Middle East to the Americas and more significantly over time from 1830 to the twenty-first century. Different regions provided different contexts as with fears of murder and grave robbing in the British Isles to supply cadavers for newly formed anatomy colleges or the ruthless repression of cholera protesters in Czarist Russia. But more astounding still are the continuities in beliefs that often defy any direct communication or imitation of one group by another[252]—cholera's propensity to divide societies by class hatred, accusations of poisoning, and attacks on the medical profession.

A CODA: EBOLA

Although Ebola is not a bacterium, the similarities it bears to cholera are striking: not only the effects of rapid dehydration, explosion of bodily fluids, and high rates of lethality of 50 per cent or greater (at least in Africa for the former, and before dehydration kits for the latter), but also the socio-psychological reactions they share, as witnessed with the Ebola virus disease (EVD) in Guinea, Liberia, and Sierra Leone in 2014.[253] Mirroring cholera's long European history, EVD sparked attacks on health workers and clinics, destruction of medical equipment, distrust of disinfectants, and beliefs that medical professionals intentionally spread the disease. In an unidentified village in Guinea around 11 February 2014, a Red Cross team burying EVD victims and taking blood samples provoked the funeral party to attack them. The villagers threw rocks and beat and trampled several workers. According to the *New York Times*, resistance was already 'evolving' from one region to the next, following the path of the virus. The reported rumour behind 'the resistance' recalls suspicions undergirding hundreds of cholera revolts in Europe: 'the Red Cross is spraying Ebola into the schools'. In Macenta, Guinea, on 5 April urban youth attacked the town's first EVD clinic, constructed a week earlier, and threatened fifty or more of the centre's personnel. Protesters claimed EVD did not exist or was purposefully spread by outsiders. On 29 August, EVD hospital and health workers spraying disinfectants through a busy market in Nzérékoré were attacked, with twenty-two wounded. Sometime before 27 July, villagers in Wabengou blockaded roads and attacked officials. According to Doctors without Borders, the villagers 'banged on' Red Cross vehicles and brandished machetes. On 16 September, Africa experienced its worst EVD atrocity in Womey, Guinea, when eight members of a high-level delegation of doctors, politicians, and journalists were murdered and their bodies dumped in a latrine. Eleven were arrested and sentenced to life in prison. The general level of violence was, however, more

[252] Even today in West Africa, not only isolated villagers, but sophisticated European health workers believe that the 2014 attacks on clinics and health workers were unprecedented and unique to Africa; communication with Dr Ruth Kutalek, WHO health worker, Liberia, 2014 to July 2015.

[253] Based on *Attacks on Health* (WHO), 18 May 2015; Bellickfeb, 'Red Cross Faces Attacks'; Fairhead, 'Understanding Social Resistance'; and references cited in Cohn and Kutalek, 'Historical Parallels'.

pervasive than the international press reported. In Guinea alone, attacks against Red Cross volunteers averaged ten a month in the last six months of 2014.

Although no violence comparable to Womey's happened in Liberia or Sierra Leone, EVD sparked open and collective attacks in these two countries. In Monrovia, Liberia, on 16 August, 'an angry mob' attacked the quarantine centre in the township of West Point. In Matainkay, east of Freetown, Sierra Leone, on 20 September, similar to incidents in Guinea, villagers assaulted health workers burying EVD victims, and in December, the Red Cross reported further violence to burial teams and damage to their vehicles. In Liberia farmers became desperate when roadblocks prevented them from travelling to Monrovia to sell their goods. Resistance flared against quarantine in homes and the reporting of sick relatives. In the poor township of West Point in Monrovia, inhabitants violated quarantine; the government retaliated, and a policeman killed a young man. As with rumours purporting Red Cross poisoning, other protests and slogans link nineteenth- and early twentieth-century cholera distrust and unrest to EVD in 2014, despite great distances and differences in social, economic, and cultural contexts: 'Ebola is a lie!' 'Here, if the people come in [the hospital], they don't leave alive.'[254] We turn now to another disease rich in social loathing: smallpox, whose history contrasts sharply with the patterns seen in the previous four chapters.

---

[254] Cohn and Kutalek, 'Historical Parallels'.

11

Smallpox Cruelty
The Case of North America

Despite the vast literature on smallpox—'the deadliest dermatological ailment' in history[1]—its social violence remains understudied. Attention has been given to anti-inoculation movements in colonial America[2] and later anti-vaccination campaigns of the second half of the nineteenth century.[3] In addition, historians have compiled stories of smallpox as a biological weapon, most famously Lord Jeffrey Amherst's (1717–97) gift of blankets smeared with smallpox pus distributed to Amerindians during the French and Indian War (1754–63).[4] Reputedly, Francisco Pizarro (c.1471–1541) beat Lord Jeffrey to the punch 205 years before with his presents to Peruvians in the 1530s.[5] Such sinister weapons continued to be used during the American Revolution.[6] Subsequent governments engaged in comparable savage practices, such as failing to supply vaccination material for Amerindians, or worse, Secretary of War Lewis Cass's refusal to allow vaccination in the 1830s so as to annihilate the peaceful Mandans.[7] In addition, at the end of the nineteenth century, second-hand clothiers infected 'the colored' in Richmond, Virginia, when

---

[1] Simmons et al., 'Smallpox', 482.

[2] Winslow, *A Destroying Angel*, vi. Attacks against Dr Boylston's introduction of inoculation in 1721 led to the firebombing of Cotton Mather's house because of his support for inoculation. According to Fenn, *Pox Americana*, 36–8, anti-inoculation sentiment sparked 'riots and other crowd actions' from the 1760s until after the Revolution. But she lists none. For smallpox riots in Colonial America, see Chapter 12.

[3] See Chapter 13 for the anti-vaccination campaign in Britain after 1868 and Leicester's peaceful mass demonstration in March 1885. For India, see Arnold, 'Smallpox and Colonial Medicine'; Satya, *Medicine, Disease and Ecology*, when people of the Melghat drove out vaccinators. For the US, Colgrove, 'Between Persuasion and Compulsion', 367–8: for a police raid and ensuing scuffle at the end of May 1894. For a summary of the anti-vaccination movement, see Blume, 'Anti-Vaccination Movements'. For anti-inoculation in Mauritius (1792), Vaughan, 'Slavery, Smallpox, and Revolution'. She cites no examples of collective protest. For resistance to vaccination in late nineteenth- and early twentieth-century Senegal, Ngalamulume, 'Smallpox and Social Control'; again no collective violence is reported. For anti-vaccination revolts in Rio de Janeiro, 1904, Echenberg, *Plague Ports*, 174–5; Aberth, *Plagues in World History*, 86; Tuells, 'La "Revolta da vacina" en Río'; and Chapter 12, n. 106. For Canada, see Jones, *Influenza 1918*, 94–8.

[4] Among other places, see Kelton, *Cherokee Medicine*, 102–4, 108, 136; Fenn, *Pox Americana*, 88–9; Reeds, 'Smallpox in Colonial North America', 664; Oldstone, *Viruses*, 72; and Duffy, 'Smallpox and the Indians', 324.

[5] Bollet, *Plagues*, 78.

[6] Fenn, *Pox Americana*, 89, 91, 131–2; Duffy, *Epidemics in Colonial America*, 244–5. For similar tactics by the British during the American Revolution, see Alchon, *A Pest in the Land*, 111.

[7] Robertson, *Rotting Face*, 309.

they were recklessly sold cheap wares from the smallpox-afflicted in northern states.[8] But almost wholly missing from analysis has been the multitude of small-scale incidents of vigilante violence and brutal neglect of smallpox victims by neighbours, along with collective violence from gangs of ten to riots of thousands. Historians have even claimed smallpox was akin to typhus, influenza, dysentery, and tuberculosis, diseases supposedly so common they 'lacked the shock effect' seen with cholera or (reputedly) yellow fever, and therefore failed to spark fear, panic, or mass violence.[9]

Given the reasons for blame and violence in the literature on epidemics, the history of smallpox violence cuts against what we should expect. When smallpox was new, mysterious, and a big killer in the New World, blame, prejudice, and violence did not appear.[10] Nor did such social toxins develop when the disease mysteriously mutated in the sixteenth century,[11] producing a variant that killed much greater proportions than at any time during the Middle Ages, and which by the seventeenth century began to replace plague as Europe's 'most efficient controller of population'.[12] Moreover, the disastrous waves of pestilence, the Antonine Plague of 165–80 BCE[13] and the pestilence of 312–13,[14] with astonishingly high mortality rates, now believed to have been smallpox, also failed to produce conspiracies, blaming of others, or social violence.

Except for four instances in colonial America of anti-inoculation riots—the firing of Cotton Mather's house in 1722, an incident spurring tar-and-feathering at Marblehead, Massachusetts, and two riots at Norfolk, Virginia (confined to members of the elites), in the early 1770s—blame and prejudice against victims of this disease blossomed only in the 1870s in Britain and the 1880s in the US—that is, at a time when the medical breakthroughs of the 'laboratory revolution' were progressing.[15] By this time, smallpox was hardly a new disease, and with Edward

---

[8] *Daily Dispatch*, 8 February 1892.

[9] See McLean, *Public Health*, 1; Emias, 'Yellow Fever', 791–2; Ackerknecht, *Medicine and Ethnology*, 141; Pierce and Writer, *Yellow Jack*: 'Dysentery, typhoid, smallpox, and many unnamed or unrecognized diseases killed many more people [than yellow fever]...yet people learned to live with them' (2). Also, Humphreys, *Yellow Fever*, claims that smallpox, like tuberculosis or typhoid, might kill as many as yellow fever, but it 'failed to stir the public from apathy' (2), and Duffy, 'Social Impact', ranked smallpox 'a poor third' after cholera and yellow fever in its capacity to shock populations (805).

[10] According to Alchon, 'A Pest in the Land': 'When smallpox first appeared in Brazil in 1562 a messianic movement attracted many Indians with promises of turning masters into slaves' (661). Yet no violence against masters or blame is reported. According to Cook, 'The Smallpox Epidemic of 1797', Indians rioted against quarantine (768), but he does not specify when or where the riots occurred.

[11] See Carmichael and Silverstein, 'Smallpox in Europe'.

[12] Crosby, 'Smallpox: "There Never Was a Cure"', 76–7; in eighteenth-century Europe, 10–15 per cent of all deaths and 80 per cent of those under ten were due to smallpox; see idem, 'Smallpox'. According to Oldstone, *Viruses*, by the seventeenth century, 'smallpox was the most devastating disease in the world' (63), killing 400,000 a year in Europe, and during the last two decades of the eighteenth century, almost one in ten in London and nearly a fifth in Glasgow. Nine of every ten were children under five (68).

[13] Nutton, *Ancient Medicine*, 24; and Stathakopoulos, 'Plagues of the Roman Empire', 536.

[14] Stathakopoulos, *Famine and Pestilence*, I, 95, 181.

[15] Campaigns and resistance to vaccination increased only by the last quarter of the nineteenth century, despite earlier mandatory legislation; Harden, 'Smallpox', 648.

Jenner's discovery of cowpox vaccination at the end of the eighteenth century, it became the first epidemic disease that could be effectively controlled through medical intervention. Yet, this disease's cultural toxins developed after these break-throughs. From the epidemic of 1881–2 to the second decade of the twentieth century, its social violence cut deeper rifts through the fabric of communities than any other disease in US history, cholera included.

Like cholera, smallpox violence spawned suspicion, hatred, and blame along class lines. But with smallpox, the instigators and victims switched sides: smallpox's rioters were rarely the poor or the marginal. Instead, they were the well-heeled, ascending as high as a son of a former US Vice President. On the other side, the victims of blame were not the police, 'medical gentlemen', or governors, but the poor—blacks, immigrant Chinese, Jews, and tramps. Smallpox cruelty in late nineteenth-century America and Britain finally fulfils an expectation professed in the current literature: the butts of blame were the weak and marginal, the outsider, and often victims of the disease thus became doubly victimized. With smallpox, rioters rarely attacked health workers or state officials and never imagined them-selves as the diseased victims' 'liberators', parading them triumphantly on shoul-ders from quarantine or hospital back to their homes.

Compared to cholera and plague riots, smallpox violence tended to be on a smaller scale. Instead of crowds in the thousands, individual acts of cruelty limited to individuals or small groups of vigilantes commonly characterized smallpox protests. Unlike with any other disease, epidemic or chronic, stories of individual- and small-group prejudice and cruel neglect of the sufferers gripped US newspapers by the 1880s. The pandemic of 1881–2 was certainly not the most severe smallpox epidemic of the century;[16] at least four others scored higher mortalities: one a decade earlier in 1871–2; another in 1852–4, which wiped out 13 per cent of Hawaii's population; the 1836–8 epidemic that decimated Amerindian populations in the upper Missouri territories;[17] and a fourth at the beginning of the eighteenth century. From my searches, the earlier epidemics failed to spark riots or the plethora of small attacks and acts of cruelty reported in 1881–2, which continued into the twentieth century.

Numerous papers available from 'Chronicling America' recorded this pandemic as it moved across the world, from its origins in the Far East to Europe and Latin America and into urban neighbourhoods and rural towns of the US by the winter of 1881. Keyword searches of 'smallpox' produce 2361 results during this year, an increase by two-thirds over those found during the previous more deadly epidemic of 1871–2 (1558 hits).[18] One reason for the higher number, no doubt, reflects the growth in US newspapers. A second reason might indicate a sudden change in journalistic fashion to script lively stories of personal tragedy and horror. Yet, if a

---

[16] Hopkins, *The Greatest Killer*, describes 1881–2 as merely 'another smaller series of smallpox epidemics' (283).

[17] Robertson, *Rotting Face*.

[18] Conditions during the Franco-Prussian War in 1870 may have set off this pandemic; Bliss, *Plague*, 49–50.

change in fashion had occurred, it did not affect any other epidemic disease during that decade or later.[19]

This chapter concentrates on these stories of prejudice and blame by individuals and trusted public institutions beginning with the earliest ones I have found in 1876. To be sure, earlier smallpox stories might be captured, as with one retold in 1895 remembering events in 1856, but Chronicling America's and Readex's newspapers show no substantial traces of such a tradition emerging before the epidemic of 1881–2. In addition to prejudice, fear, hate, violence, and cruel neglect, the newspapers after 1880 also illustrate a general failure by individuals to show compassion in the face of smallpox adversity. I cite or paraphrase a selection of these stories below:

Headline: 'Chinese Inhumanity', San Francisco 1876:

At a few minutes before 6 o'clock, four 'Chinamen' carried a large bundle down to the dock and pitched it into the river. Minutes later, yard men at the depot noticed a 'Chinaman crawl up from the bank…covered with scabs resembling…smallpox'. The yardmen then ran off in the opposite direction. The Health Officer and a physician later found the sick man concealed and delirious. The Chinese companies had paid $300 to three men 'to throw him into the river'.[20]

A colored man in Louisa Co., Virginia, infected with smallpox was repulsed from the hospital at the muzzle of a shotgun. He returned home, 7 miles away, on foot, carrying 'in his hand an improvised smallpox flag as a warning to people not to approach him'.[21]

Eagle, an old Nez Perce Indian with smallpox, was deserted by his tribe. Calmly, 'he dug his grave, lay down in it, and died' at Lewiston, Idaho.[22]

'A Hard story to believe comes from the Christian town of Jersey City': a man, seized with a malignant type of smallpox was refused admission to the police station and died on the sidewalk.[23]

'In Minnesota a Norwegian who lives a mile-and-a-half from that place, and in whose family are two cases of small-pox, made his appearance on the streets and caused a stampede.' A physician drove him out of town by threatening to shoot him.[24]

'In Jackson township last Thursday a case of smallpox was discovered. A colored girl named Holiday recently came from Pittsburgh to visit her uncle and was discovered with smallpox and quarantined. Dr. Barnes of Massillon was about to take charge of the case but was prevented from doing so by the expostulations of his neighbors.'[25]

'There is great excitement in El Paso at present on account of smallpox'. Fifteen cases are known in town, 'some patients are sitting around the streets on dry goods boxes, etc, and are shunned by everybody'.[26]

---

[19] As the previous chapters illustrate, acts of cruelty against cholera victims were rare.
[20] *San Francisco Chronicle*, 10 June 1876, 3.   [21] *National Republican*, 2 January 1881, 2.
[22] *Evening Critic*, 2 January 1881, 4.   [23] *Columbus Journal*, 4 January 1881, 2.
[24] *New Ulm Weekly Review*, 4 January 1881, 2.
[25] *Stark County Democrat*, 12 January 1881, 5.   [26] *Arizona Weekly*, 15 January 1881.

Pittsburgh: 'A smallpox hospital is on a boat kept anchored on the river. People living on the bank opposite object to its proximity and a conspiracy to cut it lose and sink it has been unearthed. The newspapers are now moralizing as to whether or not such measures would be justifiable.'[27]

'The prevalence of smallpox throughout the country has caused some strange exhibitions of fright and selfishness. Only nine miles out of St. Louis a negro lay sick with the disease on a pile of straw at the roadside. The next morning he was discovered badly frozen, but nobody went to his aid. He was left to die all alone, and did so after another night of exposure.'

'An Indian woman was left to herself in a suburb in Cincinnati. After her death the shanty in which her body remained was set on fire by throwing blazing wads of straw on it.'[28]

'Three children were abandoned by their parents at Selma, Tennessee. And in this case there was not the excuse of real danger, for the father and mother had been protected by recent vaccinations.'[29]

'The body of a five-year-old child found Saturday in the South Fordham Woods New York City was covered with sores and is supposed to be that of a smallpox victim, thrown out to avoid the quarantine that would follow.'[30]

Honolulu, Hawaii: 'In the search for nurses for the smallpox patients a well-known native woman was requested to act, as she had had the disease. "No," she replied, "go and get those Lunamakauuinanas who were so anxious to introduce the Chinese!" '[31]

'For several weeks smallpox has raged with great fatality in Jefferson Union County, Dakota.' Of ninety cases thirty-two have died. 'In many instances the dead are left unburied for days through fear and from inability to obtain help to inter them'. Jefferson (Alberta) is a 'French-Canadian settlement'.[32]

Cuba, Illinois: The father and mother of Miss Ball fled the house when it was discovered she had smallpox. 'For two days she was without medical or other attention save that rendered by a faithful brother.'[33]

The Washoe Indians have received orders from the city authorities to leave Carson, Nevada, and remain outside the city limits during the hot season. This plan has been decided upon to guard against the possibility of smallpox breaking out and spreading among the whites. The Piutes of Storey County[34] have been expelled from Virginia City because of smallpox. 'As with their neighbors the Washoes they are not specially clean in their habits—the same causes may lead to the same results.'[35]

James Hughes entered the First Precinct Station at Newark yesterday morning and said he was sick. When it was discovered that he had smallpox, he was sent to

---

[27] *Waco Examiner*, 24 January 1881, 2.   [28] *Highland Weekly*, 26 January 1881.
[29] Ibid.   [30] *Cambria Freeman*, 27 January 1881, 2.
[31] *Hawaiian Gazette*, 9 February 1881, 3.
[32] *Perrysberg Journal*, 11 February 1881, front page.   [33] *Daily Globe*, 19 February 1881.
[34] One of two Indian tribes in Nevada in the 1880s; *Sacramento Daily Record-Union*, 9 May 1881, 4.
[35] Ibid., 17 May 1881.

the office of the Board of Health. Health Inspector Mead sent him back to the station, where 'for nearly two hours Hughes lay in an alley next to the station'.[36]

Mrs Echert was sent to the Riverside Hospital; 'her two children, one ten, the other eighteen months, both more than half-starved, were turned adrift; neither the matron at the Central Office nor the Society for the Prevention of Cruelty to Children would accept them. At length, they were offered quarters by the health officers in the Smallpox Hospital and were fed in Eldridge St Police Station till morning.'[37]

'George Hoff, having the smallpox, walked fifteen miles in Somerset County from a farm house, where they would not keep him, to his home, where he arrived in a drizzling rain storm in a delirious condition.'[38]

'They have enlightened quarantine ideas at Austin [Texas]. Two children were attacked with smallpox and the city authorities resolved to isolate them. So they pitched a tent on the bank of the Colorado, outside the city limits, hoisted a yellow flag over it, and that tent is Austin's smallpox hospital. A wet norther, which is liable to ensue any day, would test the humanity of such hospital arrangements.'[39]

Louisa Courthouse (Louisa, Virginia): 'Christmas-day a case of smallpox was announced on the plantation of County-Court Judge Woolfolk, which the county physician examined. This was a colored man engaged as a labourer. On Monday he was removed to the hospital, but upon arriving was forbidden entrance by Judge Woolfolk, who declined to allow a smallpox patient to be forced upon him. He exhibited his determination by taking in hand a double-barrelled shot-gun. The physician repaired to town to obtain a warrant for the arrest of the unruly party; but the warrant was not obtained. The patient escaped through a rain storm, reached home at nightfall seven or eight miles away and was found the next morning in a feeble condition.'[40]

More than with any other disease, fear and social loathing of smallpox made its sufferers victims twice over. Moreover, smallpox inhumanity targeted 'others'— social and geographical outsiders, the poor, the tramp, the Chinese, the 'redskin', and the 'negro'. But outsiders were not always the victims. In a case from Mississippi, the victim was of the same race and church of those who tortured and murdered her: 'A negro woman supposed to have smallpox goes to church; she is run off and the next day her dead body is found. Ann Hughes, suspected of having smallpox, was brained with a bed slat by panic-stricken negroes at Columbus, Mississippi.'[41] Finally, permutations of the following story that usually did not make headlines or law courts were probably common: 'A breach of promise' case in Illinois: the plaintiff was 'a good-looking girl when the engagement was made. The smallpox disfigured her face and the defendant declined to marry her. He claims that in view of her deterioration in personal appearance since he made the promise, he is not, in law or honor, bound to keep it.'[42]

---

[36] *New-York Tribune*, 11 August 1881, 8.   [37] *New-York Tribune*, 31 August 1881, 7.
[38] *New Bloomfield Times*, 6 December 1881, 4.
[39] *The Waco Examiner*, 24 December 1881, 2.   [40] *Daily Dispatch*, 30 December 1881, 2.
[41] *Gazette*, 18 September 1897, 4.   [42] *Lancaster Daily*, 2 January 1882.

Further pitiless examples can be citied for the 1881–2 epidemic and afterwards. However, I close with a conversation between a citizen and doctor in 1881. With smallpox in decline around Johnston, Pennsylvania, a citizen asked his doctor, 'What is this smallpox?' The doctor replied: 'It is nothing except the neglect of the requirements of common decency.'[43]

* * *

What about stories reflecting the opposite—tales of self-sacrifice, compassion, heroic action? In comparison with yellow fever, influenza, and even cholera, such cases are extremely rare. Moreover, unlike community-spirited volunteers establishing soup kitchens during yellow fever or cholera epidemics, or teams of schoolteachers and debutants crossing class and racial boundaries to sweep the floors of indigent influenza victims during the deadly and highly contagious pandemic of 1918–19, the smallpox stories appear restricted largely to efforts by isolated individuals and their reportage used to foil the cases of selfish cruelty. Moreover, that compassion and courage was often restricted to the victims themselves:

'The entire Foster family were down with smallpox at Lexington, Illinois. The house was burned in the night. Rather than seek refuge with any of their neighbours, and thus spread the disease, they walked eight miles in the cold to a pesthouse.'[44]

'Smallpox has appeared among the immigrants in Cabarrus County, North Carolina. With local physicians refusing to attend, the Richmond & Danvile Railroad has supplied medical assistance. Who says corporations are soulless?'[45]

'Two deaths from smallpox at McCauleyville, Minnesota, and three others are in critical condition. Two physicians from Breckenridge, who entered town on an errand of mercy, are detained by armed guards.'[46]

'Smallpox is sweeping off the Indians of Northern Michigan, twenty having died out of the tribe located near Northport. The quarantine established cut off all medical aid, and a Catholic priest gave up his life in battling for the red men.'[47]

'Miss Teresa Harshberger, of Franklin borough [Cambria, Pennsylvania] is a Christian in act as well as in name. The children of Mr. John Hoy were down with the smallpox, a nurse could not be obtained and the mother was worn with watching and waiting. In this emergency Miss Harshberger, who had never had smallpox, went to the sick room and became the children's nurse. When the baby died, she prepared it for burial, and she faithfully attended the other children until they had recovered. Her action is in refreshing contrast with the conduct of the people who drove away two men who had buried a woman who died of smallpox.'[48]

'William Cook, sharing a single room with his wife and babe, was dying of smallpox. No one had visited the house for days. Mrs Cook gave a lighted candle to her husband, while she prayed at his bedside. Overcome by fatigue she fell asleep. The candle burned through the rigid fingers of the dying man, setting the bed clothes on fire. At the sight, Mrs. Cook fainted. A crowd of neighbors gathered at the window and looked in, but refused to cross the threshold of the

<hr>

[43] *Cambrian Freeman*, 29 July 1881, 3.   [44] Ibid., 1 April 1881, 2.
[45] *Anderson Intelligencer*, 26 May 1881, 3.
[46] *New Ulm Weekly Review*, 7 December 1881, 2.   [47] *Iola Register*, 30 December 1881, 6.
[48] *Cambria Freeman*, 6 January 1882, 3.

plague-stricken house. Finally, two men more courageous than the rest burst open the door and carried out the suffocating mother and child.'[49]

'In a Wisconsin lumberman's camp three men with smallpox were left by their companions with food and water for only three days. They would have starved to death, had a man, who heard of their plight, not gone to their succour.'[50]

Finally, an earlier story of heroism in the face of violent disregard for life, even of children, occurred in 1856, but was not reported until 1895. Immediately, it became a newspaper sensation, reflecting the current romance of the pioneering West and the dark side of smallpox that had become acute in the 1890s. Reverend Thomas Carlton with his wife and three children (an eight-month-old baby and two girls, aged six and three) left the Eastern United States for Grand Rapids. On reaching Grand Rapids, Mrs. Carlton died of smallpox. After the burial, the village was 'exceedingly anxious to have them move on', despite the road being impassable from deep snow. Carlton then aimed for Eastmanville, where he knew a minister of his denomination. But 'news of their exposure to smallpox preceded them'. Cold and worn out, the children nearly famished, the family, instead of a kind welcome, were met by the brother minister at the head of a mob, commanding them 'to continue on their journey'.

'The oxen wallowed on through the snow followed at a safe distance by the mob; when one of the oxen gave out Carlton gave up all hope of keeping his children alive.' Fortunately, they had stopped near the cabin of the trapper old Bill Nick, who, in spite of protests from settlers 'took the party to his humble home, threatening to shoot the first man who interfered'. The remaining ox died during the night, and Carlton was unable to proceed on the journey. He and his children were soon taken down with smallpox, 'and old Bill Nick watched over them for weeks without a soul to assist him'. The little boy died and then Mr Carlton. The little girls recovered, and in the spring, 'Old Nick sent them back to their people in Eastern New York'.[51]

Perhaps the reader might conclude that such stories were merely a fiction of contemporary journalism—sensationalism mixed with horror to enhance newspaper sales. Yet, to repeat, these stories were unique to smallpox and fail to appear with any frequency before 1881. By contrast, another disease that reached epidemic force, spreading panic during these same decades—yellow fever—filled these same newspapers with another side to be examined: individual and community abnegation in comforting the afflicted. Of the 2361 newspaper pages containing the keyword 'smallpox' during the 1881–2 epidemic taken from hundreds of newspapers, only two notices appear that praised individual altruism without stressing the opposite—the neglect and inhumanity of neighbours, relatives, clergy, state officials, the medical profession, and even charitable institutions. Moreover, unlike those in praise of yellow fever's secular martyrs featured in editorials and syndicated across papers, the two pieces on smallpox were brief notices only: 'The genuineness of the philanthropy of Mrs. Elizabeth Thompson has just stood a severe test.

[49] *Lancaster Daily Intelligencer*, 21 January 1882, 2.
[50] *Highland Weekly*, 26 January 1882, 10.   [51] *Omaha World Herald*, 28 March 1895, 2.

Smallpox having broken out in Stamford, Ct., where she spends a large portion of her time, she at once volunteered as a nurse, thus showing that she values her life no more than her money when the interests of humanity are at stake.'[52] And more telegraphic: 'A Catholic priest of Ellevue, Iowa, died of smallpox caught while visiting sick members of his flock.'[53] This near absence of compassion and courage was not peculiar to press notices in 1881–2. Searches for 'martyr' or 'martyrdom' associated with 'smallpox' through numerous smallpox epidemics across millions of newspaper pages contained in the 'Chronicling America' archive, from its earliest papers in 1836 to its endpoint in 1922, produces not a single hit, contrasting sharply with headline news from 1853 to 1905, celebrating those who gave their lives comforting utter strangers during epidemics of yellow fever.

In addition to exposing smallpox's power to engender selfishness and cruelty, the various stories cited here also expose racial and anti-foreign prejudices, as with the stories of afflicted blacks desiring assistance for their children rebuffed at the barrel of a shotgun, 'redskins' expelled from their homes from fear of smallpox spreading to whites, or callous neglect of medical assistance and supplies of vaccine to Amerindians, followed by blame because of their supposed 'unclean habits', then punished by eviction. Others blamed Hawaiians, the Chinese, tramps, and overwhelmingly the poor, victimized even by respected judges.

Despite condemning such neglect and inhumanity—sometimes subtly by solely presenting the 'facts'; sometimes blatantly with headlines such as 'Dastardly Work of Mob', 'Ignorant Cowards', 'Fiends in Human Form'—newspapers also broadcasted their prejudices of class, race, and ethnicity, as well as those of the public and the state regarding smallpox's origins and spread. Such expressions are visible across a wide range of newspapers from East Coast metropoles to small towns of the western territories. Their prejudices pointed in several directions: first against immigrants, and most prominently, the Chinese; then, native populations, Amerindians and Hawaiians. These varied by region. Most marked and the earliest were newspapers of western states and Hawaii, blaming the Chinese. Below are examples:

Headline: 'Chinatown Condemned: The Health Board's Investigating Committee Reports' [1880]. 'Sentiments of several physicians regarding the breeding of smallpox...were incorporated as being the views of the Committee...a severe condemnation of the manner in which the Mongolian inhabitants of the city live. The report adopted and unanimously declared Chinatown a nuisance.'[54]

In *The Daily Astorian* of Astoria, Oregon, a long, double-column article entitled 'A Pessimistic View' laid bare its anti-Chinese sentiment: At present, Chinese immigration to America is 'the size of an unchecked invasion', and 'if unchecked' is 'capable of an indefinite expansion': 'The Chinese bring with them customs and systems which displace our civilization...and in addition bring contagious disease. There have been already outbreaks of the smallpox on Chinese account in several parts of the country.... We hear of the smallpox first in those places where Chinese

---

[52] *Iola Register*, 29 July 1881, 2.   [53] *Daily Globe*, 2 December 1881.
[54] Ibid., 22 February 1880, 5.

are congregated—the Sandwich Islands, Peru, California, Cuba, and Australia. When it breaks out among them they are crafty enough to conceal it...They take no effective precautions...[making] many doomed to death by a loathsome disease.'

'When the smallpox makes its appearance on the Chinese immigrant steamers, it makes the round of the world....The mechanism for its dissemination throughout the country is now furnished by the Mongrel nucleus in every state...We cannot induce the vast mass of the Chinese nation to give up inoculation. They will, therefore, for generations continue to breed smallpox at regular intervals. As they move outwards they bring their disease with them.'[55]

Similar prejudices filled Hawaiian papers with cries for racial embargoes and hints of direct action and violence: 'The Lydia with some 700 Chinese...that she brings smallpox...requires no comment; nearly every coolie ship has had it which has come to us from China...another vessel with coolies is on its way...what powers are for stopping the inflowing tide of Chinese when the "Decima" arrives, let there be no hesitation as to what ought to be done with her.'[56]

With less rhetorical flourish, other papers presented their case more simply: Chinese in overcrowded steamers were the source of smallpox, and their 'so-called doctors' and communities habitually employed tricks to conceal cases.

Headline: 'The Case of the steamer Cassandra'. 'Every emigrant ship, especially those carrying large numbers of low-class Chinese, should be most scrupulously inspected....Here we have a youth of thirteen, who complains of being ill on the third day out, and his ailment is recognizable as smallpox three days later...The Chinese doctor takes the boy, locks him up in his own cabin, and succeeds in keeping captain and officers ignorant of what is going on. On arrival at this port, more than a fortnight later, the Captain is still deceived and answers "no sickness on board"....Some days later this youth is smuggled on shore at midnight and conveyed to a lodging in a populous quarter of the town...the police misled by the Chinese (so-called) doctors...owing to the criminal concealment practiced by the Chinese and the negligence of the captain of the ship.'[57]

Honolulu's *The Saturday Press* criticized the unregulated trade of Chinese labourers, which initially appears as an attack on traffickers and sympathetic to the Chinese but then launches into racist innuendoes about Chinese doctors and Chinese deception:

> Should it ever again become a necessity to bring over more Chinese, we hope that our Government may have a trustworthy representative in China, who may be able to prevent private individuals, Chinese or other, from chartering vessels, crowding them with the cheapest labourers to be got in the slums of Canton, and shovelling them down here, smallpox or no smallpox...Another thing to be thought of before importing Chinamen...is the appointment of a competent *white* physician for each ship. The Chinese doctors take an interest apparently in the speedy landing of the survivors of their passengers, and to effect this, do not hesitate to resort to endeavours to

[55] *Daily Astorian*, 8 January 1882, 2.   [56] *Hawaiian Gazette*, 23 March 1881.
[57] *Saturday Press*, 1 January 1881.

blindfold both the officers of the ship and the officers of the port...this kingdom is overburdened with Chinamen.[58]

When extended to Hawaiians, the racism could become more blatant:

> We have already called attention to the persistent practice of concealment amongst the natives and Chinese...We know for certain that the ignorant, uneducated natives, without any qualification whatever, are tampering with smallpox patients, helping to conceal them, treating them after their own fashion.[59]

Other papers pointed to native Hawaiians spreading smallpox because of their habits, ignorance, and deception, while excusing whites of any role in its transmission. Had the editors forgotten that Europeans carried this Old World disease to the islands in the first place, reducing Hawaii's pre-colonial population by 94 per cent in the century following Cook's landing in 1778?[60] Papers rewrote that history, blaming the natives themselves for their own disastrous decline:

> [The Hawaiian government] labored earnestly without stint of personal exertion or of money to which the foreigners as taxpayers were very far the largest contributors, this being, let us remember, a visitation [the present smallpox epidemic] that scarcely affected the whites. Abundant medical aid was provided, a large portion of the town population was supplied at the public expense and hospitals were built as fast as required. The danger of infection was urged on the community...How did the natives act? They hid their sick away, thus greatly adding to the difficulties the government officials had to contend...helping largely to spread the disease...Thus it appears that the decline of the race is owing to causes maintained in operation by the natives themselves.[61]

White settlers in Hawaii were not alone in blaming smallpox on the Chinese. According to an Oregon paper, '"China measles" is what they call the smallpox up at Dayton [Oregon]'.[62] A California politician, Dennis Kearney, who organized his campaign on anti-monopoly grounds, also played the race card, claiming that 22,000 Chinese who landed at San Francisco in 1881 'brought smallpox to the eastern states'.[63] Other places pinned other immigrants as carriers responsible for spreading smallpox. For New York City, Chicago, and St Louis, it was Bohemians, Germans, and 'the lowest of the Italians', because of their 'ignorance', 'prejudice', and allegedly 'hostility to vaccination'.[64] New York City's *Sun* focused its blame on Italian immigrants: 'A month ago a shipload of Italians again brought the disease to us and it is now more prevalent than we have known it in five years.'[65] A Dallas newspaper charged Russian Jews who had landed in New York with responsibility for the 1881 epidemic in Texas, even though they had been quarantined in New York for a month.[66] Other papers branded 'foreigners' more generally, because

---

[58] Ibid., 5 March 1881, 2.   [59] Ibid., 23 April 1881, 2.
[60] Crosby, 'Hawaiian Depopulation', 176–9.   [61] *Hawaiian Gazette*, 23 November 1881, 2.
[62] *Daily Astorian*, 5 November 1881, 3.   [63] *Waco Examiner*, 29 January 1882, 2.
[64] *Sun*, 12 December 1881, 2.   [65] Ibid., 20 January 1881.
[66] *Waco Daily Examiner*, 12 January 1882, front page.

'as a class' they are 'hostile to vaccination'.[67] The *Sacramento Daily Record-Union* claimed that smallpox had become epidemic in Chicago because it 'raged furiously in the uncleanly haunts of the foreign population', and 'these stupid people' could not grasp the importance of vaccination. The paper continued: 'No doubt filth and frowsy ways of living have much to do with it ... The clothing is habitually distributed among the relations ... If the tenement houses could be "flushed" as the sewers are, such a process would also tend greatly to the diminution of danger'.[68]

Other papers focused on 'immigrants' in general, citing statistics of those arriving in harbours such as New York's and assuming that the 'dreaded disease was amongst them'.[69] Others proclaimed that 'many physicians of great experience' confirmed that smallpox's source is the emigrant.[70] Still others mixed immigrant prejudice with religious bigotry. *The Omaha Daily Bee* attributed its city's cases to 'the newly arrived Mormon emigrants'.[71] Some members of Congress went further, establishing an inquiry that held Mormons were in collusion with the tribes of the Piutes and Navajos as smallpox spreaders, 'inciting' the smallpox outbreak in 1881, along with ordering the assassination of President Garfield that year.[72]

Notions of the immigrant were not limited to those arriving from foreign nations. In California, anyone from outside the state was labelled an immigrant. A Sacramento paper asserted that the disease's origins were 'immigrant trains', and the State Board of Health proposed stopping them at the American River Bridge to be examined by surgeons before allowing them to continue.[73] At the end of 1881, the same newspaper reported: 'Chicago is talking of quarantining against New York ... and we should think that New York ought to quarantine against Chicago. In fact, the evidence all points to the latter city as being the focus of contagion.' The paper then reiterated its plea of a month earlier: 'no relaxation of vigilance should be permitted at our frontier'.[74] Even different cities within the same state attempted to 'quarantine' those from other cities: 'Seattle has quarantined against Tacoma'. It is also 'rumoured' Steilacoom will soon follow Seattle's example.[75]

Finally, the internal migration that received the most heightened prejudice and alarm was one that coupled class with movement. The major bugbear of smallpox in the US in 1881–2 as well as of later smallpox epidemics was the tramp, who was not just impoverished, idle, and a wanderer, but often was also a 'negro'. Papers blamed them for their 'spirit of movement that infests this country ... little caring whether they spread disease or fall victims. ... The prevalence of disease can be traced to this method of transmission, their movement.'[76] The *Nashville Banner* predicted: 'If we could keep out tramps [which it defined above as Negroes], we

[67] *Somerset Herald*, 11 January 1882.
[68] *Sacramento Daily Record-Union*, 18 October 1881, 2.
[69] *Nebraska Advertiser*, 29 December 1881, front page; also, *Iola Register*, 24 June 1881, 2; *New Ulm Weekly Review*, 15 January 1881.
[70] *Sacramento Daily Record-Union*, 3 November 1881, 2.
[71] *Omaha Daily Bee*, 13 July 1881. [72] *Salt Lake Herald*, 28 January 1882, 4.
[73] *Sacramento Daily Record-Union*, 9 November 1881, 2. [74] Ibid., 8 December 1881, 2.
[75] Ibid., 14 November 1881, front page; *Los Angeles Times*, 16 July 1892, 4.
[76] *Columbian*, 3 February 1882, 3; and *Milan Exchange*, 4 February 1882, front page.

never more would hear of it in Tennessee…no one knows in these days of rapid transit when we may push up against a tramp with it.'[77]

Of course, as known from frequent flying today, rapid mass movement carries diseases and creates pandemics, which in earlier civilizations would have remained in isolated enclaves. Perhaps we should give credence to the various reports and accusations above: foreigners and immigrants carried the disease to America and were the agents of its epidemic force, even if the papers' jingoistic, often racist, rhetoric might be softened. However, one paper, which had supported the connection between Chinese immigrants and the spread of smallpox, recorded statistics compiled by the physician at San Francisco's Smallpox Hospital in the epidemic of 1876, and these failed to corroborate the general belief among journalists as well as physicians: '71 cases of smallpox have been admitted this month: 51 white males, 11 white females, 5 Chinese males, 3 colored males'.[78] By the epidemic of 1882, medical reports and counts of smallpox cases became more exacting, especially as discovered on ocean vessels carrying Russian, Jewish, Italian, Chinese, and other immigrants. In the very papers that earlier alleged that these vessels had been the bearers of smallpox epidemics, the statistics told a surprising story. At a medical convention in Chicago, doctors and Health Board officials declared that immigrants from Germany had spread smallpox through the city and then throughout America.[79] Yet among the attendees, the head of Chicago's Quarantine Hospital presented statistics from examinations of all passengers arriving at Chicago's harbour: of the thousands to have arrived during the present epidemic, only one case of smallpox had appeared, and, in that case, a man had caught it after his arrival.[80]

These statistics were not exceptional. At the ports of Milwaukee, Baltimore, and Port Huron, Michigan, over 10,000 immigrants were arriving monthly, but only three cases of smallpox had been detected.[81] In February 1882, *The Hawaiian Gazette* analysed smallpox cases on the islands since its disastrous epidemic of 1853. Although it may have exaggerated the impact of the 1853 epidemic,[82] it paid scrupulous attention to the statistics at its fingertips during the present epidemic. The evidence should have silenced other editorials published by this paper that year:

The idea so commonly current among the natives and even among a large portion of the foreigners, that the disease was brought into the country on this particular occasion [1881–2] by the Chinese is effectively disposed of. The smallpox was *not* brought in by Chinese passengers but by the officers and the crew of the *Quinta*. We understand

[77] Cited in *Milan Exchange*, 4 February 1882, 4. Southern papers were not alone in fixing smallpox on the 'tramp laborer'; see *Perrysburg Journal*, 14 October 1881, front page; and *Omaha Daily Bee*, 14 February 1882, 6.

[78] *San Francisco Chronicle*, 26 July 1876, 2.   [79] *Baltimore Sun*, 25 June 1881, 4.

[80] Ibid., 25 June 1881, 4.   [81] *Chicago Daily Tribune*, 30 June 1881, 9.

[82] The paper concluded that this epidemic levelled a third of Hawaii's population. According to Crosby, 'Hawaiian Depopulation', 191, the epidemic was the worst in the islands' history—6405 cases, 2485 deaths; the decline, however, was 13 per cent, from 84,000 (1850) to 74,000 (1854).

that the government officers have traced back the cases and they find three centres from which the disease was disseminated, and not one of these was Chinese.[83]

Towards the end of the epidemic in late October, Honolulu's *The Saturday Press* published further statistics from Hawaii's hospitals during the 1881 epidemic, divided into 'Chinese', 'native', and 'white' populations of the islands. The Chinese were neither the reservoirs nor spreaders of smallpox. Of 575 cases treated, forty-nine afflicted the Chinese, 8.5 per cent of cases, and only nine of 202 died from it, less than 5 per cent. The Chinese lethality rate was about half that of natives and lower still than that of the more privileged and supposedly more hygienic white population.[84] Yet into the twentieth century, physicians and papers continued blaming the Chinese as more susceptible and responsible for smallpox.[85]

With the epidemic on the decline, the New York *Sun* published statistics on its front page, which undermined its previous claims and those of papers across the US:

> Since January 1 a little over 100,000 immigrants have arrived at Castle Garden and [it is] said there have been twenty cases of true smallpox...The rarity of sickness among the immigrants has been so noticeable that the health officials have been led to give special attention to the incoming steamships in order to assure themselves that cases of sickness were not being overlooked by the inspecting officers. There was not one case of sickness among the 1,550 steerage passengers who arrived last Sunday in the steamship 'City of Paris'.[86]

Newspapers rarely print stories of non-events even if they might serve as correctives to prevailing myths. Occasionally, however, such stories surface as with one from the *Evening News* of Sault Ste. Marie, Michigan, in 1888, when smallpox raged in Hong Kong. Its headline admitted: steamers landing at San Francisco with passengers from Japan and China without any cases of smallpox were 'contrary to all expectations'.[87]

* * *

Although cholera in continental Europe continued to trigger massacres in Russia and Italy into the second decade of the twentieth century, it occasionally produced

---

[83] *Hawaiian Gazette*, 16 February 1881, 2.
[84] *The Saturday Press*, 22 October 1881, 2.

Smallpox Cases, Hawaii's hospitals, 1881

Cases	Deaths		Percentage
Whites	17	4	23.53
Chinese	49	9	18.37
Natives	509	188	36.94
Totals	575	201	34.96

[85] Echenberg, *Plague Ports*, 262–3.
[86] *Sun*, 30 April 1881, front page. For a week the following year, *New York Times*, 14 May 1882, reported 17,392 immigrants passing through Castle Garden and only four smallpox cases.
[87] *Evening News*, 25 February 1888, 2.

stories of altruism and self-sacrifice. In addition to those highlighted in Italy from the 1860s to 1880s, they appear elsewhere as with one from Berlin that singled out its Jewish community for praise during a cholera outbreak in 1837:

> This religious community [that of the Jews], always benevolent, have at the present alarming crisis, not only contributed handsomely to the municipal commission in aid of the sick poor, but have made the most liberal arrangements in their own hospital, so that the infected, whether of the Jewish or the Christian faith, meet with prompt and gratuitous admission.

As with the rare smallpox examples of altruism, this story too had a sting in its tail:

> Such conduct [of the Jews] is the more commendable, from contrast with the selfish intolerance of the general sanatory [sic] committee, which scarcely, if at all, admits sick Jews, but refers them to their co-religionists. So narrow a policy is everyway unworthy of Berlin, which pretends to stand forward eminently in philanthropic designs. Notwithstanding the inhumanity of this exclusion, the Jewish families are acting nobly towards their Christian domestics, tending the most dangerously affected at their own residences with untiring solicitude.[88]

Moreover, with cholera, the self-sacrifice of groups such as mayors, town counsellors, the clergy, and especially physicians is patent. Despite the double danger—the perceived contagion of cholera made worse by crowds calling them murderers, destroying their ambulances, and on occasion ending their lives with extreme brutality—these professionals usually persevered often without compensation. To be sure, some such as the surgeons of Paisley in 1832 or those in Parma in 1887, resigned in protest because of the threats. But others continued risking their lives, some travelling from one cholera hotspot to the next, as related in Thomas Shapter's eyewitness accounts in Exeter in 1832[89] and those of an anonymous English physician in Ireland in September 1832, who treated cholera patients in at least nine different regions.[90] Moreover, ceremonies of thanksgiving and public appreciation for these sacrifices could celebrate the end of a cholera epidemic, as in Exeter when 'the poorer classes deeply regretted' their previous 'unhappy prejudice' and 'inveterate hostility' towards the medical profession. They made subscriptions to fund a lasting memorial to Exeter's doctors,[91] and the Corporation for the Poor presented physicians with certificates of praise and monetary awards.[92] Similarly, after Philadelphia's trial by cholera in 1832, various Christian denominations organized a day of thanksgiving to recognize the sacrifices of the Sisters of Charity and thirteen physicians, who had entered the city's

---

[88] From the *Hamburgh Nachrichten*, translated in the *Guardian*, 7 October 1837, 2.
[89] Shapter, *Exeter*, 255–64.　　[90] *The Literary Gazette*, 9 October 1832.
[91] Shapter, *Exeter*, 258–60.
[92] Ibid., 261–2. Also, see the obituary of Rev. W. Nelthorpe Hall, *Chinese Recorder*, 1 November 1878, 460, for his visitations 'night and day' to cholera patients in Tienstsin in 1862.

hospital at the epidemic's height, after nurses had died or abandoned their posts.[93] By contrast, at the end of smallpox epidemics, I have yet to find any hints of gratitude, even from medical professionals to themselves. We now turn to the bloodier consequences of smallpox fear and hatred, from cruel neglect and vicious blame to collective violence.

[93] Watson, 'The Sisters of Charity', 13. Also, during the 1832 epidemic in Quebec, residents of Saint Roche and Saint John honoured a blacksmith who risked his life assisting cholera victims; Bilson, *A Darkened House*, 30.

12

Smallpox and Collective Violence

Despite the wide array of smallpox prejudice—racist, anti-foreign, anti-immigrant, anti-Chinese, anti-Mormon, anti-Italian, anti-Semitic, anti-indigent, and above all, against the victims of the disease—its fear and hatred sparked few large-scale incidents of collective violence, at least compared with cholera's or plague's. Nonetheless, I have found seventy-two incidents of collective protest in North America. Yet despite the vast literature on historical smallpox, scholars have mentioned only a few.

During the eighteenth century, controversies over inoculation gave rise to several riots. In response to Cotton Mather's support of Dr Zabdiel Boylston's inoculation campaign in Boston, crowds firebombed Mather's house on 14 November 1721. When inoculation hospitals opened in Salem and Marblehead in 1773, residents destroyed the one in Marblehead in January 1774, and closed the other.[1] In addition, a procession of a thousand men tarred and feathered four men suspected of carrying smallpox, 'drummed' them out of Marblehead, marched them to Salem, and paraded them through town.[2] Two more violent smallpox protests, both in Norfolk, Virginia, can be added, in June 1768 and May 1769 respectively. They concerned pro- and anti-inoculation factions, where both sides were comprised of elites in colonial plantation society, and some even from the same family, as with the Calverts, opposed one another. Unlike later smallpox riots, the divisions here concerned political ideology, not class, with the anti-inoculationists as patriots and those sponsoring inoculation, sympathetic to the Crown. The first riot consisted of 'organized mob attacks' on the plantation of Dr Archibald Campbell, who conducted inoculations for the wives and children of friends. Two days later, his house was torched. The second involved mostly the same individuals, but with the provocation now stemming from inoculating black slaves, exposed to smallpox in the West Indies. Mobs appeared at the plantations of three pro-inoculationists and damaged their houses. Unlike future smallpox riots, both the victims and targets were the elites.[3]

---

[1] Fenn, *Pox Americana*, 36 and 38; Toner, 'History of Inoculation', 180–1. For the incident at Marblehead, see *Massachusetts Spy*, 26 November 1800.

[2] A retrospective essay in the *Boston Journal*, 24 November 1901, 4, explored the burning of Cotton Mather's house (1721) and the attack on Essex Hospital, Cat Island (1773).

[3] Dewey, 'Thomas Jefferson's Law Practice', 40–1 and 43–4; and Henderson, 'Smallpox and Patriotism'. Maier, *From Resistance to Revolution*, 4–5, only mentions the Marblehead riot and one in Norfolk.

Beyond these, few smallpox riots have been investigated in the secondary literature.[4] Surprisingly, the mass destruction of the quarantine hospitals on Staten Island of 1 and 2 September 1858 has yet to receive serious analysis, despite the demolition of the thirty-two buildings—hospitals and shanties holding smallpox and yellow fever patients—the death of at least three smallpox patients and another with yellow fever, and the murder of the chief doctor's stevedore, shot in the back by the mob. A four-page article published in 1926 relied principally on judicial records that acquitted the two wealthy ringleaders of the September riots—Ray Tompkins, son of a former Vice President, and Jacob Vanderbilt.[5] No other mob violence in the US set off by concerns over infectious diseases resulted in more costly destruction to property or greater loss of life than this anti-quarantine violence directed in large part against smallpox sufferers.[6]

Despite the absence of recent historical research, a wide variety of newspapers across America reported the attacks.[7] Moreover, these lived a long time in the collective memory, one unequalled by any other US riot connected to any disease. New York's *Sun* ran retrospectives on the riots in 1868[8] and in 1897.[9] The capital's black newspaper, *Washington Bee*, 'celebrated' the thirtieth anniversary of these riots with a long description of the major events, terror, and damages inflicted.[10] A trial of New York City's police superintendent charged with malfeasance in 1898 sent journalists to their archives to review the precedent set in 1858, when the chief of police was arrested for failing to heed the governor's call to send forces to quell the riot.[11] In 1901, the *New-York Tribune* praised New York's Eighth Regiment for suppressing the riots. In 1906, from across the country, the *Albuquerque Evening Citizen*, listing the most 'Interesting Events in American History', gave the quarantine riots pride of place for 1858.[12] Finally, in 1921, three generations later, the *Evening World* revisited the events to reflect on Guy Walzer's candidacy for the New York assembly. His grandfather was the health officer at the quarantine at the time of the riots, when he chased 'the mob' away with 'his old flintlock'.[13]

Should we include these riots as smallpox collective violence? Even if these buildings housed principally smallpox patients (as reports in September make clear),[14] 1858 was not the year of a smallpox epidemic and the quarantine buildings also held patients taken from steamers in New York City harbours with yellow fever. Yet fears of smallpox were certainly behind the better-off citizens' ruthless

---

[4] For Milwaukee—Leavitt, 'Politics and Public Health'; Craddock, *City of Plagues*, 87 and 108. For Montreal—Bliss, *Plague*. And several at the end of the nineteenth century—Willrich, *Pox*.

[5] Garrison, 'The Destruction', justified the exoneration of the elite mob.

[6] These events received attention in Britain and in Latin America: *Panama Star*, 16 September 1858, 2; and *Royal Gazette*, 21 September 1858, 3.

[7] For instance, *Daily Dispatch*, 6 September 1858, and *Burlington Free Press*, 10 September 1858.

[8] *Sun*, 9 July 1868, 2.   [9] Ibid., 14 March 1897, 4.

[10] *Washington Bee*, 6 October 1888, 2.

[11] *Sun*, 27 March 1898, section 3, 7; *Daily Press*, 12 May 1898, 2.

[12] *Albuquerque Evening Citizen*, 30 August 1906, 2.

[13] *Evening World*, 28 October 1921, 17, from its archive, 4 September 1858, 2.

[14] *Daily Dispatch*, 6 September 1858.

attacks that were fuelled by their principal concern—property values. They railed against the governor and commissioners in charge of New York's quarantine for imposing a quarantine hospital on their island, and the first of the thirty-two buildings to be torched was the largest of them—the smallpox hospital.[15] Unlike the prejudice and cruelty seen in Chapter 11, Staten Island's mobs did not attack patients directly. However, they cared little for them, and several died as a result of the rioters' arson.

The anti-quarantine sentiment is better seen in Staten Island riots the previous year, after the state placed a temporary hospital at Sequine's Point. Two occurred, which drew blueprints for the 1858 conflagration and probably involved many who rioted a year later. In contrast to 1858, the riots of 1857 were not stirred by new cases of smallpox, yellow fever, or other diseases carried by foreign vessels. Instead, they were angered by the placement of New York State's principal quarantine hospital in their backyard. The first of these violent protests occurred on 6 May just before midnight, when 'a mob' of forty destroyed new quarantine buildings just purchased by the Quarantine Commissioners.[16] A picture of Mafioso *omertà* ensued: Governor King offered a reward of $5000 for the incendiaries, but as soon as the proclamations went up, they were torn down. 'The oyster dealers say no man on the Island would dare betray any of the parties engaged in that affair'.[17] However, as with the larger riot of 1 September 1858, commandeered by a Vice President's son and the brother of Commodore Vanderbilt, 'the mob' made no attempt to disguise themselves.[18] The police was 'scarcely less flagrant' than the rioters; they refused to protect the new buildings, and the mayor supported the police's inaction.[19] In the second week of July 1857, a larger 'gang of 150 disaffected inhabitants' attempted another assault on what remained of the quarantine ruins; now the police acted. Shots were fired, an officer was wounded, and several 'assailants' may have been killed.[20] The social dimensions of these riots had much in common with later collective violence that arose from smallpox. We turn to that history.

*   *   *

No smallpox riots came close to the scale of those on Staten Island until after the 1880s. Some, however, were arguably more brutal in terms of their intentional torture and murder of individual smallpox victims. No correlation linked the severity of smallpox epidemics to the frequency or size of the riots. My newspaper searches reveal no incidents of collective violence connected with probably the worst pandemic of the nineteenth century, that of 1852–3. After the colonial smallpox riots, only one riot appears before the anti-quarantine riots of 1857–8,

---

[15] Ibid. Also, see Chapter 18.
[16] *Daily Dispatch*, 9 May 1857, 2; *Burlington Free Press*, 15 May 1857, 2. *New York Times* did not report it.
[17] *Evening Star*, 14 May 1857, front page.   [18] *Burlington Free Press*, 15 May 1857, 2.
[19] *New-York Daily Tribune*, 19 May 1857, 4.
[20] Ibid., 5; *Wheeling Daily Intelligencer*, 14 July 1857, 3, maintained the assailants were oystermen 'and others'.

despite thousands of newspaper pages reporting smallpox, and it derives from a single oblique sentence in one paper alone: 'A mob in Cleveland, Ohio, week before last [around 14 August 1845], attacked and totally demolished the City Hospital that had just been erected for small-pox subjects.'[21] Moreover, between the Staten Island riots and the epidemic of 1881–2, only two smallpox riots surface. In Oakland, California, in 1868, a pesthouse placed near the properties of the privileged sparked the first of these riots, and the single paper reporting it supported the citizens, whom the paper took pains to distinguish from a mob of 'noisy' lower classes. As with most smallpox riots, no arrests were made.[22]

The second of these comes during the epidemic of 1871. At Cadiz, Ohio, 'a young gentleman from Troy was suddenly attacked with varioloid',[23] which 'the hotel people' at once decided was smallpox. A 'mob of townspeople' seized the victim, tied him up in a sack, threw him through 'his chamber window in a driving rain storm', then carted him to a deserted cabin on the outskirts, where he was 'put in charge of a half-lunatic negro' and ordered to remain there. 'Uncared for and neglected medically', he died. To add further injury, the town's authorities ordered his body to be buried in an open field. A journalist then questioned: 'If the comparatively common malady, smallpox, can demoralize a community, what shall we witness when cholera comes among us!'[24] But no one to date has spotted much more than a handful of cholera riots in the US. The journalist's point underlies assumptions in the historiography that diseases without cures and preventative measures are the ones to 'demoralize' societies, leading to blame and violence. America's experience with smallpox calls these assumptions into question.

As with stories of prejudice and cruel neglect, smallpox riots mounted only with the 1881–2 epidemic, despite the 'laboratory revolution' being in full swing. These crowds differed from those in cholera riots. In the main, smallpox rioters were solid indigenous citizens or propertied white farmers. Before the Montreal riots of 1884, the exceptions to this rule occurred aboard immigrant steamers with passengers resisting compulsory vaccination. In April 1881 a steamship from London landed at New York City with several smallpox patients aboard. The passengers, nearly 1000 of them, were removed to a quarantine centre for vaccination. While those in cabin class consented, 150 'Russians and Poles' in steerage 'made strenuous objections'. A 'Polander' knocked the syringe from the doctor. 'Men shouted, women screamed' and threatened the doctor and crew. Eventually, 'the combined crews and doctors' forced those who refused vaccination to board a quarantine boat for Dix Island.[25] A riot aboard another steamer that arrived in San Francisco from Hong Kong on 6 May 1882 was larger and more threatening. Immediately, the quarantine officer boarded the ship to vaccinate the immigrants. Faced with mandatory vaccination, 'a howling mob' of 750 'enraged Mongolians' (e.g.

[21] *Times Picayune*, 28 August 1845, 2.   [22] *San Francisco Chronicle*, 24 November 1868, 2.
[23] Believed to be of a weaker strain of smallpox.   [24] *New-York Tribune*, 9 September 1871.
[25] *Sacramento Daily Record-Union*, 26 April 1881, 2; also in Britain: *Leicester Chronicle*, 4 June 1881, 4.

Chinese) 'armed themselves with sledge-hammers, capstan bars, axes, and every conceivable form of weapon', besieged the sides of the captain's 'hastily improvised fortress', and attempted to kill the ship's surgeon.[26] These were defensive riots and unlike cholera riots did not express fantasies about the medical profession or anyone else poisoning immigrants or the poor.

Several others on land followed similar patterns of resistance. During the 1881 epidemic in Brooklyn, the sanitary inspector ordered a sick boy showing signs of smallpox and living in a crowded tenement to be removed to Flatbush hospital. The boy's mother resisted. When the ambulance arrived, neighbours assembled and barricaded the door. Only with a reserve force could police remove the boy 'amid the hisses and jeers of a large crowd of sympathizers'.[27] Eleven year later, a similar neighbourhood riot occurred in Brooklyn. On 10 April 1892, a father resisted health officers, who tried to remove his son who was infected with smallpox. The father fired a revolver at the doctors but missed. The neighbours defended the father and rioted against the doctors until reserves arrived and carried the boy to the hospital.[28]

More often, however, the poor were the victims, not the perpetrators, of smallpox social violence. In addition, the prime object of assault was the smallpox pesthouse. In June 1881 in Kansas City at around midnight 'an armed mob' surrounded tents containing ten quarantined smallpox patients and 'at the point of loaded guns drove the suffering patients into the woods'.[29] During the same epidemic, the placement of a smallpox hospital on the outskirts of Topeka, Kansas, prompted elites to mob action. The Board of Health hired a building on the outskirts of town, but before the city could take possession, Topeka's businessmen rented the building, informed the Board it was no longer available, and warned that any attempt to transport smallpox victims into town would be met with force. Fearing bloodshed, the mayor revoked his order establishing a pesthouse.[30] Less than two months later, across the country in Maine, smallpox provoked similar 'excitement' at Saint Croix, New Brunswick. Across the river, more than a hundred workers had been exposed. By nightfall, all the bridges were under guard with no one allowed to cross.[31] Brutality against the infected could take a variety of forms. In May 1882, a train passenger was sick with mountain fever, but rumours spread that he had smallpox. At Emporia, Kansas, where he was to arrive, 'a shrieking, yelling mob of 800' lined the platform to prevent him from getting off. 'Afraid to land him', the train carried him to the next siding, where the conductor 'sidetracked him on the prairie'. The paper concluded that he would probably 'die of neglect'.[32] In addition to smallpox stirring collective violence from citizens, democratically elected governments engaged in attacks against smallpox victims through legislation and expulsion. By June 'several' Nevada towns had banished 'the redskins from

---

[26] *New York Herald*, 25 May 1882, 4; *Times Picayune*, 2 June 1882; *San Francisco Chronicle*, 17 May 1882, 3.

[27] *New-York Tribune*, 4 September 1881, 12. [28] *Baltimore Sun*, 11 April 1892, 5.

[29] *Kansas City Star*, 7 June 1881, front page. [30] *Iola Register*, 27 January 1882, 6.

[31] *National Republican*, 2 March 1882. [32] *Jackson Weekly Citizen*, 9 May 1882, front page.

their midst', ordering them not to return until fall. 'Fear of smallpox epidemic was the alleged cause for the ukase [a Czarist proclamation]'.[33] Indians were not the only ones expelled. With the next smallpox epidemic a decade later, municipal governments in Idaho targeted the Chinese and Japanese, forcing them to leave 'on the first train'.[34]

*   *   *

The epidemic of 1881–2 was a watershed in North America's history of disease, setting in motion a new trend in collective violence with new levels of brutality, focused on expelling or murdering smallpox victims. Afterwards, these incidents came in rapid succession. In October 1885, placement of a pesthouse again triggered a smallpox riot. This quarantine was on the smallest of scales, built 5 miles from Winchester, Kentucky, to house a single inmate—a 'colored' prisoner. As carpenters were finishing the construction, 200 farmers armed with rifles appeared in force. The sheriff and his posse tried to defend the carpenters but were driven back, and at night, the farmers torched the pesthouse and guarded all the roads leading into town to ensure the prisoner would not contaminate their neighbourhoods.[35] As with most of these riots, no arrests were made. Instead, the rioters succeeded: the town agreed not to send further cases to the country.[36]

The next reported riot came during the epidemic of 1893–4, when a 'mob' of twenty-five masked citizens of Rockford, Illinois, assembled at midnight at the town's pesthouse. The leader warned the health officer not to keep the patients in the building. The health officer assured them there was no danger of the 'spread of contagion'; every precaution would be taken. The crowd refused to disperse and threw rails at the chief of police. Law enforcers fired into the air; the crowd dispersed. As with other citizen mobsters, none was arrested.[37]

Further smallpox riots at the end of the nineteenth century reinforced the patterns seen above: crowds of elites or middling sorts, almost always white and male, besieged pesthouses that were ready to open in their neighbourhoods. They attacked minorities and the vulnerable, victims of the disease, and law enforcers if they intervened to defend the sufferers. The victims were often blacks, generally more susceptible to smallpox than whites. Smallpox may have been a factor heightening racism at the end of the nineteenth century. Often the newspaper entries were brief, giving few clues about the 'mob', other than that they were white. On 4 May [1894] at Miles Switch, near Eldorado, Arkansas, 'a mob' burnt a hut, where a doctor had isolated 'a negro', ill with smallpox, and 'cremated' the 'colored man'. According to some reports, the mob shot him before his cremation. At least seven papers reported the case, but none speculated on the rioters'

---

[33] *Nebraska Advertiser*, 23 June 1882, 7.

[34] *Evening World*, 28 July 1892, 2.   [35] Among others, *New York Times*, 6 October 1885.

[36] *San Francisco Chronicle*, 5 May 1895, 13.

[37] *Evening World*, 6 June 1893. *Rockford Daily Register*, 6 June 1893, 2: the rioters were from the city's west side, which may have socio-economic implications.

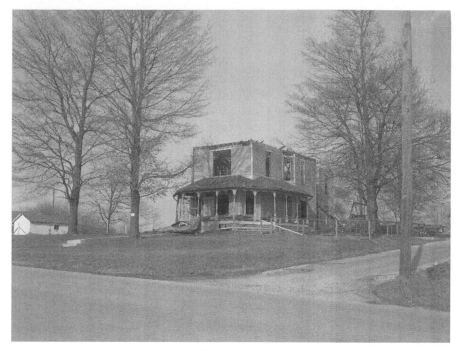

Figure 12.1. Smallpox pesthouse, Indiana, 1898.

identities, stating only that they were 'unknown', and no arrests were made.[38] Two years later, another racist riot ensued: William Haley, a 'colored' man, lay in a Memphis hospital, badly beaten and wounded with bullets in three places. Because of a case of smallpox in his family several months earlier, twenty 'whitecaps', had 'mobbed' him, 'clubbing him with guns and shot him before the eyes of his wife and children'.[39]

A year later, white farmers attacked another pesthouse. To accommodate thirty cases, nine-tenths of whom were 'negroes', a pesthouse was immediately built three miles from Bessemer, Alabama.[40] A day after its first patient—a 'negro'—arrived, a mob, composed of farmers from 'the neighborhood' came at night and 'riddled' the pesthouse with bullets. The guards, nurses, and patient fled. The mob justified their action 'as the best and quickest means of ridding themselves of [smallpox's] presence'.[41] Such incidents were not confined to the South. In 1896, at Grand View, a suburb of Kansas City, Kansas, a mob of 200 men, armed with guns, but 'urged on by a number of women', destroyed a pesthouse and scattered all its lumber

---

[38] *Alexandria Gazette*, 5 May 1894, 2; and at least eight others describe it. *Daily Herald*, 16 May 1894, 2, charged that the riot was a fiction of northern propaganda, since no southern paper reported it. But *Alexandria Gazette* and *Richmond Planet*, 12 May 1894, 3, certainly did.

[39] *Austin Weekly Statesman*, 9 April 1896, 9.   [40] 15 miles south-west of Birmingham.

[41] *Birmingham State Herald*, 27 July 1897; *New-York Tribune*, 28 July 1897, front page.

over a 10-acre site. The builders left the scene. As in many other cases, the 'angry citizens' prevailed without arrests.[42]

In January 1898, two further incidents arose, both in Wilmington, near Raleigh, North Carolina. For the first one, the notice is so brief as to obscure the motives and even the sides of the contestation. The Baltimore *Sun* simply stated that 'excited negroes' burnt down their pesthouse. With the second, the paper provided more detail. A 'colored' stevedore (James Harge) was being removed to another house 3 miles from town while the first pesthouse was being repaired; 'excited negroes' burnt the second one as well.[43] A local Wilmington paper changed the complexion of these protests. Three incidents occurred. The first, unrecorded by the larger-city papers, appears to have had the standard smallpox plot. The initial site to isolate the first black smallpox sufferer (not the stevedore but Stephen Johnson) was chosen in a sparsely populated area in the southern part of town, where white citizens resided. Between twenty and thirty armed white men gathered in front of the pesthouse and threatened that if Johnson arrived, they 'meant business'. Without hesitation, the mayor and the city's health officials changed their plan, housing him in a densely populated, predominantly black neighbourhood in the north-east of the city.[44] The story then changed colours. Three hundred black residents, armed with pistols, shotguns, and Civil War muskets, blocked all entrances to the proposed site, mounting guards of a hundred along the adjacent railroad tracks. Not only were they more numerous than the whites, the composition of the crowd differed, distinguishing it from most other smallpox protests. First, as with cholera riots, men, women, and children resisted, but more extraordinary still, white citizens joined in, making it one of two bi-racial smallpox riots that I have found. As with the earlier white protest, this one succeeded. No ambulance carrying Johnson arrived and, contrary to the Baltimore *Sun*'s report, no pesthouse had yet been burnt. The next day, however, a rumour spread that officials still planned the move, and the house was set ablaze. The health authorities decided Johnson would remain in his own house. As for the stevedore's case, after the health officials had removed him to the site 3 miles from the city, no rioting ensued.[45]

Another case that year was more straightforwardly one of racial brutality. In April, Henry Harris, an Afro-American suffering from smallpox in White Rock, South Carolina, was put under quarantine. When the attending physician returned, he found the house burnt, with no sign of the patient. During the night, 'a mob' had visited, forcing Harris to leave or be shot. 'To hasten his going, they set fire to the house. The man is supposed to have crawled off into a field.'[46]

Four years later, smallpox's usual pattern of elites inflicting physical violence on minorities or the poor resurfaced, but now with a change in geography and the

---

[42] *San Francisco Chronicle*, 30 March 1896, 2.   [43] *Baltimore Sun*, 17 January 1898, 7.
[44] Wilmington papers do not appear in 'Chronicling America' or the Readex collections. Their reports are summarized in Willrich, *Pox*, 85–6.
[45] Ibid., 86.
[46] *The Charlotte Observer*, 5 April 1898, 4, and five other out-of-state papers reported it. The state's *Edgefield Advertiser*, 15 June 1898, 3; and *Anderson Intelligencer*, 11 May 1898, front page, did not mention this incident.

race of those persecuted. Smallpox afflicted Calgary's small Chinese community, and those who were infected were removed to a quarantine camp outside town. Even so, a mob turned on the community within the city, ransacking a residence and burning it to the ground. Chinese men were attacked and their queues (waist-long ponytails) cut off. For weeks, stones were thrown through their windows, their doors kicked in, and laundries vandalized. Eventually, the entire community left. The mayor, who afterwards became the first president of the town's Anti-Asian League, refused to arrest any of the perpetrators.[47]

* * *

The Milwaukee riots, which lasted from 6 to 29 August 1894, appear as a defining moment in smallpox collective violence in North America. Crowds grew to the thousands, the composition of the rioters changed, and the police and health boards were forced to admit defeat. For a month, state and city officials lost control over an entire precinct of a major city. These events are among the few to have been studied but not in a wider comparative context of smallpox's social violence. The first Milwaukee smallpox riot of 6 August on the south side 'resulted in a decided victory for the mob'. Health officers arrived with their wagon to remove a second son of Fred Kellser, his first having died in the city's pesthouse three weeks before. A crowd gathered, declaring the child would not be removed. The police, forced to summon reinforcements, found a larger crowd of '300 excited men and women', blocking the streets and shouting loudly, 'the child should not be moved'.[48] To avoid a riot, the officers withdrew, but 'the mob', fearing their return, placed pickets to sound the alarm if they did, and remained assembled until the early hours of the morning.[49] 'The mob', estimated now at 3000, was comprised of 'men, women, and boys'. The police 'were powerless' and had to abandon their mission.[50] Thirty were injured, and women appear to have played a central role. First shouting in German, 'Down with the police'; 'Hang them'; 'Kill them'; 'They want to rob our homes', the women urged the men to throw stones, while others 'like German amazons' and 'demons' clubbed and stoned the officers.[51]

Two days later, a second 'rebellion' against smallpox ordinances struck the south side's eleventh ward. Again, crowd numbers exceeded those of any previous smallpox riot, and again included women and children. 'Assured of police protection', a Health Department van came to remove a child suffering from smallpox. When the van appeared, neighbours sounded the alarm. 'Inside of ten minutes' a mob of 'fully two thousand' arrived. With screams and threats against the officers, stones flew, but officers managed to break into the house, put the child in their van, and speed through the mob. A 'mass-meeting' was held that night, attended by 3000, 'a great many' of whom were women. Inflammatory

[47] Burnett, 'Race', 369–70, taken from Calgary's two newspapers.
[48] *Chicago Daily Tribune*, 10 August 1984, 2.   [49] *Morning Call*, 7 August 1894.
[50] *Evening World*, 7 August 1894.   [51] *Chicago Daily Tribune*, 10 August 1894, 2.

speeches were made against the Health Department and its commissioner.[52] Other newspapers put the crowd at 4000.[53]

Finally, on 28 August a third revolt occurred without a settlement in sight. With bold headlines, papers announced Milwaukee 'Abandoned to a Mob'. Women attacked and badly hurt the Chief Health Officer, when he attempted to remove a smallpox victim from the eleventh ward. It took fifty policemen and 'a pitched battle' to disperse the mob. Over a hundred policemen patrolled 'the riotous district', but without success. Pomeranian and Polish women, 'armed with baseball bats, potato mashers, clubs, bed slats, salt and pepper, and butcher knives', lay in wait all day for hospital vans to arrive.[54] By nightfall of the 29th, the Health Department abandoned the south side, leaving the ward in 'the hands of angry people', who marched through the streets hunting for quarantined houses.[55] The people's victory did not end Milwaukee's woes: two further riots of significant numbers followed, yet to be recorded in the historical literature. The following week, the removal now of the smallpox dead sparked a fourth riot on the south side. The Health Department ordered a quick night funeral, but when the undertaker carted off the body of a smallpox victim, 'a mob of five hundred' greeted him and his assistants with showers of stones, chasing them off without the body and then 'utterly demolish[ing]' the vehicle.[56] A month and a half later, when the police attempted to remove another smallpox sufferer, a 'mob' surrounded them, and a man with an axe struck at the chief inspector three times.[57]

Two months earlier, in Chicago, a similar riot occurred, though with scant attention from newspapers beyond Chicago and none from later historians. Another group of recent European emigres mobilized against health officers and smallpox control. As in Milwaukee, attempted removals of smallpox cases mobilized mobs, here comprised of 'Bohemians'; six health officers were injured. Patrol wagons arrived, but the officers gave no assistance, leaving a doctor 'half dead'; a health officer knocked down with a crowbar, with his face kicked in, jumped on and internally injured; another doctor knocked down by a club; an interpreter kicked and beaten, with facial cuts and a scalp wound; the driver of the ambulance stoned by the mob; an officer beaten, kicked, and bruised; and a second health officer flattened with a brick, his scalp torn and face cut.[58] As in Milwaukee, the 'mob' was comprised principally of women; here 500 were armed with clubs, assisted by men with pokers and crowbars and boys with rocks. As in Milwaukee, the mob won a temporary victory: two shots were fired; the police ran for their lives.

[52] *New-York Tribune*, 10 August 1894.
[53] *Big Stone Gap Post*, 16 August 1894; and *Vermont Phoenix*, 17 August 1894.
[54] Leavitt, 'Politics and Public Health', 406; *Chicago Daily Tribune*, 29 August 1894, 3 and 30 August 1894, 3.
[55] *Sun*, 29 August 1894; *Jasper Weekly Courier*, 7 September 1894; and *Fair Play*, 8 September 1894.
[56] *Chicago Daily Tribune*, 4 September 1894, 18.
[57] Ibid., 18 October 1894 and 12 September 1894, 4. The riot occurred on the night of 2 September.
[58] *Kalamazoo Gazette*, 1 June 1894, 6.

Instead of ending on 29 May, the conflict widened. Violence and distrust did not revolve solely around the 'ignorant classes among the Bohemian people' as papers labelled it.[59] The next day, the city staged a counter-attack, unreported by papers outside Chicago. Now, the more usual smallpox pattern of elites inflicting violence on the poor gained the upper hand. A hundred police accompanied health officers, raiding suspected tenements of Bohemians, smashing down doors, wrapping victims in bedclothes, throwing them into ambulances, and snatching infants as young as one and a half from their mothers. The police formed 'a formidable' block-long column and marched southward through the city's Bohemian neighbourhoods.[60]

Several days later, the community responded with collective action. This time, however, it was peaceful: two community leaders—Dr Julius Von Bernauer and the Reverend Vanek of the neighbourhood's Jan Huss Parish Church—held mass meetings. They provided damning testimony against city health officers and formed 'a vigilance committee' to protect the community from further outrages. Witness statements were collected on 'brutality beyond necessity', which included indictments against health officers intoxicated while on duty, others who solicited bribes to conceal cases, and careless fumigation, when officers suffocated an infant. In addition, the above-mentioned interpreter seriously injured a woman by striking her with the butt of his revolver. The committee used this evidence of terror and maltreatment to explain why the community had concealed cases. Had they been treated humanely, their Czech paper, *Dennu Hlasatrel*, maintained, 'none would object to vaccination or inspection to their premises'.[61] This final phase of Chicago's smallpox revolt was unique for smallpox violence in assuming a political phase that united a community's intellectual elites with its poor. With plague of the Third Pandemic, as we shall see, such configurations and ideologies were instead the rule.

* * *

Towards the end of the nineteenth century, at the settlement of Rocky Mount along the Norfolk and Carolina railway, two riots of a yet another character erupted. The first was rare in that it mobilized blacks when health authorities attempted to remove smallpox victims from their community to a pesthouse. Two hundred 'of their friends, well-armed, assembled and swore they would not allow the negroes to be taken'. Immediately, a second group of protesters combatted the first, reflecting smallpox's usual configuration of perpetuators and victims: whites armed with rifles and shotguns attacked blacks, clubbing several 'severely' and crushing the skull of one.[62]

From 1899 to 1904, a spate of large riots followed, mobilizing hundreds and, in at least two cases, thousands, with serious damage to property and life. As for reported collective action triggered by an epidemic, no period of North American history can compare, and outside the US and Canada, no country in Europe or Asia experienced similar violence with smallpox. In 1899, another part of the US showed

---

[59] *Chicago Daily Tribune*, 1 June 1894, 7.
[61] Ibid., 3 June 1894, 3 and 11 June 1894, 4.
[60] Ibid., 1 June 1894, 7.
[62] *Washington Post*, 26 June 1899, 3.

class alignments similar to the Milwaukee riots. Those from the lower classes attacked officers ordered to enforce quarantine and health measures. However, racism, first against Mexicans, then against blacks by Mexicans, continued as a factor.[63]

At Laredo, Texas, on 19 March 1899, the removal of ten Mexicans to a pesthouse provoked 'a mob of Mexicans' to assemble and attack health officers. The chief of police was called; the crowd, hurling stones and firing shots, successfully resisted the arrest of its leaders. A marshal was severely beaten before he could be rescued. 'About twenty shots were fired' and 'a dozen arrested'. The health officers resumed their work, but soon were confronted by another armed mob of 500 or 600 Mexicans. The health officers retreated and opened communication with the governor of Texas, who instructed the War Department to send troops. According to papers, one cause of the resistance was the Mexicans' 'contempt for the negro US soldiers'.[64] Two days later, violence erupted again over the removal of Mexicans to the smallpox quarantine. 'A Mob of 500 Mexicans' opposed US troops from Fort McIntosh sent to enforce the quarantine. Two more were killed and a captain of the State Rangers wounded.[65]

The following year (1900), an even larger riot momentarily seized a small Pennsylvania town. Various newspapers reported the events with dramatic headlines such as 'Mob Ruled a Town'. It lasted over two days, but I know of no historians to record it. Sparked by the Health Board attempting to convert an abandoned schoolhouse into a pesthouse, 'a mob of men and boys, numbering about 2,000' took possession of Turtle Creek, 8 miles from Pittsburgh. 'The citizens' blocked the entry of six smallpox patients to the new hospital. Twenty-five special officers were sworn in, 'but could do nothing'. The fire department turned their hose on the crowd, but the crowd cut the hose, pelted the firemen, and beat them with clubs.[66] To prevent the mob firing the building, the police drew revolvers and beat them back with the muzzles of their guns.[67] 'In the mayhem', a smallpox guard killed a patient.[68] After two days, 'excitement and anger' still smouldered.[69]

The same year produced a curious twist on smallpox protest at Centralia, Washington. Instead of the usual protest against the placement of a pesthouse, 'a mob of indignant citizens' pelted the Health Officer of a neighbouring town with eggs, sticks, and stones and chased him to the city limits. He had come to release a doctor who had spent a week in Centralia's quarantine because of suspected smallpox. The intervention incensed citizens, not because of fear of contamination but because the announcement of smallpox had stopped travel to Centralia, placing the residents under suspicion.[70]

---

[63] Willrich, *Pox*, 226.

[64] Numerous papers followed the story; for instance *San Francisco Call*, 20 March 1899; and *Detroit Free Press*, 20 March 1899, 3.

[65] *Idaho Statesman*, 20 March 1899, front page; and numerous other papers across the country.

[66] *Scranton Tribune*, 14 May 1900.

[67] *The Times* (Washington, DC), 15 May 1900, front page.

[68] *Biloxi Daily Herald*, 15 December 1900, front page; *Morning Herald*, 14 May 1900, front page; *Times Picayune*, 14 May 1900, 8.

[69] *Little Falls Herald*, 18 May 1900, 7.   [70] *San Francisco Chronicle*, 7 March 1900, 5.

In 1901, two smallpox riots erupted at Omaha, Nebraska. The first conforms to smallpox's usual pattern: 200 masked men armed with guns attacked police protecting a pesthouse in South Omaha on its opening day and attempted to burn it down. The following night, they succeeded: 'a crowd of men' of greater strength overpowered the guards and kept firemen at bay, who were forced to watch the building burn. As usual with 'citizen' mobs, no arrests were made.[71] In the same year, two further riots were reported widely in newspapers from Oregon to South Carolina. A 'mob' of 300 or 400 Italians[72] attacked the smallpox hospital in Orange, New Jersey, 'overpowering' a police guard. As with the Omaha riots, the Italians' first attempt failed. Two days later, armed with axes, crowbars, and other 'efficient instruments of destruction', they regrouped and razed the structure to the ground. These attacks were 'planned with great care and secrecy'. At 1 o'clock a pistol was fired, signalling men 'to pour out' from the surrounding tenements. In moments, the building was completely destroyed.[73] On first impression, the riot may appear to have resembled the kind of social conflicts typical of cholera— foreign emigres against authorities. The riot's social dynamics were not, however, the same. Instead, elites appear as the driving force behind the scenes. They supplied the Italians with weapons and fired the shot to begin the revolt. In addition, papers claimed the Italians had been paid $2 apiece 'for their services'.[74] Nonetheless, a residual fear and frenzied hatred of the Health Board's placing of a pesthouse in their midst seeps through. A day after the conflagration, the Italians attacked the pesthouse ruins, burning the debris.[75]

Less than a month later, 'a crowd of over three hundred men and women' destroyed another pesthouse in Pennsylvania, now at Bradford.[76] Again, plans to convert a building into a pesthouse provided the trigger. Surrounding the building, the leaders grabbed the night watchman, while 'the incendiaries' set the place ablaze. 'As the flames rolled and crackled, the mob howled its delight'. No arrests were made,[77] suggesting the usual pattern of rioters enjoying privileged status.

The following year, three further incidents flared up. The first at Bangor, Pennsylvania, mobilized 400 and recalls cholera protests of the Irish, resisting Health Board prohibition of wakes. 'A serious riot' followed the Health Board's attempt to bury an Italian woman who had died of 'malignant smallpox'. Four hundred Italians attacked the police, fatally injuring a police officer sent to disperse them. They brought the woman's body into their Catholic church and guarded it closely,[78] insisting that she had not died of smallpox and that her body should remain open to view for three days.[79] A week later, a smallpox riot showed that the characteristic pattern of double victimization had been resumed. The incident

---

[71] Ibid., 20 January 1901, 9; *Washington Post*, 21 January 1901, 4.

[72] The estimates varied: *Daily Journal*, 11 March 1901; *Albuquerque Daily Citizen*, 11 March 1901; and others.

[73] *New York Times*, 10 March 1901.   [74] Ibid., 12 March 1901.

[75] Ibid., 13 March 1901; also, *Kansas City Star*, 10 March 1901, front page; and others.

[76] *Scranton Tribune*, 12 April 1901; *Grand Forks Daily Herald*, 12 April 1901, 11.

[77] *The Times* (Richmond), 12 April 1901; *Stark County Democrat*, 16 April 1901; and others.

[78] *Scranton Tribune*, 20 January 1902, 8; *New-York Tribune*, 20 January 1902.

[79] *Fort Worth Morning Register*, 20 January 1902, front page; *Patriot*, 20 January 1902, front page.

erupted after police had chased and captured a man and wife suffering from smallpox. First, the wife was arrested and then her husband, in Greentown, Indiana, 10 miles east of Kokomo. He was housed with a carer, who had had smallpox and was judged immune. Soon a mob formed outside the house, threatening to burn it down and lynch the two, if the patient did not leave town immediately. The two opened fire and a night policeman, sent to quell the disturbance, was shot. The mob threatened to return to lynch the victim, but papers do not report if it did.[80] The third riot occurred in a region previously unseen hosting smallpox violence. It was probably on a smaller scale and, as with many others, revolved around fear and persecution of a single victim—an outsider, geographically and socially. In St Albans, Vermont, a crowd armed with clubs chased a tramp afflicted with smallpox from town.[81]

Two years later, a smallpox riot again occurred in small-town rural Pennsylvania. Although the number of participants was not large, the riot was planned and equipped with a new weapon of protest, dynamite. Unlike earlier smallpox disturbances, this was the first when relatives may have attempted to free victims from a smallpox hospital. But even if this were the case, it mentions no myths of 'liberating' patients and carrying them home triumphantly on shoulders. Instead, the instigators' motives remain unknown. In Shamckin, Andrew Sweitzer led an armed gang of ten against the Coal Township Emergency Hospital, where his wife and two children were suffering from smallpox. However, a patient seized a gun and with others went after 'the raiders'. The gang threatened to dynamite the hospital; the patients retreated. Later, 'a Pole', whose wife was a patient, tried to enter the hospital but was driven back at gunpoint. Sweitzer was arrested, and the hospital's guard increased.[82]

Two further smallpox riots appear at the turn of the twentieth century, reflecting different fears and objections from the majority of those encountered above. The first harks back to burial restrictions violating a community's beliefs and rituals. 'A mob of young men' prevented the burial of a smallpox patient in the village of Clyde, New York, after the local health officer ordered the body to be interred without delay.[83] Diverging from smallpox's general pattern, the second occurred in a large city—New York—and the rioters were the underclass. Here condescension and impositions from elites and the state provoked destitute 'negroes' and Italians to riot. But again cholera-like fantasies were absent. Instead, the police's heavy-handed tactics of forced evacuation were the cause. A cordon of police 'hedged in as completely as if in a pen...a mob of frantic negro and Italian residents', who tried to escape to safety. They appear to have been frightened by the removal of sixteen children, mostly under five, afflicted with smallpox, from a tenement.[84]

No further smallpox incidents of collective violence appear until 1920, and it was described as only a 'near riot'. Once again, a town's 'best-known citizens' comprised the 'mob'. Yet, its targets were not victims of the disease or the poor.

[80] *Evening Times*, 27 January 1902. At least five other papers reported it.
[81] *St. Albans Daily Messenger*, 16 June 1902, 2.   [82] *Washington Times*, 10 May 1904, 12.
[83] *Daily People*, 20 July 1900, front page.   [84] Ibid., 1 December 1900, front page.

Instead, the mob ordered the state commissioner of health to leave town. Similar to plague riots in turn-of-the-century India, this riot concerned enforcement of health laws.[85] The citizens objected to the commissioner's 'strong-arm methods' to vaccinate all citizens of Georgetown, Delaware, by entering businesses and demanding a census of those who had not been vaccinated. The citizens 'stormed' the hotel, where the commissioner was staying and drove him from town.[86]

* * *

To these North American smallpox riots, another cluster can be added from across the border during the epidemic of 1885 in Montreal. These show the same shift in smallpox riots seen in Milwaukee and Chicago. Within a three-month period, 28 September to 31 December, four major riots with crowds numbering over a thousand and a series of smaller ones occurred, amounting to at least eight separate protests in and around the city. Most of these received international attention.[87] Because of the anti-French-Canadian press in Montreal, papers such as *The New York Times* depicted the events as though they were in Italy or Spain in the grip of cholera.[88] The press sympathized with Montreal's elites (mostly of English origins) against the less privileged French-Canadian Catholics. Montreal's English papers, especially the *Herald*, with its 'PRO BONO PUBLICO' article published on the eve of the first major riot of 28 September, blamed the disease on French-Canadians because of their 'filthy customs', 'ignorance of vaccination', and the 'venality of their priests'.[89] New York's *Sun* followed, describing Montreal's two conflicting classes as different races, and, before any rioting erupted, charged the French community with 'harboring and breeding the smallpox'. Indifferent to its effects 'on the English population', the French population was accused of resisting vaccination and not complying 'with any sanitary measures' and fighting the disease only 'by pious observations and ceremonies'. The paper placed further blame on the 'backward' clergy, who preached that 'the plague' was sent as punishment for neglecting religious duties. There was no surprise, the paper concluded, 'that the believers in St. Roch...and those in St. Vaccination...soon fell to saying unpleasant things of one another'.[90] Moreover, tensions between French and English Canadians had escalated since the 1870s. A rebellion against the dominion in the north-west led by the ultramontane Catholic Louis Riel in the same year as the riots sharpened hostilities in Montreal.[91]

These confrontations pitched the French-Canadian Catholic working classes, who suffered the highest cases and casualties of smallpox,[92] against health authorities, the police, mayor, and eventually, the military. Compulsory vaccination sparked the riots on 28 September,[93] when 'a howling mob' surrounded the east-end branch

---

[85] *Evening Public Ledger*, 14 January 1920, 4.   [86] Ibid.
[87] *Scotsman* reported these in detail, 30 September 1885, 9 and 2 October 1885, 3.
[88] See Bliss, *Plague*, 120.   [89] Ibid., 126 and 131.
[90] *Sun*, 27 September 1885, 9; *Springfield Globe-Republic*, 28 September 1885, front page.
[91] On these 'two wars', see Bliss, *Plague*, ch. 3 and 262–6.
[92] Ibid., 259: Officially, 3614 died of smallpox in Montreal; 2887 were French-Canadians, 91.2 per cent.
[93] Ibid., 163: 'Compulsion' began on 28 September; yet nobody was to be vaccinated by force.

health office and wrecked the building. They then marched on the city hall, 'smashed' the central office, broke all the windows of the central police station, and 'wrecked' the windows of the *Herald* newspaper office, which had first published the derogatory caricatures seen above.[94] Smaller but 'serious' riots ripped through the city the same day. Protesters blocked the sanitary police from removing twenty-two cases from a tenement at the corner of Gasford and St Louis. Reinforcements arrived 'but the whole squad was driven from the premises'.[95] The events of the 28th produced smaller ripples the next day: two were arrested when a 'mob' attacked the sub-chief of police and his detachment near Bonsecour market.[96] A day later, French-Canadians were reported tearing down smallpox placards and beating isolated militiamen.[97] On 1 October, a 'crowd' in Marsonneuve Street with men swinging planks of wood and a woman armed with an ironing board threatened health workers affixing placards. When the officers returned with constables, the neighbourhood had mobilized 1600 of 'all sexes and ages', who jeered the constables, chased them away, and tore the 'obnoxious placards' 'into a thousand pieces'. The chief of police and medical health officer returned but 'had to beat a dignified retreat'.[98]

A week later, a riot arose with mixed motives. After the Health Board passed unanimously rigorous sanitary laws and made vaccination compulsory, 300 rioters attacked the Exhibition grounds, where a hundred carpenters had been 'working day and night' to complete a new pesthouse. The protesters threw stones at the cavalry protecting the site, wounding two and the guard's lieutenant. A full guard of mounted garrison artillery was dispatched.[99] Finally, three months later, at the end of 1885, another riot of major proportions erupted: because of the prevalence of smallpox in the adjacent village of Sainte Cunégonde, Montreal's health officials barricaded the village's exits. A mob of 2000 destroyed the barricades and drove the police back to Montreal; the military was summoned.[100] Fifteen minutes before New Year, 1886, the two communities negotiated a settlement. Montreal agreed to withdraw its quarantine, if the village enforced the city's health legislation.[101] But by then Montreal's reputation had been tarnished. Papers now called smallpox riots 'Montreal Pastimes'.[102]

The British press relying on news agencies and correspondents in Montreal reported only the initial riots in September and presented them narrowly as a revolt against compulsory vaccination, perhaps reflecting their own preoccupations in the 1880s.[103] Clearly, these riots combined a number of grievances with varying political agendas, which did not concern vaccination exclusively: some reflected

[94] *San Antonio Light*, 29 September 1885, front page; *Bismarck Weekly Tribune*, 2 October 1885, 2; and *Scotsman*, 30 September 1885, 3.
[95] *Perrysburg Journal*, 2 October 1885, front page.
[96] *Evening Star*, 1 October 1885, 3.   [97] *Abilene Reflector*, 8 October 1885.
[98] *Chicago Daily Tribune*, 2 October 1885, 2.
[99] *San Francisco Chronicle*, 7 October 1885, 3.
[100] *Daily Evening Bulletin*, 2 January 1886; Bliss, *Plague*, 254–5.   [101] Bliss, *Plague*, 255–6.
[102] *Daily Evening Bulletin*, 2 January 1886.
[103] On the anti-vaccination movement in the 1880s, see Bliss, *Plague*, 211; for Britain and internationally, Biggs, *Leicester*.

citizens' anxieties regarding where smallpox hospitals were placed as with Longue Pointe's 700 citizens, who in mid-October resisted Montreal's decision to build a smallpox hospital at their Christian Brothers epileptic home. As a result, these citizens (like protesters south of the border) threatened to burn the facility down.[104] In other cases, the social composition of crowds and tactics resembled more closely plague riots in India, by resisting the sanitary police's heavy-handed tactic of removing their children to smallpox hospitals. With the finale at Sainte Cunégonde, the conflict turned on political questions of municipal boundaries and sovereignty against threats by the metropolis. Finally, two riots reported by only one paper from my sample are difficult to fathom. With the initial uprisings on 28 September, working-class Catholic French-Canadians planned an attack on the convent of the Sisters of Providence. Several days later, 'working men from surrounding districts' attacked the convent of the Grey Nuns, forcing the city to summon 1500 troops. The paper made no attempt to explain why Catholic men would besiege their nunneries.[105]

Scholars have yet to ask why such frequent and ferocious smallpox violence was peculiar to North America and why it suddenly soared in the late nineteenth century. From French, British, Australian, Indian, Chinese, and US papers, I have spotted only a handful of smallpox riots beyond North America—Rio de Janeiro in 1904,[106] Kolkata in 1935,[107] and, as Chapter 13 will show, several in England. Despite the diligent and frequent reporting of the cholera riots throughout Europe and Asiatic Russia by hundreds of newspapers, only one story of smallpox collective violence emerges from my searches in continental Europe, and that story, covered by a single paper, was short and vague. In an unspecified 'Italian village', on an unspecified date in 1887, a 'mob' attacked 'some officials' trying to disinfect their homes to prevent the spread of smallpox.[108] As we shall see, such antagonism towards smallpox patients and the presence of pesthouses in people's neighbourhoods also increased in London at the same time. In England, however, as we shall see, the 'violence' differed.

* * *

In summary, North American smallpox riots varied widely in size, from gangs of ten with dynamite to organized crowds as large as 4000, who wrecked government buildings, successfully resisted the police and military, and took over districts of major cities. Towards the end of the nineteenth century, several of these began to resemble cholera riots in the composition of crowds, numbers assembled, and scale

---

[104] Bliss, *Plague*, 167.   [105] *Scotsman*, 2 October 1885, 3.

[106] According to Low, 'The Incidence of Small-Pox', 85–6, it was 'an open revolt' with barricades erected, tramcars burnt, and military law imposed for more than a month afterwards.

[107] This riot, which may have involved thousands, differed from any disease-fuelled violence seen in the Americas or Europe. A government order prohibiting self-torture as a penance when worshipping Mariamman, the goddess of smallpox, provoked it during a ceremony involving 10,000 to 15,000 participants, who pierced themselves with large hooks. The police were pelted with stones, the magistrate and sub-magistrate fled into the temple, were found and beaten, and the head constable was killed; *Straits Times*, 15 October 1935, 19.

[108] *New York Times*, 31 December 1887.

of violence. In US history no cholera or plague riots could compare. The trajectory of smallpox riots is, moreover, almost the opposite of what we might have expected from the literature on disease. Common and recurring diseases that were both endemic and epidemic, such as measles, whooping cough, dysentery, scarlatina, and smallpox, no matter how deadly, are perceived as the ones *not* to spark hatred and violence. Smallpox is doubly problematic: not only was it common, scoring deaths every year and recurring periodically with epidemic force, it was the only disease before the laboratory revolution with a well-founded practice of prevention—vaccination. Yet, by the epidemic of 1881–2, presently unnoticed by historians, smallpox had become America's disease par excellence of cruelty and blame. Except for five protests during the colonial period and the anti-quarantine riots of 1857–8, smallpox's social toxins lay largely dormant until the epidemic of 1881–2, despite the fact that earlier epidemics scored far higher mortalities.

Journalists of the late nineteenth century, in fact, posed the question: why had smallpox provoked so much social violence in comparison to other diseases such as diphtheria or tuberculosis, which had become bigger killers?[109] A Philadelphia journalist commented on a panic of Virginia state legislators during the epidemic of 1881–2. His speculations were the opposite of those now proposed by scholars to explain stigmatization of AIDS victims or of epidemics more generally:

> Consumption carries off yearly many times the number of smallpox victims, and the world resignedly bears the infliction—simply because it sees no help for it.... So of other great devastators of the race, such as cholera, yellow fever, scarlet fever, and diphtheria, smallpox losses are as nothing compared with the result of these scourges; yet medicine is practically hand-tied in all those diseases, while in the case of smallpox it has an absolute, undeniable cure—or at least preventive which is better than cure.[110]

So instead of the mysteriousness of a disease and physicians' inability to prevent it, medical success had led to smallpox's anxiety, fear, and hatred because 'others' refused the cure. As we have seen, blame for the 1881–2 epidemic in New York City, Chicago, and St Louis turned against 'Bohemians, Germans, and the lowest of the Italians', because of their supposed 'ignorance' and hostility to vaccination. Yet, against these expectations,[111] only several of the seventy-two smallpox riots I have found concerned inoculation or compulsory vaccination: four of the five protests in the colonial period, two against compulsory vaccination aboard immigrant vessels, and only three further cases, involving vaccination on US or Canadian soil. Moreover, vaccination was only one element of protest in several of these as with the Montreal riots or the attack on Georgetown's health officer.

Utilizing Chicago's Health Board statistics from 1870 to 1881, another journalist attempted to explain smallpox's tendency to arouse hatred and violence, compared with diphtheria and scarlet fever. He speculated that the age distribution

---

[109] Duffy, 'Social Impact', 798, argues that populations had grown accustomed to endemic big killers such as diphtheria and become fatalistic about them.

[110] Cited in *Daily Dispatch*, 19 January 1882, 2.

[111] The recent literature on conflict and smallpox has concentrated on vaccination; see Willrich, *Pox.*

of victims could explain the difference: smallpox 'rages among people of all ages', while diphtheria and scarlet fever were limited to children.[112] Yet, children were disproportionately spared by the influenza pandemics of 1890–2 and 1918–20, which as we will see did not ignite waves of violence, and the same goes for yellow fever.[113] Nonetheless, contemporary journalists of the nineteenth century (as with historians today) assumed that cholera's threats to public order were far worse than smallpox's or any other disease.[114] These reflections, no doubt, derived from Europe, whose waves, as John Duffy noted almost fifty years ago, dominated US papers.[115] But cholera violence in North America was much less frequent and on a far smaller scale, with only riot (and that one in Canada) drawing crowds which numbered in their thousands.

Not all epidemics had the same characteristics or socio-psychological consequences. For cholera riots, the protesters were usually outcasts—the poor, Irish immigrants, tribal Sarts, Pugliese fig-pickers, Venezuelan crabbers, and most recently, homeless earthquake victims in Haiti. Often their crowds comprised impoverished women and children and their targets, physicians and agents of state power. These rioters rarely turned on the victims of the disease; instead, they pictured themselves as the victims' liberators. For smallpox, it was generally the opposite. 'The respectable classes', the 'best-known' citizens, small-town merchants, or propertied white farmers comprised the 'mobs' that could be led by judges and shotgun-toting physicians and even include a brother of Commodore Vanderbilt. On the other hand, smallpox social violence targeted victims of the disease, making them doubly victims. They were also usually the underclass—the immigrant, the Chinese, the tramp, the 'colored'. Only a few assumed the class configurations of cholera, with health officers or the police as the principal victims. More strikingly, none of the seventy-two smallpox riots I have found carried conspiracies typical of cholera: fears of poisoning or a disease invented by physicians to cull the poor. Smallpox myths instead turned on racism, hatred of foreigners, and fears of the lower classes, expressed in individual and collective acts of intolerance, neglect, and cruelty against victims of the disease and rarely in riots in the thousands.

In addition, smallpox's social violence began late, gathering force only with the epidemic of 1881–2 with the laboratory revolution already in progress. Such violent victimization of 'others' and especially the diseased victims appears far less frequently with other epidemic diseases than historians presently presume. And in our time, the victimization of those afflicted with AIDS, certainly in the US and Europe, cannot compare with smallpox's record for cruelty with gunpoint mass expulsions of Amerindians, the torching of 'pesthouses' that cared for the afflicted, numerous murders, and the cremation alive of smallpox 'coloreds'.

---

[112] *Weekly Kansas Chief*, 2 February 1882, 4.
[113] Other journalists made more bizarre speculations, such as one in 1882 who argued that smallpox left 'no lingering seeds for subsequent diseases to start'; *Stephens City Star*, 4 March 1882, 3.
[114] See Chapter 11, note 9.
[115] Duffy, 'Social Impact', 800.

13

Smallpox Violence in Victorian Britain

To what extent can America's smallpox story of victimization be generalized? This chapter turns to England and concentrates on the same 1880–2 pandemic examined for the US.[1] The decision was not predetermined. Rather, 1880–2 appeared from my searches as equally pivotal in the emotional history of smallpox in England, even though, as in America, this epidemic proved less deadly than many previous ones in British history. Nevertheless, fundamental differences arise between the American and English experiences. First, in contrast to the US, stories of individuals' selfishness, neglect, prejudice, inhumanity, and violence against smallpox victims are almost wholly missing from the British papers. For the epidemic of 1882, the closest story I have found to hundreds readily gleaned from US papers comes from Arbroath, when the Board of Health quarantined a sailor in a ship in conditions the paper described as subhuman. He was forced 'to lie, in this broiling midsummer weather... under the deck of a small schooner, the temperature unbearable, with no ventilation...'. It was not, however, the cruelty of neighbours, as often seen with smallpox sufferers in the last decades of nineteenth-century America; instead the sailor's local community on land and the seas roundly denounced it: 'This callous treatment of a seaman is the subject of conversation amongst all... all seamen are loud in their denunciation of such heartless conduct.'[2]

The British press is filled, however, with collective actions of communities which sought to obstruct local health and asylum boards responsible for isolating and caring for the smallpox patients. Unlike the cruel direct action taken in the US, these communities did not employ Winchesters, break windows, burn buildings, or organize assaults that resulted in the cremation of smallpox victims alive. Instead of the streets, the arena of the British actions consisted of public meetings, occasional mass gatherings, but above all, legally constituted committees, such as the Boards

---

[1] For smallpox epidemics in nineteenth-century Britain, see Hardy, *The Epidemic Streets*. With 44,500 deaths in Britain and nearly 8000 in London alone, the epidemic of 1870–2 was the worst of the century (26). Yet, the 1880–2 epidemic produced almost as many newspapers articles as in 1870–2 (*Nineteenth Century British Library Newspapers*). According to Creighton, II, 615–26, England's smallpox epidemic of 1837–40 was 'the great' one. However, 1870–2 produced as many deaths in two years as the 1837–40 one did in four. Moreover, the epidemic of 1870–2 focused on London, towns, and industrial counties, whereas earlier ones primarily afflicted villages and agricultural counties. The outbreak of the 1870s struck young people and adults rather than children or infants, and therefore, given theories explored earlier, should have aroused more blame and violence, but this was not the case. By contrast, Creighton hardly mentions the epidemic of 1881–2: only that two-thirds of its deaths were in the capital.

[2] *Dundee Courier*, 30 June 1881.

of Guardians of local boroughs, whose weapons consisted of letters to newspapers and representation in law courts and even in Parliament. Nonetheless, the British reaction was similar to responses seen in America in one essential regard: the perpetrators of this legal violence were solid citizens and elites, including the medical profession. On the other hand, those primarily targeted were not smallpox victims directly but other committees and branches of government, especially the municipal boards of health and asylum, which were mandated to end the epidemic and provide care for smallpox sufferers. Yet those ultimately to suffer from the onslaught of legal actions brought about by elites, which closed hospitals and interrupted care and provisioning, were smallpox victims, who were overwhelmingly the poor. Elected leaders, such as Mr Dobson, head of the Metropolitan Asylums Board, which coordinated smallpox control in Greater London, were caught in a judicial ambush orchestrated by local elites in places such as Hampstead and Fulham and doctors, politicians, and members of parliament. The collective legal assault on government directives for treating smallpox victims may have endangered more lives in London in 1880–2, both among the healthy and the afflicted, than all the individual acts of cruelty and collective violence against smallpox victims in the US.

This public assault on government control and provision for smallpox in 1880–2 was largely a London story with much the same goals as the illegal brutality in the US—dismantling and banning hospitals for smallpox in one's own backyard. In England, the rationale was more often articulated. Their fears turned on theories of miasma and notions of the long-distance possibilities of contagion cast by infectious smallpox bodies, dead or alive (effluvia). During the last half of the nineteenth century, such notions of contagion were on the rise.[3] Prevailing views among the medical profession and educated elites held that smallpox infected not only by touch, clothing, and breathing, but by its presence in the local atmosphere, transmitted by the stench and vapours of infected patients, especially when conveyed in open ambulances from impoverished neighbourhoods, where the majority of smallpox cases arose, to asylums across London, especially in the wealthier suburbs.

In late 1880, citizens of London's north-western suburb Hampstead led the way in assaults against the Metropolitan Asylums Board and its policy of allocating city-wide smallpox hospitals. By the beginning of 1881, its citizens had issued an injunction against the Board 'rendering its managers severally and jointly liable to a penalty of £20,000', if they continued using the smallpox hospital at Hampstead or purchased or built other sites to isolate smallpox patients. By this action, the board found itself 'severely hampered in constituting their design for providing protection to the whole of London...by timely isolation of the infected and the effectual vaccination of those liable'. According to the Board's chairman, Mr W. Brewer, 'it must be obvious...that we are paralyzed'.[4] By early March, citizens' pleas came

---

[3] Among other places, see Hamlin, 'Predisposing Causes'; Baldwin, *Contagion*. For Ackerknecht, 'Anticontagionism', theories of contagion triumphed over anti-contagionism in mid-century. For criticism of his thesis, see Pelling, *Cholera*, 295–310. For the persistence of miasma theories into the 1890s in Germany, see Evans, *Death in Hamburg*.

[4] *The Times*, 5 January 1881, 11.

before the House of Lords. Hampstead's elites won, and their jubilation rang with upper-class entitlement:

> Hampstead is spared the risk and annoyance of a permanent smallpox hospital. The spirited action of the residents, backed up by what we cannot but feel is an equitable judgment, has released this delightful and constantly improving suburb from an infliction, which would always be a detriment and a source of public danger. It was argued, and we grant with some show of justice, that other suburbs had as much right to object to a small-pox hospital as Hampstead. But there are localities in the environs of London, where the risk of contagion would be limited to the traffic of the immediate neighbourhood; whereas Hampstead, being a resort of thousands for health and recreation, ought certainly to be exempt from such an establishment as the small-pox hospital. A beautiful spot... is surely not the place to make a hotbed of disease.[5]

Hampstead's verdict soon provided a valuable precedent for other wealthy neighbourhoods, desiring to dispense with their responsibilities of caring for smallpox victims, but at the same time, it created conflicts among the wealthy. By early May, neighbouring Highgate's smallpox hospital became full as a consequence of Hampstead's hospital closing.[6] By the beginning of June, with smallpox cases steadily increasing, even those in Hampstead were feeling the pinch of inadequate facilities to provide for their residents, and its citizens petitioned the Local Government Board to appropriate the workhouse at Holloway (outside Hampstead's boundaries) as a smallpox hospital. The proposal was greeted by some of Hampstead's citizens favourably.[7] Outside criticism, however, rose against Hampstead's self-centred opportunism: now that 'the disease was upon them', 'these selfish people' refused to provide for their own poor, and sought to thrust them on others.[8] But the criticisms were not needed: less than a week later, Hampstead citizens cried out against the proposed conversion. Despite being beyond Hampstead's borders, Holloway's workhouse was too close for comfort.[9]

During the late winter and spring with the epidemic waxing, the testing ground over London's jurisdiction and planning of hospital services turned from the suburbs to the capital's wealthy central districts—Kensington, Fulham, Hammersmith, and Chelsea. As in Hampstead, fear of contagion ignited the wealthy's zeal to rid their communities of smallpox patients or at a minimum to restrict hospital admissions to their residents alone. The key battleground was Fulham. Unlike Hampstead, its inhabitants showed no reversals in sentiment. They carried out their protests in public meetings chaired by their MP, Mr Firth, in the town halls of Chelsea, Kensington, and the West End, in law courts, and, in one instance, at a mass rally outdoors. Initially, in February 1881, they objected to proposals to construct an extension to Fulham Hospital.[10] However, emboldened by Hampstead's injunction

---

[5] *Era*, 12 March 1881.   [6] *Standard*, 4 May 1881, 3.
[7] *Hampshire Advertiser*, 1 June 1881.   [8] *The Times*, 15 June 1881, 15.
[9] *Standard*, 13 June 1881, 3.
[10] *The Times*, 16 February 1881, 10; 1 March 1881, 11. As early as 12 February, the Asylums Board proposed adding sixty beds to Fulham Hospital to accommodate growing numbers of cases, but residents in public meetings and lawsuits, 'energetically' protested; *Morning Post*, 12 February 1881, 3. For further meetings of ratepayers protesting extensions, see *Pall Mall Gazette*, 21 February 1881 and 22 February 1881.

ratified by the House of Lords, Fulham's residents sought to prevent smallpox patients from entering or being hospitalized in their district altogether. The ratepayers immediately used their political clout in local tribunals as well as within national politics to block Metropolitan Board plans for extensions. When the Board attempted to house the afflicted in temporary sheds and tents because of the rapidly deteriorating conditions in Fulham Hospital and within London generally due to the spread and worsening virulence of the disease, Fulham deployed its protests and legal acumen to stop even makeshift measures.[11] Residents argued that patients brought into their borough from other districts spread the disease: victims' bodily fumes contaminated the city when conveyed in ambulances along the 4–6-mile journey from the East End through the West End's crowded streets. The Metropolitan Board's policy of distributing smallpox hospitals, Fulham argued, had led to a criss-cross transport of patients, inflicting 'a permanent curse' on Fulham, Chelsea, and Kensington, endangering their residents and 'especially' their children, 'who in large numbers attended the schools in the immediate vicinity of the building'. As in Hampstead, Fulham's citizens emphasized non-medical concerns: the hospital damaged their reputation and property values.[12] They argued that every district should care for its own: the wealthy districts owed the rest of the city nothing.

With smallpox cases mounting from late April to June and all six of London's smallpox hospitals 'overcrowded and incapable of dealing with the emergency',[13] the Board abandoned plans to extend the number of beds at Fulham and attempted what it thought would be less contentious—erecting temporary wooden buildings.[14] By the end of April, the residents' legal actions defeated this plan as well. The Board then sought to pitch tents for the afflicted on a piece of wasteland on the banks of the Thames, 'surrounded by a high wooden paling', and separated by gas works with the nearest building 300 yards away.[15] But despite placing the tents as far as possible from high-density housing, the residents sought to scuttle the measures. First, they organized a mass meeting on Belbrook Common, Walham Green, presided over by their parish priest, and rallied citizens to protest 'against being saddled with those [smallpox patients] of the metropolitan generally'.[16] The residents then brought their challenges to the High Court of Justice and won an injunction restraining the defendants.[17]

By 14 May, the Attorney-General intervened, forcing the Asylums Board to dismantle the tents and temporary wooden structures and dismiss all remaining smallpox patients as soon as they became convalescent.[18] Nonetheless, the structures remained in place, and at the end of August, the residents embarked on strategies

---

[11] *The Times*, 25 March 1881, 10.

[12] Ibid., 22 February 1881, 12; 28 February 1881, 6; *Morning Post* 12 February 1881, 3; and *Pall Mall Gazette*, 24 February 1881.

[13] *The Times*, 6 June 1881, 6.   [14] Ibid., 28 April 1881, 12.

[15] Ibid., 6 May 1881, 10. News of ratepayers' resistance reached northern Scotland: *Aberdeen Weekly*, 7 May 1881.

[16] *Lloyd's Weekly*, 8 May 1881.   [17] *The Times*, 11 May 1881, 6.

[18] Ibid., 14 June 1881, 6.

learnt from Hampstead: they threatened Asylums Board managers individually with lawsuits in the High Court, charging them with damages inflicted on Fulham by 'the nuisance and mismanagement' of the Fulham smallpox hospital. In response, the defendants filed affidavits from the hospital's physicians 'to show that [the hospital] was carefully managed' and cases of smallpox near the hospital could be traced to various causes and not from the fumes of patients.[19] But their medical knowledge and statistics were ignored, and on 6 October, the residents of south-west London won the case. No longer would Fulham Hospital be obliged to admit smallpox patients from beyond its borders.[20] During these legal battles, hints circulated to the press that the ratepayers might resort to actions beyond rhetorical flourishes in newspapers or mass meetings in town halls. In late February, a Mr Tattersall wrote to *The Times*, threatening: 'If the Local Board will not listen to the voice of the inhabitants . . . I fear that other steps will be taken to try the right of any board to inflict a permanent curse upon a populous neighbourhood'. But throughout the epidemic's duration, no evidence points to inhabitants of Kensington, Fulham, Hammersmith, or Chelsea engaging in street demonstrations (other than their lawful meeting in May). Without rioting or other forms of extra-legal activity, this privileged group had won all its demands at the expense of smallpox victims and public health.[21]

London's less fashionable neighbourhoods where smallpox hospitals had been built also protested: at Homerton in Hackney, Stockwell, south of the Thames in Lambeth, and Deptford near Greenwich. These were not, however, sustained legal battles or conducted in the press as in Hampstead and Fulham. The pleas of these poorer Londoners failed to reach the courts; no injunctions were awarded to terminate hospital extensions; none from outside were turned away from care in their hospitals. In early February, a deputation from Hackney protested to the Asylums Board against proposed increases of smallpox patients at Homerton. The Board's chairman rejected the request, arguing that Hackney and Greenwich were the very districts 'where the disease had sprung up, and where it had continued to increase'; Hackney, Bethnal Green, and Greenwich showed the highest returns of smallpox cases, and Hackney, the highest unvaccinated population in the metropolis.[22] No more is heard of Hackney's protest. In May, when the Local Government Board approved a proposal to send all fever cases to Stockwell and to appropriate Homerton Hospital entirely for Hackney's smallpox patients, Stockwell's inhabitants objected but also to no avail.[23]

Residents of the districts adjoining Deptford lodged concerns twice during the epidemic. At a public meeting in April, they passed a resolution soliciting the Vestry to take steps to move its hospital to a more suitable site. They also charged that nurses, workmen, and other hospital employees had been negligent in disinfecting themselves and were contaminating surrounding neighbourhoods.[24] But the press gives no sign that their pleas reached the courts or that negotiations followed.

---

[19] Ibid., 12 August 1881, 12.   [20] Ibid., 3 October 1881, 6.
[21] *Pall Mall Gazette*, 28 February 1881.   [22] *The Times*, 8 February 1881, 10.
[23] *Standard*, 16 May 1881.   [24] Ibid., 4 May 1881, 3.

In August, residents of Camberwell living near the hospital pleaded to close it once the patients had been discharged, or that it be used only for cases from the immediate neighbourhood.[25] No injunctions or lawsuits followed; the hospital remained subject to the London-wide catchment.

With smallpox cases on the rise, the closure of Hampstead's hospital, and Fulham's prerogative to refuse patients from outside its district, the Metropolitan Board was forced to conceive new plans to isolate and treat London's growing numbers of cases. One was to isolate smallpox patients in converted ships to be moored on the Thames. At the end of May, the Board received permission from the Admiralty to convert a ship into a temporary hospital docked at Chatham and began work on the screw battle-steamer, the *Atlas*.[26] Within two weeks, however, complaints challenged the *Atlas*'s right to become a hospital, despite patient numbers increasing daily. Papers outside London now began carrying the capital's story, portraying London as a 'disgrace'.[27] But the capital's citizens continued their protests. In July, workers at a shipbuilding firm in Greenwich, near the *Atlas*'s moorings and the *Endymion* floating hospital, lodged a complaint against the proximity of these ships. But unlike their better-off counterparts in Hampstead, Chelsea, and Kensington, nothing more was heard of it.[28]

Ratepayers protested against more than just the sites of smallpox hospitals or workhouses for temporary isolation. In July, the Board arranged to build a smallpox ambulance station in Hackney, near London Fields, to convey patients within the surrounding parishes and as far as Islington to the appropriate hospitals. The arrangements provoked 'indignant protests' from ratepayers, who united in opposition with their local Board of Guardians.[29] Yet, despite local governmental support and again unlike the wealthier boroughs, Hackney's ratepayers were unsuccessful.

* * *

During this epidemic, nothing akin to the Hampstead or Fulham legal revolts to hamper smallpox control was seen elsewhere in Britain, except for one town, Romford, twenty miles east of the capital. At the end of May, the wider Rural Sanitary Authority proposed building a new infectious diseases hospital in a field adjoining its workhouse hospital. Its local board met and resolved not to cooperate. However, no vitriolic letters justifying the town's position or condemning the opposition appeared in the press or galvanized support from MPs to issue court injunctions.[30] One disturbance, however, shows different tactics from those staged by London's well-heeled. In the Black Country of the West Midlands, the epidemic of 1881 sparked an extra-legal protest. Like cholera, rumours mobilized the lower classes. Here, for the first time, even the Malthusian myth of elites inventing an epidemic to cull the poor was heard. An 'epidemic of unreason' spread through 'nearly a dozen towns and villages' north and west of Birmingham. These recall

[25] *The Times*, 5 August 1881, 6.
[26] *Jackson's Oxford Journal*, 28 May 1881; and *Liverpool Mercury*, 28 May 1881.
[27] *Leeds Mercury*, 13 June 1881.   [28] *The Times*, 25 July 1881, 11.
[29] Ibid., 19 July 1881, 7.   [30] *Essex Standard*, 28 May 1881, 8.

early modern fantasies of plague spreaders. The story, taken from the *Birmingham Mail*, was reproduced in full or in part by at least twenty-five newspapers across Britain.[31] For some days, the papers reported, 'silent rumours' spread of 'ever foolish ingenuity invented or stupid credulity swallowed': 'three black doctors' had been sent 'ostensibly to carry out the Vaccination Acts'. 'In reality', their mission was to murder 'all the infant children'. As a consequence, nearly all the schools in the district lay empty, and 'hundreds of mothers' went about 'as though possessed'. These actions spread to Oldbury, West Bromwich, Willenhall, Dudley, Coseley, Holly Hall, Bilston, and Kate's Hill: 'In the morning a rumour reaches Bilston that the "three black doctors" are coming...in the afternoon the schools are destitute of pupils', their parents 'having forced their way into classrooms and dragged off their offspring'. They believed 'that the Government, finding the population of the country to be too rapidly increasing, have decided to kill off the budding generation' under the pretext of smallpox prevention. At Holly Hall, there were rumours among 'the people' that the 'black doctors' had kidnapped and eaten a child; yet 'no disconsolate mother' came forward 'to publicly bemoan the loss of her child...No relics of the cannibals' horrible feast—not so much as a knickerbockery button— have been found.' Yet the rumours persisted.[32]

Other papers added details of the mothers' organization and actions. They approached the schools 'armed with various ready missiles', and 'in a few instances' broke windows.[33] 'In pursuit of the never-seen three American black doctors', they marched to Northampton and bombarded the School Board with insults and missiles, forcing teachers to close schools.[34] The mothers' cries and missiles, however, do not put this one isolated case on a par with the violence across America during this epidemic.

* * *

No equivalent onslaught by the wealthy against smallpox hospitals in earlier epidemics appears in the vast collection of *Nineteenth Century British Library Newspapers*. Dating back to 1800, smallpox riots and even protests against building or converting older public buildings into smallpox hospitals fail to appear until the epidemic in 1870–2.[35] This one was far deadlier than the outbreak of 1880–2 with smallpox fatality rates climbing from a norm of 35 per cent to as high as 77 per cent in places. Unlike 1881–2, when cases were concentrated overwhelmingly in London, the 1870–2 epidemic spread throughout the British Isles. Yet the protest that accompanied it paled by comparison with the less serious epidemic of 1881. In London, the Asylums Board smallpox hospitals—Stockwell, Homerton, and Hampstead—endured the 1870–2 pandemic without protest, injunctions, or

---

[31] BNA, searched on 23 April 2013. As of 8 April 2016, no Birmingham paper for this date had been downloaded.

[32] *Northern Echo*, 16 May 1881.   [33] *Bucks Herald*, 28 May 1881.

[34] *Reynold's Newspaper*, 29 May 1881.

[35] With double keywords 'smallpox' and 'protest', I searched the entire database until 1853, then the epidemic of 1862–3—the last one before 1870; see Hardy, *Epidemic Streets*. On the severity of the 1862–3 epidemic in London and Manchester, see *Preston Guardian*, 21 March 1863.

forced closures. When Stockwell's smallpox hospital was opened at the beginning of February 1871, the reaction was strongest—but the panic led to the desertion of residents, not open protest in the streets or courts against the Metropolitan Asylums Board's authority. Instead, some mothers took their children from schools bordering the hospital.[36] No public meetings of ratepayers here or elsewhere challenged temporary accommodations or closed hospitals to outsiders.

Beyond the capital, however, the first smallpox protests that I have found sprouted in the British Isles. In February, the ratepayers of West Derby Road in Liverpool met and passed a unanimous resolution, challenging the conversion of Starfield House into a smallpox hospital. No further reports, however, mention whether the resolution succeeded or continued through public meetings or legal procedures.[37] A month later, citizens in the market town of Ormskirk, north of Liverpool, convened their Health Board to object to a Poor Law resolution to build a smallpox hospital near the workhouse.[38] With cases in decline, the headmaster of the town's grammar school led inhabitants petitioning the Board of Health to cancel its plans.[39] In a suburb of Leicester, a third protest began on 1 April, the first I have found to threaten legal injunctions. But in this case, they remained only threats. A solicitor on behalf of his client, a resident of Leicester's suburb, Newfoundpool, reported that 'a rumour' circulated of plans to build a smallpox house on Freake's Grounds. If true, the solicitor argued that it would 'prove a serious nuisance to the residents', and his client would oppose it 'by all lawful means'.[40] Nothing further was heard from the client or lawyer in the newspapers. A fourth case came from the north-east which anticipated the moves made by London's privileged a decade later. Grimsby Town Council voted to place a temporary smallpox hospital in the suburb of Cleethorpes by transforming a large building in its Pleasure Gardens. Cleethorpes' citizens protested against Grimsby transporting its smallpox victims into their jurisdiction. Similar to Hampstead's later pleas, Cleethorpes pinned their case on the suburb's importance as a 'great bathing resort': a smallpox hospital in its midst would deter 'the numerous excursions' from Sheffield, 'seriously' damaging the town's livelihood. But unlike Hampstead's, Cleethorpes' objections were unsuccessful.[41] From keyword searches in two million-plus pages of the *Nineteenth Century British Library Newspapers* archive, I discover no further protests.

Except for the possible but limited violence of the Black Country's mothers, who may have broken schoolhouse windowpanes, I have found only two further incidents of threatened collective violence relating to smallpox in the British Isles, both of which occurred after the 1881–2 epidemic. The first, which appears in a US newspaper, was about to produce 'mob' action when police surveillance nipped

[36] *Morning Post* 2 February 1871; *Pall Mall Gazette*, 3 February 1871; *Fife Herald*, 16 February 1871. On the epidemic of 1870–2 as a deadly strain of smallpox, see Prinzing, *Epidemics*, 16–17, and for Berlin, 230.

[37] *Liverpool Mercury*, 20 February 1871.   [38] Ibid., 18 March 1871.

[39] Ibid., 24 March 1871; and *Preston Guardian*, 25 March 1871.

[40] *Leicester Chronicle*, 1 April 1871, 3.

[41] *Sheffield & Rotherham Independent*, 10 June 1871, 11.

it in the bud. It occurred in Hackney in May 1884 with a thousand cases already recorded and the disease on the rise. While bodies of the dead 'were being carted away in the middle of the night, a mob, terrified by the death wagon's visits, assembled and threatened violence'. The police intervened, isolating the district.[42]

The second incident arose twelve years later in Stroud, near Gloucester. It was more successful and assumed the usual smallpox pattern seen in late nineteenth-century America with the respectable as the mobsters. At midnight a 'mob' barred an ambulance carrying 'the first smallpox patient' to Bisley's hospital, 'which is extremely well isolated', and was forced to return to Stroud and deposit the 'unfortunate patient' in a lodging house, where he died. The following night, the mob 'besieged, wrecked, and burnt down' the hospital. Afterwards, 'a large body of police' guarded its remains. According to the *Lancet*, 'a number of respectable men' were responsible, but unlike similar cases in the US, the Bisley men were convicted and sentenced to imprisonment with hard labour. The medical journal ended its analysis by claiming the 'terror of small-pox in this non-vaccinating union' resembled 'the terror which the ignorant Russian peasants have of cholera'.[43] It was, however, mistaken: the perpetrators of the violence were not peasants or of the lower classes; they were the elites.

In addition, from 1868 to 1889, the campaign against compulsory vaccination legislation resulted in 6000 persons being 'hauled' before the courts for refusing vaccination in Leicester alone.[44] On 23 March 1885, that city organized an international anti-vaccination demonstration with delegates from across the British Isles and internationally from Switzerland, Belgium, France, Germany, and America.[45] The anti-vaccination advocate, who was on Leicester's Town Council, its Board of Guardians (for poor relief), and its Sanitary Committee, estimated the crowd size to be between 80,000 and 100,000.[46] The demonstration, however, was peaceful. Instead of firing buildings, distinguished delegates made fiery speeches, and its attendees formed a peaceful procession, displaying handcrafted anti-vaccination banners. No violence or confrontation with police ensued. Like J. L. Biggs, the long-time anti-vaccination activist, organizer and historian of the movement, the organizers and delegates were government officers or elected representatives.[47]

In conclusion, Britain's fear and loathing of smallpox and its victims differed markedly from the North American experience. In Britain, direct action against the victims of smallpox seldom occurred: no shotgun quarantines, vigilante gangs

---

[42] *Trenton Evening Times*, 29 May 1884, 2.

[43] '"Antagonism" to smallpox'. A London letter to the *American Practitioner and News*, 21–2 (1896), 141, estimated the crowd 'at several hundred'. The burning occurred in the presence of 'a number of' constables. 'Eventually, several arrests were made' with twelve-month prison sentences imposed. Foley, *The Last Irish Plague*, assumes that 'violence and tumult' occurred regularly with smallpox epidemics in nineteenth- and early twentieth-century Ireland but mentions only one: at Athenry, County Galway, in 1875: 'townsfolk' attacked and burned a workhouse van used to transport sufferers, 82. Searching the BNA for the epidemics of 1870–2 and 1881–2, I have found none for Ireland.

[44] Biggs, *Leicester*, 102.   [45] *The Times*, 24 March 1885.

[46] Biggs, *Leicester*, 116. *The Times*, 24 March 1885, reported it positively but estimated the crowd at just over 20,000.

[47] Biggs, *Leicester*, 101–30. I thank my student Kate McColm for this reference.

refusing patients entry to towns, burning of hospitals, or gruesome murder of sufferers. In other respects, however, the British protests paralleled those in America: ratepayers and elites, not peasants, the poor, or despised outsiders, comprised the crowds, and the protesters' targets were ultimately the sufferers, making them doubly victims of disease and social violence. As this chapter has suggested, the British use of the courts as opposed to street violence may in the end have proved more deadly to smallpox victims than the physical cruelty inflicted by individuals or groups in America. These smallpox experiences also possess a third similarity. On both continents, little protest appears against smallpox victims, health boards, or state agencies before the epidemics of 1880–2, that is, before the laboratory revolution, despite smallpox pandemics raging through the eighteenth and early nineteenth century with higher rates of mortality. Searching the 'Burney Collection of Seventeenth- and Eighteenth-Century Newspapers' reveals that no smallpox protest or earlier anti-inoculation protest triggered collective violence as it had in colonial and early Republican America. Strides in medicine that dispelled the mysteries of these epidemics failed to soften smallpox's social violence; instead, the trend ran in the opposite direction.

PART IV

MODERNITY: PLAGUES OF POLITICS

14

Plague since 1894

India

Another disease to provoke social violence and serious riots at the turn of the twentieth century was plague (caused by the gram negative-immobile bacterium that was christened *Yersinia pestis* in 1954). In India, it sparked revolts that inflicted mass destruction on quarantine centres, called segregation camps, but also on hospitals and government offices. With insurgents in the thousands and two drawing crowds of over 10,000, they surpassed in magnitude, duration, and numbers killed the largest cholera protests in Russia and Italy. A plague revolt in Kolkata and its suburbs at the beginning of July 1897 was quashed only after British and Indian troops had killed an estimated 600 rioters.[1] Such death tolls far exceed any single cholera riot, where numbers were estimated—even those crushed by Czarist troops and Cossack reinforcements. Plague rebels were able temporarily to occupy entire districts of India's two largest cities, Kolkata and Mumbai.

During the 1980s and early 1990s David Arnold, Ian Catanach, Ira Klein, and Rajnarayan Chandavarkar[2] studied Indian plague riots, and monographs have been devoted to the great Honolulu conflagration of 1900[3] and to prejudice against the Chinese during San Francisco's plague epidemics.[4] But scholars have yet to place plague's social violence in larger contexts, first within the years of modern plague itself. No one has collected these disturbances, analysed their variety, or compared their participants, targets, causes, and ideologies across the globe from 1894 on[5] or with other epidemic diseases. Did reactions to modern plague differ fundamentally from its medieval and early modern predecessors? Was it more akin to the socio-psychological consequences of yellow fever or influenza, diseases that readily ignited panic but led to collective compassion and heroic acts of self-sacrifice on behalf of victims? Or were the reactions to the modern plague determined by disgust, hatred, and fear of its rapid progression and high rates of lethality[6] such

---

[1] *Advertiser*, 8 July 1897, 5; *Barrier Miner*, 9 July 1897, 2; *Kalgoorlie Miner*, 8 July 1897, 2; and others.

[2] Arnold, *Colonizing the Body*; Catanach, 'Plague and the Tensions'; Klein, 'Plague'; Chandavarkar, 'Plague Panic'; and Sarkar, 'The Tie that Snapped'.

[3] Mohr, *Plague and Fire*.

[4] Craddock, *City of Plagues*, ch. 4; Echenberg, *Plague Ports*, ch. 8; Shah, *Contagious Divides*; and Risse, *Plague, Fear, and Politics*.

[5] Echenberg, *Plague Ports*, presents an excellent comparative analysis of plague across the globe but pays little attention to plague's social violence.

[6] Before the diffusion of antibiotics (1946), the lethality of bubonic plague ranged between 60 and 90 per cent; with septicaemic and pneumonic plague it was 100 per cent; see Twigg, *Bubonic Plague*, 19, 32, 77.

that mass violence was unleashed against its victims as with smallpox, or against modern medicine as with cholera?

Plagues of the Middle Ages certainly engendered disgust as seen from the mid-fourteenth-century verses of the Welsh poet Llywelyn Fychan, who lamented the death of his children by plague in the 1360s, transfixed by the disease's rapid transformation of human beauty into hideous sores:

> A shower of peas giving rise to affliction,
> messenger of swift black death;
> parings from the petals of the corn-poppy,
> murderous rabble, evil omen;
> black plague, they don't come with any good intent,
> halfpennies, seaweed scales;
> a grim throng, humble speech,
> berries, it is painful that they should be on fair skin.[7]

Such disgust, copiously seen with medieval plague, cholera, typhus, syphilis, yellow fever, and especially smallpox, in newspapers, common parlance, and literature is, however, surprisingly absent with modern plague. While newspaper and medical accounts often described the unpleasant physical environments of the plague-infested—their clothing, cesspools, 'filthy mud huts',[8] garbage, and the general accumulated filth of their neighbourhoods—no examples come to mind of descriptions in the press, novels, or poetry that portrayed the signs or symptoms of modern plague as especially horrifying and disgusting.[9] Perhaps the visible horror was lessened because in most outbreaks of modern plague it is a rarity to find pneumonic plague, with the coughing and spitting of blood; and unlike late medieval and early modern bubonic plague, when buboes, carbuncles, and black pustules often spread across plague-infested bodies in full view of the public, with modern plague only one bubo forms in 95 per cent of cases, and between 55 and 70 per cent of these are in the groin or armpits and thus usually concealed.[10] On the other hand, like cholera and medieval and early modern bubonic plague, modern plague was a quick killer, causing death within a week in its bubonic form, twenty-four hours or less if pneumonic, and in a matter of hours if scepticaemic. But, as we have seen, quick killers were not the only epidemic diseases to spark violence and blame. Smallpox, often a long-lingering illness whose sores marked victims for life, gave rise to the greatest waves of cruelty and blame of any disease in North American history. And while yellow fever, for example, and influenza in its most virulent form in 1918–20 could kill in a matter of days, these rapidly fatal diseases failed to spread deadly social toxins, and, as we will see, often united societies.

What then were modern plagues' socio-psychological consequences? Did plague lead to persecution of its victims or conspiracy theories and mythologies of mass

---

[7] *Galar Y Beirdd: Marwnadau Plant*, 56–8.
[8] *Advertiser*, 8 July 1897, 5; and Christos Lynteris's ERC project on photographing plague.
[9] See, for instance, Weiss, *Georg Letham*.
[10] On differences in skin disorders between the 'Second' and 'Third Pandemic', see Cohn. *The Black Death Transformed*; and idem, *Cultures of Plague*, ch. 2.

murder as with cholera, targeting the medical profession and the state? Were high fatality rates of over 50 per cent before antibiotics (or rehydration kits with cholera) the critical factors provoking social violence? With both diseases, crowds believed that those sent to hospitals or segregation camps did not return alive.

First, plague riots and protests appearing in the foreign press concentrated on India and principally on the Presidency of Bombay and Calcutta. Furthermore, weekly extracts, summaries, and translations of hundreds of Indian newspapers add much material about plague protest and especially peaceful demonstrations, but do not increase significantly the number of large violent confrontations seen in the foreign press.[11] Of 111 reported riots, disturbances, and large-scale demonstrations across the globe that I have uncovered for the Third Pandemic, sixty-three, just under a third of them, occurred in the Indian subcontinent and these clustered within four or five years. This survey challenges the conclusion that riots and violence were 'remarkably rare occurrences', providing 'the least frequent manifestation of such resistance' against colonial plague policies.[12] However, given that as much as 95 per cent of plague deaths since 1894 arose in India,[13] perhaps we should conclude the opposite of what the absolute numbers suggest. As a ratio of plague deaths, plague-related disturbances were comparatively fewer in India than elsewhere. But in the subcontinent, many more riots are suggested in the press than can be easily quantified, such as reports of an unspecified number of disturbances in villages. Moreover, in Kolkata, Mumbai, Seringapatam, and Kanpur these often lasted several days with different nuclei, probably constituting separate riots.

Certainly more Indian riots occurred than I have found. For instance, in 1944 Sir Leonard Rogers, a founder of the Royal Society of Tropical Medicine and pioneer in cholera treatment, referred to riots by people resisting inoculation, which spread through the Punjab at the turn of the twentieth century and led to 'bloodshed' with doctors losing their lives.[14] However, he doesn't specify any, and I have not found any mention of anti-inoculation riots here in the native or foreign press. Certainly, riots occurred in the Punjab but these were provoked by other causes, as in Garshankar in April 1898,[15] Sialkot in May 1901,[16] and

---

[11] According to Arnold, *Colonizing the Body*, 211, these extracts provide 'unprecedented access to contemporary attitudes' about plague. However, they rarely described riots—their movements, targets, and number of participants, those killed, wounded, or arrested. Here, foreign papers provide much more.

[12] Chandavarkar, 'Plague Panic', 220, mentions only three riots.

[13] Twigg, *Bubonic Plague*, 9 and 69, calculates from Hirst's figures, between 1894 and 1938, over 95 per cent of plague deaths occurred in India: 12.5 million in India and 652,000 in the rest of the world. These percentages have not shifted significantly since Hirst's calculations: although plague deaths in the Indian subcontinent reported to WHO constituted only 27 per cent (1910 of 7019) globally from 1954 to 1997, the subcontinent's share remains just below 95 per cent; my calculation from *Plague Manual* (1999), table 1, 18–25.

[14] Rogers, 'Cholera Incidence in India', 91.

[15] *South Australian Register*, 3 May 1898, 5, said little about this riot, and *West Australian*, 3 May 1898, 5, misidentified 'Garshauher' as near Bombay City, but reported it as serious: the police fired on the rioters, killing nine and wounding twenty-seven, with twenty-six police officers injured. Pune's *Mahrátta*, 8 May, refers to it obliquely on lessons the Indian government should learn from 'the fatal whims of individual officers'. L/R/5/153, week ending 14 May 1898.

[16] L/R/5/156, week ending 18 May 1901, no. 30 *Prabhát*; week ending 1 June 1901, no. 36. *Prabhát*.

Tehsil[17] in the Sialkot district, which was perhaps the most serious, requiring a military force of 1600 to restore order.[18] Moreover, plague riots spread to twenty-five villages in Sialkot with several medical assistants killed or wounded,[19] but resistance to inoculation is not given as the cause. The only disturbance to mention it occurred at a village, Bajaha, on 11 March 1898, and the single paper reporting it called it a 'petty riot'. As with most Indian plague riots, theirs was an attack mostly against stringent enforcement of anti-plague measures and measures such as evacuation and inoculation were only mentioned in passing.[20] Other historians have pointed to resistance against Haffkine's inoculation enterprise in the Punjab after the Malkowal incident in October 1902,[21] leading to Haffkine's sacking in 1902.[22] But it is unclear whether the reaction to Haffkine spurred rioting in villages as Sir Leonard claimed. Nonetheless, he was an eyewitness in the Punjab and could well have known of anti-inoculation riots that may not have been reported in the papers. In addition, descriptions of other Indian plague riots pointed to outbreaks that spread through numerous villages, which newspapers failed to specify—some supposedly fanned by religious fanaticism in February 1898 within the Scinde [Sindh], a province of the Presidency of Bombay,[23] others in unspecified villages near the Persian border, and the twenty-five unnamed riots around Sialkot.[24]

More importantly, the dimensions of the Indian plague riots were on another scale from elsewhere. First, only in India did they spread across regions, like the contagion of cholera revolts across Europe and the Americas in the 1830s or later in Russia and Italy until 1911. Second, outside India, only two assembled crowds greater than a thousand, and few were followed by shop closures and strikes as in India. In India's earliest plague riot (October 1896), only weeks after the plague's first appearance, 'a mob of three thousand' destroyed a plague hospital in Mumbai.[25] In Kolkata in early July 1897, 5000 rioted against plague measures.[26] In November 1898, at Srirangapatnam [Seringapatam] in Mysore, a crowd estimated at more than double the size of Kolkata's rioted, despite the southern city's much smaller population.[27] A plague protest in Mumbai on 9 March 1898 was larger still: 'thousands' rioted over several days followed by a general strike.[28]

---

[17] An administrative unit in the Punjab consisting of several villages.

[18] L/R/5/156, week ending 8 June 1901, *Gujarát Mitra*.

[19] *San Francisco Chronicle*, 5 May 1901, 3.

[20] L/R/5/156, week ending no. 70: *Rághav Bhutsham*.

[21] Cueto, *The Return of Epidemics*, 14; Arnold, *Colonizing the Body*, 234; and Catanach, 'Plague and the Tensions', 160, describe the Malkowal debacle (see note 22), but mentions no riots arising from it. On Haffkine's career, see Catanach, 'Plague and the Tensions', 154–60; for Haffkine's work on inoculation first with cholera and then plague, see Harrison, *Public Health in British India*, 144 and 153.

[22] There were plague riots in the Punjab as in Garhshankar in April 1898; Arnold, *Colonizing the Body*, 230, and my note 156. But should these be linked to tragedy of Malkowal? The Chief Plague Medical Officer, Wilkinson, in his meticulous report on the incident, mentions none (*Report on Plague*, 12 and 45–6); instead, Mulkowál [Malkowal]'s people 'behaved admirably throughout' (12).

[23] *Wagga Wagga Advertiser*, 3 February 1898, 2. Presently the province around Karachi.

[24] *Le Temps*, 2 February 1898.   [25] *New York Times*, 29 October 1896.

[26] *Guardian*, 3 July 1897.

[27] At the beginning of the twentieth century, Kolkata was India's largest city with well over a million inhabitants; see Kidambi, *The Making*, 155.

[28] See notes 125–31.

Plague riots and large demonstrations by region

Country/ Empire	No.	Dates	Village/City/Region	No.
Austria	1	1898	Vienna	1
China	25	1921	Aschho, nr Harbin, Manchuria	1
		1894	Canton	2
		1918	Fengchen	1
		1920	Hailar (Manchuria)	1
		1911	Hankow (Wuhan)	1
		1893, 1894	Hong Kong	3
		1911	Kirin (Jilin City), Manchuria	1
		1911	Kharbin (Harbin), Manchuria	2
		1920	Harbin	1
		1911	Mukden (Shenyang, Korea)	1
		1910, 1911	Shanghai	7
		1894	Shuk Lung	1
		1894	Taluk, Namhoi District	2
		1911	Manchuria (numerous unspecified riots)	1
Egypt	1	1900	Port Said	1
Hawaii	2	1900	Hilo	1
		1900	Honolulu	1
India	63		Ahmednagar	(2)
		1899	Shop closures	1
		1899	*Mofussil* towns	1
		1901	Bajaha (Nashik)	1
		1898	Bangalore	1
		1898	Balouctchistan, villages along Persian border (unspecified number)	1
		1897	Bhávnagar	1
		1901	Bihta (near Patna in Bihar), Bengal	1
			Bombay (Mumbai):	(12)
		1896	Arthur Road	3
		1896	Falkland Road	1
		1896	Juma Masjid	1
		1897	Muslim cemetery riot, March	1
		1897	Muslim cemetery riot, June	1
		1897	Riots and strikes 16–17 April	2
		1898	Julai riots	2
		1898	Plague strikes	1
			Calcutta (Kolkata)	(7)
		1897	Tchittor suburb	1
		1897	1 July	1
		1898	Numerous assaults, May	1
		1898	Segregation camps attacks, August	1
		1898	Bhowanpur, suburb	1
		1899	March	1
		1899	'Tucca-wallah' riots	1
		1900	Kanpur, Uttar Pradesh	3
		1901	Chhapra, Bihar (several riots)	1
		1898	Chikkballapur (region of Bangalore)	1
		1903	Coimbatore (Tamil Nadu)	1
		1900	Danapur, unspecified villages	1
		1906	Fatehgarh, Uttar Pradesh	1

(*continued*)

Continued

Country/ Empire	No.	Dates	Village/City/Region	No.
		1898	Garhshankar	2
		1897	Ghoti, Nashik	1
		1897	Hyderabad, 'monster' demonstration	1
		1897	Jejuri Pune	1
		1901	Katteshwarpur, near Danapur, Bengal	1
		1899	Kolhapur	1
		1901	Lachmipur (Jharkhand, Bengal)	1
		1902	Patiala, Punjab	1
		1902	Patna, Daldali bazar	1
		1897	Pune	2
		1901	Ramispur (Rampur) Uttar Pradesh	1
		1897	Rander, Surat Province	2
		1898	Scinde Province, Bombay Presidency	1
		1898	Seringapatam, Mysore (several days)	2
		1900	Shakpur [Sheikhpura]	1
		1901	Sialkot, Punjab 25 villages, Tehsil	3
		1900	Simla region	1
		1898	Sinnar, District of Nishik	2
		1897, 1994	Surat	2
		1901	Varanasi [Benares], Uttar Pradesh (Dashahwamedh and Sigre)	1
		1897	Versova, near Bandora[29]	1
Indonesia	1	1933	Tegal (Java)[30]	1
Mexico	2	1903	Villa Union	1
		1920	Veracruz	1
Persia (Iran)	3	1899	Bushire (Būshehr)	1
		1906	Nasirabad	1
		1906	Seistan	1
Portugal	4	1906	Madeira	1
		1899	Oporto	3
				4
Russia	1	1911	Vladivostok	1
Saudi Arabia	5	1898	Jeddah	1
South Africa	1	1901	Port Elizabeth strikes	1
USA	1	1900	San Francisco	1
Vietnam	1	1898	Cholon[31]	1
Total	111			

[29] *Pioneer* (Allahabad), 23 March 1897, 5.
[30] *Straits Times*, 18 April 1933, 12: Provoked by anti-plague measures, a 'furious mob' stoned Java Health Offices, killing one; seventy were arrested.
[31] *Le Temps*, 4 December 1898.

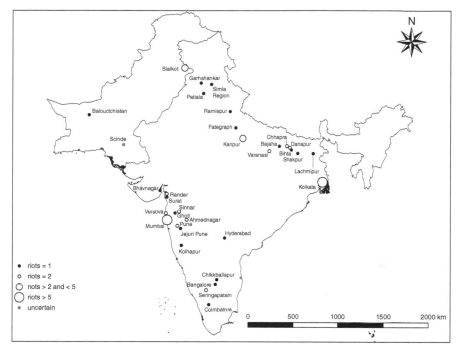

Map 14.1. Plague riots, India, 1896–1909.

Other forms of plague protest in India, moreover, drew crowds in the thousands without leading to widespread violence, such as when 3000 sellers of fruit, vegetables, and grain threatened to go on strike in Mumbai during the week of 24 October 1896.[32] Mill- and dockworkers engaged in further non-violent actions against plague measures on 6 and 7 April 1897.[33] On 11 February 1897, a peaceful plague protest approached the size of the largest of cholera riots, when 5000 Muslims opposed Mumbai municipality's closing of a Muslim graveyard.[34] In the first week of April 1898, 'no fewer than four thousand' Sunni Muslims of Mumbai held 'a mass meeting'. Instead of rioting, they passed resolutions urging Bombay's Plague Committee not to confine these Muslims in general segregation hospitals and camps.[35] As with almost all non-violent forms of plague protest none of the above was reported in the foreign press.

Furthermore, government anti-plague operations provoked numerous mass meetings and rallies throughout the subcontinent that resulted in letters, petitions, and resolutions delivered to municipal corporations and plague commissioners, such as General W. F. Gatacre in Mumbai, Walter Rand in Pune, Mr Moore in Surat, and the Governor of the Presidency of Bombay, His Excellency Lord Sandhurst.[36]

---

[32] L/R/5/151, week ending 24 October 1896, nos 24 and 25.   [33] See note 36.

[34] L/R/5/152, week ending 13 February 1897, no. 29.

[35] Ibid., 153, week ending 10 April 1898, no. 24.

[36] These fill 'native' papers but foreign ones largely ignored them. For an exception, see *Guardian*, 7 July 1897. On Lord Sandhurst's conciliatory attitudes before the 'Tragedy of Poona', see Catanach, 'Poona Politicians', 3.

For instance, on Thursday night, 25 March 1897, the Bohras of Surat called a public meeting to consider a letter from the Collector of Surat. Instead of rioting, they debated: (1) whether to accept or protest against the removal of plague patients to the municipal isolation hospital; (2) whether to follow the prescriptions to bury their plague dead in the *Begamwadi* outside of town or persist in burying them in their traditional cemetery; and (3) whether to prohibit the Plague Committee's new policy of pouring quicklime into plague victims' graves. On all three, they concluded that the Collector's policies violated their religion and the Queen's Proclamation of 1858. But no violence ensued.[37] Several weeks later in Hyderabad in Sind Province, 'a monster meeting' comprised of Hindus and Muslims of all denominations, 'high and low', protested 'strongly but respectfully' against compulsory segregation of the healthy to huts and especially the segregation of pardah ladies. Segregation, they argued, violated their religious rites and social customs. The meeting's first resolution even recognized the good intentions of the government's plague measures.[38] In Rander in the Surat district, plague legislation limiting those attending a funeral to fifteen and forcing plague burials to be removed from the city caused 'a scene of much excitement'. In opposing the law, 3000 Muslims joined a funeral procession and carried the body to their sacred cemetery (a Masjid). The next day, more Muslims assembled in their mosques and closed their businesses to oppose the funerary limit but no violence resulted.[39] Nor were these peaceful petitions and demonstrations limited to elites or middling sorts. In protesting anti-plague measures and abuses in Mumbai in April 1897, millworkers first drafted petitions to the government, and when these were not answered, 8000 dockworkers struck, closing down Mumbai's shipping commerce for a day.[40] Again, despite the numbers involved, the international press did not report these protests.

Other mass meetings resulted in actions that went beyond recommendations respectfully delivered to the Plague Commissions, but these usually developed only after the District Collectors or Plague Commissioners had refused to consider resolutions debated in general assemblies. Rarely did protest emerge spontaneously as it seemingly did with many cholera riots, without prior meetings, resolutions, or attempts to negotiate. Moreover, the few to have arisen without reports of previous efforts at reform may reflect the absence of in-depth reportage in places further removed from capitals, or journalists may have imputed violence when none had occurred. A case in point comes from conflicting reports of actions taken in Bhávnagar

---

[37] L/R/5/152, week ending 20 March 1897, no. 36, *Gujarat*.

[38] Ibid., no. 34, *Kathiawar News*. Other examples are easily found: in the week ending 13 March 1897, no. 46, *Jam-e-Jamshed*, 'a large meeting of the Mohamedans' of Surat met in the palace of the city's Nawab to oppose the Collector's unannounced practices of burying plague victims with quicklime and preventing recitation of funeral prayers over the dead. Similarly, on 23 April 1897 a public meeting occurred in Karachi to discuss segregation, detention, and disinfection, which gave the government concern; ibid., no. 21, *Phoenix*. From neither did riots arise.

[39] Ibid., week ending 13 March 1897, no. 47: *Praja Pokár* and *Deshi Mitra*. Arnold, *Colonizing the Body*, 217, also cites it.

[40] Sarkar, 'The Tie that Snapped', 185. For strikes of millworkers in Kanpur, protesting anti-plague measures, see note 178.

on 11 March 1897, prompted, according to one paper, by rumours of plague patients being deliberately poisoned at the town's segregation hospital. According to *Deshi Mitra*'s correspondent, 8000 met and proceeded to the house of the state's chief medical officer 'with the intention of mobbing that gentleman', but after 'a slight disturbance', the military moved in and the crowd dispersed. According to the *Káthiáwár Times*, a paper published the day before and closer to the scene, the crowd comprised 3000, and the protest was peaceful. The Muslims assembled in front of the house of the town's local leader (Diwán) to obtain assurances that compulsory segregation would be discontinued. No rumours of poisoning or actions against the chief medical officer were reported.[41] Other mass meetings could, however, lead to organized violence, especially after governors had long refused to negotiate. In Sinnar in Nassik Province, frustrations exploded on 23 February 1898. After a series of 'noisy meetings', in which villagers expressed discontent over forced segregation of those reputedly exposed to plague victims, a 'mob' of 600 burnt segregation huts and attacked another plague camp.[42]

'THE POONA TRAGEDY'

Given their outcome and worldwide reportage, the most significant of frustrated mass meetings, plague petitions, and recommendations were those of the first half of 1897 in the Presidency of Bombay's second city, Pune. At the Jubilee Day celebrations in honour of Queen Victoria, Lieutenant Ayerst was mistaken for Lieutenant Lewis and assassinated. More egregious as far as the British government and press were concerned was the assassination of the city's Collector, Mr Rand, who three months earlier had also become Pune's first Plague Commissioner. Quickly, he achieved notoriety for the severity and insensitivity of early-morning plague searches and his policies of isolation. Certain foreign newspapers alleged that India's 'native' press was responsible for the assassinations by defying colonial efforts to end plague. An Australian paper claimed that 'every day' Indian newspapers had grown 'more seditious' and had falsely accused British troops of 'violating women, polluting mosques, and generally insulting the Hindu and Mohammedan religions'.[43] Other papers alleged that native intellectuals had invented the abuses by Rand's officers to rouse a revolt against modern science and medicine. Such criticisms entered 'native' papers.[44] However, India's press hardly spoke with a single voice, and its divisions sharpened with the assassinations. Newspapers that were in English, a wide variety of Indian languages, and bilingual blamed other native newspapers, especially those in Pune, accusing the city's Brahmin caste of 'cowardly and dastardly deeds'. One of the earliest papers to

[41] Ibid., week ending, 13 March 1897, no. 50; the military was called to disperse the crowd.
[42] *Guardian*, 23 February 1898; and *Singapore Free Press*, 17 February 1898, 111; Arnold, *Colonizing the Body*, 230, refers to the 'disturbances' at 'Sinnat' in January but does not describe them.
[43] *Kalgoorlie Miner*, 2 July 1897, 3.
[44] For British denial of wrongdoing, see *Sheffield Daily Telegraph*, 24 July 1897, 6, alleging that stories of plague officers attacking Indian women at Pune were myths.

comment on the assassinations, the bilingual Anglo-Gujuráti *Rást Goftár*, called them a 'conspiracy' and pinned them on the 'inflammable writings' of the Deccan press.[45] 'For some time past', it alleged, Pune's papers had made threatening accusations against plague officials, publishing 'anonymous letters against their lives' which confirmed 'the general belief of Pune as a hotbed of sedition'. The paper appealed to the governor to adopt 'effective measures for the timely suppression' of Pune's native press, which happened a few days later, when Lord Sandhurst also imposed a new 'punitive' force of over a thousand police officers on the city at the native population's expense. Meanwhile, arrests and criminal charges mounted against journalists and editors. Most notable was the arrest of journalist, newspaper owner, and future independence fighter, Bal Gangadhar Tilak, imprisoned because of his articles in the Anglo-Maráthi *Sudhárak* and his own two papers, *Mahrátta* and the Maráthi *Kesari*.[46]

Other papers in native languages supported *Rást Goftár,*'s views. The Anglo-Maráthi *Dnyánodayá* claimed 'the violence of the Pune press must also be held responsible' for the assassinations.[47] English papers joined the chorus: the *Champion* declaring that 'such conduct merits one reward, the hangman's noose'.[48] Another tarred the Maráthi press with 'openly exhorting to violence': 'Native papers have been indulging in a perfect orgy of sedition'.[49] The *Bombay Gazette* 'exculpated' Rand of any wrongdoing, asserting that the 'clamour against him' arose from 'seditious newspapers conducted by the Poona Brahmins'.[50]

Pune's papers stood by their earlier editorials but did so in tones hardly bathed in 'blood-soaked violence'.[51] On 27 June, the Maráthi *Gujaráti* led the defence, first commenting on the lot of journalists of all political stripes, for their 'thankless tasks'. Instead of justifying the assassinations, the paper branded them 'tragic and deplorable'. Unlike papers outside Pune, however, it questioned the government's treatment of Pune's people, asking if it had 'acted wisely in ignoring the loud and universal chorus of disapproval' of the decisions imposed by Pune's Plague Committee. Their questioning cannot be simply labelled as anti-colonialist or anti-European. As with articles before 'Poona's Tragedy', the paper contrasted Pune's Plague Commissioner with Mumbai's, General Gatacre, praising the latter's 'admirable tact, magnanimity, and forethought'. In contrast to Mumbai, where a dialogue developed between the native population and the Plague Commission, the paper recalled its earlier appeals to Mr Rand and Lord Sandhurst, which were ignored. Yet the paper ended with the same call as those outside the city: 'The immediate question of the moment...is the detection of the murderers'.[52]

The following day, Pune's English-language *Dnyán Prakásh* made similar appeals, sending condolences to the wounded Rand (who died a week later), saying that

---

[45] The plateau region of south-central India with Pune as the centre.
[46] L/R/5/152, week ending 10 July 1897, no. 10, *Gujaráti*. On Tilak's anti-plague measures, see Arnold, *Colonizing the Body*, 212–13. On the significance of plague for his subsequent career, Catanach, 'Poona Politicians', 2–3.
[47] L/R/5/152, week ending 3 July 1897, no. 17, *Dnyánodayá*.
[48] Ibid., no. 22, *Champion*; also ibid., no. 19, *Indian Spectator*.
[49] Ibid., no. 20, *Kathiawar News*.   [50] Ibid., no. 38, *Vartahar*.
[51] Ibid., no. 20, *Káthiáwár News*.   [52] Ibid., no. 25, *Gujaráti*.

Indians felt great sympathy towards him, even though the paper had criticized 'his persistent refusal to listen to their complaints'. It held that their suggestions had been restricted to legal and constitutional methods and refuted the stereotypes pinned on Indians, that in the words of India's sanitary commissioner, Robert Harvey, they were 'suspicious of innovation, extremely conservative, very ignorant, full of prejudices and superstitions and of amazing credulity'.[53]

Were the dissidents' comments merely attempts to shield themselves from British repression, which did, in fact, unfold immediately after the 'tragedy'? What had been their record in the months leading up to the Jubilee murders? Had they, like cholera protesters across Europe, opposed all interventions made in the name of medical science, spreading rumours about hospitals and medical carers? Colonial surveillance over these papers has preserved these previous reactions, along with reports on the attitudes of large swathes of the populace. By 1897 the Presidency of Bombay alone was surveying weekly over 200 native papers in English and indigenous languages, even though their print runs ranged from only 110 to 4300 copies, with most counting less than a thousand. Their readership was thus limited to a thin layer of the intelligentsia, even if the papers might have been read aloud at public gatherings or at work. However, the papers claimed to reflect popular sentiments as when Puna's Maráthi *Dnyán Prakásh* (with 450 copies) on 28 June expressed the city's sympathy for the victims and their families attacked in Pune.[54]

The first notices in these papers of plague in Pune came in the week ending 16 January 1897.[55] Within three weeks, the papers began criticizing the ways in which government anti-plague operations had been implemented, but given later condemnations, their complaints were not what we would have expected. They did not berate municipal officials and British authorities for imposing new forms of quarantine and methods of search and seizure, or for dumping massive amounts of disinfectant on native property as had been British practice since 1896.[56] Instead, it was the opposite: *Káthiáwár News* warned the municipality to end 'its lethargy' in imposing restrictions 'and to take all possible precautions in time to keep the city clean'.[57] Another defended compulsory segregation, attacking fears that patients removed to isolation hospitals were 'killed by poison' and corrected other, less far-fetched beliefs about visitation rights at Pune's segregation hospital. It supported government anti-plague operations, even claiming that Pune's plague patients received 'the best possible treatment and nursing'.[58]

Only during the first week of March did these papers take a different tack, and it coincided with Rand's appointment as the district's first Plague Commissioner.

[53] Cited in Arnold, *Colonizing the Body*, 232; and L/R/5/152, week ending 3 July 1897, no. 29, *Dnyán Prakásh*.

[54] The weekly entries begin by listing the papers, divided by language and indicating print runs. For the most part, articles from thirty or so papers appear in weekly reports. For the rapid growth of the Indian press in the late nineteenth century, see Arnold, *Colonizing the Body*, 211.

[55] L/R/5/157, week ending 16 January 1897, no. 16, *Rajahansa*.

[56] Arnold, *Colonizing the Body*, 204; Chandavarkar, 'Plague Panic', 207; Catanach, 'Plague and the Tensions', 153.

[57] L/R/5/157, week ending 16 January 1897, no. 36, *Káthiáwár News*.

[58] Ibid., week ending 20 February 1897, no. 28, *Sudharak*.

Yet their message was not inflammatory. Instead, they regretted his approach to segregation operations and beseeched him to adopt more humane and effective procedures. *Dnyán Prakásh* advised: if the people were to accept segregation, it had to be voluntary, 'gently impressed on the popular mind by the leaders of the people'. The paper called for property destroyed by plague search parties to be compensated and hospital accommodation improved. If such steps were not adopted, it argued, concealment of plague cases would continue, 'giving firm root to the disease'.[59] Maráthi *Vártánidhi* disapproved of the burning of the poor's bedding and clothing and demolition of their houses, leaving them in a miserable condition. But it made clear that it was not opposed to the government's principles of sanitation.[60]

For the remainder of March and April, Pune's papers pointed to other violations and insults inflicted on them, documenting specific excesses. Their criticisms were presented in a spirit of negotiation, proposing reforms without challenging European medical principles. In the week ending 13 March, a native paper agreed that search parties' visitations were necessary but pleaded for women's privacy to be respected, that competent women doctors examine them, not foreign men, and that search parties include natives 'of position and influence'.[61] The Maráthi *Nyáyá Sindhu* pointed to the consequences of Rand's plague policies on the economy: they had caused a mass exodus with others 'fast leaving the city'. Gujarati grocers had closed their shops and returned to the country.[62] According to one account, three-quarters of Pune's native population had fled, not from fear of plague but from the government's harsh implementation of anti-plague controls.[63] Pune's press alleged that Rand's soldiers entered any part of the house, 'even the kitchen or rooms where the family idols are kept', picked locks, and appropriated property as they wished.[64] Still the papers remained conciliatory, maintaining that they did not object to the policies, only to the soldiers' unwillingness to 'behave with kindness, decency and respect'.[65]

From March to the assassinations, excerpts from Pune's papers continued cataloguing government abuses. On 19 March, several reported a sudden rise in military searches.[66] Two hundred cavalry and a hundred infantry invaded the neighbourhoods of Budhuwár Peth and part of Shukrawár to uncover cases; streets were blockaded and shops broken into. *Dnyán Prakásh* compared Rand's plague measures to an enemy 'sacking of a conquered town'. But the paper continued making suggestions such as asking European soldiers 'not to spit around while moving about in the houses. Spitting is considered a filthy habit by the Natives', and that it would be better to inspect the entire city at the same time, instead of by district. By scattering people from one neighbourhood to another, the practice accelerated the spread of the disease, believed by most to be highly contagious.[67]

[59]   Ibid., week ending 6 March 1897, nos 23 and 24, *Dnyán Prakásh*.
[60]   Ibid., no. 26, *Vartanidhi*.
[61]   Ibid., week ending 13 March 1897, no. 23, *Kesari*.   [62]   Ibid., no. 25, *Nyáyà Sindhu*.
[63]   Ibid., no. 43, *Dnyan Ohakahu*. Between the first appearance of plague and February 1897, 380,000 of Mumbai's population of 850,000 fled; Arnold, *Colonizing the Body*, 207.
[64]   Ibid., no. 25, *Nyáyà Sindhu*.   [65]   Ibid., no. 28, *Dnyán Prakásh*.
[66]   Ibid., week ending 20 March 1897, no. 24, *Sudharak*.   [67]   Ibid, no. 23, *Dnyán Prakásh*.

Other papers continued documenting violations to privacy, stolen and damaged property, and affronts to dignity, as when soldiers strip-searched men and women alike in public. They charged that soldiers broke open shopkeepers' boxes and safes 'with the absurd suspicion that a plague patient' might be lurking inside. Sewing machines and glass chandeliers were burnt along with account books as harbouring the disease. 'Even women in childbed' were dragged off to the segregation camps.[68] Papers complained of inadequate provisions at segregation camps, contaminated water (which the papers feared could spark cholera, then rampant in the region), and that milk was not given to infants.[69] By June, with the rainy season approaching, the papers feared the segregation camps were 'sure [to become] more unhealthy than the worst housing' in the city.[70] Reports continued of inhabitants being marched off to the camps without plague symptoms, even with medical certifications that they were uninfected.[71] Complaints surfaced 'every day' of soldiers' rudeness, insults, thievery, and rough treatment.[72] Yet the papers repeatedly emphasized that they did not oppose Rand's plague controls in principle[73] and contrasted his implementation of them with Mumbai's Gatacre.[74]

In late April, new allegations arose of soldiers burning sacred images taken from private houses and shrines.[75] On 29 April, they entered a Máruti temple in Pune's Nána Peth district, uprooted two images, painted them red, cut the legs off the idol of Garud, and burnt the temple's sofas, carpets, and other furnishings. The temple's tenants were removed to the segregation camp, along with those who came to worship there, and daily worship was outlawed.[76] At the same time, they disinterred the corpse of a Gosai (ascetic), burnt it on 'the verandah of the math', and destroyed the shrine's furniture.[77] Finally, from March to June, citizens presented letters and petitions to Rand and Sandhurst, with specific objections to military excesses.[78] After the 'Tragedy of Poona', Pune's *Dnyán Prakásh* claimed that 'hundreds of petitions and memorials' had been sent.[79] Native papers of various political and religious stripes repeated that their petitions had been ignored,[80] and accused Rand of making decisions behind closed doors without entrusting the native

---

[68] Ibid., week ending 3 April 1897, no. 19, *Kesari*.

[69] Ibid., no. 21, *Jagadhitechchhu*. Also, see week ending 15 May 1897, no. 18, *Prabhát*.

[70] Ibid., week ending 12 June 1897, no. 18, *Mahratta*.

[71] Ibid., week ending 10 April 1897, nos 16–20; 24 April 1897, no. 14; and many others.

[72] Ibid., week ending 10 April 1897, nos 12–14, 16–20; week ending 24 April 1897, no. 14, *Dnyán Prakásh*, and many others.

[73] Ibid., week ending 10 April 1897, no. 12, *Mahratta*.

[74] Ibid., week ending, 3 April 1897, nos 13–15; 17 April, nos 11, 14, and 16; 24 April, no. 9; week ending 3 April 1897, nos 13–15; week ending 24 April 1897, no. 9; and week ending 5 June, no. 11. Pune's papers also thanked city officials such as the Honourable Mr Ollivant for abolishing military house visitations; ibid., week ending 3 July 1897, no. 48, *Jagadhitechehku*.

[75] Ibid., week ending 24 April 1897, no. 14.

[76] Ibid., week ending 1 May 1897, nos 12 and 15.

[77] Ibid., 26 April, no. 12. According to the Anglo-Maráthi *Sudhàrak*, such assaults were being reported all over town; ibid., week ending 1 May 1897, no. 12. Also, week ending 15 May 1897, no. 13.

[78] Ibid., week ending 27 March 1897, no. 24; 17 April 1897, no. 11; 1 May 1897, no. 11; 5 June 1897, no. 10; 3 July 1897, no. 25.

[79] Ibid., week ending 3 July 1897, no. 29, *Dnyán Prakásh*.

[80] Ibid., week ending 5 June 1897, no. 10. On Rand's 'Triumvirate' Plague Commission, see Arnold, *Colonizing the Body*, 228.

educated population.[81] Even the English-language *Champion*, which two weeks earlier had raised no objections to Mr Rand's treatment of residents, drew attention after the 'tragedy' to the letters and petitions drafted by prominent native figures, which he 'had thrown into the waste-basket'.[82]

By May, some of the papers' pleas could be judged as inflammatory. Several recalled examples from Indian history when its inhabitants had not tolerated tyranny or had overthrown oppressive regimes.[83] They taunted: the Hindus had not always been 'cowards' as when they had thrown off 'the yoke of the Monguls'. They asked whether citizens 'should meekly endure' their present 'zulum' (tyranny).[84] After reviewing the atrocities of soldiers' house visitations, the Anglo-Maráthi *Sudhárak* chided its readers: 'still we calmly look on and show not the least sign of resistance'.[85] The Maráthi *Dnyán Prakásh* targeted Pune's Brahmins, saying they 'richly' deserved the treatment they now received from their oppressors. It came close to prodding for insurrection: 'What opposition do you offer to the high-handedness of the soldiers but your cowardly meekness?'[86] When it came to specific action, however, the papers stopped short. With Rand's forces set for house inspection in villages surrounding Pune, the *Sudhárak* called its readers to action: 'Citizens of Poona! Are you going to do anything?' But that call was entirely constitutional and advocated communication through colonial channels: 'Go to Lord Sandhurst to curb the barbarous brutes'.[87]

Moreover, despite this thundering of news and protest, not a single plague riot arose in Pune during this period. The 'tragedy' was not a riot but an assassination, a 'conspiracy' ultimately pinned on two men alone. Nonetheless, Pune and plague continued to dominate native papers of the Presidency into the following year with the outside press shaming Pune's editors and Brahmins, holding them responsible for the assassinations. Pune's notoriety even played itself out on an international stage: letters and articles reached London papers and debates at Westminster on whether the fines against an entire city and press gagging were justified. During the 'Third Pandemic', no non-violent campaign of meetings, strikes, and struggles by a local press had been as intense or protracted as at Pune. Nor had such efforts to negotiate with a colonial government principally by peaceful and constitutional means ever been met with such repressive force.

India was not unique in organizing cross-class, peaceful protest against unjust and abusive policies during the Third Pandemic. Most striking was Chinatown's struggle in San Francisco in 1900. Its merchant elites, Chinese and Caucasian, relied on mass rallies, shop and business closures, petitions and negotiations, and the courts to contest national discriminatory decrees that quarantined Chinatown alone, then inoculated the Chinese as the only source and carriers of plague. Unlike Pune's struggles, however, San Francisco's did not dominate even its local press, much less an international one, for months on end.[88]

[81] Ibid., week ending 27 March 1897, no. 17; 24 April, no. 17.
[82] Ibid., week ending 17 July 1897, no. 22, *Champion*.
[83] See, for instance, ibid., 17 April 1897, no. 14.
[84] Ibid., week ending, 8 May 1897, no. 15.   [85] Ibid., week ending 15 May 1897, no. 13.
[86] Ibid., no. 16.   [87] Ibid., week ending 8 May 1897, no. 14.
[88] Their struggles do not appear in *San Francisco Call*.

KOLKATA

Pune's protest and the assassinations failed to deter the government from pursuing overzealous, counterproductive measures to segregate plague cases and relentlessly search for suspected plague victims in a manner that only encouraged the concealment of plague cases. Nor did it dampen plague protest or large-scale riots elsewhere in India. A week after Pune's assassinations, one of the largest plague revolts in the subcontinent erupted in Kolkata. For several days, gangs roamed its wealthier suburbs attacking any Europeans they met. More serious protests against plague measures began on 30 June in the suburb of Tchittpor (or Chitpor),[89] and on 1 July, a crowd of 5000 'most determined men' protested against search parties, segregation, desecration of Muslim shrines, and destruction of the mud huts surrounding them.[90] As with other Indian plague riots, the outrage united Muslims and Hindus. By the end of the day, rebels had taken control of the north-eastern portion of the city. Clashes with police on the following days resulted in casualty figures outstripping the worst cholera riots in Russia. By one account twenty-one,[91] by another, twenty-four[92] officers had been severely wounded, with most expected to die. But the government's retaliation produced a more extraordinary massacre: reputedly, the police killed over 600 natives.[93] Citing *Le Temps*, the *Guardian* compared it to the Mumbai revolt of 1893 (though on that occasion fewer had been killed or wounded: eighty and 530, respectively[94]). The *Guardian* feared a repeat of a much larger catastrophe, the Indian Mutiny of 1857.[95]

Despite the slaughter (and unlike at Pune), the rebels won concessions. Authorities reversed their decision to destroy the mud huts, and over a hundred Muslims offered prayers of thanksgiving, celebrating their 'moral victory'.[96] But the compromise failed to end Kolkata's revolts. In May, the following year, 'numerous instances of murderous assaults' were directed against those engaged in the city's inoculation programme. Four months later (4 August), *Lancet* correspondent, Frank Clemow, then involved with Kolkata's sanitary corps, reported that 'wild and gross rumours' circulated through the city, resulting in 'some very terrible consequences', including murders with 'many others' 'severely mauled merely because the cry had been raised that they were *ticeamallons*—the native word for inoculators'. Then came the 'ambulance scare'. Any appearance of a municipal ambulance provoked 'the collecting of a crowd of excited natives'. On two occasions, 'the mob' attacked them and injured those in charge. Reminiscent of European cholera riots (which Clemow had earlier reported), protesters destroyed the vehicles and set them ablaze. From then on, armed police guards escorted patients to hospitals, and it became unsafe for Europeans, 'whether connected with the plague operations or not', to walk about the city without a revolver.[97]

---

[89] *Le Temps*, 3 July 1897.   [90] *Scotsman*, 3 July 1897, 9.
[91] *Guardian*, 8 July 1897.   [92] *Launceston Examiner*, 6 July 1897, 5.
[93] *Argus*, 8 July 1897, 5; *Scotsman*, 3 July 1897, 9.   [94] Kidambi, *The Making*, 118.
[95] *Guardian*, 8 July 1897.   [96] *Launceston Examiner*, 6 July 1897, 5.
[97] Clemow, 'The Plague at Calcutta'. Arnold, *Colonizing the Body*, 225–6 and 230, analyses this riot but does not mention the larger one of 1897. He presents the May riot as against inoculation but, as Clemow showed, it also concerned isolation and searches.

The incidents came to a climax on 21 May in the Kolkata suburb of Bhowanpur, when a doctor selecting an isolation site for those suspected of plague 'was mobbed'. Armed with a pistol, he killed a rioter and wounded two others, then fled to safety at the municipality's health office. A mob formed, demanding the doctor's surrender.[98] From a Kolkata correspondent, *The Times* reported that 3000 revolted. Negotiations followed and again resulted in successes for the native population. Nine days later, referring to the 'unrest' of May, the *Scotsman* concluded: 'We believe that the plague measures were modified because of pressure they [the native population] brought on the Government'.[99] Yet plague disturbances continued in the subcontinent's largest conurbation. In March 1899, with cases on the rise, unrest now concerned disinfection.[100] At the end of the year, the *Lancet* reported that 'the wildest stories' circulated about the 'horrors of inoculation' in Kolkata. Then, the cry, 'ticca-wallah' (inoculators) led 'on several occasions' to 'riotous mobs, and more than one innocent individual', taken as an inoculator, was killed 'by the people'. The programme to inoculate the entire native population by Haffkine's method proved a failure: only 2490 of over 700,000 came forward.[101] These incidents of violent protest and more passive resistance occurred, according to the *Lancet*, after authorities for almost a year had 'practically abandon[ed] all active measures' of sanitation and plague control. Now plague patients were allowed to be treated in private and caste hospitals, and families were no longer forced into the camps: of the former plague operations, only disinfection remained'.[102] However, despite supposed 'capitulation to native violence', government conciliation ultimately proved successful. After the inoculation policy ended in 1899, no further plague disturbances were heard from Kolkata, even though plague rose sharply here and throughout India, peaking in 1907 and persisting as a major health threat until at least 1918.[103]

MUMBAI AND THE PRESIDENCY OF BOMBAY

Despite initial qualms over the colonial government's selection of a general to direct the Bombay Plague Commission, the native press quickly changed its tune, heaping praise on General Gatacre.[104] A week after taking office, he convened

---

[98] *Scotsman*, 23 May 1898, 7, from a Kolkata correspondent; *The Times*, 23 May 1898, 7; and Clemow, 'The Plague at Calcutta', who identified the doctor as Ronald Laing, a district medical officer, and justified Laing's firing on the crowds.

[99] *Scotsman*, 2 June 1898, 6. [100] 'Notes from India', 1899(a).

[101] Ibid., 1899(d). It had not, however, been the case in other districts as in the Punjab at the end of 1898 (L/R/5/153, week ending 31 December 1898, no. 22, *Rasik Ranjani*) or in Pune in 1901 (L/R/5/156, week ending 8 June 1901, no. 28, *Deccan Herald*).

[102] Ibid., 155, 12 May 1900, 1402.

[103] See Klein, 'Plague'. On the decline of plague riots, see Kidambi, *The Making*, 67; Arnold, *Colonializing the Body*, 201; and Catanach, 'Plague and the Tensions', 165.

[104] L/R/5/152, week ending 3 April 1897, no. 13, *Akbár-e-Islam*; no. 14, *Muslim Herald*; week ending 10 April 1897, nos 24 and 25, *Muslim Herald*. Intellectuals were not alone in holding the General in esteem. After his retirement, *Kaiser-e-Hind*, L/R/5/153, week ending 15 January 1898, no. 29, claimed that 'everybody' desired his return, calling him 'the idol of the populace'.

meetings with community groups, and by the end of March allowed the building of special hospitals for Muslims and treatment of their sick by private doctors to avoid violating caste sensibilities. Further, he listened to complaints against house searches, sanitary officers' abuses, and violations of women's privacy, and modified policies accordingly.[105] Against the desires of Mumbai's citizens, the General demitted as the city's Commissioner at the end of July.[106] The native press responded with regret and raised monies to erect a monument for his services.[107]

Yet Mumbai and its suburbs experienced more plague riots and demonstrations against anti-plague measures than any place in the subcontinent or elsewhere during the 'Third Pandemic'. India's first plague disturbance occurred on 10 October 1896, when Mumbai's millhands and others, comprising 'a mob of 3,000',[108] rioted against segregating plague patients from their families by attacking the isolation hospital on Arthur Road.[109] On 5 November, they assailed the hospital again, because of 'tyrannical' rules segregating patients. News that a supposedly 'healthy and innocent' female worker had been forcibly removed to the hospital triggered the riot. Fifty workers assembled demanding her release. The following afternoon, about a thousand mill operatives from surrounding districts converged on the hospital in 'an organized attempt' to destroy it and liberate the patients. Rumours spread that not a single patient returned from the hospital alive; something 'diabolic' about it had 'claimed so many victims'; blood was being drained from patients' feet.[110] These papers, read mainly by indigenous elites, attributed the rumours to the 'ignorance' of the lower classes. Yet they also chastised 'authorities' for refusing to listen to public opinion or confide in Mumbai's native leaders. The failing, papers charged, rested with the Anglo Indian administrator, Mr P. C. H. Snow, Municipal Commissioner of Bombay, who was responsible for plague policy. Papers repeated: 'Examples do not teach him'.[111] Yet later that week, Snow, unlike Rand a year later, responded positively, ruling that 'no cases, where proper segregation and treatment can be carried out on the premises will be sent to Arthur Road'.[112]

In less than a month, however, another disturbance erupted among 'the lower classes' with an unspecified disturbance on Falkland Road; again, the provocation was colonial segregation of plague patients.[113] At the beginning of 1897, the municipal government redoubled its efforts at sanitary control by wholesale burning of slum property and closing graveyards. On 11 February 5000 Muslims assembled in the Juma Masjid district to contest the city's closing of its graveyard.[114] *Mumbai Vaibhave* protested against the burning of infected huts in the city centre at the

[105] Ibid., week ending 3 April 1897, no. 14, *Muslim Herald.*
[106] Ibid., week ending 24 July 1897, no. 45, *Rást Goftár.*
[107] Ibid., week ending 10 July 1897, no. 3, *Rást Goftár.*
[108] *New York Times*, 29 October 1896.   [109] Echenberg, *Plague Ports*, 64 5.
[110] L/R/5/150: week ending 7 November 1896, no. 12; and Mumbai's Anglo-Gujarati *Kaiser-e-Hind*, 1 November 1896.
[111] L/R/5/151, week ending 7 November 1896, nos 12–14. On Snow and his plague policies, see Arnold, *Colonizing the Body*, 204, 206–8.
[112] Ibid., nos 14–15, *Gujaráti.*
[113] Ibid., week ending 12 December 1896, no. 45, *Akhbáre Islám.*
[114] Ibid., week ending 13 February 1897, no. 29.

foot of Malabár Hill and condemned 'the folly and heartlessness of the authorities', warning Europeans not to burn further human habitations, 'lest some disastrous consequences might follow'.[115] Yet, despite the scale of the protests, far larger than any plague riots or peaceful demonstrations outside India, no foreign press appears to have reported them.

Though smaller in scale than the Muslim demonstration above, riots in March and June gained international exposure, perhaps because now they were violent. By 1897, the lessons learned at the end of 1896 had been forgotten. In March, the civic authorities decided to segregate plague patients once again with serious restrictions on family visitation. On the 23rd, Muslims rallied forces against hospitals and sanitation services. A 'small riot' destroyed three hospital vans. The Muslim community sought exemption from the policies but were 'firmly refused'.[116] In June, two officers employed by the municipality to control plague were shot and remained in a critical condition. The one paper to report the shooting does not clarify whether it occurred during a riot, but allegedly it stemmed from a 'seditious leaflet...widely circulated in India', accusing sanitary officers of polluting temples and mosques under the pretext of controlling plague.[117] A seventh plague riot in Mumbai broke out a week later, again as a consequence of plague controls that offended religious sensibilities; the protesters' actions, however, were not recorded.[118]

The high point of plague rebellion in the subcontinent lasted from late June 1897 to around 4 July. In addition to Pune's 'Tragedy' and British threats of mass repression to an entire city, gang attacks in Kolkata's streets, the riots and mass repression that swiftly followed,[119] and Mumbai's riots, further disturbances flared up against plague policies and the excesses of military search parties.[120] At Jeepore [sic], 'southeast of Poona' (which must be Jejuri) residents attacked 'nearly all the plague inspectors'. Their violations of women, 'polluting [of] temples and mosques', and generally insulting behaviour towards the Hindu and Muslim religions 'sent the population into a frenzy'. By 1 July, troops reoccupied the town, but the Indians swore 'to avenge themselves for the profanation of the mosques'.[121]

Despite modifications in policy, riots continued the following year during the plague's upsurge in the cooler winter months. In the Presidency of Bombay, these first struck towns and cities outside Mumbai. The themes and targets were much the same as earlier. On the first day of Ramadam, 24 January, 'natives' attacked a segregation camp at Sinnar, killing a hospital attendant, burning the camp, wrecking the post office, and cutting telegraph wires. The police fired on the 'mob', wounding several.[122] Afterwards, the chairman of the Sinnar Plague Commission

[115] Ibid., no. 30, *Mumbai Vaibhave.*

[116] *Launceston Examiner*, 24 March 1897, 5: from London, 23 March; *Wagga Wagga Advertiser*, 25 March 1897, 3; and *Le Temps*, 24 March 1897, front page, reported much the same with the 'crowd' breaking an ambulance to bits, but the police arrived in time to prevent rioting.

[117] *Sydney Morning Herald*, 26 June 1897, 8.   [118] *Barrier Miner*, 3 July 1897, 2.

[119] In the House of Commons, Mr S. Smith maintained that 600 was a low estimate of those killed, while Lord Hamilton claimed only seven died with twenty wounded; *Morning Post*, 10 July 1897, 6–7.

[120] *Kalgoorlie Miner*, 3 July 1897, 5.   [121] Ibid., 2 July 1897, 3.

[122] According to *South Australian Register*, 31 January 1898, 5; and *Mercury*, 1 February 1898, 2, the riot occurred at the district capital, 'Nasik'. According to *Guardian*, 30 January 1898, 5; *Scotsman*,

was found murdered in a nearby field; 150 were arrested.[123] A second riot, referred to above, erupted in the same place for much the same reasons less than a month later, after health authorities converted other hospitals to segregate plague patients. This time, however, the mob—600 villagers—came from outside, burnt the segregation huts, then went to a second site—Dr Gwyther's camp—burning his tents and everything inside. The villagers attacked a government dispensary, where they 'brutally murdered' an elderly Brahmin assistant, then pillaged the post office, burnt its books, and destroyed telegraph equipment. Finally, they marched to the city's treasury and hacked a Brahmin pleader to death.[124]

A week later (9 March 1898) a plague riot at Mumbai provoked the widest international coverage of any uprising of the 'Third Pandemic' and has been one of the few to receive attention outside plague histories. The historian of late nineteenth- and twentieth-century Mumbai, Prashant Kidambi, placed it alongside the massive textile revolt of 1893 as the two revolts to reshape social and political relations between the populace and police, leading to the Police Act of 1902 and a new social order for Mumbai in the twentieth century.[125] The immediate cause was the discovery of an ill twelve-year-old 'Mahometan Julai' girl, suspected of having plague but later found to have been afflicted by another disorder. She and her family refused to allow the search party to examine her by an inexperienced European male medical student. 'An enormous crowd of caste men gathered' and attacked the search party and plague authorities.[126] A Parsee magistrate intervened to persuade the crowds to disperse and was gravely assaulted.[127] In addition, a British doctor and a member of the inspection party were stoned to death.[128] Police were called in; four Muslim protesters were killed and tensions escalated. Hindus and Muslim united, and attacks against Europeans moved to the wealthy suburbs. One section of the mob attacked the Victorian buildings in the suburb of Byeulla. According to the British press, 'No Christian is safe'.[129] The following day, two soldiers from the Shropshire Regiment were murdered as they walked along a quiet street, and Europeans were beaten and stabbed in the bazaar. Ambulances used to transport plague victims to hospitals were burnt, and attempts were made to set hospitals ablaze, including the Jamsetjee hospital, which was defended by staff and students. European nurses narrowly escaped with their lives.[130] It took two days for the police and military to restore order but not until casualties and arrests had

31 January 1898; *The Times*, 31 January 1898; and *Le Temps*, 30 January 1898, it was at Sinnar. Also, see week ending 2 February 1898, no. 33, *Indu Prakásh*.

[123] *Scotsman*, 31 January 1898, 6; and 1 February 1898, 5; and *The Times*, 1 February 1893, 3. Native papers of the Bombay Presidency attributed the riot to the stringency of segregation and Dr Gwyther's orders to demolish housing at Sinnar; L/R/5/152, week ending 5 February 1897, no. 33, *Indu Prakásh*; no. 34, *Native Opinion*, 29 January; no. 35, *Gurákhi*; and no. 36, *Mumbai Vaibhav*.

[124] *Guardian*, 23 February 1898, from *Bombay Gazette*; and *The Times*, 19 February 1858, 7.

[125] Kidambi, *The Making*, ch. 5.

[126] *Guardian*, 10 March 1898, 11 March 1898, and 12 March 1898. Papers across the globe covered it.

[127] *The Times*, 10 March 1898, 5; and *Guardian*, 10 March 1898, 5.

[128] *Scotsman*, 10 March 1898; *Manchester Courier*, 10 March 1898, 5; and many more. The inspector was Mr Dawes, not the doctor.

[129] *Guardian*, 10 March 1898.   [130] Among other places, *Argus*, 11 March 1897, 5.

mounted to levels seen only during the worst of the Russian cholera riots. In addition to the two Shropshire soldiers, a sergeant, who accidentally shot himself, and a police inspector were killed, two constables were seriously wounded, and thirteen other 'European' officers and five native policemen received less serious injuries. Seventeen European members of the public were 'injured and roughly handled', including a nurse. Nine of the protesters were killed, twenty-two seriously injured, and 109 arrested.[131] We will return to the significance of this riot as influencing a fundamental change in plague policy, not only for Mumbai but for the subcontinent as a whole. For now, these riots, initiated by the Chinese-style search parties that had become standard throughout India, had not ended. The following days of non-violent mass protest by the city's working classes may have been more effective in prompting the abrupt change in Sandhurst's strategies of plague control: workers and small merchants of Mumbai's piece-goods markets closed their shops, with larger shopkeepers shutting theirs in the city bazaars, and 15,000 dockers, labourers, and cartmen employed at railway goods stations joined the protest by striking.[132] The international press claimed that Indians considered this riot to have been the most alarming disturbance of any sort to have 'occurred for years amongst the native population'.[133]

This was, however, the Presidency's last major plague riot, and only two further disturbances transpired further south in central India. These occurred within a month of each other in 1899; neither was mentioned in foreign newspapers, but the *Lancet* reported them. The first would be better described as a combination of threats and passive resistance than a plague riot. In early September in Ahmednagar, Indians refused segregation and inoculation and closed their shops in protest. Police and troops were ordered to guard the Collector's house and the city gates. According to the *Lancet*, the resistance here and in surrounding *mofussil* (small backward) towns resulted from the indigenous peoples' fatalism and belief that modern medical precautions and interventions were useless, and for this reason villagers evaded colonial controls and inoculation.[134] On 27 September, a second incident erupted in Kolhapur in southern Maharashtra. By contrast, this was a major riot. Three thousand 'malcontents' marched on the plague hospital, wrecked the homes of two plague officers, smashed dispensatory rooms, and set fire to a portion of the hospital where no patients were present.[135]

* * *

Certainly, David Arnold is correct: government compromises, slackening of segregation and quarantine policies, and curbing military excesses such as the brutal destruction of shrines and the property of the poor account for the virtual disappearance of plague riots in India by 1902.[136] But, as we have seen, already a

---

[131] Numerous papers tallied the casualties, such as *Guardian*, 12 March 1898 and *Scotsman*, 19 March 1898, 10.

[132] *Scotsman*, 19 March 1898, 10; and others.

[133] *Argus*, 11 March 1898, 5; *Singapore Free Press*, 17 March 1898, 165 and 180; *Straits Times*, 18 March 1898, 2; and *Mid-Day Herald*, 19 March 1898, 2.

[134] 'Notes from India', 1899(b).   [135] 'Notes from India', 1899(c), 1197.

[136] Arnold, 'The Rise of Western Medicine'; idem, *Colonizing the Body*, 200–39.

year earlier General Gatacre had initiated such compromises, with newspapers praising him for 'his extreme courtesy',[137] 'tact and kindness,[138] and 'patience'.[139] *Rást Goftár*, even criticized him for becoming too lax and pleaded that he reinstate plague searches and visitations at least for the monsoon season.[140]

Yet plague riots continued in other areas of India and returned to Mumbai when Gatacre left. As native papers chided, it took time for the British to learn simple lessons such as not allowing male doctors to examine girls, and the dangers of over-zealous quarantine, unnecessary segregation, and abusive and arrogant behaviour by doctors, even native ones. In May 1898, the *Mahrátta* pointed to the recent riot in Garhshankar as confirmation of the British failure to learn.[141] Still later that year, with employees leaving work in the city of Hubli at the Presidency's south-western tip (today, Karnataka) and with riots seeming inevitable, the *Gurákhi* thought it 'strange' that the government had yet to learn from their 'plague operations at Mumbai, Poona, and Calcutta', that such stringent measures only 'create[d] hatred against the Government'.[142] At the end of May 1901 with riots spreading through the region around Sialkot in the Punjab, the *Prabhát* was astonished that the gov-ernment still had not learnt 'an object lesson': 'coercive measures . . . are highly offensive', and 'the people should not be lashed into such madness'.[143] Papers closer to the scene were more specific. Despite experiences in Mumbai and Kolkata over several years, the lessons—'Touch not their religion and women'—had not been learnt further north: male doctors examined native female villagers; rioting followed. Here, however, native doctors, not the British, were those guilty of 'insuf-ficient tact', sparking attacks on magistrates and police. One thousand six hundred soldiers were called to quell the revolt. As a local paper commented, this was a 'most serious affair'.[144]

Finally, with pressure from London and fears of plague spreading to other parts of the subcontinent and Europe, new plague legislation published in the *Bombay Government Gazette* on 7 May 1901 mostly repeated the measures enforced for the Presidency in 1897, only now, they were 'more drastic', reinstating 'the hated disin-fection and detention camps', endless medical examinations, and without providing 'lady doctors'.[145] In exasperation, numerous native papers responded: how could the government have profited so little from experience?[146] It was as though the lessons of the last five years were now lost.[147] This time around, however, the government's lapse in memory was shorter. In mid-June Lord Curzon clarified that the letter of new regulations was not what it seemed; the spirit of the laws was more important:

[137] L/R/5/151, week ending 17 April 1897, no. 11.
[138] Ibid., week ending 24 April 1897, no. 9.
[139] Ibid., week ending 5 June 1897, no. 11. He yielded to the objections voiced by the city's Muslims; ibid., week ending 3 April 1897, nos 14 and 15; and 5 June 1897, no. 11.
[140] Ibid., week ending 17 June 1897, no. 17.
[141] Ibid., week ending 14 May 1898, *Mahrátta*.
[142] Ibid., week ending 6 August 1898, no. 30, *Gurákhi*.
[143] Ibid., 156, week ending 1 June 1901, no. 36, *Prabhát*.
[144] L/R/5/27, Part II, week ending 25 May 1901, no. 1556, *Amrita Bazah Patrika*. Also, see ibid., week ending 4 May 1901, no. 1435, *Bengalee*.
[145] Ibid., 156, week ending 25 May 1898, no. 41, *Sudárak*.   [146] Ibid.
[147] Ibid., week ending 1 June 1901, no. 36, *Prabhát*.

'no new departure in the policy...would occur'; instead, every effort would be made to ensure tolerance and kind treatment towards the afflicted.[148]

Factors other than British fear of riots and their inconveniences contributed to the decline of rioting. One factor was a shift in medical awareness of the disease. Whether or not the pathogen was the same as the Black Death's, it had proven not to have behaved in the same contagious fashion. Already, by 1898, reports gathered from hospitals in the Presidency from the first outbreak in 1896 revealed surprising observations: nurses and doctors attending the plague-stricken and victims' relatives, despite close contact, crowded conditions, and customs such as passing sputum from one relative to another, rarely caught the disease. Repeatedly, hospitals discovered, 'the safest place to be during times of plague was the plague ward'.[149] As a hospital reported in 1897: 'Of about 400 people..who either visited their sick friends or remained constantly by their bedsides . . . in not a single instance did any of these persons contract the plague'.[150]

Yet at the end of 1898, with plague spreading through the Punjab to Bengal and the Himalayas, plague riots continued and in places approached levels of violence and crowd estimates seen in Mumbai and Kolkata. Moreover, in southern India, the first signs of plague disturbances erupted at Bangalore at the end of November, fuelled by native distrust and anger seen earlier in central India. When a Muslim was removed to a plague hospital, a crowd attacked the health officers, stabbing some and 'murderously handling others'. The *Guardian*'s description of the riot does not estimate the crowd size, those injured, or killed, but reports eighteen arrested.[151] In the same week, riots broke out in Chikkballapur, north of Bangalore, in opposition to segregation measures. Forty-nine natives were arrested, deported to Bangalore, and imprisoned for six months. The measure proved insufficient. Soon afterwards, 'fresh riots' appeared, when 800 Muslims attacked a local official (*Tahsildar*), threatened to kill him, burnt the region's segregation camp, and took over the town until troops from Bangalore arrived.[152] A third riot in the south, this one at Seringapatam near Allahabad in the district of Mysore, with crowds estimated over 10,000, was of a different order of magnitude. It began by uniting a thousand Muslims and Hindus, mainly from the city's fishermen class, but by the second day galvanized 10,000 villagers from the surrounding region. Armed with guns, swords, and axes, it lasted several days, freed prisoners, captured the city's fortress, and took control of the city. It ranks among the largest and most violent of plague riots anywhere and received wide coverage in Britain, the US, and Australia. Again, it arose from military searches and plague segregation.[153]

---

[148] Ibid., week ending 22 June 1901, nos 22–4.

[149] Cohn, *The Black Death Transformed*, 123.

[150] Gatacre, *Report on the Bubonic Plague*, 94; also see Bannerman, 'The Spread of Plague': at the plague hospital of Parel which had 533 cases in 1896–7, plague did not infect any nurses or other attendants (180).

[151] *Guardian*, 22 November 1898, 9, from *Times of India*.

[152] *Scotsman*, 24 November 1898, 5; and *The Times*, 24 November 1898, 5.

[153] See, for instance, *New York Times*, 22 November 1898, from Allahabad; *The Times*, 22 November 1898, front page and 3; *Guardian*, 15 December 1898, np; *Scotsman*, 23 November 1898, 9; *The Times*, 22 November 1898, 3; and *Argus*, 23 November 1898, 5.

Yet in the south, these plague riots failed to spawn the same riotous contagion seen in central India in 1897–8. Only a hint of one further riot ensued, and failed to appear in foreign papers. In November 1903, because of 'precautionary measures' an attempt was made at Coimbatore to torch the town's plague camp. Evidently, it failed; no injuries or arrests were recorded.[154] Otherwise, the plague riots across vast regions south of Maharashtra were confined to a single week in late November 1898. When plague spread further south into Sri Lanka (Ceylon) in 1914 in septicaemic form that kills 100 per cent of victims within eight hours, no plague riots appeared.[155] Furthermore, for southern India, the international press does not report any myths accusing doctors, governors, or foreigners of disseminating plague, seizing body parts, or using poisons to exterminate the poor.

As plague spread in northern and north-west India—the Punjab, North-Western Provinces, United Provinces of Agra and Ould, Uttar Pradesh, and Bihar— where plague mortalities would reach their highest levels in the subcontinent, a greater number of social disturbances erupted than in the south but not with the frequency or scale seen in Mumbai or Kolkata. We have mentioned riots in Garhshankar in April 1898 and in the district of Sialkot in May 1901, where foreign papers and the *Lancet* reported only one of twenty-five. Provoked by the medical examination of women, a 'mob' beat hospital assistants and a local officer (*Naib-Tahsildar*), and ignited his huts. They overpowered the local police, and the cavalry from Sialkot had to be called to restore order.[156]

At the same time (May 1901), 'troubles' spread to Chapra in Bihar, because plague regulations 'exasperated the people'.[157] A sergeant, the Superintendent of the Salt Revenue, and the District Magistrate were roughed up and the plague camp was attacked.[158] Despite the violence, native newspapers hardly touched these riots, while the international press did not mention them at all. 'Several riots' provoked by plague operations in the same district led to attacks on Europeans: rioters drove the Collector out of the district and assaulted the Plague Officer, who with his wife hid in an indigo factory. A plague riot of 200 also assaulted a Salt Revenue officer at Ramispur (Rampur) in the state of Uttar Pradesh.[159] Finally, four small riots in northern India, for which no crowd numbers or arrests are mentioned, occurred in 1901, without any notice from foreign papers. In February, two plague riots erupted within days of one another in different parts of Bengal. Both were fuelled by fear and distrust of European disinfection, aided by false rumours. At Bihta near Patna (Bihar), villagers assembled with sticks (*lathis*) to intercept the disinfector assigned to their houses, but because of the police's 'timely arrival', no injuries occurred.[160] The second incident at Lachmipur, further east,

---

[154] 'Notes from India' (1903).
[155] On these plagues, see Hirst, *The Conquest of Plague*, 148ff.
[156] *Evening Star*, 27 April 1901, 2. 'Notes from India' (1901) adds that 'only one European', an assistant commissioner, was attacked.
[157] L/R/5/156, week ending 1 June 1901, no. 35, *Moda Vritta*.
[158] L/R/5/27, week ending 1 June 1901, no. 1608, *Bengalee*, reporting from *Pioneer*; ibid., no. 1609, *Hindoo Patriot*.
[159] L/R/5/156, week ending 1 June 1901, no. 35, *Moda Vritta*.
[160] L/R/5/27, week ending 16 February 1901, no. 538, *Bengalee*.

proved more violent. Villagers imagined that a man from Arrah on business had thrown disinfectants into a well and thrashed him for it.[161] Less than a month later, 'rowdies' armed with sticks from Dashahwamedh and Sigre in Varanasi (Benares), Uttar Pradesh, reflected another rare instance of rumours of intentional plague spreading. According to a local paper, lads guarded their streets expecting to discover a 'scape-goat', spreading plague from the town's neighbourhoods of Gola Dinanath and Chetganj, but no violence or arrests were reported.[162] A fourth riot appears more consequential. As with the first two, the anger and distrust were provoked by the use of disinfectants. Villagers at Katteshwarpur, near Danapur, attacked a party of disinfectors and the Subdivisional Officer of Danapur. A paper partially justified the attack, pointing out that 'many qualified medical men are doubtful of the efficacy of chemical disinfection alone', and that plague in previously disinfected houses 'makes excusable the belief among commoners that the process of "throwing water" only spreads the disease'. No more is heard of the 'attacks'.[163]

Despite this smattering of small-scale disturbances in villages and towns across northern India, only one plague riot spurred extensive violence, and it received international coverage. In Cawnpore (Kanpur), a major city of Uttar Pradesh and the site of a key battle during the Mutiny of 1857, 'thousands of rioters' in mid-April 1900 besieged a segregation camp and set it ablaze along with the hospital and a ginning and pressing mill. The rioters beat twelve constables, killed the head constable, and threw five native ones, alive, into the camp's raging fires. Businesses remained suspended for days afterward, and troops patrolled the city, guarding mills and factories.[164] On the other side, ten or eleven[165] rioters were killed, twenty rebel leaders sentenced to death, and another transported.[166] *The Times* speculated that the riot was set off by 'unprincipled natives' disguised as doctors or sanitary inspectors, who blackmailed 'rich and poor alike'. They visited the sick and threatened to remove them 'to an unknown place', where the government would 'do away with them', unless a certain fee was paid.[167] Two months later, the riot still captivated international attention. London's *Pall Mall Gazette* and the *Scotsman* concluded that organizers had planned it by spreading 'the wildest rumours' about mysterious disappearances among the Hindu and Muslim lower classes. Rumours of a child kidnapped and brought to a plague segregation camp to be burnt were claimed to have triggered the riot, and the *Scotsman* asserted that '[T]he lower classes would sooner die like flies than submit to the sanitation measures.' In the

[161] Ibid., week ending 16 February 1901, no. 591, *Amrita Bazah Patrika*.

[162] L/R/5/78, week ending 16 March 1901, no. 31, *Bharat Jiwan*.

[163] L/R/5/27, 1901, week ending 30 March 1901, no. 1080, *Behar Herald*. I find no trace of it in the *New York Times* Archive, 'Chronicling America', BNA, or Trove.

[164] *New-York Tribune*, 3 June 1900, 4; *New York Times*, 28 May 1900; *San Francisco Call*, 13 April 1900, 4; *Morning Post* 14 April 1900, 3; *Guardian*, 14 April 1900, 5; *Scotsman* 14 April 1900, 9; *The Times*, 14 April 1900, 3 and 16 April 1900, 4.

[165] *The Times*, 14 April 1900, 3. Native papers such as *Indian Daily Telegraph*, L/R/5/77, week ending 24 April, no. 24, reported 'ten or eleven'. *Times of India*, 13 April 1900, 7, reported 'eight or ten'.

[166] *South Australian Register*, 25 August 1900, 7; *Bunbury Herald*, 25 August 1900, 3.

[167] *The Times*, 14 April 1900, 3.

end, the paper, however, admitted that at Kanpur (as earlier at Pune and other places) the sanitation orders and officers had been overzealous, giving 'secret agitators a text for their seditious discourses'.[168] The *Lancet* went further: 'the people' had been ill-informed about plague regulations, and the police, 'utterly useless', 'apathetic and ignorant' of 'the state of feeling among the populace'. In addition, leading natives failed to lend any assistance and 'gave covert support to the agitators', and those blackmailing rich natives had not been just any 'natives' but were members of the police.[169]

Despite the crushing of the rebels by the Fifth Bengal Cavalry, the colonial government immediately made compromises in plague policy following a script enacted two years before at Kolkata. Again, the *Lancet* felt the government had capitulated to native demands, abandoning 'all active measures', and called the government's about-face a farce. After the riots, 'isolation' was allowed in private homes; caste hospitals could be arranged; families would no longer be separated; the police would have no power in determining 'suspected cases'; and people could choose not to undergo European treatment.[170] Whether relaxation of sanitary controls fuelled plague's later spread might be open to debate, but there is no doubt that government compromise succeeded in ending popular outrage. Plague riots in the thousands, with numerous injuries, arrests, and killings, vanished from the north.

Like the foreign press, at least one native paper, Kalakankar's *Hindustan*, explained the violence at Kanpur as sparked by the 'most foolish and mischievous rumours', circulated 'among the ignorant masses'. The paper claimed that some believed doctors were poisoning plague patients and that six bags of snakes and other poisonous worms had been ground and dissolved in the pipe-water to bring on the plague. It concluded: 'India is a land of superstitions and false beliefs'; 'the fault of the riots…was king Mob [which] is impervious to reason'.[171] These myths, however, appear to have materialized after the riots and were not their spark.[172] In neighbouring Allahabad, where the conciliatory intervention of the District Magistrate averted plague riots at the time of Kanpur's,[173] native papers did not mention popular fantasies; instead, they stressed bitterness towards incompetence, abuses, and unnecessary inconveniences as the riots' causes.[174] Even more so, they stressed a factor not mentioned in the foreign press: the remarkable extent to which plague measures had created a new spirit of sympathy, cooperation, and political unity between otherwise embattled communities of Muslims and Hindus: the impositions

---

[168] *Scotsman*, 15 April 1900, 8; 'Notes from India', 1900(c), while stressing the compulsory removal of cases to segregation camps, also pointed to a false rumour of a boy forcibly removed to be burnt.

[169] 'Notes on India', 1900(c).   [170] 'Notes from India', 1900(a).

[171] L/R/5/77, week ending 1 May 1900, no. 12; also see ibid., week ending 24 April, no. 24, *Oudh Akhbar*.

[172] Ibid., no. 13, *Prayag* (Allahabad), 26 April; and no. 21, *Oudl Punch*.

[173] Ibid., no. 16, *Almora Akhbar*.

[174] Ibid., week ending 17 April 1900, no. 23, *Hindustani* (Lucknow); ibid., no. 24 *Indian Daily Telegraph*; week ending 24 April 1900, no. 8, *Hindustani*; ibid., no. 23, *Shahna-i-Hind* (Meerut) 16 April; week ending 1 May 1900, no. 15, *Nasim-i-Agra* (Agra); no. 16, *Almora Akhbar*; ibid., week ending 17 April 1900, no. 22, *Cawnpore Gazette*.

and prejudices of plague policies created 'brotherly relations and amity' between the two at Kanpur and Allahabad. This mutual respect caught several Anglo-Indian newspapers by surprise, and they made little secret of their disapproval.[175] On the day of Bakr-Id, 20,000 Muslims and Hindus gathered. First, Muslims out of respect for the feelings of their Hindu neighbours resolved not to sacrifice cows at the festival, and at the conclusion of prayers, two Muslims and two Hindus 'made the crowds swear by the Qoran and the Ganges water not to allow plague doctors to enter their houses'. Later that day, the police seized two boys and declared them plague victims. Two to three hundred men left the Idagh to set the plague camp on fire. The crowd increased 'to several thousand';[176] the plague riots of Kanpur had begun.[177]

In addition, about 3000 workers in the cotton, wool, and jute industries held a meeting on the eve of the riots and went on strike, protesting plague measures.[178] In a mocking cartoon, Lucknow's *Oudh Punch* illustrated the Kanpur riots as having worker–artisan origins: butchers and shoemakers are depicted holding a meeting under a tree 'promoting mutual sympathy and concord', while a butcher on the side kicks an unwelcome policeman.[179] As the text makes clear, the sketch was hardly sympathetic: 'Ignorant shoemakers and butchers combined, and crowds of people proceeded to the plague camp, and set it on fire.'[180]

More than any other plague riot, except Mumbai's of 9 March 1898, this one lingered on, first in the courts, then in recollections of the press. Yet less than ten days after the riot, compulsory segregation, forced inspections at railway stations, and other plague regulations ended or were modified, and the Secretary of State for India was asked in Parliament why these changes had not been made earlier.[181] Court cases against twenty-five men condemned to death for 'unlawful assembly, riot and murder' dragged on until December, when the decisions were appealed, first to District Magistrate Macdonnell, and, after his refusal to grant pardons, to the Viceroy of India, Lord Curzon, who did the same. On 11 December, seven of the convicted were executed.[182] Details of the cases reached papers as far away as Mexico.[183] With subsequent protests against plague measures and abuses, native papers from May 1901 to June 1911 recalled the lessons that should have been learned at Kanpur.[184]

In the international press only four further plague disturbances appear for northern India. Most were little more than criminal incidents or acts of civil disobedience against sanitary regulations. The most serious of these occurred in mid-April 1900,

[175] Ibid., week ending 1 May 1900, no. 19, *Hindustani*.
[176] Ibid., week ending 1 May 1900, no. 19, *Almora Akhbar*.
[177] Ibid., week ending 24 April 1900, no. 11, *Oudh Akhbar*, also highlighted the significance of the Hindu–Muslim 'union'.
[178] Ibid., week ending 17 April 1900, no. 24, *Indian Daily Telegraph*.
[179] Ibid., week ending 24 April 1900, no 16, *Oudh Punch*.
[180] Ibid.   [181] *Times of India*, 21 April 1900.
[182] *Pioneer*, 22 July 1900, 4; 23 September 1900, 5; *Amrita Bazar Patrika*, 4 December 1900, 4; 13 December 1900, 4.
[183] *Mexican Herald*, 23 August 1900, 2.
[184] L/R/5/156 1901, week ending 1 June 1901, no. 32, *Kál*; ibid., week ending 8 June 1901, no. 28, *Deccan Herald* (Pune); and week ending 15 June 1901, no. 17, *Phoenix*; *Amrita Bazar Patrika*, 2 September 1901, 2: *Indian People*, 15 April 1909, 3; *Leader*, 6 June 1911, 8.

along a dirt track at the village of Shakpur (Sheikhpura). 'A large crowd' attacked three soldiers, mistaken for plague officials, and wrecked their carriage. Near Danapur, villagers barred a disinfecting party from entering their houses. But to avoid unrest, the magistrate withdrew the disinfecting party.[185] The *Lancet* was the only journal to report these events.

At the time of the Kanpur riots, the *New York Times* reported 'serious riots and disturbances, arising from plague prevention' in the Punjab region of Simla. It maintained that 'the people' were convinced that to control the plague, government doctors were ordered to poison patients—'no one who goes to a Government plague hospital ever comes out alive'. Yet the only specific riot or disturbance the paper mentioned was the well-reported one at Kanpur.[186] Finally, in 1902 at Patiala in another part of the Punjab, a particularly fiendish riot against compulsory segregation erupted: 'a large mob attacked the chief medical officer and his native staff with bricks, stones, and sticks, wrecked the dispensary, and set the plague camp on fire, leaving plague invalids dying'. According to one report, the medical officer was fastened down, pelted with stones, then carried off and 'thrust into a mass of filth'.[187] He survived, despite nine wounds mostly to the head. But the *Lancet* concluded, such 'disturbances' were no longer common.[188] My survey of foreign and native papers confirms the journal's impression. Compared to the Presidency of Bombay and Calcutta, far fewer plague riots troubled other parts of India. From the plague's first appearance in the north in 1898, little more than one incident a year occurred in the vast territories of the Punjab, Bengal, Bihar, and regions further north through present-day Pakistan, although plague mortality in the Punjab would rise to its highest rates anywhere in the subcontinent.[189] After Patiala, the only disturbance to appear in northern India cannot be called a riot. Only one paper reported it, and it was brief: on 1 April 1906 in the 'jungle town' of Fatehgarh, Uttar Pradesh, foreign missionaries were accused of being plague spreaders. Exactly who spread the rumours is unstated, but unlike Europe in the seventeenth century or China into the twentieth, no injuries, destruction of property, trials, or murders followed.[190]

* * *

Plague riots and their relation to anti-plague policies show no straightforward history in the learning curves of colonial or municipal governments.[191] Instead, from the arrival of the disease in Mumbai in 1896 to 1902, profound reversals occurred with forgotten lessons and repeat performances of practices that regenerated violence. At least three major shifts can be traced in anti-plague operations in

---

[185] 'Notes from India', 1900(b).   [186] *New York Times*, 28 May 1900.
[187] 'Notes from India', 1902.   [188] *Guardian*, 12 March 1902, 7.
[189] Arnold, *Colonizing the Body*, 202; an estimated 3.5 million died of plague before 1914.
[190] *Omaha Daily Bee*, 3 April 1906, 18.
[191] This also included the Governments of Native States, not directly under British control. On 31 January 1898, *Indu Prakásh* (L/R/5/152, week ending, 5 February 1898, no. 33) attributed the plague riot at Sinnar to 'segregation and similar innovations'. It claimed these operations had been unknown there until recently but by the eve of the riot had become 'far stricter' than those imposed in British territories; ibid., week ending 5 March 1898, no. 49, *Baroda Vatsal*.

Mumbai over a short seven-year history. At the same time, however, one major transformation determined Indian attitudes towards plague policy, and historians have yet to notice it. Throughout the 'Tragedy of Poona', the 9 March riots of Mumbai, and the Kolkata riots of 1898, even the most vehement and damning criticisms of anti-plague operations were consistently pitched in a divided fashion. As hundreds of native newspapers reveal, protest against plague policies before June 1898 did not lash out against Western ideas about infectious diseases or question plague's contagious potential. Instead, they objected to the 'tyrannical' means by which these operations steeped in corruption, ignorance, or indifference to native customs had been implemented. The Indian press and intellectuals wholeheartedly endorsed the principles behind quarantine, segregation, and even military searches for plague victims. As the *Indian Spectator* stated in early March 1897, 'Segregation is good, but not without reasonable provision... proper treatment and diet'.[192] Moreover, they argued that the manner in which governments enforced segregation could be counterproductive. Fear of humiliation and hardship caused by cruel and corrupt implementation of sound plague operations encouraged Indians to conceal cases and flee, thereby fanning the contagion. These papers even hammered governments for being too lax in their measures to protect Indian communities.

As early as April 1898, native papers began lodging criticisms not only against government practices but against a key concept behind them—that modern plague was a highly contagious disease. Their doubts did not derive from Eastern folklore, superstition, or fatalism; instead, the latest Western science along with their own observations over several plague seasons had changed their minds. Bal Gangadhar Tilak's paper, the *Mahrátta*, that had ardently defended the anti-plague principles of quarantine and segregation, while opposing their tyrannical enforcement, sounded a new note: 'The surest and the best method of arresting the progress of plague, recommended by both Western and Eastern writers of scientific fame, is the temporary abandonment of the infected area'. Such practices had already been pursued and 'had brought plague under control at Belgaum, Sátára, Sholápur and Nagar'.[193] With the growing consensus that the rat was the disease's principal carrier in India, plague doctors and scientists began seeing the disease as one of place rather than person-to-person transmission.[194]

By May, the divided voice that persistently defended the government principles of plague control began to crack. Karachi's *Phoenix* criticized current plague policy, calling it 'a mistake' to remove plague patients to hospitals against their wishes. Their argument was no longer based on the poor physical conditions of plague camps, violence of military searches, or the principle often invoked in the past—for segregation to work it had to be voluntary. Now, the criticisms questioned the policies' theoretical foundations: 'Four English doctors say that segregation does no

---

[192] L/R/5/152, week ending 13 March 1897, no. 16, *Indian Spectator*.

[193] L/R/5/152, week ending 16 April 1898, no. 23, *Mahrátta*.

[194] From newspapers of the Presidency of Bombay, killing rats as an anti-plague measure appears only in July 1898. The Hindu *Poona Vaibav* (week ending 16 July 1898, no. 13) disapproved of the policy, not because of religion or denial of the rodent's role in spreading plague but because the presence of rats warned residents when to leave.

good'.[195] A week later, the paper was more emphatic, calling notions of segregation 'absurd'. The argument rested on recent historical observation: 'In our city, notwithstanding disinfection, quarantine, segregation, hospitals, public and private, and other various means...the disease is on the increase'. It then analysed plague mortality figures in Mumbai after the 9 March riots, when 'people began nursing their own relatives in their homes'. Contrary to notions of strict segregation, 'the plague declined'.[196]

Governments' opinions soon followed, even if their practices lagged behind the science of their medical advisors. In July, the Supreme Government of Bombay ordered the municipality to abolish all quarantines and sanitary cordons, declaring them 'of no use in stamping out the plague or diminishing its intensity'.[197] Yet the city continued its rigorous, unpleasant cordons and examinations at railway stations on the city's outskirts well into 1901, and at other places, through 1902 and beyond, despite repeated complaints and petitions for their repeal.[198] By 1901,[199] the chorus of criticism against the old approaches and theories of plague control, many reaching back to the late Middle Ages, was nearly universal across the Presidency of Bombay's newspapers. As Sàtàra's *Skubh Suchak* declared, government measures 'for preventing the progress of plague' had proven 'their absolute futility'.[200] Pune's *Kál* condemned the theory and practice of segregation and burning clothes: 'Nobody requires any more of these measures'. 'The People are disgusted with these troublesome and futile rules' that 'gave rise to riots in Bombay, Calcutta, and Cawnpur, and now are doing the same in the Punjab'.[201] Wai's *Moda Vritta* claimed that 'Hundreds of instances can be cited showing plague regulations, however severe, are absolutely inefficient against the disease and are only a fruitful source of trouble both to Government and the people'.[202] The following month, bilingual papers concurred. In reviewing the recently published Bombay Plague Commission report, Mumbai's *Native Opinion* concluded: 'The gist of the whole report is that almost all the measures that have been up to this point adopted for the repression of plague have been found...to be more or less of very little practical use'.[203] By the end of the nineteenth century, outrage against principles of segregation, examinations at railway stations, and quarantine based on the old assumptions of plague as highly

---

[195] Ibid., week ending 14 May 1898, no. 24, *Phoenix*.
[196] Ibid., week ending 21 May 1898, no. 54, *Phoenix*.
[197] Ibid., week ending 16 July 1898, no. 12, *Bombay Samáchár*.
[198] Ibid., 156, week ending 16 February 1901, no. 53, *Satya Vijay*; week ending 7 September 1901, no. 16, *Mumbai Vaibhav*, 4 September; week ending 14 December 1901, no. 36, *Mumbai Vaibhav*. Other Collectors continued these cordons and inspections in other parts of the Presidency as in Hubli (ibid., week ending 19 October 1901, no. 26, *Dhárwár Vritta*; and other papers). Mumbai also continued its segregation policies as well as in the Punjab; Wilkinson, *Report on Plague*, part 1, 7; part 2, 7, 9. In 1902, native papers reported numerous complaints from Hyderabad (Sind) and neighbouring towns such as Tondo on compulsory segregation in huts, quarantine of passengers, medical inspections at stations, and other measures they argued were useless, incurred wasteful expenses, and contravened 'the express wishes of the Government of India'. For Hyderabad: L/R/5/156, week ending 1 February 1902, no. 36 *Prabhát*; and numerous other papers.
[199] Extracts from the Presidency of Bombay are missing for 1899 and 1900.
[200] Ibid., 156, week ending 1 June 1901, no. 34, *Skubh Suchak*.
[201] Ibid., no. 32, *Kál*.   [202] Ibid., no. 35, *Moda Vritta*.
[203] Ibid., week ending 14 July 1898, no. 12, *Native Opinion*.

contagious spread to other parts of India. As early as October 1899, Bangalore's *Suryodaya Prakasika* protested against plague policies such as fumigating railway passengers and confiscating their clothes for 'only a little bit of cloth'. Such rules created hardship and humiliation, particularly for native women.[204] In August, the paper railed against the 'uselessness of segregation' and other plague measures at Bangalore;[205] and in October, against quarantine in general, maintaining that it contravened the latest medical findings.[206] For the next two years, their criticisms continued against the Mysore government, which maintained its restrictions, steeped in outdated notions of plague transmission.[207]

From theories of prevention, native papers also began questioning Western medicine's record in treating plague. The challenges did not derive from fears of poisoning, superstition, or fatalism, but from observation. By calling to account Western medicine's plague record, local papers attacked the Punjab government's decision to prohibit patients from consulting native *hakims* (doctors): Instead of manifesting scepticism clouded in fatalism, as health authorities such as Harvey asserted, these papers sought improvement.

There were exceptions. In the opening years of the twentieth century, with rising rates of plague mortalities and the failure of Western medicine to prevent plague or discover a cure, papers in the North-Western Provinces questioned the efficacy of any scientific, medical, governmental, or personal initiative, native or European, in preventing the disease. *Rohilkhand Gazette* of Bareilly, Uttar Pradesh, considered plague a matter of divine intervention: 'no human efforts can possibly combat it...death has its fixed time'. [208] But such voices were rare. A year later, a paper from the same region turned the divine-intervention argument on its head: 'If the plague is a divine lesson, it is a lesson to teach us better rules of sanitation, and to induce us to make more intelligent provisions for the preservation of health in our crowded cities.' It then called for sanitary reform 'all over the Empire'.[209] Those crying for sanitary improvements also blamed municipal and colonial governments for their apathy in not attending to filth in cities and villages and their failure to provide modern drains, latrines, fresh water, and proper burials for animals and humans.[210]

---

[204] L/R/5/108, week ending 31 May 1899, no. 58, *Suryodaya Prakasika* (Bangalore).

[205] Ibid., week ending 15 August 1899, no. 72, *Suryodaya Prakasika*.

[206] Ibid., week ending 15 October 1899, no. 72, ibid.

[207] L/R/5/110, week ending 19 October 1901, no. 15, ibid.; L/R/5/109, week ending 30 September 1899, ibid.; and ibid., week ending 15 November 1900, ibid.

[208] L/R/5/77, week ending 1 May 1900, no. 11, *Rohilkhand Gazette* (Bareilly). *Dacca Prakash* (L/R/5/25, week ending 25 March 1899, no. 18) criticized the British government for failing to eradicate plague. Instead of proposing reforms, it questioned, 'Can anyone expect that any human agency will be able to stamp out the plague?' and saw the cause in the 'growing irreligiousness of the people'. An Oriya paper from Bengal, ibid., week ending 28 August 1899, no. 38, *Utaldipika*, accused the government of wasting money on plague defence: plague 'like other mortal diseases should be allowed to take its natural course'.

[209] L/R/5/78, week ending 27 April 1901, no. 11, *Oudh Times* (Lucknow).

[210] Citations in the native press of criticisms of sanitary conditions and suggested reforms fill pages. Here are several examples from the Punjab, the North-Western Provinces, and Bengal: L/R/5/188, week ending, 8 July, no. 13, *Tribune* (Lahore); L/R/5/77, week ending 3 April 1900, no. 9, *Hindustani*; week ending 17 April 1900, no. 25, *Tihfa-i-Hind* (Bijnor); L/R/5/79, week ending 18 April 1903, no. 19, *Hindosthan* (Kalakankar).

Instead of 'fatalism', native papers sought new solutions. An editorial in the *Indian Spectator* on 20 October 1901, anticipated the international plague reports and massive experimentation and accumulation of data that began five years later.[211] Calling for action, the paper declared it was 'strange in the midst of all scientific and medical activity, no systematic commissions... to investigate the causes and methods of treatment of plague' had been organized.[212] Half a year later, Lucknow's *Advocate* made similar pleas for empirical analysis of recent plague records to decipher what factors caused some communities to be devastated by plague, while others escaped or were only slightly scathed. It pleaded for scientific studies into the conditions of life, 'modes of living', food consumption, and preventive measures to explain the divergences, and advised that committees be appointed to compile surveys. Far from being fatalistic, it preached that only through 'constant enquiries' and 'science' could plague's present mysteries be unravelled.[213]

By a strange shift in fate, the city that now led new approaches to control plague was Pune, previously so battered by overzealous and punitive procedures of segregation. With Mr Cappel's appointment as Collector in mid-1901, it leapfrogged Mumbai, the city the press had earlier urged Pune to emulate. Pune now adopted the latest scientific theories: (1) inoculation; (2) destruction of rats; (3) disinfection; and (4) evacuation, with government building at its own expense temporary huts for the poor. The old principles—isolation hospitals, segregation, quarantine, border controls, cordons, and detention of passengers—no longer figured.[214] Native papers praised the change, saying it reflected, 'nearly six years of close acquaintance with this enemy'.[215] Yet the old plague paradigm of controls and quarantine died hard with some colonial governors. Useless segregation measures, compulsory plague camps, railway detentions and inspections of passengers, death certificates demanded by health officers while plague corpses dangerously piled up, and other infringements against the new anti-plague laws of India continued to the end of 1902, even at Pune (with railway inspections) and in other places such as Válvé Táluka (Sàtàra District), Kalyán, Neral (District of Kolába), Braoch City, Surat, Allahabad, and especially Hyderabad.[216] Contrary to the memorandum of Mumbai's sanitary commissioner issued in 1898, government 'conservatism' and reluctance to break with ideas of plague control reaching back to the Middle

---

[211] From 1906 into the second decade of the century, these included thousands of pages of temperature and humidity charts and correlations with plague outbreaks, mapped across vast regions of the subcontinent, cases analysed by caste, religion, race, social class, occupation, and housing, down to types of masonry; see Cohn, *The Black Death Transformed*, 26–33.

[212] L/R/5/156, week ending 26 October 1901, *Indian Spectator*.

[213] L/R/5/80, week ending 16 May 1902, no. 11, *Advocate*. Similarly, *Naiyar-i-Azam* (ibid., week ending 15 November 1902, no. 35) advised collecting statistics to distinguish plague mortalities by religion to see if diet and modes of living affected resistance to plague. During plague at Allahabad in 1902, *Amrita Bazah Patrika* (L/R/5/27, week ending 29 March 1902, no. 513) berated government officials for fleeing: not only had they reneged on their duties, they had failed 'to take advantage of the occasion' to gather statistics that would 'add to the stock of knowledge on plague'.

[214] In districts such as the Punjab, the transition from segregation to evacuation was not so immediate. Wilkinson, along with other scientists, thought the 'Infection was chiefly due to human agency though rats were observed to die before the epidemic broke out among people in almost every village that became infected'; *Report on Plague*, part 2, 20, 22–3, 27, 36; citation 20.

[215] L/R/5/156, week ending 22 June 1898, no. 26, *Sudharak*.   [216] See note 198.

Ages—not 'native fatalism' or 'superstition'—determined India's zigzag path in adapting scientific and forward-looking measures.

* * *

Unlike the history of riots and violence provoked by plague in early modern Europe from the 1530s to the 1660s, or smallpox in late nineteenth- and early twentieth-century America, or especially cholera from 1830 to 1911, India's plague riots of the 'Third Pandemic' were short-lived, clustering into a mere four or five years and ending a decade or more before the pandemic reached its peak. The only exception came eighty years later. With the recurrence of plague at Surat in pneumonic form, panic sprang forth again. Initially, mass migration was its expression, marking the largest wave of human movement in the subcontinent since the 1947 partitioning. With only two plague deaths, 300,000 fled Surat.[217] By the time the plague ended, a quarter more of Surat's half-million had departed,[218] alarmed in part by rumours that 'Muslim terrorists' had poisoned the city's water supplies, although these rumours failed to provoke sectarian violence, despite the city's deadly sectarian riots two years earlier.[219] Soon, however, panic erupted into popular violence but with motives strikingly different from fears of poisoning or mythologies about Western medicine. Similar to the Neapolitan cholera riots of 1973, the poor, instead of fearing doctors and hospitals, felt entitled to the benefits of modern medicine and rebelled because these services, if delivered, were inefficient and corrupt. As *The Times* pictured it: 'Every morning the hospital is a bedlam of people demanding check-ups, families visiting patients, and slum-dwellers appealing for supplies [such as] tetracycline antibiotics that have assumed an almost mystical reputation'.[220] The flight of four doctors from the city ignited the poor's resentment: 'angry mobs' ransacked doctors' offices and set four dispensaries ablaze. Crowds broke into pharmacies, not because of suspicions of poisoning, but because of profiteering. Four hundred reserve police officers dispersed the crowds.[221]

This late twentieth-century plague riot might lead us to conclude that its trajectory paralleled cholera's: both progressed from suspicions of modern medicine to demands for its most advanced procedures. Scattered rumours of blood sucked from patients' feet, doctors poisoning patients, or, in China, foreign missionaries accused of spreading plague might lead us to conclude that reactions to plague during the 'Third Pandemic' even replicated early modern accusations of plague spreaders. To assume such continuity across place and disease, however, would misconstrue what was central to the vast majority of Indian plague riots. Few were predicated on 'superstition' or distrust of Western medicine, and instead of dividing societies by class, religion, or ethnicity, as with cholera, plague in India often unified communities, easing even rising tensions between Hindus and Muslims. While the poor may have comprised the bulk of plague rioters, artisans and shopkeepers supported

---

[217] By the plague's end, there were 5000 suspected cases, of which 238 were confirmed with fifty-six deaths; Barrett, 'The 1994 Plague', 49.

[218] *The Times*, 28 September 1994, 11.   [219] Barrett, 'The 1994 Plague', 49–50, 57, 63.

[220] *The Times*, 28 September 1994, 11.   [221] Ibid., second article from Reuters in Surat.

them with shop closures and general strikes; and native intellectuals, instead of insulting them from the sidelines, rallied to their defence with mass assemblies, written resolutions, petitions to the highest authorities, and editorials decrying the backwardness and counterproductiveness of British measures steeped in medieval ideas of quarantine and segregation. In contrast to the bulk of cholera and smallpox riots, plague riots in India assumed another dimension, one centred on political protest and change. To what extent did plague protest beyond India's borders replicate these patterns?

15

Plague Beyond India

CHINA

The first scene of modern plague to fall under the international spotlight was Hong Kong in May 1894. Soon those at the forefront of biological science—the German–Japanese coalition under the direction of Shibasaburo Kitasato, who had studied at Berlin under Robert Koch, and Swiss-born Alexandre Yersin, trained at the Pasteur Institute under Émile Roux—converged on the city, racing to discover the pathogen of the ancient disease that caused the sixth-century Justinian Plague, the Black Death, and the plagues of early modern Europe. This race not only made headline news in 1894; ever since, it has fuelled eulogies to these micro-hunters and stimulated debates among historians and medical scientists over the nature of the disease.[1] Yet other than clashes in medical culture between the Chinese and the West, study of the plague's resurgence in China has uncovered far fewer examples of violence than were experienced in India. The near absence of violence in the plague's initial incursion is surprising given current perceptions about epidemics and their power to induce hatred and blame: the expectation that the sudden appearance of a mysterious pandemic should produce not only fear and panic but persecution of the 'other'. Such violence was doubly expected from a disease with such a pedigree, given its connections in the popular imagination with the Black Death massacres of Jews and plague spreaders in early modern Europe.

Early traces of social upheaval and protest, however, can be detected from the *Lancet* and archival sources such as the British Colonial Office correspondence.[2] With the arrival of plague in China in the autumn of 1893, 'considerable excitement' and threats of violence erupted against the British and their 'sanitary' impositions. According to a telegram posted in the Shanghai Club in late May 1893, the 'Chinese' in Hong Kong had tried to prevent plague inspection: 'many houses [were] blockaded, sanitary officers stoned, mob dispersed by police'. By Monday, however, inspections resumed under police guard; no further troubles were reported.[3] Quickly, British authorities agreed that Chinese doctors from 'an independently instituted plague hospital' would conduct the searches. Yet, a year later, Hong Kong recorded a second riot and this time the 'excitement' was more serious. The colonial government,

---

[1] See Cohn, *The Black Death Transformed*, 1–3; Benedict, *Bubonic Plague*.
[2] Solomon, 'Hong Kong, 1894'.
[3] *North-China Herald*, 25 May 1893, 786; and *Singapore Free Press*, 5 June 1894, 340. I find no notice of this disturbance in the Hong Kong collection of online English-language papers, despite articles on plague daily by June 1894.

critical of Chinese medicine and their plague facility, Tung Wah Hospital, closed it and removed patients to Canton. Violent mobs mobilized. Western doctors had to carry pistols for protection; a gunboat was summoned to restore order.[4] Yet no injuries, destruction to property, or arrests appear to have been made. Had widespread violence erupted, the international press would have reported it, as happened two years later in India.[5]

Nevertheless, the British Plague Commissioner, James Lowson,[6] fully believing that modern plague, like its medieval/early modern predecessors, was highly contagious, initiated policies later exported to India—digging up floors, flooding houses and streets with vast quantities of disinfectants, and allowing house searches to be conducted by soldiers with no knowledge of indigenous customs or religions. Lowson even employed the same Shropshire Light Infantry for these operations that four years later contributed to one of the largest, most violent mass protests of the 'Third Pandemic', Mumbai's riots, strikes, and shop closures of March 1898. He would also move to Bombay in 1897 to become a chief advisor of plague operations through British India.[7] According to the English press, the feeling at Hong Kong was 'bitter' against the 'foreign devils' (that is, the British), who 'were at work boldly entering the hovels, seeking out and burying the dead, removing the sick, disinfecting the hotbeds of disease...'.[8] Yet neither in 1893–4 nor later did enforced plague searches or other controls trigger disturbances approximating those in India.

Newspapers, especially Chinese ones, reveal further incidents. Yet these remained few and did not spread contagiously from city or region as would happen in central India. The Chinese protests, moreover, differed in another respect: consistently, they blamed the foreigner. In the last week of June 1894, two incidents erupted in Canton that were almost carbon copies of one another. First, a 'Chinaman' at Honam passed out in the street in front of two American women attached to a Presbyterian mission (Miss Fulton, a qualified medical practitioner, and Mrs Noyes). Miss Fulton applied smelling salts to the man, who soon died of plague. A 'crowd of natives' gathered, attributing 'his demise to the machinations of the ladies' but the two were rescued by the 'timely arrival' of a customs officer.[9] The second disturbance received wider coverage. Again, it involved two American women missionaries in Canton, this time from the China Inland Mission; both were doctors (Misses Bigler and Halverson). Lying on their mission's doorstep was a 'Chinaman' dying of plague. Halverson searched for a boat to take him to the hospital, but a 'mob' followed her,

---

[4] Solomon, 'Hong Kong, 1894'; *Hong Kong Telegraph*, 11 June 1894, 2 and 19 June 1894, 2. With the appearance of plague in Hong Kong in May, incidents occurred but it is difficult to judge their seriousness, as when a court sentenced three older women on 21 May 1894, charged with assaulting a sanitary official and inciting 'a mob' against him while inspecting a house; see Platt, Jones, and Platt, *The Whitewash Brigade*, 36.

[5] Benedict, *Bubonic Plague*, 144–8, does not mention this incident but discusses recriminations over hospital care and plague measures between Chinese and English-language papers, Hong Kong's colonial government, and the Chinese directorate in 1894.

[6] On Lowson, see Catanach, 'Plague and the Tensions', 152–3.

[7] Harrison, *Public Health in British India*, 142.

[8] *Yorkshire Evening Post*, 28 August 1894, 2, exposes its prejudice and blame of the Chinese for plague.

[9] *North-China Herald*, 22 June 1894.

shouting 'devil woman', and accusing her of carrying the man away to be killed. Her appeals to shopkeepers for protection were refused. She was dragged from a shop, 'savagely struck', doused with dirty water, and whisked to a place where the crowd 'intended to kill her'. She escaped to the house of an English captain, which the mob 'assaulted' with stones. When Bigler searched for her friend, she too was stoned. In her case, a Christian 'Chinawoman' rescued her.[10] Given their easy escapes without serious injuries, the crowd (which none of the papers estimated) must have been small, and no arrests were reported.

The same week, similar episodes appear to have been spreading. The American consul wired concerns over Americans' safety in Canton to the Marine Hospital Bureau: 'The natives are trying to blame foreigners for the plague and have gotten up riots in Canton and the surrounding country'.[11] Placards were posted across the city accusing foreigners of importing plague to poison all the Chinese.[12] At Shuk Lung (near Tungkun), north of Hong Kong, the threats materialized. On 20 June, a 'mob' demolished the American Presbyterian Church, killing one person, and the Roman Catholic Church had to be heavily guarded. Two rioters were arrested.[13] The British were not the only targets. At that moment in Macao, then plague-free, placards in streets and markets accused French missionaries of poisoning wells and distributing packages allegedly spreading a smell that 'causes instant death'. Placards called on 'people' to kill with explosives the lawyer and editor of the *Independente*, Sr José da Silva, denounced as the poisoners' agent, who desired to 'bring about desolation'.[14] At Kuangfung, 'libellous stories' targeted doctors, the police and military, and also foreigners. According to the paper, anti-foreign sentiment, 'always pretty high', was 'now at boiling point'; the slightest collision with anyone in the narrow streets led to 'outrage and violence'. Yet no riots flared up. After the attacks on the lady doctors of the American mission, 'happily', the paper added, 'no chance had been afforded'.[15] The foreign press also reported that rumours spread with the plague, such as 'civilized physicians cut up bodies both live and dead to secure organs and tissues, which they convert into medicine'.[16] At least one further plague riot occurred in 1894 but not in a major city or reported by a foreign paper. Yet, it may have been the most violent plague riot in 1894 or possibly afterwards in China. In the village of Taluk, Namhoi district, where sixty Christian families resided and were 'hated for their religion', outsiders seized on rumours of foreigners treating plague patients badly. On 16 June, a band of about

---

[10] Ibid., 29 June 1894, 1030; and a three-column article with interviews of the two doctors and translations of the placards, *Hong Kong Telegraph*, 14 June 1894, 2. The incident was reported widely in small-town British papers, such as *Shields Daily Gazette*, 23 August 1894, 3. For other Chinese assaults on missionaries during plague, see notes 12, 14, 27, and 28. Waves of cholera in China provoked similar reactions; see, for instance, *North-China Herald*, 14 October 1892, 555 and 9 August 1895, 218.

[11] *San Francisco Chronicle*, 7 August 1894, 3.

[12] *The North-China Herald*, 22 June 1894 and 29 June 1894, 1003 and 1030; and Benedict, *Bubonic Plague*, 145–6. After the attack on the two American missionaries, the British outlawed placards and advised missionaries to discontinue medical aid in Chinese neighbourhoods.

[13] *China Mail*, 25 June 1894, 2.

[14] *North-China Herald*, 6 July 1894, 15, and *China Mail*, 25 June 1894, 2, translate the placard.

[15] *North-China Herald*, 6 July 1894, 15.   [16] *San Francisco Chronicle*, 19 August 1894, 16.

100 armed men invaded, beat the villagers, smashed their furniture, and looted valuables. Their appetite whetted by booty, they attacked other villages: 'some lives were lost'; the Viceroy sent a gunboat to restore order.[17]

Neither the *Lancet* nor foreign or English-language Chinese papers report further plague-inspired violence until November 1910, when trouble broke out in Shanghai. Except in its scale of violence, arrests, and destruction of property, it appears more akin to Indian riots.[18] *The Times* of London commented on the protesters' 'abysmal ignorance and credulity made to serve the political element' but admitted that the incident was hardly 'serious'.[19] The *Scotsman* alluded to rioters' 'suspicions of foreigners' but failed to report any anti-foreign actions. Instead, plague measures imposed by British and Chinese authorities had aroused popular anger. With the first plague death at the end of October, the Municipal Council of the International Settlement imposed emergency plague prevention measures that cut off the Hongkou district. The government sent in sanitary investigators to inspect houses and forcibly removed residents suspected of plague to an isolation hospital. Soon, they evacuated an entire housing block, where the first cases were discovered, removed ceilings and foundations and fumigated the neighbourhood.[20] 'Not surprisingly', as in India, the measures provoked violence: bands of Chinese pelted foreigners with stones, beat sanitary inspectors with bamboo poles, and smashed disinfecting vans and equipment.[21] Chinese elites and members of their Chamber of Commerce negotiated with the Council to temper the destructive sanitary measures and on 13 November agreed to hold a public meeting with the Council to 'educate' Chinese residents, organized with Chinese and foreigners on the platform to explain anti-plague measures.

Based on its Beijing correspondent, the *Lancet* attributed the riot entirely to 'rumours' by 'the lower classes who resented the house-to-house visitation'. The *North-China Herald* concurred, concentrating on the 'many wild rumours among the lower classes of Chinese about sanitary measures'. Some said that those taken to the isolation hospital were 'at once exterminated'; others thought the patients had not died from plague which was why the authorities refused to send the bodies to relatives for proper burial.[22] A week later, the paper elaborated on the rumours and held that they came from 'the better classes of the Chinese', who were 'as gullible as the most ignorant coolies'. Supposedly, the municipal council seized women and children and forced them into the isolation hospital, 'whence they never emerge alive'. Others alleged children were killed, either for production of vaccines or to light electric lamps.[23] Later, it was said that children had been kidnapped to take their eyes and hearts to manufacture medicines to treat foreigners then afflicted

[17] *North-China Herald*, 6 July 1894, 15.

[18] 'Plague in the Far East' reports cases and fatalities. Plague caused a third of the population of Pakhoi to flee. This bubonic pandemic may have been a source of the pneumonic plague in Manchuria in the winter of 1911. Already by autumn 1910, the *Lancet* reported the spread among tarbagan trappers in Manchuria; see ibid.

[19] *The Times*, 8 December 1910, reported the riots almost a month after their occurrence.

[20] Goodman, *Native Place*, 154.   [21] Ibid.   [22] *Scotsman*, 16 November 1910, 7.

[23] Ibid., 18 November 1910, 392; and *Straits Times*, 21 November 1910, 7.

in Manchuria.[24] But unlike cholera riots, this demonstration showed solidarity across class lines, at least within the Chinese community, and achieved political objectives. Afterwards, Chinese representatives modified the Council's plague measures, and the Chinese press celebrated the changes as a 'popular nationalist victory'.[25] This political dimension is attested in further descriptions of the protest. The Health Board had attempted to explain its anti-plague measures to the public at an auction warehouse (*godown ewo*) but opened its doors only to well-dressed elites. A crowd estimated at a thousand gathered outside, broke past the police into the hall, interrupted the speeches, and shredded the summaries of them. Those outside bolted the *godown*'s doors and held their own stump oratories. They stoned the thirty foreign guards, and a company of Volunteers and Sikh constables armed with bayonets had to be called to free the caged health officials and their audience.[26]

In December, further plague disturbances spread through Shanghai. Rioters demolished numerous buildings, including the American Presbyterian Church, its hospital, and college. They then tried to massacre missionaries, but with the gentry's assistance, they escaped on boats to Canton.[27] Marines from various foreign powers were called to patrol the streets, along with 'large bodies of Chinese troops'. Gatling guns were positioned on street corners, and 'a number of sharp engagements took place between the soldiers and mobs'. From the paper's interview with a returning missionary, the cause appears again to have been 'the stringent sanitary measures used by the Chinese quarantine officials'. Yet another element was added. According to the missionary: 'The Chinese believed the quarantine authorities were stealing little babies to make medicine, and when officials went around fumigating houses, the natives hurled stones at them.'[28] The *Lancet*, nonetheless, concluded: 'It is now confidently expected that the measures taken will permit the routine work of disinfection and supervision to be carried on as before.'[29] Their prognosis was incorrect. In August the following year, 200 to 300 rioters threw stones at municipal police who were erecting a corrugated iron barrier to isolate a Chinese neighbourhood and supposedly to keep out rats. The crowd destroyed the barrier and Sikh police armed with carbines and fixed bayonets charged the 'mob'.[30]

A further riot occurred in another region of China, but it was not a protest against plague measures; in fact, it is difficult to call it a plague riot. Nonetheless, it provoked the largest demonstration even vaguely connected with medicine in my sources. In Hankow (Hankou, presently part of Wuhan), the municipal police took a nearly dead 'ricshaman' to the surgery of one of the city's leading physicians.

---

[24] Recounted in praise of Shanghai's chief-of-police; *North-China Herald*, 25 March 1936, 533.
[25] Goodman, *Native Place*, 156.
[26] *North-China Herald*, 18 November 1910, 395. Also, ibid., 20 May 1930, 309, celebrating Dr C. N. Davis's retirement as Shanghai's public health commissioner. Further disturbances erupted in other parts of Shanghai. A woman's foot and bloody dressings found in a vacant lot spread rumours of foreign doctors 'mangling Chinese'; crowds gathered at the Railway Hospital and police station. The following day, Chinese merchants threatened to cease shipping cargo in foreign-owned steamers. Ibid., 18 November 1910, 397 and 385 reported attacks on individual foreigners in Shanghai's 'ghetto' (Hongkou), but considered these prompted by plague measures and not as 'riots'.
[27] *Weekly Sun*, 17 December 1910, 9.   [28] *Detroit Free Press*, 18 December 1910, 8.
[29] 'Appearance of Human Plague'.   [30] *Straits Times*, 26 August 1911, 10.

En route, the ricshaman died. In the 'Chinese version' of the story, the police officer escorting the patient had instead murdered him. As a result, the dead man's
fellow 'ricshamen' rioted, took strike action against driving policemen on their
beats, and stoned the police station. The next morning, a crowd of 20,000 that
increased to what must have been 30,000 'at one time during the day' stoned
buildings, looted businesses, 'bombarded' shipping offices, and 'pulled up trees'
until naval authorities arrived and fired on the crowds. The article concluded: 'There
is also a great deal of fear with the common people regarding the plague'.[31]

During the frigid winter of 1910, plague began spreading in Manchuria, leading
to the most deadly wave of pneumonic plague ever recorded. Much has been written on the Manchurian plagues in 1911 and 1922, the most noteworthy account
being by the Cambridge-trained plague doctor and director of the Chinese commissions to combat them, Wu Lien-Teh, an eyewitness.[32] Furthermore, in English,
interest in them has recently been rekindled with at least two scholarly articles and
a monograph.[33] Only one of these hints at any social unrest.[34] The contemporary
sources, however, describe several riots with serious damages to property, grave
injuries, loss of life, calls for military intervention, and in two cases declarations of
martial law.[35] In addition, without specifying towns, villages, or exact dates, US
papers reported that the 1911 plague sparked 'numerous' industrial protests[36] and
bread riots.[37]

Of those dated or described with any specificity, the first conflict broke out in
Harbin on 14 January 1911 and was unlike any seen in our database of disease-
induced violence. With panic came the common instinct of masses to flee the city,
but troops were sent to prevent people leaving. 'Mobs' formed, and troops patrolled
the streets with orders to kill any who resisted. When the 'terrified people' fought
back, martial law was declared in the suburb of Fudiziandan, the zone worst hit by
plague.[38] A month later around Vladivostok (Russia, 800 km south-west of Harbin),
an equally deadly riot erupted; however, the one paper I have found reporting it
was telegraphically brief: against 'sanitary regulations', Chinese residents clashed
with Russian troops, leaving six dead and twenty wounded.[39]

At the same time in Kirin (Jilin City) in Manchuria, presently North Korea,
two or three riots may have erupted. In February, the government in Beijing dismissed the commander of the 23rd division of the Chinese army for resisting

---

[31] *North-China Herald*, 3 February 1911, 244. According to a second account, the officer escorting
the patient was a foreigner, ibid.

[32] Wu Lien-Teh, 'First Report'; idem, 'Historical Aspects'; and idem, *Plague Fighter*.

[33] Gamsa, 'The Epidemic of Pneumonic Plague'; and Summers, *The Great Manchurian Plague*.

[34] By contrast, Lynteris, 'Epidemics as Events', citing Nathan, *Plague Prevention*, 68, describes a
riot in Hailar at the epidemic's beginning: an ambush on health authorities killed the local police chief
and injured the leading medical officer; skirmishes against inspection squads also arose at Harbin.

[35] *Iowa State Bystander*, 17 February 1911, 2.   [36] *Iron County Register*, 2 March 1911, 2.

[37] *Keowee Courier*, 8 March 1911, 3.

[38] *Washington Times*, 19 January 1911, 8. Over 200 newspapers in Trove reported the spread of
pneumonic plague through Manchuria 1911, but I have found none to report this or other plague
riots in January.

[39] *Iowa State Bystander*, 17 February 1911, 2; papers in Trove reported plague around Vladivostok
but not this conflict.

implementation of quarantine regulations. What was behind the commander's refusal is not stated.[40] Several weeks later, matters deteriorated. Terrified of contagion, peasants in the surrounding districts refused to bring their produce to town, threatening a famine. According to *The Times*, '[t]he authorities are said to be at the mercy of the mob'. Whether this was a figure of speech or mobs had in fact assembled and rioted is unclear.[41] A week later, a second disturbance occurred in Harbin that clearly was a riot. As with several Chinese cholera and plague riots, anti-foreign hatred was at its core. A 'Chinese mob' attacked the Japanese police, killing two of them on the Antung Railway. The account in *The Times* stated that Chinese officials incited the anti-Japanese riot. But in addition to anti-foreign sentiment, Japan's sanitary measures had aroused mob anger.[42] Finally, in mid-March, perhaps the most serious of the Manchurian riots erupted; yet it too seems to have included few protesters, and is found in a single paper, this time an Australian one. Again, anti-foreign sentiment appeared at its core, but this time a Japanese population attacked Chinese authorities. As with other Chinese plague riots, it hinged on discontent over anti-plague measures, but instead of protesting against the imposition of harsh, unfair, prejudicial, and inconvenient measures, the local community defended an earlier agreement on quarantine regulations. A small body of Chinese police attempted to break the quarantine in Mukden (Shenyang), north of the Korean border. On being opposed, they killed a Japanese sentry. A Japanese crowd assembled and attacked the police, who numbered twenty, 'killing or wounding most of them',[43] making this small plague riot possibly the deadliest of the 'Third Pandemic' anywhere in China. In summary, in less than two months, from mid-January to early March, at least six plague riots spread through Manchuria and into adjacent Russia, without counting the alleged waves of industrial and bread riots sparked by the plague. These events marked this pneumonic plague as producing China's worst plague violence, outstripping the social disturbances provoked by the intial shock of bubonic plague in China in 1893–4. Yet few historians of the pneumonic plague have investigated its social toxins. No doubt, study of indigenous sources will produce more in-depth reportage and further violent events.

A final riot came from a less-studied wave of pneumonic plague at the end of World War I, in January 1918. The events at Fengchen in Shaanxi Province, central China, despite their small scale, attracted a greater variety of sources than any other Chinese plague riot. According to US papers, four 'American doctors' were sent to investigate it. 'A mob' threatened, forcing the doctors to request a special train to escape. The one contemporaneous account found in my searches reported no damages or injuries to the doctors or anyone else; nor did it estimate crowd numbers or explain the reasons for the threats.[44] A month and a half later, the *El Paso Herald*, for no apparent reason, updated the story on its back pages. Again, the dual characteristics of Chinese plague riots come to light—a 'superstitious aversion

---

[40] *Le Temps*, 15 February 1915, 2.   [41] *The Times*, 3 March 1911, 5, from St Petersburg.
[42] Ibid., 28 February 1911, 5.   [43] *Argus*, 21 March 1911, 8, from Mukden.
[44] *New-York Tribune*, 16 January 1918, 2 and 4, from Peking.

to foreign investigators' and the 'inception of the quarantine campaign'. This paper presented the mob as more than 'threatening': the doctors had been 'besieged in their quarters for several days'. By the time of this report, however, local opposition had evaporated.[45]

Chinese sources provide greater clarity with a telegram published from the doctors and an interview conducted almost two weeks after they escaped. On 10 January, a 'mob' of eighty, organized by an elderly man whose son died of plague under the doctors' care, invaded their railway wagon and stabbed a missionary who barred the gate. Instead of four American doctors, two doctors, O. Eckfeldt and the famous Manchurian physician and plague commissioner, Wu Lien-Teh, were removing the spleen of the boy in a post-mortem examination. The father screamed, 'You cut my son's heart out! Cut mine also!' Although the doctors were able to save their missionary friend, they were confined to their quarters for the next nine days. According to the *North-China Herald*, the military had a hand in it,[46] and the sentiment in town was 'that the foreign doctors were cutting up and killing people'.[47] Finally, in his long autobiography, published forty-one years later, Wu presented new details. First, before the doctors arrived, the local population and even the 'insufficiently educated' had opposed health workers.[48] Second, Wu judged the doctors sent by the Ministry of the Interior as 'inexperienced'. Third, the American doctor, Eckfeldt, was to blame. Unaware of the 'susceptibilities' of bereaved Chinese families, his carelessness provoked the riot. He did not even bother cleaning up the post-mortem 'mess'. After absolving himself of guilt, Wu admitted he 'had so many sleepless nights after these events' that he left his present duties and returned to his newly constructed laboratory at Harbin.[49]

The last Chinese plague riot came from a village near Harbin in Manchuria (Aschho), and except for its scale might have resembled a cholera riot as much as any of the Chinese plague disturbances. Because of the anti plague policy of removing the sick to hospitals and isolating contacts, doctors for over a week faced protesters with 'revolvers and knives in the course of their duty'. Around 10 March, 'a mob of sixty' entered the isolation station, liberated two patients, and chased away the doctor in charge.[50]

After India, China presented the greatest number of plague disturbances. None of them, however, received the global or foreign front-page coverage accorded to numerous Indian ones. Except for the protest at Hankow, that involved a plague victim but was not a plague riot, only one comprised crowds of more than a hundred, and in only three was anyone killed, quite unlike the scores seen at Kanpur or the 600-plus killed at Kolkata. More than in India, anti-foreign phobias against the US, British, French, and Japanese and fantasies of gruesome indecencies and murder underlay the Chinese riots. Yet in contradistinction to the bulk of cholera riots, Chinese plague riots cut across classes and showed prior organization. Most significantly, like the Indian protests, the Chinese ones were united by concrete

---

[45] *El Paso Herald* 30 March 1918, 11.   [46] *North-China Herald*, 19 January 1918, 129.
[47] *Shanghai Times*, 24 January 1918, 12.   [48] Wu Lien-Teh, *Plague Fighter*, 104.
[49] Ibid., 106–7.   [50] *Shanghai Times*, 21 March 1921, 12.

objectives to change policy and practices at the core of colonial anti-plague measures; once these were lifted, the riots receded.

OTHER REGIONS OF ASIA, AFRICA,
AND THE MIDDLE EAST

Beyond China, fewer plague disturbances emerge. In other regions of Asia no further plague riots, even small incidents of violence, appear from my searches, despite plague raging through the Mekong Delta of Cambodia and Vietnam and into Asiatic Russia in the very places that had spurred violent cholera revolts less than a decade before and would do so again during cholera's last major sweep of the early twentieth century.[51] On the other hand, various newspaper archives and articles in the *Lancet* point to plague riots in the Middle East. The most significant ones were in Saudi Arabia (then part of the Ottoman Empire) at the pilgrimage site of Jeddah, gateway to Mecca. As one paper put it, Jeddah was 'the port of Mecca', a halfway house between Europe and farther East, 'a place for pilgrims and a place of exchange for all infectious diseases'.[52] But from various newspaper collections—the US, British, French, and Australian—with thousands of pages on plague across the globe, only four mentioned these 'serious disturbances'[53] and only obliquely without describing a single incident.[54] However, two articles in the *Lancet* analysed them. In 1899, the population at Jeddah became 'excited' against sanitation measures and rioted: pilgrims were ill-treated; stores and shops plundered; physicians had to hide.[55] The health controls were not, however, the same as those that provoked either European cholera or Indian plague riots—in the first, fears of the state and hospitals; in the second, military excesses, the abuses of segregation camps, and humiliating searches. At Jeddah, the riots' leaders were the military and the sheriff's employees, and, despite the religious significance of the place, their rationale appears purely economic: quarantine spelt losses to the pilgrimage trade. Furthermore, similar riots had erupted the previous year during the pilgrimage season.[56] A London paper reporting it pointed briefly to religious rather than economic causes: 'All attempts to regulate the Mohannedan pilgrimage to this holy city are met by protests against the interference with religious sentiments'.[57] Later, however, the *Lancet* drew

[51] For instance, at Tashkent, attacked by cholera riots in 1892 and 1910, plague struck in 1897 with no reported violence; *Scotsman*, 8 March 1897, 9, from St Petersburg.

[52] *Evening Telegraph* 18 April 1898, 4. The same regions along the Volga that sparked serious cholera riots in 1892 were hit the previous year by an epidemic of typhus, particularly severe among Germans, but without riots or blaming of Germans; see *Brisbane Courier*, 12 October 1891, 4; and *Maitland Mercury*, 13 October 1891, 4.

[53] Allusions to various plague incidents at Jeddah in 1898 and 1899 but vaguely reported from a Constantinople correspondent in the *Nottingham Evening Post*, 8 March 1899, 3. *London Standard*, 9 March 1899, 7, mentioned 'similar disorders' the previous year, when authorities tried to isolate the town.

[54] Three papers in BNA mention vaguely that disturbances occurred at Jeddah in the last years of the nineteenth century.

[55] 'Jeddah'.   [56] Ibid.

[57] *Evening Telegraph*, 18 April 1898, 4.

general connections between plague rioting and Jeddah's pilgrimage economy. It explained: Jeddah's livelihood depended on the thousands of pilgrims coming from abroad, and plague measures prevented them entering the city and spending their money: 'It will be recalled that such opposition [to these health board measures] led to serious riots in the years mentioned', that is, the years of plague at Jeddah, 1897, 1898, and 1899.[58] Yet online newspapers, including the extensive BNA, capture only one.[59]

Pilgrimage towns were not the only Middle Eastern places to arouse protest against plague measures driven by hard-headed economics. An Egyptian protest in 1900 mobilized 2000 'rioters', who assembled in front of the house of a suspected plague patient at Port Said, preventing him from being removed to a plague hospital. Despite the crowd far outnumbering the few police on duty, it did not behave violently, at least, not initially. It allowed two English inspectors to examine the patient but 'deterred' them from removing him. Later, 'the Arab part of the mob' (suggesting that Europeans had participated) smashed an empty ambulance and broke the windows of the French doctor who had diagnosed the town's first plague case. The newspaper attributed the protest to 'the lower-class complaint'. Yet that complaint reflected neither the fantasies typical of cholera protests, nor the range of Indian grievances against violations to privacy or customs. Rather, it was much the same as Jeddah's: quarantine was killing them economically.[60]

A third series of Middle Eastern plague riots received more attention in the Western press with articles from San Francisco to Tasmania. Here, the disturbances clustered in small villages and towns in and around Seistan (Zistan or Sistan), Persia. Given the character of this region—a Persian province today crossing the borders of Afghanistan, Iran, and Pakistan, and also within Russia's sphere of influence[61]— these might be classified as Indian or Russian riots. The most notable of them struck at the beginning of April 1906 and shared characteristics with cholera protests: a 'fanatical mob' attacked Seistan's quarantine station, forced its officers to withdraw, and demolished the town's plague hospital, severely beating the doctors with sticks. The crowd then attacked the British consulate and customs house. Cossack troops arrived to save the latter.[62] A month later, the *Lancet* reflected on the hospital's destruction, reporting that a crowd had destroyed temporary shelters for plague patients and a plague hospital at Nasirabad. It held that the cause lay with enforcement of plague measures.[63] But outside India, plague, unlike cholera, provoked remarkably few incidents, despite its novel spread to many places across the globe. Moreover, as witnessed in India and Persia, the first year or years of plague were not always the ones to provoke violence; nor did the rioting necessarily end after a community's first contact with the disease. For example, Mumbai's largest and

---

[58] 'The Outbreaks of Plague'.
[59] *Nottingham Evening Post*, 8 March 1899. According to *London Standard*, 9 March 1899, a plague ordinance forbidding pilgrims to enter the city caused the riots.
[60] *Morning Post*, 7 May 1900, 5, from *New York Herald* (Paris edition).
[61] *Bairnsdale Advertiser*, 3 April 1906, 2.
[62] Ibid.; from London; and *San Francisco Call*, 1 April 1906, 36, from Tehran.
[63] 'Plague Riot in Seistan'.

most disastrous plague rebellion erupted two years (and four plague seasons) after the plague's arrival in 1896. In addition, certain areas in Asia had been experiencing plague for fifty years before Yersin cultured the bacillus,[64] but for these years I have found no mention of plague uprisings. Back to Seistan, plague first struck here in November 1904 but plague rioting did not emerge until 1906.[65]

The *Lancet* article then cast another light on the Seistan riots that separates them from the majority of Indian cases and those at Jeddah and Port Said. A mullah 'sent specially from Mushad' to preach in Seistan declared that plague did not exist and incited popular unrest against plague measures. Unfortunately, the *Lancet* does not explain the motives of the mullah or the Muslims who sent him: was it for religious or economic reasons?[66] But, as with cholera riots in Persia during the 1890s, so with this plague disturbance, priests more than elsewhere were instrumental in stirring resentment to outside medicine and Western ideas about controlling disease. As early as 1899, when plague first reached Persia's major port city on the Persian Gulf, Bushire (Būshehr), reports filtered back to Western papers that the priesthood was 'instigating the people to resent the institution of preventive measures'.[67] Mullahs and 'the people' demanded that all plague measures be suspended. When their demands were not met, riots destroyed the telegraph office, and the English dispatched two gunboats.[68] Finally, in 1911, 'serious riots' occurred in Nasretabad (Nasirabad) in Seistan province and followed the region's earlier pattern. 'Instigated by priests', 'five hundred fanatics' attacked the English consulate and destroyed all its plague medicines and drugs. Suspicions emerged that had more in common with cholera than plague. According to an Australian paper: 'The misguided people could not understand why Europeans should come to their aid without reward; nor how it was that not a single European was attacked by the plague'.[69] Yet cholera's core myth of intentional poisoning was not evident.

Despite widespread waves of plague, spreading as early as the last years of the nineteenth century and continuing in places such as Madagascar and Tanzania in Africa,[70] Uzbekistan in Asia, and throughout Latin America, Peru, Ecuador, and Brazil to the present, keyword searches through thousands of newspapers have produced few instances of collective violence or even concerted peaceful protest. In Africa, after the 1900 Port Said riot, plague triggered only one further social disturbance—at Port Elizabeth, South Africa, in the summer of 1901. It was not, however, a riot; nor did it provoke accusations of blame or fears of conspiracies. With plague gaining momentum in Cape Town and Port Elizabeth, a decree required the indigenous population to be inoculated before being allowed to travel

---

[64] *Evening Telegraph*, 18 April 1898, 4.   [65] *Examiner*, 17 January 1911, 3.
[66] 'The Seistan Plague Riot'.
[67] *Morning Post*, 10 July 1899, 4; *Aberdeen Journal*, 11 July 1899.
[68] *Aberdeen Journal*, 5 August 1899, 5.   [69] *Examiner*, 17 January 1911, 3.
[70] 'Serious' plague mortalities in Madagascar were reported as early as December 1898, *Pall Mall Gazette*, 2 December 1898, 7; and *Glasgow Herald*, 15 December 1898, 6–7). Less than a year later, plague erupted in Algeria (*Liverpool Mercury*, 16 November 1899, 7) and was 'virulent' in Magude, Delagoa Bay, southern Mozambique (*Leeds Mercury*, 14 September 1899, 5; and *Edinburgh Evening News*, 15 September 1899, 2.

freely. In protest, 'many thousands' of workers went on strike,[71] and within two days the decree was revoked.[72] As in India, the protest may have hinged on the racial character of compulsory inoculation as well as on legitimate fears that the serums were experimental and had considerable risks, as seen in Malkowal that very year. Here, as in India, plague protest was organized and political.

Despite numerous waves of plague in Central America,[73] only two violent incidents surface. The first in the small town of Villa Unión, near Mazatlán in central Mexico, near the Pacific Ocean, involved 'only a hundred men or so of the lower classes',[74] over a hundred by another account,[75] and 250 by a third.[76] Nonetheless, it was 'a serious disturbance', requiring the governor to send an infantry unit along with the local police ('rurales').[77] The targets were sanitary inspectors, and one was wounded. After the crowds were dispersed, 'a mob' continued hunting two doctors held accountable for burning two houses, where Unión's only two cases occurred.[78] As with the vast majority of plague riots, even in those confined to the lower classes and which attacked doctors, no cholera-like conspiracies appear.[79] Instead, a gross error inflicted by government officials, which they afterwards acknowledged, provoked the violence. Carelessly, they took extreme measures and burnt down the victims' houses; twelve other houses caught fire and were completely destroyed. Outraged homeowners led the townsmen. The following morning the sanitary authorities promised to pay for the damages; the disturbances ceased.[80]

A plague riot in Veracruz, the second to occur in Mexico, was much larger, more threatening, and required military intervention. Well covered by the Mexican press, this riot initially resembled European cholera disturbances. On 24 June 1920 with plague spreading through southern Mexico, crowds of 3000, armed with sticks, iron pipes, and other implements, guarded the houses of the plague-stricken, preventing doctors, police, and ultimately the military from carting them to the lazaretto. Armed escorts had to accompany doctors. Yet behind the crowd's efforts to 'protect' their families and neighbours, the press did not reveal traces of cholera's core myths of an epidemic invented to annihilate the poor.[81]

---

[71] *Le Temps*, 12 June 1901, front page; *Manchester Evening News*, 11 June 1901, 5; and *Sheffield Daily Telegraph* 11 June 1901, 3.

[72] *Coventry Evening Telegraph*, 13 June 1901, 3.   [73] Pollitzer, *Plague*, 55–60.

[74] *Hawaiian Star*, 5 March 1903, 2.   [75] *San Francisco Chronicle*, 5 March 1903, 8.

[76] *San Antonio Express*, 6 March 1903, 5.   [77] *Saint Paul Globe*, 5 March 1903, front page.

[78] *San Francisco Chronicle*, 5 March 1903, 8.

[79] Also from Readex's Latin American Newspapers.

[80] These details come from *San Antonio Express*, *El Imparcial*, 5 March 1903, 2: 'Los Motines en Villa Unión: Energicas Disposiciones' reported the riot differently, attributing the cause to the rioters' 'sinister objectives', citing the crowds' chants as 'Mueran los agentos sanitarios!' and 'Death to the filthy doctors (*cochinadas de médicos*)!' Several papers in the Readex collection briefly reported it: *El Comercio*, 5 March 1903, 2, blamed the riot on the 'ignorance and prejudice of the poor, who wished to disrupt sanitary operations' and said that the crowd hunted the doctors. But no paper attributed conspiracy theories to the crowd. See *Estrella de Panama*, 8 March 1903, 8; and *La Voz de Mexico*, 7 March 1903, 2.

[81] *Excelsior*, 25 June 1920, front page and 7: 'En Veracruz Hubo Motines Ayer con Motivo de la Peste Bubonica'; and *El Dictamen*, 26 June 1920, front page.

EUROPE

Despite fears and panic over plague invading Europe with the full terror of the Black Death or of later waves dramatized by Alessandro Manzoni and Daniel Defoe, the plague that struck European ports at the turn of the twentieth century—Glasgow, Lisbon, Oporto, Trieste,[82] Hamburg, Paris, Hull,[83] Newcastle,[84] Southampton,[85] and Willesden (London)[86]—never spread significantly inland. Even in the impoverished industrial docklands, which proved fertile ground for cholera from the 1830s to as late as 1912, the 'Third Pandemic' in Europe never produced the disastrous consequences expected at the end of the nineteenth century. Cases rarely surpassed a hundred and deaths were counted in the teens, not the millions as Black Death forecasters predicted. Perhaps for this reason outbreaks of social violence were rare and on a small scale; yet fear and panic over plague remained strong in Europe until the outbreak of the Great War.[87]

The earliest threat of renewed plague violence in Europe occurred in Vienna in 1898. This incident presented a Frankensteinian horror, a disease intentionally created in the laboratory for experimental science and progress. The theatre of horror was Vienna's Institute of Pathology, which specialized in producing pathogens for sale.[88] To understand the biological basis of the plague, the laboratory had unwittingly created a virulent pneumonic strain. Four cases and four fatalities with high fever and spitting blood followed—a plague specialist, two nurses, and a laboratory assistant at the Institute and the assistant's wife. News of the deaths spread through the Western press as far as Tasmania,[89] Little Falls, Minnesota,[90] Crawfordville, Florida,[91] Ritzville, Washington (then a US territory),[92] and the Chinese papers.[93] With headlines such as 'Terror in the City', the papers anticipated more than four casualties.[94] Fears spread to England that because of the experiment an epidemic could soon erupt on home soil.[95]

The plague specialist who died, Dr Mueller, had previously worked with plague victims in Mumbai and had escaped all dangers. In Vienna, the more contagious

[82] Zavitziano and Mally, 'Turkey', 2214–15.
[83] *Manchester Courier*, 17 January 1901, 2, 6, 10.
[84] *Tamworth Herald*, 4 October 1902, 6.   [85] Ibid., 21 March 1901, 3.
[86] *Edinburgh Evening News*, 31 May 1901, 6.
[87] See Cohn, *The Black Death Transformed*, for articles on plague threatening a return of the Black Death in Europe. At the turn of the century, plague and other infectious diseases stimulated a rich novelistic strain imagining Armageddon as in Jack London's *Scarlet Plague* (1912), H. G. Wells's *The War of the Worlds* (1898), and Conan Doyle's *The Poison Belt* (1913).
[88] Sixteen years later fencing-master Karl Hopf bought typhus, cholera, and anthrax to kill his third wife and collect the insurance; see King, *Auf Leben und Tod*.
[89] *Mercury*, 28 October 1898, 3; numerous Australian papers reported it; for example, *Times and Liverpool Plains Gazette*, 29 October 1898, 2; *Sunday Times*, 30 October 1898, 8; *Burrowa News*, 28 October 1898, 3.
[90] *Little Falls Weekly Transcript*, 26 October 1898.
[91] *Gulf Coast Breeze*, 28 October 1898, 2.
[92] *Adams County News*, 28 October 1898, front page.
[93] *North-China Herald*, 31 October 1898, 802.
[94] *New York Times*, 23 October 1898.   [95] *Gloucester Citizen*, 26 October 1898, 3.

strain no doubt added to the panic and historical parallels drawn with the Black Death. The Institute had to be 'specially guarded in anticipation of an attack by a mob'.[96] But no mobs formed, even though Vienna's anti-Semitic newspapers capitalized on the tragedy, accusing Jewish doctors of intentional poisoning. With the general rise of anti-Semitic violence in the capital, correspondents feared the worse,[97] but no pogroms materialized.[98] By mid-November, the laboratory scare passed, and Vienna's plague news bore the headline 'Good News'.[99]

A second European incident occurred in Oporto, Portugal. Newspapers across Europe, Australia, and America reported here more than vague descriptions of panic or expectations of mob violence.[100] Various groups assembled and were violent, even if the 'mob' was small and constrained compared with plague riots in India or cholera protests in Europe. Similar to Vienna's disturbance, a laboratory was at the heart of the controversy. In Oporto, crowd anger focused more intently on one man and his findings, Dr Riccardo Jorge, Director of the Bacteriological Institute and Chief Medical Officer of Portugal. From laboratory evidence, he declared Oporto to be under siege by plague, triggering commercially crippling quarantine restrictions of the sort that had been plague policy in places since 1377.[101] The populace's first reaction was reminiscent of cholera riots— denial of the disease, followed by accusations of intentional 'plague spreading'. On 21 August 1899, during the funeral of an early plague victim, the 'popular classes' accused Jorge 'of inventing the plague' by injecting the poor with the bacillus.[102] Unlike with cholera, however, no riot immediately followed. The next day, however, 'several groups' formed, first near Jorge's laboratory and, when he left work under police escort, outside his home. The controversy may have opened as a scientific debate: a Dr Costa denied the plague's presence, challenging Jorge's findings. Whether Costa had organized the crowds or even appeared in the streets is unclear.[103] In these demonstrations, two protesters were injured, but only a few were arrested. Here, instead of physical attacks against persons or property, 'abusive language' was the crowds' gravest crime, and the protesters were easily dispersed. The initial opposition may have begun with the poor, but the middle classes and business leaders, fearing quarantine's economic consequences, quickly took over. On the day of Jorge's declaration, ships from Oporto had already been quarantined in places as far away as Leith (Scotland).[104] In Oporto, shopkeepers closed their stores,[105] and a photograph shows a businessman

[96] *Little Falls Weekly Transcript*, 26 October 1898.
[97] *New York Times*, 23 October 1898. Curiously, the Institute's director, Dr Nothingale, the target of this supposed Jewish conspiracy, was a noted anti-Semitic.
[98] I searched newspaper databases for such consequences through October and November.
[99] *Zeehan and Dundas Herald*, 14 November 1898, 2.
[100] Hundreds of newspapers reported this relatively small protest. For instance, *Le Temps*, 22 August 1899.
[101] Not until 24 August, after the demonstrations ceased, did Jorge order a residence burnt; see Echenberg, *Plague Ports*, 118.
[102] Ibid., 125.   [103] *Glasgow Herald*, 23 August 1899, np.
[104] *Scotsman*, 23 August 1899, 4.   [105] *Le Temps*, 22 August 1899 and 24 August 1899.

protesting the government's imposition of a national quarantine in front of Oporto's stock market.[106]

Three weeks later with several new plague cases appearing, a second demonstration arose against the city's plague doctors. Although fewer newspapers reported it, it was probably more serious. A government deputy now organized renewed attacks on Jorge.[107] But crowd violence hit other doctors arranging a post-mortem plague examination, stoning the physicians' carriages and injuring 'slightly' two of the Portuguese doctors.[108] By this time, however, the commercial classes appear to have accepted Oporto's fate. On the day of the second riot, the Commercial Association began a charitable campaign for sanitary improvement, and its first day's subscriptions were impressive.[109] Unfortunately, the papers fail to clarify the reasons for the outrage or composition of the crowd: unlike the earlier demonstration, rumours of Jorge or other doctors purposely spreading the disease are not reported.

Finally, early in 1906, a third incident to strike Portuguese territory affected the Atlantic island of Madeira. It possessed some similarities with cholera riots. Reports of plague (which were in fact misdiagnosed) prompted authorities to remove by force 'anyone showing feverish signs' to the local lazaretto. Patients returning from the lazaretto reported to their neighbours the prison-like conditions of their confinement, provoking a crowd to storm the hospital to liberate those remaining. They wrecked the hospital and, reminiscent of cholera scenes, paraded the infected 'triumphantly' to their homes. The medical officer barely escaped 'the infuriated mob' as he boarded a Portuguese warship.[110] But despite this single case of a cholera-like rescue of patients and storming of a hospital and its doctors, plague riots of the 'Third Pandemic' proved extraordinarily rare in Europe. A contagion of violence and conspiracy failed to spread, as had been Europe's fate with cholera and not only with its well-studied first wave of the 1830s. Moreover, stories like those initially reported at Oporto did not replicate cholera myths of physicians intentionally poisoning the poor that continued to swirl in parts of Europe into the twentieth century. Instead, in Austria, the new threat of laboratory experimentation led to panic and protest, and in Oporto, it was principally the economic threat of quarantine. Neither case provoked mass violence or blaming 'the other'. Even in pogrom-prone Vienna, attempts to blame Jews fell on deaf ears.

THE US AND ITS TERRITORIES

The US and its territories are the only places outside India to receive extensive analyses of the outbreak of plague and its socio-psychological consequences, and here for two cities alone—Honolulu and San Francisco.[111] Despite interpretations of prejudice against the Chinese in both cities and against the Japanese and native

---

[106] In Echenberg, *Plague Ports*, 125.   [107] *Guardian*, 21 September 1899, 8.
[108] *Scotsman*, 21 September 1899, 5; and *The Times*, 21 September 1899, 4.
[109] *The Times*, 21 September 1899, 4.   [110] 'Madeira'.
[111] Mohr, *Plague and Fire*; Shah, *Contagious Divides*; Chase, *The Barbary Plague*; Craddock, *City of Plagues*; Echenberg, *Plague Ports*, ch. 8; and Risse, *Plague, Fear, and Politics*.

Hawaiians in Honolulu, nothing points to the widespread violence seen throughout much of the Indian subcontinent or within China or the Middle East. Of the two cities and their plague crises, far less has been written about Honolulu's. Because of inadequate control and changing gusts of wind, the conflagration that engulfed Honolulu on 20 January 1900 created the worst destruction in that city's history. With the fire out of control and Chinese, Japanese, and Hawaiian men, women, and children desperate to escape their quarantine-locked inferno, white citizens armed with bats, clubs, and pickaxe handles blocked the exits. The situation was ripe for massive riots and racial violence, but they did not occur.[112] Unlike the mass of cholera and smallpox riots, or plague riots infecting Indian cities and villages, 'miraculously' neither the conflagration nor threatened social violence claimed a single life. White citizens, despite prejudices against 'the frantic horde of dirty, plague infected people',[113] refrained from attacking the helpless 'screaming women and children and men' who charged the gates.[114] Instead, 'volunteers came forward from every side and every business... ready to assist the now homeless residents of Honolulu's Chinatown'. Immediately, 'tons of food, clothing and miscellaneous goods began to arrive'.[115] A Red Cross society, formed by Honolulu's 'most prominent ladies', nursed the injured. Local physicians and clergy submitted 'to voluntary isolation to minister to the physical and spiritual needs of the stricken'.[116]

Numerous newspapers praised the charitable aid given to Honolulu and archival evidence corroborates that the kindness went beyond newspaper rhetoric. As James Mohr has concluded from a wide variety of sources, immediately, 'volunteers throughout the city began collecting household goods for distribution in the camps, while churches and other relief organizations redoubled their clothing and sewing drives, and wealthy whites donated thousands of dollars to Chinese, Japanese, and Hawaiian relief funds'.[117] Subsequent protests by the burnt-out residents were fought not in streets fuelled by conspiratorial frenzy but in courts over compensation. Newspapers and Mohr's research do not reveal a single plague riot during these populations' quarantine, which resulted in the near-complete destruction of their homes and businesses, nor afterwards with problems of rehabilitation, rehousing, and reintegrating Honolulu's natives and Asians. Instead of the cruelty to victims so often seen with smallpox, plague here spurred collective compassion, uniting the city across class, ethnic, and racial divides.

Hawaii's single plague riot, in fact, has gone undetected by historians. It occurred in the largest town on the island of Hawai'i, at the opposite end of the archipelago, less than a week after Honolulu's disaster, news of which (at least according to the papers) created 'the frenzy' and conditions for 'mob' violence. On hearing of Honolulu's conflagration, citizens of Hilo sought to bar anyone coming from Honolulu from landing on their island. On 26 January this included their sheriff returning after official business in Honolulu. An 'organized mob', armed with guns and stones 'made an ugly demonstration at the landing', barring the sheriff entry. The few papers covering the story fail to clarify exactly what crimes or violence may

---

[112] *Sun*, 18 February 1900, 2.   [113] Ibid.   [114] Ibid.   [115] Ibid.
[116] *New York Times*, 27 January 1900.   [117] Mohr, *Plague and Fire*, 148.

have been committed, but no evidence points to any wounded or arrested.[118] With assistance from a US survey ship, the sheriff eventually landed.[119]

*   *   *

Much more has been written about the two plague outbreaks in San Francisco, especially the first in 1900 and its connection to the city's legacy of anti-Chinese sentiment and discrimination towards sufferers of epidemic and endemic diseases, especially smallpox and syphilis.[120] Susan Craddock, one of the few to compare the effects of different diseases on scapegoating, has shown that blame of San Francisco's Chinese community was more pronounced with smallpox during the mid- to late nineteenth century than with tuberculosis or any other disease, endemic or epidemic.[121] Yet here, plague and the imposition of quarantine, fumigation, and compulsory inoculation by health authorities in response provoked more collective violence than in any city in the Americas, Africa, or Europe. Still, the secondary literature and my newspaper searches reveal that collective action outside the courts was limited. Certainly, medical opinions and government quarantine and inoculation were decidedly racist: they singled out the Chinese as the source and carriers of plague into the city, and these ideas reached the highest echelons of the medical profession and government authorities, including the city's chief bacteriologist, Joseph Kinyoun, a student of Koch at Berlin, and the US Surgeon General, Walter Wyman, who in 1900 pronounced plague to be 'an oriental disease, peculiar to rice eaters'.[122] Nonetheless, the crowds threatening violence from March to June 1900 were comprised largely of Chinese workers and petty merchants. No vigilante whites attacked the Chinese, despite newspaper and medical dispatches regularly blaming the plague on them. Moreover, the Chinese targeted mainly those from their own community, rarely attacking physicians or figures of authority outside Chinatown. In this way, plague protest differed radically from smallpox violence in the US or cholera in Europe. Physical violence was not aligned by class, with assaults made on victims of the disease, or against the medical profession or officials suspected of diabolical deeds.

Relying on the popular press in English, Nayan Shah has described several demonstrations by the Chinese community, but these are difficult to characterize as 'riots'. The papers he cites report no crowd numbers, no injuries, damages to property, or arrests. The first demonstration occurred after the first plague death was declared (that of Wing Chung Ging on 6 March 1900). The national Public Health Service's (PHS) snap decision to place Chinatown under quarantine provoked it, but it did not split communities by class either within Chinatown or

---

[118] This incident does not appear in Trove, BNA, or Gallica. In 'Chronicling America', it appears in three papers, but the *New York Times* gives the most comprehensive account. No Hawaiian paper in 'Chronicling America' reported it. *San Francisco Chronicle*, 26 January 1900, 3, briefly noticed it.

[119] *New York Times*, 27 January 1900.

[120] Craddock, *City of Plagues*, 10 and throughout. According to Chase, *The Barbary Plague*, 106, Surgeon-General Wyman in 1900 'endorsed the racial theory of plague as a disease that selectively attacked Asians, owing to their poverty and vegetarian diets'.

[121] Craddock, *City of Plagues*, ch. 2.   [122] Cited in Shah, *Contagious Divides*, 155.

the city at large. Crowds of Chinese merchants and shopkeepers, small and large, gathered in front of the headquarters of the Chinese Consolidated Benevolent Association (CCBA), an organization founded in 1870 by Chinatown's wealthiest businessmen, to defend their commercial interests and represent the community in political and legal battles.[123] The cross-class crowd challenged the quarantine as unfair discrimination. San Francisco's white merchant class and mainstream newspapers supported the Chinese, fearing the PHS might expand its quarantine to the entire city. Their united front brought quick success: in less than three days (9 March) Chinatown's quarantine was lifted.

The victory, however, was short-lived. In mid-May, the Surgeon General reimposed quarantine on Chinatown alone[124] and now called for mass inoculation of the Chinese community. On 17 May, large crowds assembled in opposition outside the CCBA and even larger crowds the following day, calling on Chinatown's businesses to close. This time the consensus was not, however, as solid. The CCBA was caught off guard; their leaders had instead concentrated their struggle within the courts and negotiations at Washington. Rumours circulated of white doctors spreading plague by injecting the bacillus into the veins of the Chinese poor and of health authorities inoculating fish with the bacillus fed to rats to spread plague to the Chinese.[125] But unlike cholera fantasies, the rumours did not provoke assaults on any white doctors, hospitals, and city officials. Instead, small groups harassed other Chinese who submitted to inoculation or turned to white doctors for treatment. Other rumours spread against leaders of the CCBA and Consular Ho in Washington, that they had made a pact with the white devil to poison Chinese workers and petty merchants. A San Francisco telegram reached even the British press, reporting that a secret society, the High Binders, threatened to kill any 'Chinaman' in San Francisco who agreed to be inoculated.[126]

Yet the rumours remained rumours, largely failing to spur crowds to form or engage in collective violence.[127] The worst Nayan Shah could find from his exhaustive research was several Chinese chasing across Chinatown a prominent Chinese businessman, who had submitted to inoculation. The businessman found refuge at the CCBA and remained unharmed. Another rumour spread that a white man had been spotted poisoning; a crowd formed, chanting 'Kill him! Beat him! Make him eat his own poison.' However, a white officer then appeared, explained what the man was doing, and no violence followed.[128] Myron Echenberg reports two occasions when violence amounted to more than threats or fruitless chases. On the first, 'a crowd of a thousand descended on health officers' who were attempting vaccinations. The police dispersed the crowd, who then vandalized a shop in Waverly Place, whose owner was rumoured to have collaborated with health officers. A second occurred at a Chinatown coffin shop, when a crowd of 300 scattered empty coffins

---

[123] On this organization, see ibid., 23–4 and 131–2.   [124] Ibid., 131–2.
[125] Ibid., 133–5.
[126] *Yorkshire Evening Post*, 22 May 1900, 3; and *Birmingham Post*, 22 May 1900, 3.
[127] During the four-month plague in Chinatown, *San Francisco Call* 13 April 1900, 4, reported only one plague riot and that was in distant Kanpur.
[128] Shah, *Contagious Divides*, 143 and 142, respectively.

onto the cobblestones.[129] But Echenberg neither dates nor cites the sources, and I have found no references to them.

Two incidents from newspapers, yet to be cited in secondary sources, appear more menacing. On 10 June, Chinese mobs in quarantined Chinatown attacked a physician on the Board of Health, smashed windows and doors, and threatened the lives of merchants, beating and stoning all who opposed them.[130] Another on 9 June began with a Chinese man being fumigated before boarding a ship for a Russian expedition to Siberia. Rumours spread that those departing had been inoculated. 'An angry crowd' gathered in front of the store of the recruiting agent, breaking windows and doors before the police's arrival.[131] But these two incidents hardly compare with events in India: only two months before, Kanpur's atrocities had become international news from Tasmania to San Francisco. By contrast, not even the *San Francisco Call* bothered mentioning the Chinatown riots, and according to the *San Francisco Chronicle*, only one person was arrested.[132]

While these occasional threats and acts of violence were occurring, Chinatown's businessmen took the community's battles against discrimination on quarantine, travel restrictions, and inoculation to the courts and won.[133] Chinatown's mistreatment, moreover, was fought by means that have been largely overlooked.[134] On 19 May, 'all the large Chinese stores' shut down business in protest against the Board of Health's order to inoculate the Chinese. Reports circulated that five had died from the adverse effects. Chinese merchants called it 'a great outrage' and, despite rumours that they had caved in, stood firm in refusing to abide by the national legislation.[135] These battles were not based on myths of poisoning but on concrete evidence of racial discrimination, and their successes appear to have contributed to longer-term cultural changes, re-evaluating the Chinese community as an integral part of the city's heritage, essential to San Francisco's commercial and cultural image, which became crucial to the city's reconstruction after the earthquake and fires of 1906. With the city's second plague in 1907, no question of pinning blame on the Chinese arose, despite persistent prejudice among medical professionals.[136] Secondary literature and the press reveal no further riots, not even acts of individual violence or rumours associated with plague, in San Francisco or in other US cities. As in India, plague in San Francisco was a unifying force across class and racial barriers, in marked contrast to smallpox in San Francisco and across the country during those same years.

[129] Echenberg, *Plague Ports*, 223.   [130] *Akron Daily Democrat*, 11 June 1900, front page.
[131] *San Francisco Chronicle*, 10 June 1900, 11.   [132] Ibid.
[133] Shah, *Contagious Divides*, 138–9.   [134] Ibid., 133–57.
[135] *Evening Bulletin*, 26 May 1900, front page.   [136] Shah, *Contagious Divides*, 153–5.

16

Myths of Plague

Plague terror of the 'Third Pandemic' provoked conspiracy theories, myths of poisoning, and allegations of doctors purposely spreading the disease. From the previous chapters' descriptions, such examples might be collected leading us to conclude that the overriding socio-psychological reactions to cholera and plague were much the same: that for both diseases, their social violence rested on myths of poisoning that targeted the medical profession and state. This chapter challenges that conclusion.

First, although cholera riots rarely targeted Jews, other religious minorities, or racial groups, it occurred more often with this disease than with modern plague. In Russia, examples of attacks on Jewish doctors blamed for cholera's arrival were seen in St Petersburg in 1831 and against Jews who were not doctors in Hughesovka (Donetsk) in 1892. In addition, glimpses arise of vigilante groups or governments blaming minorities like the Irish during cholera's first epidemic in English, Scottish, and US cities, or later the gypsies in Italy. In Astrakhan, cholera rioters targeted Persian merchants and Armenians in 1892.[1] By contrast, despite anti-Semitic riots raging through large portions of Europe at the end of the nineteenth century, no anti-Semitic violence seeped into the general panic and anxiety over plague on any continent. The one charge by Vienna's anti-Semitic papers blaming Jewish doctors for bringing plague to Austria in 1898 is the exception that proves the rule. Their attempt failed to stir anti-Semitic violence even in this city steeped in such hatred at the end of the century.

The failure of plague to provoke anti-Muslim or anti-Hindu rioting in India is also surprising. The most that can be seen was an occasional aside in native newspapers accusing Hindu Brahmins of whipping up anti-colonial sentiment that had led to the assassinations at Pune. But these papers, like the *Bombay Gazette* and *Times of India*, were in English with Christian editors.[2] Instead, with Muslim–Hindu hatred and violence on the rise, plague protests consistently brought the two together in mutual sympathy and support against colonial and native municipal plague restrictions that violated the religious customs of both groups. Nor did plague protests in India generally target foreigners, even if gangs during riots in Mumbai, Kolkata, and Kanpur attacked isolated Europeans in back alleys or medical officers who happened to be British. As the native papers' attacks on Pune's plague commissioner made clear, they were not against his race, nationality, or

---

[1] See Chapter 9.
[2] L/R/5/152, week ending 3 July 1897, no. 38; and week ending 10 July 1897, no. 47.

even his policies but against his insensitive implementation of those policies, which they contrasted to Mumbai's under General Gatacre. Indian cases, however, differed from those in China and to a certain extent those in San Francisco and Honolulu. While the Chinese riots were less frequent, on a smaller scale, and less violent than India's, anti-foreign violence was prominent with posted placards denouncing foreigners as poisoners and attacks on foreign missionaries and doctors, who risked their lives saving Chinese plague victims; and Westerners were not the only foreigners targeted.

*   *   *

The major source of evidence we have for plague's social violence derives from India: to what extent was it fuelled by myth-making and conspiracy theories? Certainly, the international press and to some extent the native papers pointed to the 'ignorant' and 'uneducated' as the ones stirring the 'anti-sanitary' violence. As a Mumbai paper put it, with the outset of plague in October 1896, it 'has had a most disastrous effect on the minds of the ignorant labourers and *ghâtis*[3] in the city…all sorts of rumours and prophecies are afloat among them'.[4] In March the following year, native English-language papers held that 'the people' were 'foolish, ignorant, or superstitious', which accounted for their opposition to segregation.[5] The local paper of Udváda in the district of Surat alleged that 'ignorant' villagers believed that livers of patients in segregation wards were sent to Bombay to suppress the plague in that city.[6] And the *Mumbai Vaibhav* held that the removal of a plague-stricken Hindu child to a hospital was sufficient to bring 2000 'ignorant' Hindi and 'Mohammedans' into the streets to smash a municipal ambulance to splinters.[7]

This last reference evokes European cholera scenes with crowds driven to frenzy by fears of hospital litters and ambulances carrying off their relatives. As *The Times* proclaimed in 1898, 'Hindus dread the inside of the plague van…it is a chamber of horrors on wheels…that carried them to the plague hospital…an ante-chamber of death'.[8] The *Lancet*'s correspondent in Kolkata, who six years earlier reported on cholera riots in Russia, concluded much the same describing Kolkata's plague riot of May 1898, which he says developed a specific phase, 'the ambulance scare'.[9] Yet, despite his claims, ambulances do not appear as the fetishized objects of plague violence as seen across Europe with cholera. In India, reports of smashing these vehicles were rare, and when it occurred, it was not a prime object of attack as it often was with cholera. The most significant instances of plague riots attacking ambulances came early on with 'a small riot' in Mumbai on 23 March 1897, when three hospital vans were smashed during protests against segregating plague cases.[10] The only other riot in Mumbai or its Presidency to mention them occurred during its largest

---

[3] Hindi slang for the uncultivated.   [4] L/R/5/151, week ending 31 October 1896, no. 26.
[5] L/R/5/152, week ending 13 March 1897, no. 16.
[6] Ibid., week ending 20 March 1897, no. 35, *Gujarat Mitra*.
[7] Ibid., week ending 3 April 1897, no. 16.   [8] *The Times*, 30 August 1898, 2.
[9] Clemow, 'The Plague at Calcutta'.
[10] *Launceston Examiner*, 24 March 1897, 5; and *Aberdeen Journal*, 24 March 1897, 4, which reports only one van being smashed.

plague riot of 9 March 1898. Yet the seizure and burning of ambulances was just one in a long litany of attacks on persons and objects targeted by the crowds.[11] Outside Mumbai only one further attack on a plague ambulance appears. It too was only one of many attacks on plague measures in Kolkata in 1898.[12] Beyond India, such assaults were equally rare. From my survey, only one surfaces: at Port Said, in addition to assaults on the police, coastguard, and doctors, 'the Arab part of the mob' also smashed an empty ambulance they happened to find after the riot had ended.[13]

Plague riots may have shared some common ground with cholera violence in that their targets included hospitals, doctors, medical assistants, sanitary authorities, governors, and with plague, the equivalent of the cholera lazaretto—segregation and detention camps. But did plague attacks arise from the variety of fears, myths, and conspiracy theories seen with cholera—murders for anatomy cadavers, live burials, or the general belief that the state through hospitals and medical services was culling populations of the poor? Rumours could set off Indian plague riots, as with those in Kanpur in April 1900, when, according to the *Scotsman*, 'the inflammable Hindoo and Mohammedan artisans' imagined 'the mysterious disappearance of a native here and there', and stories that a child had been kidnapped and burnt in a segregation camp were thought to have triggered the riot.[14]

Other 'wild' and 'false' rumours can be plucked from the vast newspaper coverage of the Indian plague riots. One of Mumbai's dailies claimed that in the earliest plague riot the millhands' destruction of the Arthur Road hospital resulted from their belief in stories of blood-letting from patients' feet. Other claims come closer to European cholera conspiracies or even suggest early modern fears of plague spreaders. In February 1897, a Pune paper alleged that the populace believed patients in isolation hospitals were being poisoned but then cautioned: such claims were 'too absurd' to be worthy of a response.[15]

Of sixty-three plague riots in India alone, presented by hundreds of papers from India and around the world, only a handful of reports alluded to beliefs of intentional poisoning. In March 1897, London's *Morning Post* reported that 'a number of fisher folk violently resisted' the Plague Commission's sanitary regulations in Versova, near Bandora, because rumours spread of European officers intending to poison wells.[16] The same month, a paper held that plague patients believed they had been deliberately poisoned at a segregation hospital in Bhávnagar, across the Normada Estuary, which led to thousands marching to the house of the chief medical officer. But as mentioned before, the previous day a paper closer to the incident reported nothing about poisoning.[17] Moreover, whether or not such rumours were afloat, neither paper described the allegation whipping crowds to a frenzy as

---

[11] Numerous papers provided long descriptions of this riot without mentioning attacks on ambulances; for one that did, see *Evening Herald*, 10 March 1898, 3.

[12] See, for instance, *Scotsman*, 23 May 1898, 7; and Clemow, 'The Plague in Calcutta'.

[13] *Morning Post* 7 May 1900, 5, from *New York Herald* (Paris edition).

[14] *Scotsman*, 15 June 1900, 8.

[15] L/R/5/152, week ending 20 February 1897, no. 28, *Sudhárak*.

[16] *Morning Post*, 30 March 1897, 5.   [17] L/R/5/152, week ending 13 March 1897, no. 50.

seen with the majority of European cholera riots. By both accounts, the crowd was orderly and caused no injuries or damage to property.

Another alleged rumour comes closest to the cholera mythologies. After thousands burnt the segregation camp in the city of Kanpur and fed five native constables to the flames, the *New York Times* asserted that 'the people' were convinced the government had ordered the doctors 'to poison off all patients . . . to stifle the spread of the disease', because they believed 'no one who goes to a Government plague hospital ever comes out alive'. The paper then generalized: 'it is only necessary to be known as a plague doctor to cause a mob to assemble for the purpose of murder'.[18] Yet of numerous foreign and native papers reporting this riot, the *New York Times* alone made this allegation.

At Kanpur, no attacks were made on doctors or other members of the medical profession. In fact, in the riot's immediate aftermath, the demands of the 'people' showed the opposite sentiments: 'a committee of Government and private doctors and *vaidyas* and *hakims* should be formed in every town . . . to examine the sick'.[19] As seen from numerous native newspapers, communities across the subcontinent were requesting more, not fewer, plague doctors and especially female ones to examine women.[20] Nor were these demands exclusive to metropolitan centres. The Maráthi paper in Násak suggested in July 1898 that the government appoint a committee of doctors and 'native' physicians to examine plague patients.[21] In November that year, a local paper in Sátára protested that villages were not receiving medicines quickly and argued that their high plague mortalities would be 'very greatly reduced' if the government took proper measures to ensure medicines were made available for every village in the district.[22] Three years later, another of Sátára's papers protested against government closures of its medical dispensary, putting 'to much inconvenience' those needing anti-plague medicines.[23]

In Gadag and its nearest town, Dhárwár, 400 km south of Pune, villagers requested and were granted a lady doctor to inoculate their women.[24] When plague cases increased rapidly at the end of 1898, she became overwhelmed by the demand. Through their local newspaper townsmen and villagers sought to appoint a second doctor.[25] At the time of the Malkowal disaster, a paper of small-town Hapur (east of Delhi) thanked the Punjab government for appointing European doctors to inoculate them, but expressed 'surprise and regret' that not a single lady doctor was employed. If a woman doctor were appointed, they argued, their 'ladies' would willingly undergo inoculation.[26] In 1904, Allahabad's *Citizen* led a campaign to increase medical staff to control plague. Here, it argued, the poor had no reason

[18] *New York Times*, 28 May 1900.   [19] Ibid., week ending 24 April 1900, no. 8: *Hindustani*.
[20] See for instance L/R/5/152, week ending 13 March 1897, no. 28; week ending 17 April 1897, no. 9; week ending 30 October 1897, no. 15, *Kalpatara*; L/R/5/153, week ending 5 February 1898, no. 22; week ending 9 March 1897, no. 18, *Champion*.
[21] Ibid., week ending 9 July 1898, no. 19, *Loka Seva*.
[22] Ibid., week ending 12 November 1898, no. 23, *Vritta Sudha*.
[23] Ibid. 156, week ending 23 November 1901, no. 33, *Moda Vritta*.
[24] Ibid., week ending 24 September 1898, no. 40, *Rasik Ranjini*.
[25] Ibid., 153, week ending 31 December 1898, no. 22, ibid.
[26] L/R/5/79, week ending 1 November 1902, no. 30, *Al Mulk* (Hapur).

to fear physicians: 'medical gentlemen' attending plague victims among the poor were unheard of.[27] Other papers castigated their doctors, not over alleged poisoning, but for lackadaisical care. In Karnataka in southern India, the local paper complained that its physician did not step from his carriage to examine plague patients but pronounced 'his opinion...on the strength of his subordinates'.[28]

As these cases suggest, in large cities and villages alike, hostility to Western medicine was hardly paramount as seen with cholera in the West, where I discovered no protests demanding an increase in cholera doctors or hospitals. Moreover, the Indian public clamoured for the latest medicines and Western innovations, such as the new anti-plague serums devised by Yersin, Waldemar Haffkine, Paul-Louis Simond, and Professor Lustig.[29] Local newspapers explained microbes, mechanisms of plague transmission, and the importance of sanitation,[30] and berated colonial governments for failing to introduce modern drainage, sewers, and other sanitary measures to their cities and villages.[31] Matters of sanitation and governments' failures to attend to them were uppermost in editorials across India on ways to combat plague. When communities could afford to make changes themselves, as with lower-class tenement housing ('chawls'), they proudly boasted of them, based on the latest 'scientific' information'.[32] Even after the Malkowal debacle, a local paper, instead of blaming Western medicine, lashed out against Westminster's meagre scientific response, which had been to send only two bacteriologists to India to study plague.[33] At the same time, other Punjab papers strongly endorsed the anti-plague inoculation campaign, calling for 'kindly and considerate doctors' to be posted in every district to start the operations. They argued that evidence from Sialkot had proven inoculation to have been the 'great preventative against the plague',[34] praised the Plague Commission's arrangements for inoculation, and thanked their 'eminent scientists' for 'working their brains to discover the cause of the disease'.[35]

Even opposition to doctors' 'interference' and police appointed to patrol plague did not mean that villagers or small townsmen rejected modern medicine or the

[27] L/R/5/80, Part 2, week ending 26 March 1904, no. 12, *Citizen*.

[28] L/R/5/109, week ending 31 July 1899, no. 46, *Karnatuka Kesari*.

[29] See for instance ibid., 152, week ending 16 January 1897, no. 28, Bombay's *Samáchár*; no. 29, *Satya Mitra*; week ending 13 March 1897, no. 37, *Indian Spectator*; ibid., no. 27, *Jagatsamáchár* (Thána); week ending 12 June 1897, no. 17, *Rást Goftár*; and no. 18, *Mahrátta*; L/R/5/78, 1901, week ending 18 May 1901, no. 9, *Aligarth Institute Gazette*; week ending 28 May 1898, no. 35, *Sind Times* and *Phoenix*. On 7 August 1898, ibid., week ending 13 August 1898, no. 28, *Rást Goftár*.

[30] L/R/5/78, week ending 13 April 1901, no. 23, *Advocate* (Lucknow).

[31] L/R/5/151, week ending, 10 October 1896, no. 31, *Gujaráti*; ibid., week ending 3 October 1896, nos 33–5, *Bombay Samáchár*, *Akhbár-e-Sodàgar*, *Jám-e-Jamshed*, and *Kaiser-e-Hind*. Ibid., week ending 17 October 1896, no. 15; week ending 17 October 1896, no. 20.

[32] Ibid., week ending 24 December 1898, no. 20, *Native Opinion*.

[33] L/R/5/188, week ending 24 June 1905, no. 12, *Punjabee* (Lahore). This is the earliest surviving volume for the Punjab.

[34] Ibid., week ending 23 September 1905, *Punjab Organ* (Sialkot, Urdu).

[35] Ibid., week ending 25 March, *Prativasi*. By 1902, papers across northern India supported renewal of inoculation; see L/R/5/79, week ending, 18 April 1902, no. 19, *Hindosthan*; L/R/5/188, week ending 23 April 1905, nos 13 and 14, *The Paida Akhbar* (Lahore); ibid., week ending 23 September, 1905, no. 20, *Punjab Organ*.

importance of hospitals. In May 1900, the inhabitants of Khairabad in the Sitapur district, near Nepal's present borders, held a public meeting demanding that they be allowed to make their own arrangements for treating patients and establish their own hospitals. The district's Lieutenant Government consented, and the villagers returned home, praising his governance.[36] Other communities demanded that their *vaidya*, *hakim*, and university-trained physicians not replace European doctors, but accompany them in inspection parties and at railway station examinations,[37] serve in elected committees to study the plague,[38] be allowed to treat plague patients,[39] receive comparable salaries,[40] and be respected for their long experience diagnosing this disease.[41]

A final case on popular beliefs and poison illustrates further differences in these socio-psychological reactions. In September 1898, Dhárwár's local paper reported that plague patients believed they were being poisoned at the town's hospital. The paper agreed, 'to some extent it may be true'. Patients had lodged complaints of their hands and legs being tied, against their will and the law, while nurses rammed medicines down their throats.[42] Other local papers corroborated the story.[43] A month later, another local paper called the idea of doses of poison being prescribed at the hospital 'sheer folly', but legitimated townspeople's fears of the drugs: ingredients such as eggs, brandy, and milk were mixed in the medicines, which 'do not suit all persons'.[44] Clearly and especially in regions with high levels of lactose intolerance and other food allergies, these ingredients could have proved poisonous. Yet, only complaints to the District Collector ensued; no burning of hospitals or slaughter of doctors.

Examples of 'wild rumours' and supposed poisoning were the exceptions with plague protest in India.[45] In striking contrast to newspaper coverage of cholera riots, the vast majority reporting plague in India did not describe any conspiracy theories, poisoning, diabolic dissection, or imaginary mistreatment. The rarity of myth-making with plague is well attested by Major E. Wilkinson's exhaustive reports on plague in the Punjab from 1901 to 1903. In addition to tables of cases, mortality rates, rates of inoculation, etc., he included sections divided by districts on 'attitude of the people'. From these, he uncovered only one story suggesting a

[36] L/R/5/77, week ending 1 May 1900, no. 30, *Riaz-ul-Akhbar* (Gorakhpur).

[37] Ibid., week ending 19 June 1900, no. 16, *Oudh Akhbar* (Lucknow).

[38] Ibid., week ending 24 June 1900, *Hindustani*.

[39] Ibid., week ending 1 May 1900, no. 16, *The Almora Akhbar* (Almora).

[40] L/R/5/157, 1902, week ending 9 August 1902, no. 40, *Rást Goftár*, 3 August; L/R/5/27, week ending 23 February 1901 (151).

[41] L/R/5/77, week ending 24 June 1900, *Hindustani*; L/R/5/156, week ending 15 June 1901, no. 29, *Broach Samáchár*; L/R/5/188, Punjab, week ending 22 June 1905, no. 13, *Paida Akhbar*; L/R/5/80, week ending 2 May 1902, no. 17, *Tafrih* (Lucknow); L/R/5/28, Bengal 1902: Part II, week ending 8 February 1902, no. 142, *Bengalee*.

[42] Ibid., week ending 24 September 1898, no. 35, *Rájahansa*.

[43] Ibid., no. 36, *Karnátak Patra*; ibid., week ending 15 October 1898, no. 22, *Kálidás*.

[44] Week ending 15 October 1898, no. 22, *Kálidás*.

[45] These derive principally from papers in the Punjab; also Wilkinson, *Report on Plague*. Arnold, *Colonizing the Body*, 219–20, has added further tales of plague poisoning, but these did not spark riots. As Arnold cautions: plague 'rumors are far from being an uncontaminated source'. They were employed 'to show ... naive credulity of the masses, and prove "King Mob" was "impervious to reason"' (218).

popular belief in intentional murder by doctors—'needles a yard long...were pushed in at one side of the body and emerged at the other'. This story, however, came from the Amritsar District, where plague had not reached. Instead, the 'rumours' noted in his reports concerned inoculation's side effects and villagers having been thrown out of their houses with their property destroyed. Against the general notion that 'ignorant' and backward villagers were spreading such rumours, Wilkinson found that 'certain zaildárs and other local influential officials' were abetting the resistance to inoculation.[46] Even after the Malkowal disaster, he reported no upsurge in tales of medical or governmental poisoning.[47] Instead, he praised 'the great fortitude' with which they bore their misfortune,[48] and said that the debacle had diminished trust only in cities. He backed his claims with statistics showing a rapid recovery in villagers accepting inoculation along with other governmental anti-plague operations.[49] In many districts inoculation was 'freely accepted' from the outset,[50] and where doubters existed, their opposition could be overcome 'by the exercise of tact and patience and enlisting influential locals to argue the case'.[51]

REASONS TO RIOT

When papers alleged that 'false rumours' and 'the wildest beliefs' fanned Indian plague riots, even these often differed from the myths behind cholera riots. With the 'Tragedy of Poona', the government, foreign press, and native papers outside Pune blamed those published in Pune, its elites, and especially Brahmins for their 'imbecile outcry against the Government as usual'.[52] This 'outcry' was not founded, however, on conspiracies concocted about poisons or demonic practices behind hospital blinds. Rather, it took the form of documented complaints against excesses and abuses by overzealous officials and European soldiers, who knew no native

[46] Wilkinson, *Report on Plague*, part 2, 51.
[47] Reports differed on the numbers inoculated and those killed on 30 October 1902. Recent historians have settled on nineteen inoculated and nineteen deaths.
[48] Wilkinson, *Report on Plague*, part 2, 45–6.
[49] Ibid., 25, 27, and 56. Such stories of ready acceptance of inoculation, evacuation, and other new anti-plague operations are seen in the native newspapers: for example, in Belgaum in 1902; 157, week ending 11 October 1902, no. 32, *Chikitsak*.
[50] Wilkinson, *Report on Plague*, 56.
[51] Ibid., appendix, xxxvi. Modern historians concur: according to Catanach, 'Fatalism?', 191, after the accident at Malkowal it is 'remarkable how quickly Indians accepted inoculation'. Another myth, reflecting plague and geopolitics at the turn of the century, spread near the Afghan border at Etawah. A local paper, *Al Bashir*, reported that residents believed those disinfecting their houses were sprinkling them with 'poisonous drugs...the logic being that a foreign enemy will not invade a country infected with plague'. Russians supported by the Amir of Afghanistan were believed to be planning an Indian invasion, and the British, as a countermeasure, were believed to be spreading plague; L/R/5/80, week ending 28 March 1903, no. 20. Similar myths appeared a year or two before in the Punjab and North-Western Provinces as far south as Madras: L/R/5/77, no. 20, *Hindustan* (Kalakankar); L/R/5/110, Madras, week ending 19 January 1901, no. 4, *Puduvai Mitran*.
[52] Ibid., week ending 15 May 1897, no. 16. These accusations reverberated through foreign papers; see for example *South Australian Register*, 11 August 1897, 4.

Indian languages and little about indigenous customs. Conspiracy theories could instead come from the press, native and international, in support of the government. Concerning the destruction of the Arthur Road hospital in Mumbai in November 1896, one paper concluded that the Brahmins had 'for days past' prepared the ground by floating rumours of 'the tyrannical character' of the government's sanitation and segregation policies and practices.[53] Two years later, after Mumbai's most serious plague riot in March 1898, the Chairman of the Bombay Plague Committee floated a similar conspiracy: outsiders had 'deliberately planned' the violence well in advance. Three months later, a detailed police report overturned the accusation.[54]

Instead of myths, Indian plague protesters pointed to concrete reasons for distrust. These centred on a wide range of humiliating and damaging practices— careless segregation of the healthy among the plague-stricken; prison conditions and inadequate lodging in plague camps; detention centres with provisioning at starvation levels; harassment of passengers; indifference or hostility to religious customs, with destruction of shrines and violation of sacred spaces; abuse from police, search parties, and plague commissioners; military pre-dawn strip examinations in public places; destruction of homes, especially those of the poor; and a general milieu of arrogance, corruption, and blackmail.[55]

In summarizing the events at Pune in the summer of 1897, a newspaper of Western Australia reported such complaints as though they were myths: 'The troops are accused of outraging women, insulting the religion of the natives and of general plundering'.[56] But from case reports found in hundreds of native papers, these malpractices had become the operating procedures of anti-plague control across the subcontinent. Native papers followed by international ones began to recognize them as grounded in realities.[57] For instance, soon after the assassinations at Pune the *Guardian* supported Pune's papers, citing *Mahratta* approvingly, that no measure undertaken by the colonial government 'has interfered so largely and in such a sys- tematic way with the domestic, social and religious habits of the people as the enforcement of the measures adopted for stamping out the plague'.[58]

In Mumbai and eventually throughout India, municipal and colonial govern- ments admitted that plague searches had been abusive and their ignorance of local customs a reality to their detriment. Governments drafted policies and practices accordingly, reforming searches, allowing relatives to visit plague patients, limiting the military in anti-plague operations, and allowing segregation within private

---

[53] Ibid., week ending 7 November 1896, no. 12, *Kaiser-e-Hind*.

[54] Ibid., week ending 18 June 1898, no. 25, *Indian Spectator*. On this report, see note 82.

[55] For charges of blackmail by threatening to put the uninfected in segregation camps, see L/R/5/151, week ending 7 November 1896, no. 19, *Champion*; ibid., 153, week ending 19 March 1898, no. 21, *Kaiser-e-Hind*; and *The Times*, 14 April 1900, 3. For other forms of corruption, see L/R/5/153, week ending 19 March 1898, no. 21, *Indian Spectator*.

[56] *Kalgoorlie Western Argus*, 8 July 1897, 19.

[57] For Pune, 152, week ending 24 April 1897, nos 8–16.

[58] *Guardian*, 3 July 1897; also see *Scotsman*, 15 June 1900, for Kanpur.

homes and in caste hospitals.[59] Though a year of petitions and peaceful assemblies had failed to move Lord Sandhurst, less than a week after Mumbai's Julai riot, he began reforming plague policy, first by cancelling the registration of plague deaths, which had especially offended Hindus by allowing strangers to touch corpses and which raised serious health risks with bodies having to lie unburied in homes throughout hot summer months. He also made changes to a policy whose history of native complaint stretched back to the plague's origins in 1896—that of soldiers composing plague search parties. The reversal changed public opinion immediately. The Anglo-Marátthi *Indu Prakásh* concluded, now that Indians could examine their own houses and their dead, they 'will submit to everything...without a groan' to stamp out plague.[60] Shortly thereafter, Sandhurst enacted a major constitutional change by disbanding the Bombay Plague Committee. Since Gatacre's resignation, it had been a thorn in Mumbai's side.[61] Papers claimed its abusive enforcement and incompetence had sparked the riots.[62] Others charged the Committee not only with indifference and an 'unsympathetic attitude' towards rich and poor alike but with 'stupidity'.[63] Even the usually pro-government *Indian Spectator* condemned the Committee for its abuses and policies 'as purposeless interference'.[64]

The Julai riots of March 1898 emboldened native papers to risk firing further barbs at the Committee, accusing it of mismanaging Mumbai's plague hospitals, making them 'more miserable than cattle-sheds'.[65] Other papers pointed to its vast expenditures that had brought the municipal government to the brink of bankruptcy. These criticisms mounted into June, when finally Lord Sandhurst devolved plague control back to the municipal corporation.[66]

CLASS UNITY

In contrast to the 'Tragedy of Poona', which so divided the indigenous press in their attributions of blame,[67] all native papers, regardless of language or religious orientation, spoke with a single voice in the aftermath of the Julai revolt. They began with what appears as a mandatory prelude, condemning the lower-class rioters, 'the

[59] Gatacre pioneered these compromises; he was the first to reject strict segregation and ruthless searches violating privacy and religious sensibilities. On changes after the 9 March 1898 riots, see 'Notes from India' (1898). In Kolkata, fundamental reforms were achieved in the aftermath of its most devastating plague riots, late June to 1 July 1897; see *Guardian*, 3 July 1897, 9; and *Scotsman*, 3 July 1897, 9. At Danapur in April 1900, the magistrate dismissed disinfection parties, unless unopposed, and troops were ordered to abstain from force when carrying out plague evacuation; 'Notes from India' (1900). In Kanpur, plague measures were modified and compulsory removal of plague patients to hospitals was abolished after the riot; 'Parliamentary Intelligence'.

[60] L/R/5/153, week ending 19 March 1898, no. 22.   [61] Ibid., no. 22, *Indu Prakásh*.

[62] Ibid., no. 23, *Kesari*.   [63] Ibid., week ending 12 March 1898, no. 26, *Indu Prakásh*.

[64] Ibid., week ending 19 March 1898, no. 16, *Indian Spectator*.

[65] Ibid., week ending 12 March 1898, no. 26, *Indu Prakásh*.

[66] Ibid., week ending 26 March 1898, no. 33, *Mahráttta*; week ending 23 April 1898, no. 41, *Native Opinion*; and many more.

[67] See Chapter 14.

wretched Julai',[68] for their ignorance, fanaticism, and acts of violence 'repugnant to law'.[69] Papers then concentrated on what they considered the principal causes of the 9 March violence, maintaining that the Julai and working-class residents of the impoverished Madanpura district caused it only 'indirectly'.[70] Signs of deeper causes had been apparent for at least a month.[71] It had been 'the talk of the town', but because of increased colonial control over the press, Indian papers had not recorded it. With this law (Section 505 of the Criminal Procedure), editors doubted whether their papers could ever criticize government again.[72] After the riots, the *Champion* became emboldened; pointing to the long-term policies of anti-plague defences, it accused their 'servitors' of:

> rushing into private houses when the male members were away, pestering patients down with ordinary ailments...frightening their relatives, threatening to carry off patients, catching hold of the poor in the streets and elsewhere, thrusting the thermometer into their mouths, wantonly destroying property.

It charged that 'these and other complaints, to say nothing of petty corruption' had 'filled the air for weeks' and fixed the blame squarely on the constitutional arrangements that had endowed the Bombay Plague Committee with so much power: 'no real peace' was possible until Lord Sandhurst dismissed the Committee and placed it under municipal control.[73] The *Mahrátta* called the Committee the 'author' of the riots.[74] According to *Kaiser-e-Hind*, 'discontent' was not the Julai's alone: 'everywhere in the Native town', cries of '*zulum*', scandal, and corruption, 'including blackmail' were heard.[75] *Indu Prakásh* said the cause reached higher than the Committee, implying it rested with Sandhurst himself, although, given Section 505, it was not so foolish to say it.[76] Other papers stressed that the hapless medical student's order to examine the Julai girl was only the tip of iceberg: general discontent stretched across Indian society, by class and religion, and had been mounting for some time.[77] Even after Sandhurst's about-face, papers continued to emphasize his earlier refusal to negotiate with 'the people of Bombay'.[78] By April, other native papers followed suit; the *Hindu Punch* charged: 'The Government will do nothing voluntarily'. To redress their grievance, the people will have 'to make a stir'.[79] Now, instead of castigating the rioters as the 'ignorant' poor, papers praised them: the 'lawlessness and violence' of 'the ignorant and *budmash*[80] element' had brought 'the Government to reason'. The efforts of 'their wiser brethren' (i.e. the intellectuals and journalists) with their 'milder remedies' of persuasion and reform had failed.[81] By mid-June, the government had concurred. A report by Mumbai's Police Commissioner, Mr R. H. Vincent, refuted the Plague Committee's claims of

---

[68] L/R/5/153, week ending 19 March, no. 16, *Indian Spectator*; ibid., no. 19, *Mahrátta*.
[69] Ibid., week ending 19 March, no. 16, *Indian Spectator*; ibid., no. 18, *Champion*.
[70] Ibid., no. 23, *Kesari*.   [71] Ibid., no. 20, *Gujaráti*.
[72] Ibid., no. 16, *Indian Spectator*, and no. 17, *Rást Goftár*.   [73] Ibid., no. 18.
[74] Ibid., no. 19, *Mahrátta*.   [75] Ibid., no. 21, *Kaiser-e-Hind*.   [76] Ibid., no. 26.
[77] Ibid., no. 23; week ending 15 March, no. 24, *Rást Goftár*; no. 25, *Gurákhi*.
[78] Ibid., week ending 26 March, no. 33; also see ibid, week ending 26 March, no. 33, *Mahrátta*.
[79] Week ending 2 April, *Hindu Punch*.   [80] Hindi for villainous.
[81] Week ending 11 June 1898, 6 June.

outsiders and Brahmins instigating the riots. Instead, 'universal discontent' permeated 'all classes'. The responsibility rests more with the plague 'regime with its unwillingness to show sympathy with the people and inability to read the signs of the times, than with the bellicose tendencies of the *budmash* element of the city'.[82] Other papers put it even more bluntly: 'the unpopularity of the plague measures were the sole cause of the riots, and the plague authorities were to blame'.[83] It took 'the roughs of the Muhammadan community' to 'rouse the absent-minded Government to do its duty'.[84]

CLASS AND CULTURAL UNITY BEYOND MUMBAI

Plague protest in India rested on much more than claims of blood drained from patients' feet, livers dissected for cures, or rare references to fears of doctors' poisons. Political motives—the zeal of the indigenous population to challenge government abuses and to be recognized as citizens, essential in their own plague defence—recur as the dominant causes of plague riots from Mysore to the foothills of the Himalayas. These concerns united social classes, cut across castes, and temporarily fused the sympathies of the subcontinent's two major religions.[85] Such a consensus was not exclusive to Pune or Mumbai. In another part of the Presidency, Hyderabad, 'a monster meeting' united Hindus and Muslims, 'high and low', to oppose compulsory segregation—a practice that violated their religious rites and social customs.[86] In few cholera riots or protests had any hint of a united front been achieved, except perhaps for brief moments as during the morning of Madrid's Puerta del Sol protest, before bourgeois café-goers retreated.[87] Instead, from the 1830s to the twentieth century, cholera riots ripped societies asunder, ploughing deep trenches along class lines. They failed even to unite various strata and occupations within the working class, as plague strikes achieved in India.[88] No doubt, this unity explains much of the success of India's plague riots, and why, unlike cholera riots, they lasted such a short time, vanishing well before plague's climax around 1907 or in the Punjab a decade later.[89] With momentary exceptions in places such as Kolkata in 1898 and 1899,[90] once governments modified their policies, the riots declined. Realpolitik proved a less plausible antidote against fears based on imaginary forces like cholera frenzy: discovery of

---

[82] Cited in ibid., week ending 18 June 1898, no. 25, *Indian Spectator*.
[83] Ibid., week ending 11 June 1898, no. 29, *Akhbár-e-Sodágar*.
[84] Ibid., week ending 26 March 1898, no. 33, *Mahrátta*.
[85] L/R/5/152, week ending 6 March 1897, nos 28–32; week ending 20 March 1897, no. 27; week ending 24 July 1897, no. 11; and week ending 31 July 1897, no. 36.
[86] Ibid., week ending 10 April 1897, no. 34.   [87] See Chapter 10.
[88] Also see Sarkar, 'The Tie that Snapped', 186–7, 190, 193, 202, 206.
[89] See Arnold, *Colonizing the Body*, 201–2; Klein, 'Plague, Policy and Popular Unrest', Table 1, 724. The highest mortality was in 1907 with 1,116,000 plague deaths. For India as a whole, average plague mortalities remained many times higher, even as late as 1918, than during the peak of the riots in 1897 and 1898.
[90] L/R/5/153, week ending 21 May 1898, no. 53, *Champion*; and week ending 11 June 1898, no. 29, *Akhbár-e-Sodágar*.

cholera's epidemiology and pathology along with better preventive measures failed to dampen its class hatred and violence against doctors and the state in Russia and Italy into the twentieth century.

* * *

Instead of the key words used to describe participants in European cholera riots—the ignorant, superstitious, and uncivilized—the press on occasion characterized Indian plague 'conspirators' as quite the opposite, as the ones with the 'brains'. In an editorial comparing the origins of the plague riots in India with the Sepoy Mutiny of 1857, an Australian paper attributed 'the trouble' behind both to the 'Brahims': ' "They were," as one authority says, "fanatical, and they had the brains to contrive mischief when discontented." '[91] In none of the Indian riots were crowds described as the marginal or 'untouchables'. Instead, even the rioters of Mumbai's 9 March revolt that engulfed a quarter of the city were identified as 'caste men', Bombay's 'Zulais or Musalman weavers',[92] who were among Mumbai's highest-paid workers.[93]

To be sure, some papers pointed to the 'low-class element',[94] and claimed that 'trouble' originated from 'the quarters of the low-class Hindoos and Mahammedans'.[95] Yet with the major plague riots, upper- and middle-class resentment against governmental abuses surfaced, first with peaceful protest—editorials, complaints to Plague Commissioners, petitions, and resolutions drawn in town meetings. Second, a principal criticism against anti-plague measures was an elitist one, derived from the upper castes, especially Brahmins: removal to the segregation camps forced them to mix with other religious groups and, worse, with lower castes, thus violating their 'caste prejudices and religious susceptibilities'. Native papers complained: it was 'rather queer that the authorities should make no distinction in this respect between the well-to-do classes', who could afford isolation in their own houses 'and the low unprotected, who could not'.[96] Why should natives, 'who excel the Europeans in dress, cleanliness etc. be subjected to the same treatment as the low-caste and dirty people'?[97] Yet this class prejudice rallied no reported resistance from artisans, labourers, peasants, or out-castes. Instead, unlike the great majority of cholera riots, Indian plague riots composed largely of labourers and artisans often

[91] *Kalgoorlie Miner*, 8 July 1897, 2.
[92] *New York Times*, 10 March 1898; *Guardian*, 10 March 1897, 5; L/R/5/153, week ending 12 March 1898, Bombay riots of 9 March, nos 22–8, cited from *Jám-e-Jamshed*.
[93] Sarkar, 'The Tie that Snapped', 197; and Ramanna, 'Coping with the Influenza', 89.
[94] See for instance *Rást Goftár*, 3 April 1898, ibid., week ending 9 April 1898, no. 10.
[95] *The Evening Herald*, 10 March 1898, 3; *Sun*, 10 March 1898, 3; and *The Times* (Washington, DC), 10 March 1898, front page.
[96] L/R/5/151, week ending 17 October 1896, no. 16, 11 October, and no. 17, 11 October, *Gujaráti* and *Satya Mitra* expressed the same resentment.
[97] Ibid., 152, week ending 19 June 1897, no. 23, *Sind Sudhár*. A riot in the village of Sávli (Baroda State) was one of elites. Nearly a hundred Brahmins, fifty-eight of whom were arrested, harassed a plague nurse, pelted the local judge (*Fouzdar*) and assistant Plague Commissioner, and attacked the village hospital, destroying its furniture and burning sheds housing patients (ibid., week ending 21 May 1898, no. 71, *Shri Sayáji Vijaya*).

presented a united front from Brahmins and the intelligentsia to day-labourers.[98] Finally, the composition of plague riots differed from cholera's in another respect. They were not comprised largely of impoverished women as were the majority of cholera riots. While an examination of a girl may have sparked Mumbai's largest riot, this and other plague uprisings appear to have been matters for men, outraged (among other things) by officials' treatment of their women, which insulted their masculinity and sense of decorum.

BEYOND INDIA

Plague protest outside the subcontinent did not differ radically from India's. Conspiracies with myths of 'plague spreaders' rarely mobilized plague rioters. Even at Jeddah and other holy places, plague protest railed against the excesses, abuses, and insensitivities of plague regulations. At Port Said, Jeddah, Harbin, and elsewhere, the ruinous economic impositions of quarantine together with the destruction caused by disinfection and burning homes incited revolt, not mythologies of poisoning or of physicians out to kill the poor. Conspiracy theories prevailed more in China than elsewhere with foreigners as the targets, but even here, the causes of protest were concrete and political, against government abuses and harsh and ineffective anti-plague restrictions that discriminated against the native population.

Finally, as with plague protest in India, rioters beyond the subcontinent were not restricted to the poor or minorities. Instead, they created united fronts across classes, races, religious groups, and nationalities. The Port Said riot, for instance, began as a protest that included Europeans and Arabs. The first Oporto protests combined workers with traders and the merchant class. San Francisco's protests united Chinese labourers and small shopkeepers with Chinese merchants as well as with the city's white elites against quarantine and compulsory inoculation based on race. They marched together, closed their stores, and funded lawsuits that reached the nation's capital. These differed sharply from earlier Chinatown conflicts provoked by smallpox and tuberculosis that had divided the city by class and race.

Without doubt, the 'Third Pandemic' at times mobilized suspicion, hate, and blame with gangs attacking Europeans and placards damning foreigners. In India, the numbers of rioters involved, killed, wounded, and arrested surpassed even Europe's most deadly cholera riots. Yet it would be incorrect to take the exceptions as the rule and conclude that plague and cholera riots were much the same.[99] Instead of imagined conspiracies, concrete economic and social realities spurred

---

[98] Wilkinson, *Report on Plague*, part 2, even asserted: 'Everywhere' the greatest resistance to adopting the government's plague policies came from 'the well-to-do and educated classes' (2).

[99] See for instance Klein, 'Plague, Policy and Popular Unrest': 'The majority of the people believed that doctors were the chief men who spread the plague, and this some believed they did for their own living and maintenance' (749). Also, Catanach, 'Fatalism?', suggests that rumours of well poisoning with Indian plague was similar to blaming the Jews during the Black Death (190).

the majority of plague protesters to assemble, and their protests often began with peaceful assemblies, petitions, and letters to commissioners, in which they documented their grievances. Instead of being suspicious or opposed to Western medicine, they called for more empirical and international research based on statistics. Nothing similar is found in the hundreds of cholera riots I have uncovered. Finally, plague riots had little in common with smallpox-induced violence. No plague riot I have found blamed the victim. On this score, plague and cholera social violence shared something in common.

PART V

MODERNITY:
PLAGUES OF COMPASSION

17

Yellow Fever

Stories from Philadelphia and Memphis

Historians of diseases have rarely attempted to distinguish epidemics that tend to spark blame and social violence from those that do not.[1] The few exceptions have turned to psychology rather than collecting and mapping epidemics' patterns in past time. Joost Meerloo's 'patterns of panic', drawn largely from his patients during and immediately after World War II, have constituted a model: 'mystery, unexpected danger, and unknown threats always prepare the way for collective fear'[2] and thus explain pandemics' propensities to spur violence and blame. In other words, those fanning violence would be the ones to strike suddenly then disappear for some time as with waves of plague, especially in the medieval and early modern periods, or with cholera and yellow fever in the nineteenth century. By contrast, diseases that were more or less endemic such as dysentery, typhoid, and tuberculosis supposedly did not stir panic, fear, blame, or social violence, even though over time they killed far more. Others have added smallpox to the list of commonplace diseases, ones that 'people learned to live with'.[3] Our evidence raises questions about this model. The sudden, unpredictable recurrence of plague after the Black Death and its quick disappearance in a matter of months did not lead to repeated mass abandonment or widespread massacres as seen in 1348–51. On the other hand, in places such as Mumbai and Kolkata plague recurred like clockwork biannually during the last years of the nineteenth century but also repeatedly produced widespread rioting.

For nineteenth-century America, two epidemic diseases have been most often cited as the ones provoking the greatest terror—cholera and yellow fever—and for some, yellow fever ranks first.[4] Other historians of yellow fever have emphasized the panic it caused, which they have measured by the breakdown of commerce and mass migration. Such was the chaos produced in 1853 in New Orleans, when yellow fever decimated a tenth its population, plus others who fled from their property, businesses, and family members. Moreover, John Duffy concluded these

---

[1] For a rare attempt to explain diseases most prone to generate terror, see Humphreys, 'No Safe Place', 848–9, and its implementation by Foley, *The Last Irish Plague*, for influenza in Ireland, 80.

[2] Meerloo, *Patterns of Panic*, 48–50; also cited by Smelser, *The Theory of Collective Behaviour*, 141.

[3] See Chapter 11, note 9.

[4] Pierce and Writer, *Yellow Jack*, 2; and Bloom, *The Mississippi Valley's Great Yellow Fever Epidemic*, who hails it as the 'King of Terrors', 117.

were the 'standard reactions to the threat of yellow fever'.[5] For Memphis, the terror and mass migration wrought by the pandemic of 1878, which swept through southern states from the Atlantic to Texas and as far north as Ohio, had long-term damaging consequences.[6] According to the detailed eyewitness account of the Memphis journalist J. M. Keating, 'the whole population was precipitated into a panic, surpassing all powers of description, and which deadened all human sympathy, all the kindlier emotions of the human heart, all feeling of kinship, all regard for neighbourly claims'.[7]

THE PHILADELPHIA STORY

But did a disease's tendency to generate panic, fear, and terror necessarily translate into hatred, blame, and collective violence?[8] Historians of medicine have concluded that little separated cholera and yellow fever in their propensity to produce social loathing. In his eloquent and highly influential essay outlining the dramaturgy of epidemic diseases across time, Charles Rosenberg held that 'the blaming of victims' was the same with yellow fever in Philadelphia in 1793 as with cholera in New York in 1832: 'Equally obvious is the way in which coping with randomness provides an occasion for reconfirming the social values of the majority, for blaming victims. Framing and blaming are inextricably mingled...'.[9] Other historians have tried to corroborate such an equation by singling out specific incidents in a single place during a single yellow fever epidemic. Supposed 'persistent rumours of wells having been contaminated' in preparation for a French invasion of Philadelphia in 1793 'led to threats of mob violence against the hapless refugees'.[10] But unlike

---

[5] Duffy, *Sword of Pestilence*, 124.

[6] According to Baker, 'Yellow Jack', 241–64, 260, it struck over 200 towns that year with approximately 100,000 cases and 20,000 deaths in the Mississippi Valley. Also, see Ellis, 'Businessmen and Public Health', 197–212; 197. For yellow fever's long-term consequences, the impressions of Baker, 'Yellow Jack', 263–4, are mixed: he points to Memphis's demographic decline, absolutely and relative to other southern cities, and to Memphis's loss of ethnic diversification. Yet the response to public initiatives was positive, and after 1879 Memphis was not hit by later epidemics that swept the south. For sanitary reforms in Memphis and other south-eastern cities, see Ellis, 'Businessmen and Public Health', who also gives a mixed account. The epidemic of 1878, along with those in the 1880s and 1890s, stimulated businesses to pass reforms and gave rise to philanthropic societies, such as New Orleans' Auxillary Sanitation Association. These provided better health for upper- and middle-class whites but failed to break 'the link between poverty and ill health'. Because of the growth of racial prejudice, conditions for the poor deteriorated (370–1). Carrigan, *The Saffron Scourge*, concurs with Baker: yellow fever contributed to the decline of southern cities in the nineteenth century, especially those on the Gulf and rivers, but yellow fever was only one factor. She too argues that it spurred advances in sanitary and health policy throughout the South; 113, 127, 128, 199, 378–9, 381. Finally, Humphreys, 'Appendix II', 192, saw yellow fever in the South as 'central to the origins of federal public health involvement', encouraging research and reform; see also idem, *Yellow Fever and the South*, 178 and 182.

[7] Keating, *History of the Yellow Fever*, 107.

[8] See notes 2 and 4 and Delaporte, *Disease and Civilization*, ch. 3.

[9] Rosenberg, 'What is an Epidemic?', 9–10.

[10] Pernick, 'Politics, Parties, and Pestilence', 244. However, Powell, *Bring Out Your Dead*—still the most cited work on this epidemic—does not mention this rumour.

waves of cholera that provoked mobs to endanger lives of physicians and destroy hospitals, police stations, and town halls, Philadelphia's yellow fever violence remained only a threat.[11] And unlike plagues of late sixteenth- and seventeenth-century Europe, no trials, torture, or executions of plague spreaders ensued.

Nonetheless, as with the Black Death, criticisms surfaced of cruel abandonment of family members, producing stories such as one about a woman, who cared for her dying husband and after burying him, her father refused her entry into her house.[12] The most significant outcry against a minority—Philadelphia's black community—derived from one voice alone, that of the publisher Mathew Carey. He charged 'negro' nurses with neglecting their duties in treating white yellow fever patients, pilfering property, and charging extortionate fees.[13] Yet within two months he tempered his criticisms, after members of Philadelphia's African-American community[14] soundly refuted the accusations.[15] From a rich array of concrete cases, leaders of the Free African Society documented the blacks' care of afflicted whites, often without charging fees. Prominent whites such as the city's renowned physician, Dr Benjamin Rush, and mayor, Matthew Clarkson, corroborated the blacks' counter-claims. Based on previous reports from epidemics in the West Indies, Rush and other Philadelphia worthies believed blacks possessed immunity to yellow fever and called on the former slaves William Grey, Richard Allen, Absalom Jones, and their Free African Society to nurse, bury, and provide medical services such as bleeding yellow fever sufferers. Without hesitation, they served: 'Since God had granted them special exemption, they pleaded that they had a particular obligation to come forward and attend the sick of all ranks'.[16]

In their pamphlet—the first polemic published by any black authors in the US—Allen and Jones described the horrors they faced during rounds of the city: stories of whites charging extortionate rates for care or burial,[17] neighbours refusing to care for infant orphans,[18] and white husbands who threw infected wives out of their homes.[19] But despite Carey's recriminations and Allen and Jones' counter-accusations, no race riots or even small vigilante incidents erupted. Nor did rumours provoke individual or governmental acts of persecution. Instead, Allen and Jones' account like other sources testifies to the blacks' willingness to care for white strangers, and the whites' heartfelt appreciation of the care they received. Poor black men, such as one named Sampson, 'went constantly from house to house where distress was, and

---

[11] Another rumour spread of five 'negroes' arrested for poisoning pumps, but again without consequences; Powell, *Bring Out Your Dead*, 106.

[12] Smith, *Ship of Death*, 216–17.

[13] Carey, *A Short Account*, 4th edn, first published on 14 November 1793, was the earliest history of this epidemic. It went through several editions, in which he softened his view of Philadelphia's black community; see Smith, *Ship of Death*, 230–2; and Griffith, '"A Total Dissolution"'.

[14] See the preface to the 1993 edition, Powell, *Bring Out Your Dead*, ix; and Allen and Jones, *A Narrative*.

[15] On Carey's 'instant history', see Griffith, '"A Total Dissolution"'; on Allen and Jones' rebuttal, Lapsansky, '"Abigail, a Negress"'.

[16] Cited by Powell, *Bring Out Your Dead*, 95.

[17] Allen and Jones, *A Narrative*, 7. On the background and successes of these authors and the Free African Society, see Nash, *Forging Freedom*, 95–9 and 124–33; and Lapsansky, '"Abigail, a Negress"'.

[18] Lapsansky, '"Abigail, a Negress"', 18–19.   [19] Ibid., 19.

asked for no assistance, fee, or reward'.[20] Afro-Americans took it upon themselves
to ask the mayor how they could best serve the city.[21] They transported victims to
the new emergency hospital at Bush Hill and buried hundreds while refusing wages
at the going rates or without payment at all.[22] The black community continued to
provide these services after mid-September, when it became clear that, unlike in
earlier yellow fever epidemics in the West Indies, the black population was dying in
proportions almost equalling whites.[23] Such a sudden turn in fate might have
fomented conspiracies as seen with cholera, when the poor, suddenly dying in great
numbers, blamed elites for creating the disease to kill them off.

Nor were whites in general as ungracious as the publisher Carey first appears.
Even Allen and Jones' tract (bent on rebuking Carey's claims by contrasting black
humanity with white cruelty) portrayed whites as appreciative recipients of the
blacks' charity and sacrifices. They presented the story of a black nurse who treated
a white women afflicted with yellow fever for only 50 cents a day, despite the
patient pleading that the wage was too low. When she died, she left the nurse a
life annuity.[24] At the end of their pamphlet, they printed Mayor Clarkson's letter
of appreciation sent to the Free African Society in praise of the city's black population during the epidemic.[25] One aim in reproducing it was certainly to document
their case of black sacrifice, but their decision also testifies to their gratitude for
the whites' appreciation.

The other central text produced from this epidemic, Mathew Carey's *A Short
Account of the Malignant Fever*, was also an uplifting story of unity, charity, and
self-sacrifice, despite its emphasis on white males mostly of the middling sort, near
neglect of women's sacrifices, and occasional charges against black nurses.[26] It begins
with scenes of abandonment cruelty that could almost have been lifted from Boccaccio
(although no evidence shows Carey knew that work):[27]

> Who, without horror, can reflect on a husband, married perhaps for twenty years,
> deserting his wife in the last agony—a wife unfeelingly abandoning her husband on
> his death bed—parents forsaking their only children—children ungratefully flying
> from their parents...?[28]

---

[20] Ibid., 11.   [21] Ibid., 18.

[22] One story not told by Allen and Jones concerned the black nurse Anne Saville, a member of the
Free African Society, who took over nursing and organization at the Bush Hill Hospital, transforming
it from 'a great human slaughterhouse' to 'a place where most patients survived'; Smith, *Ship of Death*,
228. To their credit, Allen and Jones, *A Narrative*, 11–12, described the sacrifices of five black women.

[23] Of Philadelphia's population remaining during the epidemic, 11 per cent of blacks and 14 per cent
of whites perished; Lapsansky, ' "Abigail, a Negress" ', 67.

[24] Allen and Jones, *A Narrative*, 11. Certainly, blacks were not the only heroes as death tolls of doctors
and stories from diaries reveal. The Quaker carpenter Samuel Garrigues nursed the sick, buried the dead,
and found shelters for orphans, He caught the disease, recovered, and returned to charitable work; Smith,
Ship of Death, 219–20; and DeClure and Smith, 'Wrestling...The Diary of Edward Garrigues'.

[25] Allen and Jones, *A Narrative*, 23–4.

[26] See Carey, *A Short Account*, chs 16 and 17, mentions the ill-treatment of Philadelphian fugitives
seeking food and shelter in other cities. But Carey counterbalances these 'scrapes' with stories of charity from other places as in Gloucester County, New Jersey, 91.

[27] Carey's narrative was influenced by plague stories from London, 1665, and Marseille, 1720;
ibid., 96–112.

[28] Ibid., 23.

Carey ends his lament with an analogy still closer to the *Decameron* with a lapdog replacing Boccaccio's 'dead goat': 'so much did *self* appear to engross…that less concern was felt for the loss of a parent, a husband, a wife, or an only child, than…by the death of a servant, or even a favourite lap-dog'.[29]

Yet the human drama that unfolds from Carey's Philadelphia in 1793 diverges strikingly from Boccaccio's Florence in 1348. Carey's description of the horrors of abandonment, which gives no names, serves solely as a prelude. Rapidly, the chapter shifts to praise named Philadelphians, who laboured 'day and night, attending the sick, and ministering relief to their spiritual and temporal wants'.[30] This chapter alone details the heroic and charitable actions of twenty-one men, 'some in the middle, others in the lower spheres of life, who, in the exercise of the duties of humanity, exposed themselves to dangers…'.[31] He begins with their dedication to afflicted family members but concludes that their actions 'dealt out with equal freedom to an utter stranger as to his bosom friend'.[32] Carey then delves into greater detail on the operations of volunteer committees such as the 'benevolent citizens' who joined the Guardians of the Poor, those founding and running orphanages, and especially, the contributions of the wealthy French merchant Stephan Girard and artisan Peter Helm who transformed Bush Hill Hospital into a place of effective care for the yellow-fever-stricken.[33] These men (and by the fourth edition also Anne Saville[34]) did more than administrate from a safe distance (unlike the bulk of late medieval and early modern plague saints). The former toiled long hours 'to comfort the sick', 'wip[ing] the sweat off their brows, and perform[ing] many disgusting offices of kindness for them, which nothing could render tolerable'.[35] In addition, these yellow fever experiences were unifying: '[We] became a band of brothers, attached to each other'.[36] As shown from the work of Allen and Jones, Benjamin Rush, Mayor Clarkson, and now from the evaluation of historians, those bonds of brotherhood, even 'if only briefly', united Philadelphia's blacks and white citizens.[37]

* * *

The yellow fever epidemics which raged in Louisiana in 1804[38] and 1837,[39] and in Alexandria, Virginia, in 1833,[40] produced responses which historians of the period can point to as resonant with sharp anxieties. Because this disease's 'differential immunity'[41] produced a situation which saw whites often dying in far greater proportions than blacks, exacerbated further by white flight from cities, fears grew that slaves might take advantage of whites' sudden weakness and mount a revolt.

---

[29] Ibid., 23.   [30] Ibid., 25.   [31] Ibid., 25–8; 25.   [32] Ibid., 25.

[33] Ibid., 31–5.   [34] Ibid., 35.   [35] Ibid.

[36] Cited in Griffith, ' "A Total Dissolution" ', 50 and 53, and Carey's autobiography, written thirty years later.

[37] See Smith, 'Comment', 154. Nash, *Forging Freedom*, 125, suggests the same: by the end of the epidemic, white opposition to building Philadelphia's African church had melted away.

[38] Carrigan, *The Saffron Scourge*, 33. The governor did not think there were signs for alarm but nonetheless strengthened night patrols.

[39] Carrigan, 'Yellow Fever', 62. Humphreys, *Yellow Fever and the South*, 49.

[40] Pierce and White, *Yellow Jack*, 50; Carrigan, *The Saffron Scourge*, 33.

[41] From McNeill, *Mosquito Empires*, 4, and throughout his book.

During the yellow fever epidemic of 1853, such fears resulted in the summoning of armed patrols and units of the local militia in New Orleans. Thirteen years after the abolition of slavery, rumours of a general uprising of blacks also arose at the beginning of the epidemic in Memphis of 1878.[42] But neither rebellion materialized; nor did any violence ensue beyond one report of a scuffle at a relief centre in Memphis.[43] The anxieties of dominant classes, moreover, differed categorically from the terror induced by smallpox, plague, or cholera in the nineteenth and early twentieth centuries. No reports surface of slaves or whites being prompted by fear or hysteria to concoct myths of poisoning or blaming one another for inventing the disease. Instead, the whites' fears were reported as cool-headed calculations: the sudden change in demographics might provide slaves with the same opportunities they seized upon when Toussaint Louverture led a successful revolt in Saint-Domingue.[44] In nineteenth-century America, however, such fears quickly dissipated.

More often, historians have pointed to yellow fever's shotgun quarantines with farm roads locked, public roads wrecked, and bridges burned,[45] seeing the cessation of commerce as evidence of the disease's social toxins.[46] An examination of these measures, however, reveals they were enacted late in yellow fever's history,[47] and more importantly were rarely illegal, imposed by non-elected vigilantes, as historians often assume and newspapers sometimes misrepresent.[48] For instance, during the epidemic of 1888, an article carried by US papers and copied in the British press cited the Postmaster General at Cairo, Illinois: '[T]he railway trains to New Orleans are stopped. The country below is in the hands of a howling mob. Quarantine is everywhere general.'[49] But none of these accounts describes any violence or blame. More to the point, those mounting the quarantine were not citizen mobs taking the law into their own hands, bent on barring those authorized from entering towns or seeking assistance in hospitals, as happened with cholera and smallpox. Instead, 'the supposed howling mobs' were legally sanctioned officials and deputized volunteers.

Towns, counties, and states instituted yellow fever quarantines through proper legal and democratic channels. In rare instances when organized violence was reported, later investigation showed that the incidents were often only acts of vandalism.

---

[42] Bloom, *The Mississippi Valley's Great Yellow Fever Epidemic*, 194.   [43] Ibid.

[44] McNeill, *Mosquito Empires*, 260. From a physician's diary, Humphreys, *Yellow Fever and the South*, 49, describes rumours of a slave revolt at Alexandria, Virginia, but makes it clear that blacks saw these circumstances as an opportunity to seize their freedom; it was not that they blamed white slave owners for spreading the disease. In contrast to tuberculosis, smallpox, and cholera, blacks possessed greater immunity to yellow fever.

[45] Crosby, *The American Plague*, 47–8.   [46] Carrigan, *The Saffron Scourge*, 67–8 and 352–3.

[47] Bloom, *The Mississippi Valley's Great Yellow Fever Epidemic*, reports a spate of them with the pandemic of 1878 in Vicksburg, Jackson, Memphis, and other places, but none before that date. His descriptions do not make clear if these quarantines, which could pitch one jurisdiction against another, were illegal; 99, 129, 146.

[48] See Price, 'A Legislative History', 14: these were 'rarely the result of vigilantes'. Instead, they 'came at the behest of mayors, town councils and other political bodies'. In fact, she gives no examples of illegal 'shotgun quarantine'. Carrigan, *The Saffron Scourge*, 152, presents Shreveport's 'shotgun quarantine' that blocked all entrances to the city by 'mounted volunteers' as though it were illegal but then mentions that Shreveport's Health Board had authorized it.

[49] *The Times*, 26 September 1888, 5; *Morning Post*, 26 September 1888, 4; *York Herald*, 27 September 1888; 29 September 1888.

For instance, on 23 October 1897, a railway bridge east of Lake Charles, Louisiana, was partially destroyed by fire. The railway's manager charged that it was an illegal act of 'self-imposed quarantine' reputedly following threats made by citizens in a mass meeting the night before. The *Times Picayune* sent a journalist to investigate, who discovered that the town meeting had not issued any threats, and no 'mob' action had ensued. Instead, the town meeting had been conciliatory, and following the bridge's partial burning, citizens held a second meeting, denouncing the destruction and agreeing to help apprehend the vandals if 'in fact an act of incendiarism' had occurred.[50]

A rare exception may have developed in Georgia, which the *Lancet* mentioned briefly in 1893 without naming the town or specifying the date: 'thousands' fled an epidemic of yellow fever, but 'were driven back by the armed resistance of terrified and indignant neighbours'.[51] 'Chronicling America' includes thirteen papers reporting a short wave of yellow fever in Georgia in September 1893 that produced only a few cases. Worst hit was Brunswick, where panic created a mass exodus, closing shops and threatening a famine due to an absence of supplies. But no paper reported the 'disgrace' described in the *Lancet*.[52] Instead, relief agencies 'made heroic efforts' to meet 'the demands of hundreds of sufferers'.[53]

Further, no newspapers among the hundreds archived in 'Chronicling America' reported cases of the leaders of so-called shotgun quarantines battling against elected mayors, governors, or health boards as seen with US smallpox epidemics during these decades. In 1888, the city of Jackson established a 'shotgun quarantine' based on one that had kept yellow fever away from Natchez in 1878, believing it could be successfully re-enacted.[54] In 1897, four southern states established 'shotgun quarantines' between one another 'and were becoming stricter' in their inspections of those arriving from infected places.[55] During the same epidemic, such quarantines were established in parts of eastern Texas,[56] and by October, they stretched across south-western Texas, but there is no evidence that any of these were illegal.[57]

In 1900, a year before *Aedes aegypti* was proven to be the disease's vector, 'yellow fever quarantines hedged in by shot guns' stretched through the states bordering the Gulf of Mexico,[58] and even after the discovery of its insect transmission, widely publicized in small-town and county newspapers, local governments still imposed quarantines.[59] From the 1901 epidemic to yellow fever's epidemic finale in 1905, these quarantines, against the new evidence in fact, became more sophisticated and

---

[50] *Times Picayune*, 24 August 1897, 8.   [51] 'Armed Resistance'.
[52] See for instance, *Evening World*, 18 September 1893, front page.
[53] *Roanoke Times*, 23 September 1893, 3.
[54] *Alexandria Gazette*, 21 September 1888, 2, from *Times Picayune*.
[55] *Wichita Daily Eagle*, 23 September 1897, 8; and Carrigan, *The Saffron Scourge*, 185.
[56] *Scranton Tribune*, 30 September 1897, front page.
[57] *El Paso Herald*, 23 October 1897, 2. The following year, 'the people of Meridian', Mississippi, elected to enforce 'a shotgun quarantine'; *Appeal*, 5 November 1898, 4, mocked it: 'Yellow Jack cared nothing for the idiotic performance, and it entered Meridian anyhow'.
[58] *Hawaiian Gazette*, 2 January 1900, 4.
[59] In 1903 those living along the Rio Grande appealed to the War Department to enforce their locally instituted quarantine; *Evening World*, 1 October 1903, 5.

extensive. They prevailed throughout the southern states of Louisiana, Mississippi, Alabama, and Texas, establishing new detention camps enforced by Gatling guns and muskets. 'Steamship transportation...extending around half a continent' was curtailed.[60] Yet, despite disapproving tones and scepticism over these measures' efficacy, no newspaper hinted that the quarantines were illegal or blamed victims of the disease for spreading it as was continuing to happen with American smallpox epidemics. My searches reveal only one clear case of a clash between different levels of government over enforcement of a yellow fever quarantine.[61] It arose between the health boards of Atlanta and the state of Georgia, when the city defied the state's attempt to stop refugees from yellow fever-stricken Louisiana entering Atlanta. But no matter how acrimonious the conflict, it was fought in courtrooms, not on the tracks or streets with shotguns.[62]

In October 1898, President Grover Cleveland (1837–1908) sent US soldiers to ensure that the recent National Quarantine Act was respected and that trains stopped by 'mob' quarantines would be kept running.[63] But here too no reports appear of violence or clashes ensuing from the President's order. On occasion, railway tracks were uprooted, once in September 1888 between Harrison and Natchez,[64] and in 1897, near Jackson, during a severe yellow fever epidemic in Mississippi, but without riots or reported injuries.

*   *   *

Few scholars have argued that epidemic diseases may present different dramaturgies or that the attitudes to yellow fever may have differed fundamentally from cholera's or smallpox's. Yet with yellow fever, persecution of the victim and blame of others were rare, and large-scale collective protest and violence almost non-existent, despite prevailing preconditions that were ready to ignite them. As yellow fever spread through the South in 1853 and in 1878–9, racism and sectional tensions between North and South were on the rise, stoked by pressures soon to trigger the Civil War, then with resentment over Reconstruction, the rise of Jim Crow laws, and a crescendo of southern lynchings. Nor do characteristics of yellow fever's aetiology, epidemiology, or its signs and symptoms suggest an easy explanation for the lack of violence. First, its epidemic waves appear as random and mysterious as those of cholera, and its mechanisms of transmission remained unsolved for almost half a century after cholera's had been discovered, with yellow fever's pathogen only being identified in 1924. Moreover, as graphically described in medical texts by the physician-novelist Ernst Weiss and others,[65] yellow fever's signs and symptoms

---

[60] *Perrysburg Journal*, 25 August 1905, 3.

[61] On 25 August 1905, the *Perrysburg Journal* claimed there were such conflicts but documented none.

[62] Price, 'A Legislative History', 32–5. Another occurred the same year in Louisiana, when its Health Board threatened to use troops against locally imposed quarantines (61).

[63] *Times Picayune*, 15 October 1898, 4.

[64] *Los Angeles Daily Herald*, 22 September 1888, 4.

[65] Weiss, *Georg Letham*, 278 and elsewhere; Pierce and Writer, *Yellow Jack*, 7; Craddock, *City of Plagues*, 66; Humphreys, *Yellow Fever and the South*, 6; Bloom, *The Mississippi Valley's Great Yellow Fever Epidemic*, 6; McNeill, *Mosquito Empires*.

could rank with cholera or smallpox in frightfulness and disgust. It developed quickly with chills, high fever, and jaundice. After a false recovery on the third or fourth day, all hell broke loose, with haemorrhaging through the nose, gums, and stomach lining, 'digested' black blood, horrific stench, and 'blazing red eyes with vividly inflamed conjunctivae'. Then black vomit erupted, not only through the mouth, but from the nose and other orifices, bequeathing the disease its Spanish name, 'el vómito negro'.[66]

Finally, the social explanation for cholera's provocation of class strife and con-spiracies of class hatred—that cholera struck mostly the poor—fails to distinguish it from yellow fever. In districts of European capital cities, cholera could be a dis-ease that afflicted the rich as much as the poor, as in Vienna in September 1831, when the 'higher classes' were 'singled out for the ravage'. For an English physician, this pattern confirmed theories of miasma: the wealthy occupied the lower floors, while the 'lower classes' lived in the 'more airy' higher floors and suburbs.[67] Certain Parisian neighbourhoods also posed similar enigmas in 1832. A French physician pondered: 'One must ask why cholera strikes more often the beautiful boulevards of the Faubourg de Saint-Germain than the narrow twisted streets of la Ponte Saint-Eustache'.[68] By contrast, yellow fever, more than cholera, was America's 'disease of strangers'.[69] Because of its patterns of immunity, it attacked previously unexposed immigrants in greater numbers and with higher rates of fatality. With the exception of blacks, these comprised the most dispossessed in America—the Irish, Central Europeans, and Russians. During the New Orleans epidemic of 1853, 7000 of the 8000 to 11,000 victims were immigrants, in the main, poor Irish.[70] Although yellow jack may not have killed as quickly as cholera, its crisis point of three or four days was extraordinarily rapid as infectious killers go and its mortality rates were generally higher than cholera's, reaching catastrophic levels among recent white immigrants. During the yellow fever epidemic of 1878, over 70 per cent of whites who remained in Memphis perished.[71] But by the nineteenth century, yellow fever's fatality rates had generally fallen significantly below cholera's, a point to which we will return in the conclusion.[72]

---

[66] Craddock, *City of Plagues*, 66; Pierce and Writer, *Yellow Jack*, 7.

[67] Blane, *Warning to the British Public*, 33.

[68] Piorry, *Clinique médicale*, 231. During the cholera epidemic in 1832 artisans were reported harder hit than the poor, native French-Canadians, or newly arrived Irish; Bilson, *A Darkened House*, 49.

[69] On its patterns of immunity and effects on immigrant populations, see Pierce and Writer, *Yellow Jack*, 15, 38, and 47.

[70] Ibid., 47–9. Bloom, *The Mississippi Valley's Great Yellow Fever Epidemic*, 39. Officially, yellow fever mortality that year was 8100.

[71] Keating, *A History*, 139–40. His figures pertain to a population of 19,600 remaining after 1 September; only 8 per cent of the black population died from the disease. Statistics from the city's charity hospital during thirteen epidemics, 1822 to 1849, report 12,913 cases and 6332 deaths, a fatality rate of 49 per cent (ibid., 33).

[72] See McNeill, *Mosquito Empires*, 37–8, 132, and 134, and his citation of other authors, especially Sloeck, 'Aedes aegypti', 249, who estimated yellow fever fatality rates as high as 94.5 per cent. Similarly, McNeill estimates mortality rates as high as 90 per cent among Europeans in Kourou (French Guiana), June 1764 to April 1765 (134), but admits that data on yellow fever fatality rates in the colonial period is 'sketchy'. He might have added that yellow fever, especially among the young, can produce mild cases, which before laboratory tests were rarely diagnosed as yellow fever; see Bloom, *The Mississippi Valley's Great Yellow Fever Epidemic*, 5, 10. In other places, fatality rates were much lower; and according

Despite these characteristics—its randomness, mysteries of transmission, grue-some signs and symptoms, widespread panic and fear, concentrations among the poorest, and the prevailing social and political contexts—yellow fever's propensity to arouse hatred and blame differed strikingly from that of smallpox or cholera. In his detailed study of yellow fever in New Orleans in 1853, John Duffy revealed a picture of this disease's social effects that contrasts sharply with what historians have come to expect, especially since the emergence of AIDS in the 1980s. Despite panic and mass migration with racism on the rise, the 1853 epidemic failed to pitch citizens against immigrants or whites against blacks. As with epidemics described by Livy, it instead united communities. Northerners sent money and supplies to the South, and the disease encouraged a new tolerance and respect across class and racial lines. Because of resistance gained from centuries of exposure to yellow fever in West Africa, blacks in general possessed greater immunity to it, whether acquired or innate.[73] When called in Philadelphia to serve the great numbers of whites who were dying, the black community agreed to do so, and the white community did not fail to express its gratitude.

The blacks' immunity might have stirred suspicion, as happened with Jews in 1348–51, when some alleged they had escaped plague in greater numbers, or with gravediggers and plague cleaners in sixteenth- and seventeenth-century Italy, who may well have gained stronger resistance because of their greater exposure to plague, or the rich during the last plague of Naples in 1656, whose rates of mortality sank far below those of the poor.[74] Molly Crosby has asserted that blacks' immunity to yellow fever 'had been fuel for racism for decades'; but she fails to supply a shred of evidence for this claim,[75] and the evidence thus far presented from Philadelphia (despite Matthew Carey's initial allegations) and New Orleans roundly refutes it. As we will see in Chapter 18, evidence from other southern cities and villages dur-ing yellow fever epidemics in the Deep South also disproves this pronouncement.

At least one historian post-AIDS has observed that 'less blame [was] attached to the victims of yellow fever than to some other diseases of the mid-nineteenth century', and explained the difference:

> Catching yellow fever seemed to depend less on behavioural factors (e.g., personal cleanliness and morality) and more on where one lived, whether one could leave, and how long one had been there. Since filth from the early nineteenth century was felt to be the principal culprit in breeding yellow fever, the blame… fell on government officials charged with sanitation rather than the unlucky of the dirtiest districts.[76]

---

to Humphreys, *Yellow Fever and the South*, 6, for late nineteenth-century southern cities ranged from 10 to 60 per cent, reflecting southern adaptation. Also, see Bloom's statistics for New Orleans, 1853, Memphis 1873, and smaller places such as Grenada and Holly Springs, Mississippi, *The Mississippi Valley's Great Yellow Fever Epidemic*, 10, 39. However, by the epidemic of 1897 and 1905 in places such as New Orleans, these rates had declined further to around 9 to 13 per cent; Carrigan, *The Saffron Scourge*, 194. On southern states' greater exposure and higher 'differential immunity' as early as the American Revolution, see McNeill, *Mosquito Empires*, ch. 6. Cholera's fatality rates were higher, ranging between 40 and 60 per cent into the twentieth century; see Chapters 8–10.

[73] McNeill, *Mosquito Empires*, 44–6.   [74] Pullan, 'Plague', 117.
[75] Crosby, *The American Plague*, 79.   [76] Humphreys, *Yellow Fever and the South*, 7.

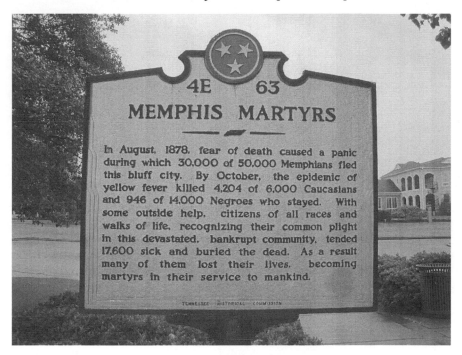

4E 63

MEMPHIS MARTYRS

In August, 1878, fear of death caused a panic during which 30,000 of 50,000 Memphians fled this bluff city. By October, the epidemic of yellow fever killed 4,204 of 6,000 Caucasians and 946 of 14,000 Negroes who stayed. With some outside help, citizens of all races and walks of life, recognizing their common plight in this devastated, bankrupt community, tended 17,600 sick and buried the dead. As a result many of them lost their lives, becoming martyrs in their service to mankind.

TENNESSEE HISTORICAL COMMISSION

Figure 17.1. Memphis Martyrs.

If this were the case, why then did the same social peace not follow from cholera, where filth and especially contaminated sources of water, even before John Snow's observations, and more so afterwards, were rightly seen as cholera's cause, combined with governments' neglect of sanitary conditions? Moreover, like yellow fever, cholera and plague have often been seen as diseases of place with the impoverished left behind and the rich and middle classes fleeing. As a result of these conditions, cholera violence continued to be directed against government officials well into the twentieth century (and in Haiti into the second decade of the twenty-first). In contradistinction to yellow fever, cholera riots in nineteenth- and early twentieth-century Europe and plague revolts in India produced the most extreme cases of social violence propelled by any disease since the Black Death. Nonetheless, in her judicious analysis of Memphis during its worst epidemic of 1878, Humphreys confirms that even the 'most violent protest' against yellow fever pales by comparison with cholera violence. The strongest protest she has found there came from a group of merchants headed by the owner of the largest cotton gin in Memphis. The merchants' tools of protest were not, however, guns or tactics of vigilante violence. Instead, they collected signatures and brought a court order to end the city's quarantine on imported cotton which was vital to their commercial interests.[77]

---

[77] Ibid., 106. Neither Humphreys nor Crosby cites the two most violent threats during the 1878 pandemic at Memphis. With the first confirmed cases of yellow fever in Memphis, 'mobs' attempted to prevent the Citizens' Committee from establishing a refuge for those afflicted at Camp Joe Williams

Similarly, after generalizing about the socio-psychological consequences of epidemics giving rise 'to the heights of generosity and heroism' along with 'the depths of callousness and depravity', Jo Ann Carrigan seems surprised by her findings from thirty epidemics in Louisiana, 1796 to 1905: 'social order held together, and one searches in vain for reports of widespread looting, debauchery, violence, or other signs of social dissolution so often associated with catastrophe'.[78]

THE STORY FROM MEMPHIS

The difference between yellow fever on the one hand and nineteenth- and early twentieth-century smallpox, plague, and cholera on the other was not only the absence of violence. The remarkable compilation of sources and commentary on the Memphis yellow fever epidemic of 1878 by M. L. Keating, editor-in-chief of Memphis's *Daily Appeal*,[79] discloses that yellow fever had entirely different social side effects from those produced by the other three infectious diseases. Keating begins by reflecting on Memphis during the twenty years preceding the epidemic: already, the city was in decline with crises and conflicts mounting. Black immigrants, who were no longer productive, poured into the city, 'adding to the ranks of the very poor as petty thieves or worthless paupers'; the city was 'plagued' by 'sectional animosity' and 'the bitterness of party politics'. The city's sanitary conditions 'were disgraceful in the extreme': privies lay stagnant; dead animals decayed in the streets; and conditions worsened 'because of the criminal neglect of the city officials'. Few funds were available for 'sanitary relief', because 'every interest was carefully guarded...save for the health and lives of the people'.[80] By mismanagement, 'the ignorance of the city legislators, and the indifference of the better classes of her people', Memphis was reduced to bankruptcy in January 1878.[81]

In the opening days of the epidemic with thirty-three new cases on 16 August, Keating continued his dismal sketch, focusing now on the populace rather than their rulers: 'the whole population was precipitated into a panic', eradicating 'all human sympathy, all the kindlier emotions of the human heart, all feeling of kinship, all regard for neighbourly claims. Men, women, and children poured out of the city...like dogs, neglected and shunned, as if cursed of God.'[82]

With yellow fever cases soaring to 3000 and after 'all had fled who could',[83] Keating recorded a remarkable shift in sentiment by the end of the month:

---

outside the city and at an emergency orphanage run by the Sisters of Saint Mary, but on both occasions violence was averted; see Baker, 'Yellow Jack', 259 and *New York Times*, 19 August 1878, 13–14.

[78] Carrigan, *The Saffron Scourge*, 28.
[79] Keating was also a member of the Citizens' Committee and possibly the Howard Association.
[80] Keating, *A History*, 101, 102, and 103.   [81] Ibid., 101.
[82] Ibid., 107–9.   [83] Ibid., 109.

Most of the white men who were not in bed...were engaged in the work of relief as physicians, nurses, as Howard visitors,[84] or as members of the other organizations which did such noble service.[85]

Numerous mini-biographies followed with descriptions of city and national organizations, all attesting to this sudden impulse of compassion that filled the bulk of his 400-page compilation of sources and commentary. The first of these tributes singled out a foreigner for praise: 'a volunteer from abroad...a trained thinker with some pretensions as a philosopher'. He 'walked the wards' of the charity hospital, 'anxious to save life', giving sufferers hope. 'He went deliberately to his death', as 'did the priests of the Roman Catholic Church'.[86]

A case of a local physician, who died treating his patients for yellow fever, followed,[87] and then cases of Catholic priests:[88] 'Every visit made by them was a step toward death—yet they went on' and 'nuns were quick to volunteer'.[89] His view did not prejudicially favour Catholics: 'all members of the Christian Church are alike in their aspirations'. He reported that Protestant pastors, with 'the same purpose as their Roman Catholic brethren' visited all in distress 'in mind, body, or estate'.[90] Mr Thomas, a German Reverend was the first to die attending the stricken of his flock. Similar examples of 'martyrdom' were recounted of Presbyterian, Methodist, Baptist, and Episcopalian ministers (even if he had to admit that the flight of a few pastors gave rise to acerbic comments in the press).[91]

He next turned to the charitable works of 'the Hebrews', lauding the work of their synagogues and, more so, their benevolent societies. He focused on members of the Hebrew Hospital Association who 'were especially notable for ardour...and unstinted charity'. Going from house to house, they asked who was in need and made no distinction based on race or creed.[92] In praising these 'martyrs', Keating set a young 'Hebrew', Louis Daltroof, apart for 'special mention'. Facing the mounds of unburied corpses, he organized an interfaith burial corps for Memphis's Howard Association and died serving. For Keating, his sacrifice, along with others of the Howard Association, recalled 'the early ages' and 'zeal' of Christian martyrs.[93]

Keating then focused on a long list of other non-denominational lay societies— Free Masons, Odd Fellows, Special Relief Committee, Memphis Typographical Union, Knights of Honor Central Relief Committee, Independent Order of

---

[84] The Howard Association was founded in New Orleans during the yellow fever epidemic of 1837. By the Civil War, it had become the richest benevolent society in the US, even though it focused on yellow fever relief alone. It attracted wealthy young men as volunteers. Various dates are listed for the society's formation between 1842 and 1853; Keating, *A History*, 133–5. Baker, 'Yellow Jack', 252–3; Carrigan, *The Saffron Scourge*, 45; and Ellis, 'Businessmen and Public Health', 202. Curiously, this American society was named after the prison reformer, traveller, and scholar who had no connections with yellow fever; see Baumgartner, 'John Howard'.

[85] Keating, *A History*, 109. [86] Ibid., 118.

[87] Keating praised few physicians. Baker, 'Yellow Jack', 253–4, maintains that many physicians without immunity persevered despite herculean caseloads, illustrating their sacrifice with the story of a Dr Armstrong.

[88] Keating, *A History*, 119. [89] Ibid., 120. [90] Ibid., 121.

[91] Ibid., 124. [92] Ibid., 126. [93] Ibid., 143–4.

Mutual Aid,[94] and others—'remarkable for an active benevolence, a sleepless vigilance', from whom he celebrated heroes and martyrs. These included civic leaders but also the unsung, 'even outcast women and men not so good in life or living', who propelled by the peril of yellow fever jeopardized their lives to engage in charity. By Keating's account, 'Heroism was the rule in all the walks of life, neglect and desertion the exception'.[95] Such judgement did not depend on his sentimentality. He collected and reprinted numerous stories and short notices of deaths from local newspapers of previously uncelebrated individuals, who lost their lives assisting the victims, such as the prostitute Annie Cook. 'After a long life of shame', she died of yellow fever, nursing her patients.[96] She converted her house of prostitution into 'a refuge for the afflicted, who she nursed herself'.[97]

Despite his racist inclinations, Keating also praised Memphis's black community, citing articles from his newspaper *The Appeal*: 'Let it be recorded to their credit that the negro militia and policemen have discharged their duties zealously and with discretion. We are proud of them, They proved their title to the gratitude of the people of Memphis'.[98] Another story recounted that:

> the [white] man in charge of the Memphis Elmwood Cemetery came to the spot where the grave was to be dug and informed the negroes that they would not receive any extra pay for the extra work they were doing after six [p.m.] ... The negroes, more humane than he, and indignant at such an exhibition of brutality before the husband and children [of the deceased] replied that sometimes they worked for friendship. They dug the grave, lowered the casket...[99]

The epidemic of 1878 also spawned concrete social, political, and economic changes for Memphis's black community, which neither Reconstruction nor a coalition of black and white politicians led by a progressive mayor in 1874 had achieved. Even with the return of a conservative city government in 1878, the epidemic finally led to Memphis's police department being racially integrated, with black officers praised for their service. They remained on the force for the next seventeen years.[100] With the diminution of yellow fever in 1878, Memphis's mayor, John Flippin, praised racial solidarity and predicted its longevity: 'common suffering should weld them [blacks and whites] together, even long after this unfortunate dispensation of Providence has passed'.[101]

Finally, as with New Orleans' experience in 1853, the Memphis epidemic eased, at least temporarily, the strained relations between North and South, now fuelled by Reconstruction as described in Keating's prelude to the epidemic.[102] At the height of the fever's mortality (14 September), he reported the outpouring of charity from northern cities to Memphis, 'money forwarded by hundreds, by thousands of

[94] His long appendices detail their charitable work—monies raised and those dying from the disease.
[95] Keating, *A History*, 126 and 129. [96] Ibid., 159.
[97] Baker, 'Yellow Jack', 258. [98] Keating, *A History*, 158.
[99] Ibid., 194; *Memphis Appeal*, 26 September 1878, front page. The following day the foreman was dismissed, ibid., 27 September 1878, front page.
[100] Rousey, 'Yellow Fever'. Memphis's police force became integrated when forces in other southern cities were being segregated.
[101] Ibid., 367. [102] Keating, *A History*, 102.

dollars' with New York City alone donating $43,800. It seemed as though 'the people of the North...could not do enough'.[103] Keating concretized his sentiments with individual vignettes. At the onset of the epidemic, Reverend Louis Schuyler, a priest from Hoboken, New Jersey, raced to Memphis to volunteer his services; by winter he paid for it with his life, and the *Memphis Appeal* gave thanks to him, celebrating his life in its pages.[104] Keating maintained Schuyler was not an isolated case. The North's volunteerism had 'erased all memories of sectional divisions or of the political animosities of the Civil War'. Neither Keating nor his paper were alone in praising yellow fever's side effects. One to miss Keating's scrutiny was Reverend W. T. D. Dalzell, who before serving in Memphis in 1878 had volunteered in Savannah during the epidemic of 1857 and then helped out in Shreveport's disastrous yellow fever outbreak in 1873.[105] Furthermore, the *New York Times* and even the *London Standard* corroborated Keating's conclusions, praising 'the courage and endurance of the people of the South during the epidemic'.[106] In response Memphis's papers printed lists of donations, often paltry sums, acknowledging the charity from the North as with a notice of late September entitled 'A thousand thanks to the generous people of New York'.[107]

Certainly, Keating's story of Memphis was not entirely rosy. He was not averse to reporting incidents of selfishness, opportunism, and inhumanity—tales of debauchery and sexual abuse[108]—'a noisy multitude of negroes each clamouring for his dole of the bounty',[109] 'a cheeky nurse'; 'an incorrigible rascal and thief';[110] and nurses (reminiscent of the greed of seventeenth-century *monatti*), who stole watches from the deceased under their care.[111] But the weight of Keating's story is clear: it was an uplifting one of individual and societal transformation, of heroism, compassion, sacrifice, and unity.

Keating was not the only figure to have published a record of yellow fever heroism in Memphis in 1878. The Catholic priest, Reverend Denis Alphonsus Quinn, drew a similar account, except that his was less catholic, celebrating exclusively the deeds of his religion.[112] Along with the myriad of newspaper articles from across the US, these stories, despite their florid presentation, contrast sharply with the hundreds of reports of individual and collective reactions to cholera and especially smallpox epidemics—often in the same newspapers. These rarely, if ever, mentioned martyrs, volunteers, or foundations of new charitable organizations to relieve suffering. With few exceptions (such as Italy during the cholera epidemics of 1867, 1884, and 1887), neither cholera nor smallpox signalled long lists of donations criss-crossing geographical divides to aid devastated regions. Instead, the stories that dominated these epidemics recounted class hatred, religious and racial prejudice, and with smallpox victimization of diseased victims. We now explore how well these stories represent yellow fever's socio-psychological reactions.

---

[103] Ibid., 115.   [104] Ibid., 181.   [105] Carrigan, *The Saffron Scourge*, 108.
[106] Keating, *A History*, 177.   [107] Ibid., 164.   [108] Ibid., 118.
[109] Ibid., 110.   [110] Ibid., 164.
[111] Ibid., 190. See similar complaints against nurses in Baker, 'Yellow Jack', 254–5.
[112] Quinn, *Heroes and Heroines*. Also, Baker, 'Yellow Jack', 257.

18

Yellow Fever

The Broader Picture

Unlike cholera riots—their mobs, violence, and conspiracies—or the abundant stories of neglect and inhumanity associated with smallpox—yellow fever presents a wall of near silence on these scores, even though the newspapers in 'Chronicling America' alone contain almost 100,000 pages with either 'yellow fever' or 'yellow jack'. For the *Lancet*, with its international network of correspondents throughout Europe, Asia, Africa, and the Americas, who produced detailed reports not only on disease but on the violent social consequences of cholera and plague, not a single article links 'riot' or 'mob' with yellow fever.[1] Similarly, in the Burney Collection of seventeenth- and eighteenth-century British newspapers with one million scanned pages and 2532 containing 'yellow fever', mobs or riots in connection with this disease fail to appear. J. R. McNeill has emphasized the importance of yellow fever in shaping and destroying New World empires from the mid-seventeenth to the early twentieth century. But despite his attention to yellow fever's quick and catastrophic political consequences—the American Revolution in the 1780s, slave and anti-Spanish revolts at Saint-Domingue in the late eighteenth and early nineteenth century, the liberation of Mexico from Spain in the mid-nineteenth century, the Cuban revolution of the mid-1890s—he shows no instances of this disease spurring hate or blame against foreigners, minorities, or elites.[2]

Linkages, however, can be found. For instance, *The Times* Digital Archive produces three associations of a riot or mob with an epidemic of yellow fever. Two of them have been mentioned—the Staten Island burnings of 1858[3] and the Post Master General's claim of 'shotgun' quarantines in 1888.[4] To repeat, neither can be depicted as a yellow fever riot. The third is the only incident of a yellow fever riot not found in a US paper and the only one I have found to have occurred outside the US. In April 1874, islanders on Portuguese Madeira threatened to revolt against the reopening of its lazaretto. In addition, *The Times* referred to a previous undated disturbance, when yellow fever infected the island, and 'the people, full of fear and fury' burnt down the lazaretto. Now, they decided to do it again. Their

---

[1] *Lancet*, ScienceDirect Backfiles, 1 January 1823 to 24 December 1994: 4389 articles on yellow fever, 1823 to 1910.

[2] McNeill, *Mosquito Empires*, ch. 7.

[3] *The Times*, 18 September 1858, 7; 20 September 1858, 7; 22 September 1858; 26 September 1858, 5.

[4] *Guardian*, 26 September 1888, 6.

action was not, however, motivated by fears of contagion. Instead, they believed yellow fever had been sent to punish their sins, and humans should not tamper with its control.[5] In contrast to hundreds of articles describing cholera riots in these same newspapers in Britain, North America, Europe, Africa, the Middle East, and Asia, no further hints of yellow fever riots appear, despite meticulously reporting of yellow fever epidemics across the globe, especially by the British, concerned by disruptions to trade and industry.

*   *   *

As historians have agreed,[6] recurrences of this epidemic in the Deep South continued to arouse panic with mass migration from cities such as New Orleans, Shreveport,[7] Memphis, and Mobile and crises in commerce and controversies over the efficacy of quarantine as seen in Chapter 17. In the first month alone of the Memphis epidemic in 1878, its city population collapsed from 47,000 to 17,000, with white flight, not yellow fever mortality, accounting for the lion's share of the loss.[8] Yet, despite recurrent yellow fever panics throughout the Deep South from the late eighteenth century to 1905,[9] only a handful of minor incidents arose and only one which might be considered a riot. Moreover, these did not begin until 1897, that is, on the eve of discovering yellow fever's mechanisms of transmission. A possible exception occurred, not in the South, where yellow fever epidemics had been confined since the early nineteenth century, but in Tarrytown, New York, in 1874, when yellow fever was not even present. Dr Lindly, an ex-Union soldier, left his home to care for yellow fever sufferers during the 1873 epidemic in Jacksonville, Florida. The following year, while treating yellow fever in Tennessee, he died. His body was shipped home for interment as a 'yellow fever martyr'. On learning of Lindly's death, a crowd gathered, chanting 'No yellow fever for Tarrytown'. By severing the ropes of the tug carrying Lindly's coffin, the crowd cut the eulogy by the Board of Health's chairman short, forcing the crew into river.[10]

From 1897 to yellow fever's final US pandemic eight years later, a new development in yellow fever fear and violence emerged, which historians have yet to register. In September, Governor McLaurin of Mississippi summoned troops 'to prevent further tearing up of railroad tracks by mobs provoked by yellow fever panic'.[11] No more details are given. A week later, a Hawaiian paper, presumably carrying the same story, posted a similar short notice, revealing that the incident took place near Jackson, but failed to comment on the mob's composition, the extent of damage, whether injuries were inflicted, or the mob's motives.[12] Two days later, another

---

[5] *The Times*, 6 April 1874, 7.

[6] Pierce and Writer, *Yellow Jack*, 2; Duffy, *Sword of Pestilence*, 124; Emias, 'Yellow Fever'; and Humphreys, *Yellow Fever and the South*, 9.

[7] For the epidemic of 1873, see Carrigan, *The Saffron Scourge*, 106, 152.

[8] Crosby, *The American Plague*, 47–8.

[9] In New Orleans, only nine years between 1840 and 1905 were without a yellow fever epidemic; Humphreys, *Yellow Fever and the South*, 3.

[10] *Memphis Daily Appeal*, 6 June 1874.

[11] *New-York Tribune*, 19 September 1897, 6: the incidents occurred are not specified.

[12] *Evening Bulletin*, 28 September 1897, front page.

short notice tells of a similar event at another southern town: a 'mob' armed with shotguns prevented a train carrying physicians from passing through Lafayette, Louisiana.[13] Two weeks later, a third small but more sinister incident erupted, this one reminiscent of North American smallpox riots: 'An unknown man', travelling from Memphis to Louisville, was 'put off' the train near St Louis and later found unconscious near a cemetery. He was dumped in a 'rude stable', where he 'raved' on about yellow fever. To stop the spread of 'the supposed yellow fever', armed men tried to burn down the stable. Its owner, however, chased off the mob.[14]

Finally, a fourth incident in 1897 showed greater potential for destruction and loss of life than the others that year or at any other time for yellow fever and again recalls smallpox unrest. On 23 September, as final preparations were being made to open Beauregard School in New Orleans to treat yellow fever patients, 'citizens' held a mass meeting and threatened 'to fire' the school. When the fire department arrived, the mob cut the hoses and damaged the building before a 'big squad of officers' beat them back.[15] The 'rabble' between 400–500 included 'some substantial citizenship'. However, unlike smallpox incidents, other prominent citizens, who had spoken out against the school's conversion to a hospital, condemned the arson as a disgrace to the city.[16] The following morning, papers across the country rallied in support of the mayor, claiming the riot had been 'roundly denounced on all sides'. Despite political divisions in New Orleans, 'every newspaper in the city' pledged support to the mayor, 'to punish the culprits' and restore the hospital.[17] The hospital's fate was not that of so many smallpox pesthouses. In three days, Beauregard had been restored and its first inmates treated without disturbance.[18] Three years later, an out-of-town newspaper returned to the incident, condemning the 'unreasoning fear' that led to the Beauregard School burning.[19] No smallpox incident received such widespread, cross-country condemnation of elite mobsters, despite many marshalling greater numbers, cruelty, and damage.[20]

Yellow fever's next provocations were its last, sparked during its final pandemic of 1905, after its mosquito vector was known and well publicized in local papers with sound advice on preventive measures.[21] Yet this pandemic (having already spread through the Caribbean and South America) produced more incidents and threats of violence than at any time. These focused on small towns and plantations in Louisiana's sugar belt, where southern Italian emigrants had recently replaced

[13] *Desert Evening News*, 30 September 1897, 3.
[14] *Evening Bulletin*, 14 October 1897. *Phillipsburg Herald*, 21 October 1897, 3, locates it in Mayfield, Kentucky. The man was later found to have had malarial fever.
[15] *Evening Star*, 24 September 1897, front page. Also, *Times Picayune*, 24 September 1897, 1, 4, 6.
[16] *Ibid.*, front page.
[17] *Desert Evening News*, 25 September 1897, 3; *San Francisco Call*, 25 September 1897, front page; *Wichita Daily Eagle*, 25 September 1897, front page; *Evening Herald*, 25 September 1897, front page.
[18] *Norfolk Virginian*, 25 September 1897, front page.
[19] *Evening Times*, 27 December 1900, 4; and Carrigan, *The Saffron Scourge*, 147–9.
[20] *Wichita Daily Eagle*, 25 September 1897, front page.
[21] As early as 1901, US Surgeon General Sternberg was delivering public speeches 'On the Transmission of Yellow Fever by the Mosquito' which circulated in newspapers; see for instance *Evening Times*, 17 April 1901, 2.

black labourers, who had emigrated to the North.[22] In the first event, which appeared small, violence was averted, but it bore similar traits to cholera and smallpox mania. In mid-August, with yellow fever rapidly spreading across plantations south and west of New Orleans, Dr Corpetat was assigned to the 'sugar belt'. On his first day, he was 'mobbed' by Italian workers who accused him of murdering a boy. To save his skin, he injected himself with a hypodermic needle, the treatment earlier given to the boy.[23] A Washington paper expressed prejudices similar to those of elites that often preceded cholera riots. 'Such fear of doctors', it claimed, arose 'through superstition and ignorance' and 'appears in every such panic, no matter what disease'.[24]

The same week, Italian sugar workers at plantations 20 miles west of New Orleans refused to go to the emergency hospital and threatened to shoot anyone who forced them. According to a local doctor, Good Hope's hundred Italians 'present a formidable set in rebellion'.[25] At nearby St Rosa, a family supported by neighbours successfully prevented health officers from fumigating their house and took oaths not to allow anyone to fumigate their premises.[26] The resistance continued for several days.[27] At Hanson City, near Kenner, the plantation of Pecan Grove[28] and another at Pointe à la Hache, in Plaquemines Parish, Italians ordered shells loaded with buckshot to oppose doctors. Local authorities considered calling the militia,[29] but as with the threats above, no violence or destruction ensued.

In the Delta, south of New Orleans, further strife against fumigators flared, and fear of doctors led Italians to hide the sick.[30] But at Patterson, the consequences were graver, receiving coverage even from the British. The *Guardian* reported a riot with hints of European cholera suspicion:

> A mob of Italians . . . attempted to burn the yellow fever hospital there, and had to be repulsed by the local militia. Feelings run very high among the Italians because so many of their relatives have died in the hospital.

It alleged that 'two or three hundred began the attack by hurling stones' and breaking hospital windows. Attendants held 'the mob' at bay by pouring pails of hot water on them from the windows, giving the attendants a chance to telephone the mayor. He summoned the militia, which arrived 'in considerable force with loaded rifles'. Moreover, ethnic prejudices—here southern hatred of Italian labourers—became pivotal. The paper claimed the 'townspeople' were 'furious against the Italians', and given an opportunity, would 'no doubt' lynch the ringleaders.[31] Before the alleged insurrection, tensions ran high between townspeople and the Italian workers, with 'whites' blaming them for the spread of yellow fever. Even on the eve of the Civil War or afterwards during the Reconstruction, neither the press

---

[22] On changes in the labour force in Louisiana's sugar fields, see *Times Picayune*, 1 September 1905, 25.
[23] *New-York Tribune*, 18 August 1905, 8.   [24] *Evening Star*, 26 August 1905, 4.
[25] *Times Picayune*, 25 August 1905, 2.   [26] Ibid., 27 August 1905, 4.
[27] Ibid., 29 August 1905, 2.   [28] Ibid., 1 September 1905, 47.
[29] Ibid., 25 August 1905, 2.   [30] Ibid., 1 September 1905, 8.
[31] *Guardian*, 4 September 1905, 7. For correctives, see *Times Picayune*, 3 September 1905, 3; 4 September 1905, 2; 5 September 1905, 2; and 12 September 1905, 4.

nor mobs had blamed the previous plantation workers—'Negroes'—or those most susceptible to the disease—newly arrived white immigrants. The 1905 pandemic brought with it a new racism and it was not restricted to the southern press. On the day of Patterson's supposed 'rebellion', an article appeared in a small-town Missouri paper, charging that Italians 'and other foreign races' were 'the bête noir of New Orleans'. They had carried the disease from the city and now were 'carrying it back and planting it in new localities'.[32] Anti-Italian sentiment provoked by yellow fever went further. Newspapers in San Francisco, Los Angeles, and Bisbee, Arizona, also blamed it on 'ignorant'[33] 'superstitious Italians'.[34] A Florida paper quipped: 'The Italians at Paterson, La., are threatening to make trouble for the yellow fever doctors. Let's see: someone was advocating the immigration of these people to this country not so long ago.'[35]

To return to Patterson's mob scene: should the *Guardian*'s story be believed? At least twenty-nine US papers in 'Chronicling America' described the threats. Yet, despite alarmist, sensational headlines,[36] none related that a mob of 200–300 assembled before the hospital, hurling stones and breaking windows, or that hospital staff poured pails of hot water on them. The town's mayor does not even appear in their narratives. The man calling the shots, instead, was Dr C. L. Horton, the head physician on Patterson's Board of Health. He telegraphed Governor Blanchard, reporting that yellow fever doctors 'had been secretly warned to be on their guard', and that he 'feared' an attempt might be made to burn the emergency hospital. Rioting by Italians may have been feared, but no riots or calls for the militia occurred. Instead, Horton requested volunteers to guard the hospital with a sheriff in charge.[37] By 3 September, no trouble had occurred, and local papers reported none was now expected. The following day, despite prejudices against 'ignorant' Italians and claims that they believed doctors were 'killing off members of their race',[38] newspapers across the country reported tensions easing[39] and praised 'the excellent work' within the Italian community that had kept the peace. The Jesuit priest, Reverend Father Widman was singled out. He had 'quietened' the community: 'all danger of trouble has passed'.[40] As we shall see, this peaceful

---

[32] *Flair Play*, 2 September 1905, front page. Moreover, ideas of human carriers of yellow fever in some quarters appear to have become more pronounced after the discovery of the mosquito vector. Patterson's officers called out guards to protect the town from 'the Italian laborers on the Bellesein plantation, who continue to bring infection'. Merchants in Bayou Sara and St Francisville 'signed an agreement not to buy goods of any kind from New Orleans'; Sun, 1 September 1905, 7.

[33] *San Francisco Call*, 4 September 1905, 3; and *Los Angeles Herald*, 4 September 1905, 2.

[34] *Bisbee Daily Review*, 3 September 1905, front page.

[35] *St. Lucie County Tribune*, 15 September 4, from *Gainsville Sun*.

[36] To take one example—'Fear Attack On Hospital'; *San Francisco Call*, 3 September 1905, 28.

[37] Ibid.

[38] *Washington Times*, 3 September 1905, front page; *Salt Lake Herald*, 3 September 1905, front page; *New-York Tribune*, 3 September 1905, front page; *Washington Times*, 3 September 1905, front page.

[39] *Los Angeles Herald*, 4 September 1905, 2; *Salt Lake Herald*, 4 September 1905, front page; *Salt Lake Tribune*, 4 September 1; *Arizona Republican*, 4 September 1905, front page.

[40] *Evening Star*, 4 September 1905, front page; *Palestine Daily Herald*, 5 September 1905, 3; and *Edgefield Advertiser*, 6 September 1905, 4. Carrigan, *The Saffron Scourge*, 190, treats events at Patterson briefly and none of the others in the bayous, 190–5.

resolution differed strikingly from cholera conflicts which were still rising in parts of Europe.

Further disturbances on sugar plantations at Pointe Celeste, 30 miles from New Orleans occurred at the beginning of September. This time, the Italians were not the dirt-poor but managed small plantations employing black labourers. Their actions were not, however, organized collective ones but limited to threats by individual families,[41] who refused treatment by physicians and barricaded their homes from fumigation. Yet, as in Patterson, the threats did not to go beyond words.[42] The health board counter-threatened to abandon their operations, forcing 'the fever to run its course among the refractory foreigners'.[43] They then went further, threatening to quarantine Pointe Celeste, 'starving the Italian into submission'. Several days later, the authorities backed their threats with criminal indictments.[44] By the end of the month, former Congressman Wilkinson, who owned the plantation, intervened; the Italians yielded and accepted medical treatment.[45]

* * *

Increased threats and resistance to doctors and health officers in the bayous during this last yellow fever epidemic might suggest parallels with cholera riots. Despite the discoveries of 1901, newspapers continued to blame Italians for spreading the disease by concealing their dead and refusing to report cases as though it were a disease transmitted person to person. An editorial in the *Times Picayune* admitted that Italians had not brought yellow fever to the plantations but charged they were 'largely responsible' for 'scattering' it, because of their 'secretive' and 'suspicious disposition'.[46] Physicians also made their prejudices clear. During the Patterson threats, the President of Louisiana's State Board of Health, Dr Edmond Souchon, explained: 'We are threatened with riot from Dagoes...we have been armed to expect trouble. I am guarding the hospital'. He then praised 'Citizens' for organizing for their own protection and endorsed their call for the governor to send arms (which, in fact, he did).[47] Yet despite elite prejudices, distrust by Italians, citizens armed by the governor, and papers predicting the worse, the threats never escalated to collective violence as they had with smallpox and cholera.

Aspects of these conflicts in 1905 suggest that even if yellow fever's puzzles of transmission had not been untangled in 1901, this disease would not have produced the hatred and collective violence still brewing with smallpox and to some extent now stirring with poliomyelitis. First, the disturbances of 1905 were

---

[41] *Washington Times*, 25 September 1905, 4; *Minneapolis Journal*, 25 September 1905, 3; *Edgefield Advertiser*, 27 September 1905, front page; and *Evening Statesman*, 2 October 1905, 6.

[42] *Times Picayune*, 24 September 105, 4. The local doctor of Plaquemines Parish claimed the Italians barricaded themselves in their houses, threatening to kill any doctor who entered.

[43] *Minneapolis Journal*, 25 September 1905, 3.

[44] *Edgefield Advertiser*, 27 September 1905, front page.

[45] *Palestine Daily Herald*, 30 September 1905, 5; *Gainsville Daily Sun*, 2 October 1905, front page. Yellow fever violence concerning burial and Italian fears of contagion also threatened at Leesville, north-west of Baton Rouge. But because of the local physician's actions and explanations, once again it subsided; *New-York Tribune*, 28 September 1905, 8.

[46] Ibid., 1 September 1905, 25.   [47] *Times Picayune*, 3 September 1905, 3.

confined to recent Italian immigrants on Louisiana's sugar plantations. Although newspaper accounts rarely mentioned their regional origins, the Italian fear of physicians and suspicion of health officers bear an uncanny resemblance to attitudes seen in cholera riots of southern Italy and several northern cities in the 1860s and 1890s. At least one contemporary in New Orleans, the social worker and progressive activist, Eleanor McMain, connected the immigrants' suspicions with 'legends' of state-backed poisoning from their homeland in Sicily.[48]

Yet, despite these underlying fears, even the most violent of Louisiana's yellow fever conflicts differed markedly from cholera's. In addition to being small, short-lived, and mostly without violence, the course of yellow fever resistance took a different path. After initial family fears and protests against fumigation and doctors, attitudes in bayou communities changed swiftly because of friendly intervention from health workers, priests, and Italian-speaking neighbours. Corinne, a plantation south of New Orleans, provides an example. Italians at first opposed fumigation 'and similar measures', but because of a campaign of 'education' and 'good neighbourly relations', their views changed from resistance to 'voluntarily' visiting doctors and asking that their houses be fumigated.[49] Dr Charles Lopez, who treated Italians afflicted with yellow fever in New Orleans and initially ridiculed their 'queer' habits, now reported (while congratulating himself) that these same Italians soon became convinced that hiding afflicted relatives would not save lives, and they began to trust their doctors.[50] At the plantation at Good Hope, a Dr Montz expected the worst from the Italians, especially when he asked them to go to the emergency hospital. Within two weeks, however, they saw matters differently; now they were 'inspired with much confidence in the Doctor'.[51]

The most reported example of this transformation came from Patterson after the governor had armed citizens to patrol the hospital[52] but violence was averted. Papers such as the *Times Picayune* attributed the change not to outside forces but to activities within the Italian community: the Jesuit Father Widman, the priest Placide, the Bendectine abbot Paul Schaeuble, several longer-term residents fluent in Italian, and the recent immigrants themselves strove to educate one another.[53] Early on, the community called in the Italian Consular Agent, Mr Rampo, to hold a meeting of Italians to allay their fears. A heavy downpour, however, cancelled his lectures.[54] The change in attitudes instead depended on door-to-door canvassing of Italian families by their own priests and Italian neighbours, several of whom publicly volunteered to stay in the emergency hospital.[55]

Patterson was not alone in turning potential violence to trust. Little appears in the papers about troubles from New Orleans' Italian community but hints of distrust of doctors and threats of violence had been evident.[56] In an editorial,

[48] Carrigan, *The Saffron Scourge*, 189.   [49] *Times Picayune*, 11 September 1905, 3.
[50] Ibid., 1 September 1905, 47.   [51] Ibid., 18 September 1905, 4.
[52] Ibid., 4 September 1905, 2.
[53] *Times Picayune*, 3 September 1905, 3; 5 September 1905, 2; 12 September 1905, 4.
[54] Ibid., 4 September 1905, 2.   [55] Ibid., 11 September 1905, 3.
[56] For instance, *Evening Star*, 26 August 1905, 4.

Gabriel Dilda, head of the Italian Relief Committee, praised the work of the city's Italians and especially of one resident, Mr Patorno, who 'personally and pecunarily [sic]...day and night' devoted himself to working within his Italian neighbourhood. He went 'house to house in the most afflicted localities' offering 'cheering messages and substantial relief to the poor and suffering', preparing the dead for burial, acting 'as a pallbearer at many a poor funeral'. Dilda, however, stressed another component of Patorno's assistance: he 'conducted a campaign of education'. He demonstrated to his compatriots that the medicines distributed by the emergency hospital were not poisons but were 'for their own good'.[57]

At New Orleans, Patorno was only one of 'a large army of volunteers' during the 'Anti-Mosquito Crusade' of 1905, which united a broad coalition of scientists, university lecturers, clergymen, and lay volunteers. From his pulpit, Reverend Dr Beverley Warner 'preached' instructions about drainage, screening cisterns, and cleaning gutters. He joined forces with several local physicians, who in one week alone visited fifty-one schools and talked to 43,000 children, distributing instructions for their parents. Reverend Paroli gave lectures on the new yellow fever science and distributed pamphlets to Italian neighbours, allaying their fears for afflicted relatives removed to emergency hospitals. By mid-August, New Orleans' Italian community had become 'cooperative' and 'amenable to reason' before social violence had threatened the plantations.[58] The city's Italians had joined the anti-mosquito campaign.[59] In addition, white middle-class women volunteered with health officials, distributing leaflets door-to-door and advising on fumigation and screening. Others canvassed black neighbourhoods and delivered lectures to black and mixed-race audiences. The health board took on new workers, organized 'gangs' of five to search cases, fumigate, and supply screening across the city. As Jo Ann Carrigan concluded, 'The medical profession was never so unified.'[60]

Neither with cholera nor smallpox do similar stories of peace missions from within the afflicted communities arise, converting potential violence and hatred to cooperation and charity.[61] Instead, the principal counterbalance to cholera or smallpox conspiracies was generally state repression for the former and turning a blind eye to the latter. While Catholic priests in cities such as Liverpool during the cholera pandemic of 1832 may have provided services and solace to communities of the poor, no programmes appeared that sought to allay protesters' fears and prejudices; no Mr Patorno or fellow residents canvassed homes or entered emergency hospitals, convincing neighbours to trust physicians and fumigators. Instead, with cholera epidemics in southern Italy and Eastern Europe, the clergy were often the ones firing their flocks with myths and hatred, leading them in the assaults against doctors and state officials.

---

[57] *Times Picayune*, 14 September 1905, 7.   [58] Carrigan, *The Saffron Scourge*, 189 and 342.
[59] Ibid., 174.   [60] Ibid., 174, and for above, 171–5.
[61] The only evidence of regret that I have spotted by those who had attacked members of the medical profession during a cholera riot comes from Shapter, *Exeter*, 258.

YELLOW FEVER ABNEGATION

Not only did yellow fever spur few incidents of blame and violence, it also exhibited another side, again missing almost entirely from cholera and smallpox. As seen from Duffy's study of New Orleans in 1853 and the sources assembled by Keating for Memphis in 1878, yellow fever crises eased pre-existing racial and class tensions. Donations from the North supported afflicted southern cities; northerners such as the Hoboken priest Schuyler travelled south and sacrificed their lives with southern papers celebrating them as 'martyrs to the fever'.[62] As the editor of New Orleans' *Times Picayune* proclaimed at the end of the 1878 pandemic, the North's charity had 'overswept all geographical and party lines, we declare that the war is over, now at last and forever'.[63]

Praise of volunteers and elevation of ordinary people to martyrdom were not particular to Memphis in 1878. As we have seen, a doctor from Tarrytown travelling south to Jacksonville died volunteering in the previous epidemic of 1873. During the 1878 epidemic, Lieutenant H. H. Brenner became a volunteer on a St Louis relief boat caring for yellow fever sufferers in that city and was celebrated as 'a martyr to his heroism'.[64] Papers praised Reverend James W. Marley, aged twenty-eight, born in Philadelphia, who served yellow fever sufferers in Whistler, Alabama, north of Mobile, and died on 18 October 1878, as a 'Martyr to the scourge devastating our Southern land'.[65] Richmond Virginia's *Daily Dispatch* sainted William Willis, who died serving the afflicted in Memphis in 1878. His remains were returned to his home in Fredericksburg, Virginia, in 1881, where his Masonic lodge paid him further honours near the cenotaph that employees of the Southern Express Company had erected for his grave.[66] Papers from 1898 to 1905 declared Colonel G. E. Waring, who died of yellow fever in 1898 'a Martyr to Duty'. With the outbreak of yellow fever in 1878 he went to Memphis and changed the city's sewage system, which papers alleged 'succeeded in checking the spread of the disease'. Later, his system of engineering was 'adopted in many cities in all parts of the world'. He died of yellow fever in October 1898 while 'making provisions for sanitary improvements in the principal Cuban cities'.[67]

After the discovery of the disease's transmission, people continued to be elevated to 'martyrdom' in the disease's last US pandemic, such as New Orleans' archbishop, who died of yellow fever in August 1905.[68] Others gained martyrdom in places further afield: the Italian Sisters of the Missionary of the Sacred Heart first volunteered to work with New Orleans' Italian population, then travelled to Veracruz,

---

[62] Duffy, *Sword of Pestilence*, 127. Carrigan, *The Saffron Scourge*, relates similar stories for New Orleans and other Louisiana towns, 1853 to 1905.

[63] For both citations, Carrigan, *The Saffron Scourge*, 357.

[64] *Waco Daily Examiner*, 23 October 1878.

[65] *Morning Star and Catholic Messenger*, 3 November 1878, 4; and *National Republican*, 7 February 1881, 2.

[66] *Daily Dispatch*, 4 February 1881, 3.

[67] *Aberdeen Herald*, 1 December 1898, 6; *Donaldsonville Chief*, 8 July 1905.

[68] *Intermountain Catholic*, 19 August 1905, 6.

Mexico, 'into the lair of the dread pest'. Seven died as 'martyrs'.[69] During the epidemic of 1878, sisters from their mother house near Bardstown, Kentucky, went to stricken Holly Springs and Yazoo, Mississippi, where more than eleven died. In the same epidemic, sisters of the Dominican house of St Catherine of Siena travelled to Memphis, then Pensacola, to battle the disease, dying as a result. A Catholic paper extolled their sacrifice: 'There were martyrs in the arena of Rome long ago, and there are martyrs today'.[70]

The clergy were not the only ones so elevated. During the 1905 pandemic, a doctor from Dakota moved to a plantation on Bayou Barataria and received more publicity for his martyrdom than any of the above. He volunteered to treat the yellow fever afflicted, 'day and night', and placed his steamboat launch at the disposal of the authorities.[71] He soon caught the fever, but with early signs of recovery, resumed his medical care and died. Papers celebrated him with headlines, 'Martyr in Fever Fight'.[72] During the same pandemic, a local paper pronounced Mrs Eugene Arbona as Pensacola's 'guardian angel' because of the many she had nursed with the 'dreaded disease' without compensation.[73] Finally, towards the end of this pandemic, a small-town Oklahoma paper proudly announced that 'Yellow Fever martyrs were on the increase' and praised them 'as truly heroic as any of the soldiers who died in the defense of their country'.[74]

With discoveries achieved from experiments on human subjects, papers praised a new species of martyrdom, those who donated their lives to science.[75] As early as February 1901, Washington's *Evening Times* celebrated Chicago's native son John Moran, a steward in the US Hospital Corps, who 'offered himself to the men of science': he died in a human experiment near Quemados, Cuba.[76] Later that year, papers from New York to Omaha, Nebraska, to Brownsville, Texas, celebrated others who gained martyrdom in Cuba by becoming human guinea pigs: men and women who allowed themselves to be bitten by infected mosquitoes, like the nurse Clara Maass.[77] Later in the twentieth century, she achieved further acclaim when Belleville Hospital (New Jersey), where she had trained, was renamed after her and in 1952 when a postage stamp bore her portrait.[78] One of these experiments involved eight subjects, three of whom died, and in another

---

[69] Ibid., 26 August 1905, 5.

[70] Ibid. According to Carrigan, *The Saffron Scourge*, 109, public recognition of yellow fever martyred priests at New Orleans originated with the epidemic of 1853.

[71] *Minneapolis Journal*, 10 October 1905, 3.

[72] *Salt Lake Tribune*, 10 October 1905, front page. Further 'yellow fever martyrs' can be culled from newspapers, such as Dr C. M. Shanley; *Omaha Daily Bee*, 10 October 1905, 9.

[73] *Pensacola Journal*, 31 October 1905, 4.

[74] *Daily Ardmoreite*, 15 October 1905, 4. See the praise fifteen years earlier of 'Yellow Fever martyrs'; *Evening Star*, 15 August 1890, 3.

[75] Numerous works recount the discovery of yellow fever's transmission; for instance, de Kruif, *Microbe Hunters*, ch. 9; Bloom, *The Mississippi Valley's Great Yellow Fever Epidemic*, 20–2 and ch. 6. Reliable scientific accounts also appeared in newspapers from 1901 to 1915. Yet, even after 1905, many continued to believe the disease was transmitted person to person and by bedding and clothing. For yellow fever's medical controversies, see Carrigan, *The Saffron Scourge*, 206–91.

[76] *Evening Times*, 4 February 1901.

[77] *Brownsville Daily Herald*, 22 August 1901, front page; *New-York Tribune*, 26 August 1901, 4, 8.

[78] Bollet, *Plagues*, 61.

of seven, three more perished including the yellow fever surgeons Jesse W. Lazear and Dr Carrol, sainted as 'martyrs to science' in numerous newspapers.[79]

In praise of yellow fever martyrs, the public went beyond words, commissioning memorials, portraits, and statues. Such an avalanche of recognition is invisible with other epidemics before HIV/AIDS.[80] In addition to the above-mentioned cenotaph erected in Fredericksburg in 1881, yellow fever memorials, publicized in overwrought prose, were raised in Memphis, not during its most disastrous epidemic of 1878–9, but rather in its lesser previous one in 1873. The Howard Association and a citizens' committee solicited donations to finance the first monument to yellow fever martyr Mattie Stephenson, who died in that year's epidemic. With gushing articles on the funding, the artistic creation, and its merit, little was said about 'the brave young girl martyr', even where she came from or what she did in 1873,[81] only that she 'went her way rejoicing in doing good'.[82]

A second 'handsome monument' was erected in Memphis's Calvary Cemetery, dedicated 'to the memory of the noble priests who died at their posts of duty during the frightful epidemic of 1873'. This one too gives barely any description of the martyrs, not even their denominations or how many were honoured.[83] In 1874 Memphis papers requested subscriptions for a third monument, this one to commemorate 'the fathers of the Catholic Church', who died of yellow fever in the autumn. Memphis's Catholic paper claimed that Protestants along with Catholics pledged money to it, and it was constructed by Memphis artists, who had gone to 'the quarries of Carrara, where Michelangelo had selected his marble'.[84] Five months on, a fourth commission celebrated further 'yellow-fever fallen', five fathers and seven unnamed sisters of St Dominic and St Francis.[85]

Sculpture was not the only medium to perpetuate these memories. The *Memphis Daily Appeal* congratulated the *New York Daily Graphic* on its engraved portraits of Miss Lulu Wilkerson and Mr A. E. Frakland of Memphis, who had volunteered and died in the epidemic of 1873.[86] Finally, during an epidemic in 1883, a portrait was commissioned of a former superintendent of a Sunday School in Austin, Texas, 'a martyr to the yellow fever at Holly Springs [Texas]'.[87] By contrast, of the thousands of news reports on cholera, smallpox, influenza, typhus, and many other epidemics, only one example has emerged from my survey of any memorial sculpted, drawn, or painted to honour a physician, cleric, or volunteer, who died combating any of the other epidemics. In the 1892 typhus epidemic, New York City commemorated 'the heroism' of Dr Mott, a house surgeon at the North Brother's Island quarantine hospital, with a bronze wall statue on the Nurses' Pavilion.[88]

*   *   *

---

[79] Numerous papers extolled these sacrifices, for instance, *Omaha Daily Bee*, 4 September 1901, 6, and pressured Congress to grant their widows pensions; *Washington Times*, 30 January 1902, front page.

[80] For cholera, I found only one attempt at funding a physical memorial; see Chapter 11, note 91.

[81] *Memphis Daily Appeal*, 6 June 1874, 4.

[82] Ibid.; *Public Ledger*, 20 October 1873, front page; and 12 March 1874, 2.

[83] Ibid.   [84] *Morning Star*, 24 May 1874, 8.

[85] *Public Ledger*, 9 November 1874, 2; *Memphis Daily Appeal*, 19 December 1875, 6.

[86] Ibid., 11 November 1873, 4.   [87] *Austin Weekly Statesman*, 6 December 1883.

[88] *Evening World*, 12 February 1892, 3.

Individuals were not the only ones extolled for heroic altruism during yellow fever's last epidemics. New and old organizations devoted their efforts and resources to battling the southern plague. As with the cases of individual martyrdom, echoes of late medieval and early modern spiritualism resonate. A single issue of the *Memphis Daily Appeal* on 10 October during the epidemic of 1873 gives a sense of the range, purpose, and zeal of these organizations. Unlike most late medieval religious confraternities, these secular organizations had networks that extended beyond cities and in the case of the Howard Association were international. The Memphis paper illustrated its own national networks, attracting donations across America, calling on fellow German immigrants and expressing the city's gratitude by publishing notices of the donations, such as gifts from Proctor & Gamble and a Memphis sewing machine company, which furnished a horse and wagon to transport provisions to homes of the afflicted. After itemizing the donations of corporations, churches, and individuals, the paper published abridged reports from relief committees: the Howard Association for organizing, recruiting, and paying for nursing and supplying whiskey and sherry-wine to patients; the relief and visiting committees of the Odd Fellows for volunteering and hiring of nurses; the Fireman's Relief Association for caring for its sick members and other families; a new Memphis organization, the Shoulder-To-Shoulder Club—an offshoot of the Scottish St Andrew's Society—which opened an office 'ready to assist sufferers'; the Masonic Relief Board; the German Relief Association; and the Mutual Benevolent Association.[89]

During the next yellow fever epidemic in 1878, probably the worst epidemic in US history before the Great Influenza, the Howard Association made use of its interregional networks and took to the rails to break the rigid, but legal, 'shotgun' quarantines that were reducing towns across Mississippi to starvation. It sponsored a Howard special relief train between Meridian and Vicksburg, carrying supplies, two physicians, and fifteen nurses, and established 'a public kitchen' to feed, nurse, and clothe the afflicted and abandoned, starving even in the capital, Jackson, because of the 'merciless' quarantine.[90]

With the US's fever finale of 1905, national and interregional relief organizations became well entrenched in other southern cities. In Pensacola, United Charities furnished 'the needy with necessary groceries, fuel, etc.' and paid the rent of afflicted families.[91] Non-charitable organizations joined relief efforts, including the New Orleans police, who delivered the sick to hospitals and orphans to shelters, despite their force being comprised of Irish and German immigrants, highly susceptible to the disease.[92] New Orleans' *Times Picayune* and local businesses offered their services. Even 'youngsters of the Columbo Bitters Baseball Club' were recognized for their 'noble actions' in relief of the poor struck down by the fever.[93] Similar civic action fanned across the South.[94]

---

[89] *Memphis Daily Appeal*, 10 October 1873.   [90] *Waco Daily Examiner*, 23 October 1878.
[91] *Pensacola Journal*, 26 October 1905, front page.   [92] Carrigan, *The Saffron Scourge*, 353.
[93] *Times Picayune*, 15 September 1905, 3.
[94] For volunteers from the Odd Fellows, Masons, YMCA, the Howard Association, the Charity Organization Society; the League of Italian Societies, Peabody Subsistence Association, Italian Sisters of the Sacred Heart, Wholesale Grocery Merchants Association, and Ladies of the Era Club in towns

Today such reports of organized charities and action may not strike us as surprising. Yet for late nineteenth-century America, the response to yellow fever was unique. The papers reflect no trace of such organizational zeal with other infectious diseases—smallpox, cholera, and typhus—then crossing America. As we shall see, influenza during the most crippling pandemic in world history would stimulate an even greater heroic response, but relief from businesses, clubs and special committees was muted by comparison with the last yellow fever epidemics from 1873 to 1905. The Great Influenza founded no special ongoing charitable societies to relieve the poor's suffering, nothing comparable to the Howard Association or the Yellow Fever Italian Relief Committee; nor did it momentarily convert previously established clubs, such as the Odd Fellows, Masons, St Andrew's Society, or a Little League Baseball Team, into organizations devoted to care of sufferers and their families for the duration and after-effects of epidemics.

Montreal's smallpox epidemic in 1885 provides a bleak contrast between the reactions to these late nineteenth-century killers:

> Nobody came to town to help fight the pestilence. No parsons from outside, no social workers, no politicians representing the province of Quebec or the government of Canada. It was a local problem, the responsibility of the local authorities.[95]

With yellow fever, individuals, charitable organizations, and local clubs were not alone. Much is heard of communities uncharitably guarding their borders in times of epidemic. In 1905, the state of Missouri, in defiance of recent scientific findings, quarantined 'all infected points' leading into the state. Historians, however, have yet to comment on two southern cities' responses to Missouri: Knoxville, Tennessee, and Mena, Arkansas, invited those afflicted or threatened by yellow fever to come and reside in their cities.[96] Nor was this the first time a municipality had acted with such altruism when faced with yellow fever. During the nation's worst yellow fever pandemic, 1878, when most still believed humans carried it, Atlanta welcomed between 1500 and 2000 refugees fleeing New Orleans, Memphis, and other cities stricken with yellow fever. Moreover, the city acted as a hub, dispensing supplies and volunteers across the south-east,[97] and afterwards continued extending her arms to yellow fever refugees from Jacksonville, Florida, in 1888; Brunswick, Georgia, in 1893; and Memphis and New Orleans in 1897, despite having been quarantined by other south-eastern cities.[98] In 1905, Atlanta defied Georgia law that barred escapees from Louisiana from entering the state, and the people of Atlanta welcomed an estimated 5000 yellow fever refugees into their homes.[99]

Given the 'stampedes' of mass exodus with 200,000 refugees pouring across the Ohio River from southern states during the summer of 1878, yellow fever produced mass panic on a scale unseen with any other disease in American history.[100] Yet panic

in Mississippi and Louisiana, see Bloom, *The Mississippi Valley's Great Yellow Fever Epidemic*, 127; and Carrigan, *The Saffron Scourge*, 173, 187, 191, 342, 344.

[95] Bliss, *Plague*, 205.   [96] *Times Picayune*, 4 August 1905, 2.
[97] Ellis, 'Businessmen and Public Health', part 2, 346–71, 347.
[98] Ibid., 369.   [99] Price, 'A Legislative History', 33.
[100] Bloom, *The Mississippi Valley's Great Yellow Fever Epidemic*, 185.

did not translate into mass violence, as scholars presume was normal with epidemics. Moreover, the few threats of violence sparked by yellow fever came not when the disease was new and mysterious but after years of familiarity and especially during its 1905 finale, after the enigmas of transmission had been resolved. Despite the worst waves of yellow fever erupting during periods of heightened tension between North and South, with racial strife on the rise, and producing refugee crises of victims believed to be spreading the disease, yellow fever ignited movements not of hatred but of charity and abnegation.

19

The Great Influenza
A Forgotten Pandemic?

On the socio-psychological consequences of influenza, historians have concentrated almost exclusively on the Great One, 1918 to 1920,[1] that worldwide killed as many as 50 million, possibly even 100 million[2]; yet has been called the 'forgotten pandemic'. Alfred Crosby invented the title for the US experience, but scholars have applied it to other places.[3] As recognized by the resounding success of Crosby's work and the flurry of publications on the pandemic that followed, the tag no longer applies. Since 1976, studies of the Great Influenza have outstripped in number any other pandemic in world history, except perhaps the Black Death and AIDS of our own time. Epidemics with more violent social ramifications such as cholera now receive less historical attention.

But was the Great Influenza as forgotten as Crosby claimed in 1976? Two years before, a fundamental work on the social history of the Great Influenza—Richard Collier's *The Plague of the Spanish Lady*—put this pandemic in a global context.[4] His principal source was a remarkable set of letters from influenza survivors he solicited via newspaper adverts in 1972. The responses came from many places across the globe. Given the ages of survivors, this was a timely work. Conceived before knowledge of AIDS or current threats from new and re-emerging diseases, Collier's work also provides a vantage point. The survivors' reminiscences portray a largely upbeat picture but not because of any hubris about the medical profession's power to conquer infectious diseases. On that score, the survivors' reflections were the opposite. Nonetheless, they recalled little of the socio-psychological horrors that since the 1980s have taken centre stage as the normal reactions to large-scale pandemics, especially mysterious ones such as HIV/AIDS.

As mentioned in Chapter 17, Margaret Humphreys is one of the few to have constructed a model predicting which diseases are more likely to trigger panic and violence. From her model, the Great Pandemic of 1918–20 should have produced

---

[1] Much less attention has been devoted to the 1889–94 pandemic: Smith, 'The Russian Influenza', concentrates on its spread and medical approaches in Britain. Also see Humphries, 'A Pandemic Prelude'; Honigsbaum, 'The Great Dread'; idem, *A History of the Great Influenza Pandemics*, chs 1–4; and Rice, *Black November*, ch. 1. None investigates self-sacrifice or volunteerism.

[2] Johnson and Mueller, 'Updating the Accounts'.

[3] See for instance Rice, *Black November*, 8–9: 'I could not recall hearing about it in school, and though I had taken a course in New Zealand history as a part of my degree...'

[4] Crosby either did not know it or chose to ignore it.

horrific social and psychological consequences. It satisfied more or less all her criteria: (1) adults rather than children comprised the majority of victims; (2) the disease killed quickly, usually within a week of the first signs and symptoms and in cases within twenty-four hours; (3) throughout the pandemic this influenza was mysterious; (4) preventive measures and remedies were questioned throughout the pandemic; (5) in contrast to the usual forms of influenza, the Great One produced unusual signs and symptoms, evoking horror and disgust.[5] Below, we examine these characteristics.

First, it was unlike most previous epidemics of influenza, where populations had been exposed to different strains of the virus for several centuries and influenza casualties clustered among the young, old, and weak. The pandemic of 1918–20 instead killed in greater proportions those in the prime of life, young adults, and the middle aged.[6] Second, the latency period for influenza is short, usually a day or two. Because of its unusual virulence in 1918–20, often triggering bronchial-pneumonic complications, its quick spread meant that a much greater proportion of sufferers died. Third, the pandemic did not follow influenza's usual seasonality; instead, it mounted in the summer in Europe and Australia, and in most places peaked in October and declined in winter. Fourth, from its beginning this pandemic was mysterious, prompting physicians to question whether it was influenza. The signs and symptoms of the early cases detected in the US army camp of Fort Devens, near Boston, in September 1918 created great consternation among the medical corps. Army doctors had never witnessed influenza with such an abrupt onset and a 'propensity for pneumonic complications'.[7] In some cases, bodies of healthy adults were transformed as quickly as with cholera. As a Midwestern doctor described: 'In one or two hours…"bloody exudate" filled the lungs and [the patient] literally drowned from fluid in their lungs…a few hours later death comes…it is simply a struggle for air until they suffocate. It is horrible.'[8] Some thought it a new strain of meningitis; some, including William Henry Welch, then 'the most distinguished pathologist', physician, and scientist in America, believed it was a new disease altogether, 'a new plague'.[9]

Similarly, US journalists claimed it was caused by a 'new hitherto unrecognized bacillus', not the old 'grip', and criticized those in the medical profession who called it 'influenza'. To back their claims, they cited opinions of Canadian army doctors, who were said to have proven that the bacillus was new: the supposed agent of influenza 'bacillus influenza' or 'Pfeiffer bacterium' was absent in all cases and its clinical course was much shorter.[10] New York City's *Sun* claimed 'most medical writers' shared this view and 'deprecated' the use of the term 'influenza'.[11] In September,

---

[5] Humphreys, 'No Safe Place', 848–9.

[6] Later, Burnet and Clark, *Influenza*, unravelled the mystery as an autoimmune reaction: the weaker immune systems of the young and old triggered insufficient inflammation to flood their lungs with fluid to suffocate them.

[7] Crosby, *America's Forgotten Pandemic*, 5–10.   [8] Bristow, *American Pandemic*, 45.

[9] Crosby, *America's Forgotten Pandemic*, 9.

[10] *Washington Times*, 6 October 1918, 22; *Sun*, 27 August 1918, 6.

[11] *Ibid.*

even before October's spectacular spike in mortalities, Philadelphia's *Evening Public Ledger* exclaimed that the pandemic had 'mystified European scientists'. On the battlefields of France, physicians had diagnosed it as the 'Black Plague'.[12] A week later, with mass death rising in Boston and the disease striking as far west as Colorado, allusions to the Middle Ages became more terrifying. The *Washington Herald* called it '"the mysterious malady", a medieval plague' that 'threatens to overwhelm the whole country'.[13] By November, it was inflicting such unparalleled death worldwide, that more physicians were drawing comparisons with the 'Black Plague': 'plagues of the nineteenth-century'—smallpox, yellow fever, cholera, and bubonic plague—paled by comparison. Front-page headlines exclaimed: 'SAYS BLACK PLAGUE, NOT THE INFLUENZA', citing in full a long declaration by Howard Eckles, who had examined 'thousands of bodies' of influenza victims collected by the Council of National Defence in Philadelphia. From the autopsies, he concluded that the disease was not influenza. Instead, its symptoms matched those 'of the Black Plague of the Middle Ages'.[14] By the end of the year, doctors attending the annual meeting of the American Public Health Association in Chicago 'disagreed radically' on the best methods to check the spread of the disease, admitting they had no way of combating it.[15] Towards the pandemic's end in the US, *Scientific American* concluded the pandemic was 'even more a disease of mystery today' than previously thought.[16] That mystery led to a turning back of the clock in medical theory and treatment with a host of dangerous therapies from ingestion of precious metals to increased reliance on bloodletting.[17]

Influenza mystified scientists in Europe. Early on, the scientific community in Switzerland and Germany saw 'Spanish influenza' as either the return of the plague or an epidemic of smallpox or cholera.[18] In Spain, 'medical men' debated whether it was a severe form of typhus or pneumonic plague.[19] As late as the end of November, English doctors questioned if it were influenza or swine fever and thought the cause was bad bacon.[20] With evidence from Australia's quarantine stations, the Acting Prime Minister argued that the disease was not 'Spanish Influenza'.[21] 'People' and physicians in China were also uncertain; here, because the symptoms resembled cholera with 'constant thirst', 'rapid loss of strength', and 'death in some cases coming in less than a day'.[22] By the end of October 1918, Richard Pfeiffer (1858–1945), credited with discovering influenza's bacterium during the previous pandemic, now questioned his 'discovery'.[23] In early November, *The Times* declared that 'discoveries'

---

[12] *Evening Public Ledger*, 15 September 1918, 12.

[13] *Washington Herald*, 23 September 1918, 2.

[14] *Times-Herald*, 30 November 1918, front page. For survivors' later association of the Great Influenza with bubonic plague, see Taksa, 'The Masked Disease'.

[15] *Baltimore Sun*, 14 December 1918, 6: 'The Influenza Puzzle'. Much the same was said two days later by the director of the state bacteriological laboratory at the University of California; *San Francisco Chronicle*, 16 December 1918, 3.

[16] *Detroit Free Press*, 9 March 1919, D2: 'The Influenza Mystery Deepens'.

[17] Hildreth, 'The Influenza Epidemic', 281–93.   [18] Witte, *Erlärungsnotstand*, 81–4.

[19] *The Times*, 8 November 1918, 5.   [20] *Guardian*, 24 November 1918, 8.

[21] *Mercury*, 12 February 1919, 5.   [22] *Shanghai Times*, 2 November 1918, 269.

[23] *Guardian*, 31 October 1918, 3. Also see Hildreth, 'The Influenza Epidemic', 280; and Tognotti, 'Scientific Triumphalism', 103–6.

of new bacteria of influenza occur daily and concluded: the 'new discoveries simply add to the mystery of the disease'.[24] Because of the rapidity of its spread, suddenness of attack, and the speed with which pneumonia developed, this influenza was called the 'mystery fever' in India.[25] After it subsided in Mumbai in mid-December 1918, the *Times of India* scoffed: 'it is not to the credit of medical science that so little is known about its origin'.[26] Even in the twenty-first century, those at the forefront of influenza research refrain from identifying the 1918 virus as simply a strain of influenza.[27]

Occasionally, health authorities and newspapers took the opposite tack. Trying to pour cold waters over fears and panic stoked by rising mortalities and the pandemic's peculiar characteristics, they claimed nothing was new. New York City's Health Commissioner, Dr Royal Copeland, ever optimistic about the case and mortality figures in his city and ever cautious not to stir panic,[28] continued to call the present influenza that 'old fashion influenza'.[29] In mid-September, the *New-York Tribune* charged that 'the term "Spanish influenza"' caused 'unnecessary alarm . . . the so-called new disease is none other than the old enemy "la grippe"'.[30] A local paper of tiny Bayou Sara, Louisiana, asserted the same: 'Spanish Influenza' was a new name for an old disease.[31] Other papers used history as a sedative, scripting long narratives of supposed influenza epidemics reaching back by some accounts to the sixteenth century and by others to antiquity, citing Hippocrates and Livy. They reassured their readers: 'Spanish influenza' was 'a crowd disease, centuries

---

[24] *The Times*, 5 November 1918, 3; 18 December 1918, 5, reported influenza's new bacilli being 'discovered with great regularity' and called them 'a great deal of nonsense'.

[25] *Times of India*, 21 October 1918, 11.   [26] Ibid., 17 December 1918, 10.

[27] See Taubenberger, Hultin, and Morens, 'Discovery and Characterization': 'Rather, the 1918 virus is an avian-influenza-like virus that appears to have been derived *in toto* from an unknown source'.

[28] Even at the end September, Copeland claimed: 'There is no epidemic in this city' and resisted school closures 'as a sign of hysteria'; *Evening World*, 26 September 1918, 12. Despite cases and deaths in October soaring, he announced that the 'Influenza situation is well in hand' and repeated his blind optimism throughout the month; *New-York Tribune*, 1 October 1918, 16; 4 October 1918, 14; 15 October 1918, 4; and *New-York Tribune*, 16 October 1918, 18. On Copeland, see Robins, *Copeland's Cure*, who has not chronicled his reactions during the epidemic. Ultimately, over 48,000 would die in New York City with well over two million cases. Copeland, however, put the death toll at 35,000 and was criticized for his underreporting and claims that his city was faring 'better than did the rest of the world'. Even according to the official figures of influenza deaths, 33,387 over twenty-seven weeks, 14 September to 15 March, New York scores the highest influenza mortality rate out of forty-five cities tabulated by Crosby with 104 deaths (influenza and its pneumonic complications) per thousand, followed by Pittsburgh with 100 per thousand (my calculations). Andrews, 'Epidemics and Public Health', uses the figure of 27,362 deaths (lower even than Copeland's), ranking New York City the seventh highest mortality rate of the eighteen cities she selected (by what criteria is not explained) and three from Canada (also not explained). The only other city to follow Copeland's laissez-faire policy, refusing to close schools, that I know of was Vancouver but here only for the pandemic's first three weeks, when the regional health board overruled Vancouver's policies. Nonetheless, it tallied the highest influenza-pneumonia mortality rate of the Canadian cities charted by Andrews, ibid., 21: table 1. More recently, two articles by two independent research groups have argued that the most important variables in reducing excess mortality rates in US cities (seventeen in the first study; forty-five in the second) were the rapid and sustained implementation of measures such as school closures and other places of public assembly; Hatchett, Mecher, and Lipsitch, 'Public Health Interventions'; Bootsma and Ferguson, 'The Effect of Public Health Measures', 7588–93.

[29] *New-York Tribune*, 17 September 1918, 9.   [30] Ibid., 19 September 1918, 9.

[31] *True Democrat*, 26 October 1918, front page.

old'.[32] Some papers had it both ways: the disease may have been the old influenza but should be taken deadly seriously. An *El Paso Herald* front-page headline proclaimed: 'Spanish Influenza: Dangerous Disease. Dr Ramsey Says Worse than Hun Army'. Yet the doctor considered the current disease the same as the one he had witnessed as a medical student in 1889.[33]

Consistently, Italian papers denied that anything was unusual about this influenza. Milan's largest circulating paper, *Il Secolo* decried 'the exaggerated and unjustified alarm' in using terms such as 'grippe' and 'febbre spagnola'. As with all previous waves of influenza, there was no need to change habits of ordinary living; all that was needed was to avoid excesses and wash hands before eating.[34] Rome's *Idea Nazionale* reported 'the illness had been around Europe since 1173 with the same symptoms'.[35] 'As in the past, it would last no longer than four to six weeks'.[36] Well into October, with cases and deaths reaching their peaks, Milan's *Il Secolo* continued to insist nothing was new.[37] The major threat of the disease was not the illness itself—'that could be quickly cured by efficacious treatment and common sense—but panic that pervaded a part of the citizenry'.[38] Behind these headlines, however, lurked disquiet. As early as September, a paper of Monza admitted: 'worthy and knowledgeable clinicians did not know how to define the disease'.[39]

The Great Influenza's symptoms of disgust compounded its mystery. At the pandemic's start, papers cracked jokes about the usual sniffles, coughs, and brief bouts of intestinal troubles, but by October the joking stopped. Papers, instead, reported those coughs spewing blood-stained sputum with masses of blood flowing from the nose and sometimes the ears, as with yellow fever or today, Ebola. From influenza's acute septicaemia, skin disorders formed, as described by surviving physicians in Collier's sample: 'Raised purple blisters, like a scurvy victim's, all over the man's back and face and chest', and 'on the right side of the man's neck, above the clavicle, was another strange factor: a pronounced inexplicable lump'.[40] Faces of victims turned blue, asphyxiated by the inability of their infected lungs to transfer adequate supplies of oxygen to the bloodstream, the same symptom seen with cholera, called cyanosis, and the lungs filled with a bloody frothing fluid.[41] A Dublin physician described one of his patients as 'drowned in her own blood, which bubbled in froth from her nose and mouth as she passed away'.[42] Often immediately after death, these bodies rapidly turned black, horrifying family members,

---

[32] *Washington Times*, 25 September 1918, 19; and *The Bismarck Tribune*, 8 October 1918, front page. The *Washington Times* claimed the present spread of influenza had 'not been as rapid as in 1889'.
[33] *El Paso Herald*, 2 October 1918, front page.
[34] *Il Secolo*, 3 October 1918, 3; and 12 October 1918, 3.
[35] *Idea Nazionale*, 8 October 1918, 2; and *Il Secolo*, 17 October 1918, 3.
[36] *Idea Nazionale*, 11 October 1918, 2; and *Il Secolo*, 10 October 1918, 3.
[37] *Il Secolo*, 13 October 1918.
[38] Ibid., 16 October 1918, 3; also see ibid., 17 October 1918, 3; 19 October 1918, 3; and 21 October 1918, 2. For confusion over the disease's character, agent, and what to call it in Britain and France, see *Edinburgh Evening News*, 28 October 1918, 2; and *Le Figaro*, 28 May 1918.
[39] *La Brianza*, 28 September 1918, 2.   [40] Collier, *The Plague of the Spanish Lady*, 20.
[41] Ibid., 131–3, based on descriptions by the Surgeon General of the US Army at Fort Devens.
[42] Foley, *The Last Irish Plague*, 98.

even undertakers.[43] Isaac Starr, a medical student serving as head nurse at a Philadelphia hospital in 1918, described his patients:

> After gasping for several hours they became delirious and incontinent, and many died struggling to clear their airways of a blood-tinged froth that sometimes gushed from their nose and mouth. It was a dreadful business.[44]

As for cures and prevention, doctors across nations felt despondent, a jolt to the optimism that had grown since the laboratory revolution's progress in discovering bacterial agents and new and effective treatments. By Crosby's account, 'doctors stood nearly as helpless in the presence of this epidemic', as Hippocrates and Galen had with their epidemics.[45]

THE HISTORIOGRAPHY

Two fundamental studies of the Great Influenza, written on the eve of the AIDS pandemic—Alfred Crosby's *America's Forgotten Pandemic*, first published in 1976 as *Epidemic and Peace, 1918*, and Richard Collier's less known but more global *The Plague of the Spanish Lady*—reveal no incidents of social violence against victims of the disease or anyone allegedly carrying it. Instead, the picture is overwhelmingly one of compassion, volunteerism, and martyrdom. Despite its rapid contagion, Crosby shows influenza uniting communities. With public services in Philadelphia near collapse and the unburied left in heaps, volunteers from elite families entered the city's ghettoes and opened soup kitchens to feed the poor; cab drivers mobilized 2000 cars to serve as hospital ambulances; organizations cut across accustomed denominational boundaries, with Catholic nuns working in Jewish hospitals. 'People of all kinds poured into Emergency Aid Headquarters' volunteering as nurses, 'thrusting themselves into the presence of lethal disease'.[46] This self-sacrifice materialized, moreover, in the absence of institutional structures and despite deep schisms then splintering this and other wartime societies.[47]

According to Collier, 'rarely in the history of mankind had so many volunteers toiled so long and so patiently in the service of humanity'.[48] No instances of riots, violent protest, or individual acts of aggression surface from his exhaustive reading of diaries, official documents, and solicited letters of at least 1706 survivors worldwide.[49] The worst that appears is people in Midwestern towns avoiding soldiers out of fear of contagion. Instead, compassion united groups which previously and long after the pandemic remained segregated, often holding one another in bitter contempt. A black survivor, Willard Bryan, from Monroe, Louisiana, recalled just before 1974 (nearly a decade after the Civil Rights Amendments): 'White and coloured worked side by side then. Had we the cooperation between races today

---

[43] Rice, *Black November*, 24 and 95.   [44] Starr, 'Influenza', 517.
[45] Crosby, *America's Forgotten Pandemic*, 10.   [46] Ibid., 82.
[47] Ibid., chs 4 and 7.   [48] Collier, *The Plague of the Spanish Lady*, 89.
[49] These are the numbers I count in Collier's book. According to Honigsbaum, *Living with Enza*, 84–5, more letters survive in Collier's Collection deposited at the Imperial War Museum.

that we had during that epidemic it would be a blessing.'[50] In Winnipeg, the capital of Manitoba, Canada, workers voluntarily and 'daily whipped up quarts of lemonade and soup, gallons of orange juice, egg-nogs and soft puddings' to care for the flu-afflicted. In Ottawa, 'two hundred' volunteers, 'busy women', nightly until 11 p.m., filled 'the capital's Council Hall sewing clothing' for the afflicted. Canada was hardly alone in exhibiting this spirit. Collier's letters of survivors from Italy, the Orange Free State, Cape Town, Johannesburg, and other places illustrate much the same—an infection of compassion and self-sacrifice.[51] In contrast to Crosby or more recent monographs on the Great Pandemic, Collier emphasized the international ties of this cooperation that cut against the hyper-nationalistic antipathies intensified by the Great War: 'National concerns gave place to international…Old grudges were forgotten'.[52]

With the eruption of AIDS in the 1980s, new works on epidemic disease have lost sight of influenza's seemingly inexplicable propensity towards abnegation and compassion. Instead, scholars have assumed that large pandemics were bent on blame, persecuting foreigners, Jews, and other outsiders. In his study of infectious diseases in America (but concentrating mostly on New York City) during the late nineteenth and twentieth century, Alan Kraut argued that a 'double helix of health and fear of the foreign-born', was 'ever present throughout American history' and especially during peaks of immigration,[53] as had been the case with the influx of refugees from war-torn, revolutionary, and famine-stricken Europe on the eve of America's entry into the First World War and the outbreak of the Great Influenza. But regarding America's most devastating pandemic, Kraut had little to say. Others, concentrating on the Great Influenza, have tried to muscle this pandemic's experience into the post-AIDS frame that epidemics of all sorts, especially contagious and mysterious ones, provoked blame and violence. Instead of pointing to the overflowing volunteerism that Crosby and Collier described, John Barry, in a work that has gone through many reprintings, ferreted out details of protest and supposed persecution. His harvest, however, was meagre, especially compared with what can be found of US smallpox atrocities or cholera riots in Europe. For influenza's 'violence', he reported that in places health officials 'placarded' the houses of the infected.[54] In Arizona a Citizens' Committee deputized a special police force and called on:

> all patriotic citizens to enforce anti-influenza ordinances, including requiring every person in public to wear a mask, arresting anyone who spit or coughed without covering his mouth…Soon the *Republican* described 'a city of masked faces, a city as grotesque as a masked carnival'.[55]

These, however, were municipal regulations, which did not lead (as far as Barry shows) to collective violence, burning houses, injuring persons, or discrimination against foreigners. By his account, the only possible marginal group to suffer were

---

[50] Collier, *The Plague of the Spanish Lady*, 88.   [51] Ibid., 88–9.
[52] Ibid., 273–5, for his example between China and Japan.   [53] Kraut, *Silent Travellers*, 256.
[54] Barry, *The Great Influenza*, 348.   [55] Ibid., 350.

dogs (and perhaps dog-lovers), but only in one small Kentucky town, where dogs were thought to be carriers and were shot. Finally, an internal American Red Cross communiqué called the 'fear and panic of the influenza akin to the terror of the Middle Ages regarding the Black Plague'.[56] Yet, as far as Barry's synopsis goes, the Red Cross did not support its analogy with any examples, let alone massacres on a Black-Death scale.

Other works, such as Eugenia Tognotti's survey, report nothing of the pandemic's propensity to draw volunteers. Instead, she characterizes the pandemic as one that blamed the victim. Her evidence, however, rests on a manual on hygiene distributed to the popular classes that instructed on matters of cleanliness and advised washing hands with warm water, not spitting in public, and covering one's nose and throat when sneezing and coughing.[57] Such advice supposedly reveals blame. Niall Johnson's *Britain and the 1918–19 Influenza Pandemic* begins with the post-AIDS paradigm of what should be expected from transnational epidemics, especially a highly contagious one that dwarfed others in absolute mortalities. In an in-depth discussion of naming diseases, their metaphors and representations, he concurs with Susan Sontag and others that this pandemic was essentially one of 'foreignness': 'What is wrong or unnatural cannot be of us, but must be of the "other"'; thus 'One of the most obvious expressions of such externalising of blame is when a geographical name becomes attached to a disease.'[58] Yet, when he turns to his subject, Britain and its 'Spanish flu', he is forced to contradict his theoretical underpinnings (though without admitting it): the naming of this disease neither blamed Spaniards nor led to any abuse of them.[59]

Moreover, the naming 'Spanish Flu' within the British Isles was not as universal as Johnson suggests. Caitriona Foley finds that in Ireland the epidemic was rarely called after the Spanish,[60] and that any blame such as holding soldiers responsible for its spread, 'never led to widespread social antagonisms'.[61] On the other hand, in the US, where papers regularly used 'Spanish Influenza' to distinguish it from previous waves of influenza, journalists not only refrained from blaming Spaniards, they correctly refuted that it had Spanish origins. As a small-town Minnesota paper commented: 'In the first place, it may be said authoritatively that this disease is not "Spanish" influenza any more than it is Irish, Hindu, or Norwegian'. It speculated that, like the pandemic of 1889–90, called 'Russian', it originated in the Orient.[62] Other small-town papers agreed: no evidence pointed to the current influenza as Spanish, in its origins or for any other reason.[63]

[56] Ibid.　　[57] Tognotti, *La 'Spagnola'*, 53.

[58] Johnson, *Britain*, 152–3.　　[59] Ibid., 153 and 159.

[60] Similarly, Australia papers consistently called it 'Pneumonic Influenza', not after the Spanish.

[61] Foley, *The Last Irish Plague*, 169.

[62] *Warren Sheaf*, 9 October 1918, front page. Many small-town newspapers questioned the Spanish origins of the 1918 pandemic; see for instance *Pullman Herald*, 18 October 1918. Later, virologists argued that the 'Russian' pandemic of 1889–90 originated in China; see James, *The Chinese Labour Camps*, 559.

[63] *The Citizen*, 10 October 1918, 5; *The Coconino Sun*, 11 October 1918, front page.

BLAME

Authors, including Collier,[64] have pointed to incidents of international blaming during the pandemic regarding poisoning and biological warfare: 'Citizens of many Allied nations accused Germany of creating influenza as a biological weapon during the First World War'.[65] Some went further, asserting that 'Anyone of German origin was suspect and in at least one case a man was murdered after being accused of being a spy and spreading the disease'. Yet, in this case, not even the country where the incident supposedly occurred is documented.[66] Caitriona Foley has found that the butt of this name-calling extended beyond the Germans. In Britain, Chinese labourers were blamed for carrying the disease to its shores. Americans 'were happy to call it the "German Plague"'; Poles called it the 'Bolshevik disease'; and in Ceylon, it was 'Bombay fever'.[67] But again, no specific cases are brought to bear; nor in this excellent study or in others have historians sought to investigate the extent that such terms had entered public discourse, as with, for example, the regularity and duration of their appearances in newspapers. And except for the one undocumented murder above, none of these studies has cited any examples of such naming-calling spawning individual or collective violence. Collier's is the only work to cite a source identifying who said what in these allegations of blame: Lieutenant [sic][68] Philip Doane of the US Emergency Fleet Corporation went on record: 'the Spanish influenza was the Kaiser's secret weapon, spread by agents sent by submarines to the eastern seaboard'.

Such a remark, however, does not necessarily implicate public opinion. From the newspapers in 'Chronicling America', the significance of this conspiracy theory can be estimated—the extent of its circulation and whether it sparked direct action. First, papers across the US and its territorial possessions do not support claims that Americans were 'happy to call the Great Pandemic the "German Plague"'. While stories of the pandemic fill at least 25,306 pages in these newspapers, with many containing multiple articles on the pandemic, only one refers to 'German plague', and it appears in an advertisement requesting subscriptions for the Third Liberty Loan without any connection to influenza.[69]

On the other hand, claims that the Germans spread influenza as a biological weapon received some attention. Even before the first victims at Camp Devens received widespread publicity, a US paper claimed:

> that the appearance of the disease represents one of the fantastic methods of the German warmakers, who are supposed to have developed the menace with weird

[64] Collier, *The Plague of the Spanish Lady*, 83.
[65] Irwin, 'Scapegoats', 619; also, Tognotti, *La 'Spagnola'*, 135.
[66] Quinn, *Flu*, 141.
[67] Foley, *The Last Irish Plague*, 75. James, *The Chinese Labour Camps*, 556, asserts that the Chinese Labour Corps in northern France were blamed for introducing the pandemic into Europe; however, he provides no evidence for it. Also, see Langford, 'Did the 1918–19 Influenza Pandemic Originate in China?'.
[68] He was a lieutenant colonel.
[69] *New-York Tribune*, 15 April 1918, 3; also, no papers in BNA or Trove called it 'German Plague'.

dreams of prostrated armies laid low and surrounded after the disease had been spread by shells charged with it.[70]

But, as its language suggests, the paper took such claims as little more than madness. A few days later, however, after sharp rises in mortalities along the eastern seaboard and more importantly because of the official pronouncement by Lieutenant-Colonel Philip Doane, head of health and sanitation of the Shipping Board, matters changed. From the capitol, he advised 'all shipyards to use special precautions... the disease germs might have circulated here by German agents':

> It would be quite easy for one of these German agents to turn loose Spanish Influenza germs in a theatre or some other place where large numbers of persons are assembled. The Germans have started epidemics in Europe, and there is no reason why they should be particularly gentle to America. Of course, there is no way of proving that the epidemic was started by German submarine agents...[71]

During the week, two further papers carried the story, though with less sensational headlines. The *Washington Times* cautioned that the 'Foe may have spread germs of influenza along the coast'.[72] Arizona's *Bisbee Daily Review* conjectured, 'German cunning and ruthlessness' might have had a hand in it', claiming 'the propagation of disease germs' had been 'a speciality of German bacteriologists and chemists'. Yet the paper had its doubts: 'of course, it is probable as well as possible, that the disease was started here from ordinary and natural causes'.[73]

More significantly, the U-boat speculation proved to be a story without legs: it appeared in fewer than a handful of papers, failed to cross the country, or fuel new stories pointing to nefarious German submarines or their spies furthering influenza's assault on America. A week after Doane's speculation, only the *Washington Times* entertained the possibility that it might 'have been intentionally disseminated by the German Government' but argued against the speculation. It stuck instead with the standard story: the pandemic's American origins were from a neutral country that favoured the Entente—the landing of the Norwegian *Bergensfjord* at New York City on 12 August.[74]

From my keyword searches only three more papers—a minuscule appearance among the thousands reporting the pandemic—referred to the supposed German operation. Two saw it as implausible. A small-town Midwestern paper ridiculed the accusation: how could a 'mysterious infection of a new kind' have appeared 'so suddenly and extensively across the country by such means'; the 'theory' was 'not only entirely groundless but really absurd'.[75] The second paper made a joke of it. Commenting on a recent decision to close Philadelphia's saloons to fight the

---

[70] *Evening Public Ledger*, 15 September 1918, 12.
[71] *New-York Tribune*, 19 September 1918, 9.
[72] *Washington Times*, 19 September 1918, front page.
[73] *Bisbee Daily Review*, 26 September 1918, 4; and *New York Times*, 19 September 1918, 11. In addition, see *Boston Globe* [not included in 'Chronicling America'], 19 September 1918, 14.
[74] *Washington Times*, 6 October 1918, 22. On passenger casualties, see *New-York Tribune*, 14 August 1918.
[75] *Coconino Sun*, 4 October 1918, front page.

pandemic, it quipped, 'the spread of the influenza germ has been libelled. Since the germ has a bone-dry tendency, no one can ever say again that it was "made in Germany"'.[76] The single exception may have occurred in Boston during the last week of September, when influenza deaths suddenly soared. A Washington paper alleged that the U-boat story reached 'terror-striking proportions'.[77] If true, it is surprising that neither Boston's papers nor any others reported it.

A few newspapers considered other theories involving Germans and influenza but used the stories to crack jokes. Before Doane floated his U-boat speculation, the *Evening World* mocked the idea of blaming the disease on the Kaiser:

> The best thing we can do with this Spanish Influenza is to change its name and blame it on the Kaiser. That bird is responsible for everything that is happening in this corrugated vale of sorrow, moths and celluloid collars. And tossing old Castillian influenzy would make everyone happy except the birds who are suffering from it...[78]

Two decades later, a dim remembrance of these theories seeped into the conversations of Denver journalists in Katharine Anne Porter's *Pale Horse, Pale Rider*, but the imagery had changed. Instead of a U-boat, a supposed camouflaged German ship brought the germ to Boston Harbour. One of journalists jests, 'Maybe it was a submarine, sneaking from the bottom of the sea'. The group agrees that that sounds better. Another laughs, 'they think the germs were sprayed over the city' and an old woman saw it: 'a strange, thick, greasy-looking cloud float up out of Boston Harbor'. The journalists then brushed off the story: 'they always slip up somewhere in the details'.[79]

Two stories of influenza's war origins appear in two Australian papers but neither attributed blame. The first, derived from Cape Town, South Africa, alleging the disease could be traced to poisonous gas used by the Germans.[80] It was not, however, a theory of biological warfare; instead, it was believed to have been a side effect of poison gas. A second paper reported an American story of German conspiracy, no trace of which is found in US papers: 'Spanish Influenza' had attacked a convoy

---

[76] *Evening Public Ledger*, 5 October 1918, 8. *Clayton's Weekly*, 12 October 1918, 12, dismissed the importance of speculating 'whether it was brought over in German submarines...More practical' was how to combat it. Keywords—Kaiser and Influenza—produced forty-eight results; only one relates to a supposed German influenza plot (the one below).

[77] *Washington Herald*, 23 September 1918, 2.

[78] *Evening World*, 28 August 1918, 10. At Camp Dix, Wrightstown, New Jersey, the cook at the army barracks, a supposed 'German sympathizer', was arrested for attempted poisoning. His alleged poison was flour, but despite influenza's rapid spread at Camp Dix, no allegation was made of intentionally spreading the pandemic; ibid., 14.

[79] Porter, *Pale Horse*, 206. *Baltimore Sun*, 8 October 1918, 5, alluded to 'absurd rumours' regarding alleged incidents at Camp Meade: a doctor and nurse were caught poisoning soldiers, and a German spy distributing propaganda was killed by a doctor and nurse. Another in the *Chicago Daily Tribune*, 7 October 1918, 17, reported a rumour of several medical officers at Camp Grant having been 'shot at sunrise for deliberately causing the deaths of epidemic victims'. The head of intelligence at the Surgeon General's office immediately branded the rumours false, saying the same stories had come to them 'from four or five other camps'. A faint appearance of the German U-boat conspiracy in America reached the Australian press. But only two papers reported it: *West Gippsland Gazette*, 5 November 1918, 2; and *Queensland Times*, 23 September 1918, 6.

[80] *Myrtleford Mail*, 10 October 1918, 5.

of American troops en route to England, leading to rumours of 'wholesale poisoning by enemy agents'. The paper, however, reassured readers that the US Surgeon General had dismissed the allegation.[81] By contrast, reports in the Australian press had shown empathy for German civilians as the pandemic spread through Germany's industrial belt in the summer of 1918, exacting horrific death tolls that by October had claimed the lives of 8000 children in Berlin alone.[82]

Perhaps more surprising, thousands of papers in the British Library's BNA thus far downloaded fail to refer to Lieutenant-Colonel Doane's allegation or others accusing Germans of spreading influenza on British soil or elsewhere, even though U-boats were a much greater threat to British coastlines than to America or Australia.[83] The closest any British newspaper came to connecting German infiltration with influenza had nothing to do with intentional disease spreading. A paper reporting a parliamentary committee's investigation on whether alien enemies had gained government positions during the pandemic was convinced it would find nothing: neither Lloyd George nor successive home secretaries had been so criminal or imbecilic.[84] In summary, the one conspiracy to appear in more than a single newspaper, linking influenza to a fiendish German plot, came not from ordinary citizens or the lower classes but from the highest echelons of the US military. Its scant appearance in papers, however, suggests it had little influence on popular opinion; the little attention it received mostly consisted of ridicule.[85]

* * *

More recently, three monographs on the Great Influenza grounded in meticulous research from diaries, medical bulletins, and archival sources in specific towns and regions, have reported blame and stigmatization, but these incidents were slight, infrequent, and failed to spark collective violence. Foley's study of the pandemic in Ireland finds only one incident—a relative of a flu patient was refused service in a local shop[86]—and concludes the pandemic created surprisingly little panic.[87] She explains it by 'an evolution in popular understandings of sickness and the body', in particular 'the more material form of microbes and germs'.[88] Yet as Nancy Tomes, Martina King, and others[89] have shown, popular awareness of germs and microbes had already filtered through the media and into popular romances during the last two decades of the nineteenth century, when, as we have seen, stigmatization of

---

[81] *Queensland Times*, 8 October 1918, 5. [82] *Cootamundra Herald*, 15 July 1918, 2.

[83] Keyword searches for 'influenza and German' and 'influenza and Kaiser' produced ninety-four pages of results (*c*.940) for 1918 without a single suggestion of influenza as German biological warfare.

[84] *Burley News*, 6 July 1918, 5.

[85] In Germany and Switzerland ideas of influenza caused by poisonous military gas do not appear widely reported, and no riots or persecution are mentioned; see Witte, *Erlärungsnotstand*, 81. Other papers show even less evidence of blaming Germans than in the US. Out of Canadian papers I searched, Toronto's *Globe and Mail* (30 November 1918, 6) alone reported a story circulating in Spain of the disease carried there by German submarines, but the paper disbelieved it. The major Italian papers— *La Stampa*, *Corriera della Sera*, *L'Idea Nazionale*, and *Il Messaggero*—report no U-boat stories or other conspiracies. *Guardian* (19 November 1918, 12) reports a Soviet conspiracy theory from the paper *Izvestiya*: 'Imperialists' were spreading influenza 'to exterminate the proletariat'.

[86] Foley, *The Last Irish Plague*, 76. [87] Ibid., 68 and 82.

[88] Ibid., 82–3. [89] Tomes, *The Gospel of Germs*.

victims, blaming others, and collective violence spurred by epidemics were at their peak, with smallpox in the US and cholera in Italy and Eastern Europe. Furthermore, these tendencies continued into the early twentieth century in varying degrees with plague in San Francisco, tuberculosis called the Jewish disease, and the polio epidemics of 1907 and 1916 blamed on dirty Italians.[90] Far more horrific was the Nazi branding of typhus in the 1930s and 1940s as the *Judenfieber* that supplied further justification to gas Jews as the supposed disease carriers.[91] Certainly, these Germans were profoundly aware of germs and microbes.

Similarly, in an analysis of the Great Pandemic in the US, Nancy Bristow finds influenza capable of stirring controversy and conflict in several communities. However, these failed to provoke any traces of physical violence and were mild-mannered compared to the acts of hatred seen in previous chapters in this book. In small-town Globe, Arizona, citizens brought health officials to court against closing schools. Their case was dismissed, and the protest disappeared. In some places, individuals refused to comply with compulsory wearing of masks in public, and in San Francisco, an anti-mask league formed, to which we shall return in Chapter 20.[92] But Bristow concludes: 'In most cases citizens ultimately accepted the decisions of local authorities'.[93] She then explains the absence of bitter confrontation by turning to US experience alone, alleging that by 1918, 'few broad-based and organized efforts to demonize immigrants' remained. One might ask about the Sacco and Vanzetti trials, their execution, and the country-wide media frenzy and popular rage it stirred up against Italians and other recent immigrants; or the blame placed on Jews, Italians, and other impoverished ethnic groups in New York City only two years before for a polio epidemic;[94] or the effects of internal migration and race from 1918 to the early 1920s in Tulsa and East St Louis that produced the longest and bloodiest race riots in US history. But even if we accept Bristow's US- or Foley's Irish-centric explanations, how do we then explain what appears as a global pattern? At present, we can observe: this pandemic failed to spark collective persecution anywhere in the world; nor has any social violence yet to be found with earlier epidemics of influenza. Instead of riots that cremated blacks, destroyed hospitals, or murdered physicians, the Great Influenza produced unprecedented levels of volunteerism, compassion, and self-sacrifice to be explored in the remaining chapters on the Great Influenza.

Finally, in her study of Winnipeg in 1918, Esyllt Jones argues that the influenza crisis emboldened workers to organize a general strike but maintains that it never led to violent confrontations, certainly nothing approaching cholera's terror.[95] Any fear that may have accompanied flu's fierce contagion certainly did not deter

---

[90] Kraut, *Silent Travellers*, chs 4 and 6.

[91] Weindling, *Epidemics and Genocide*, 70–1, 106–7.

[92] Bristow, *American Pandemic*, 112–18.   [93] Ibid., 115.

[94] Risse, 'Revolt against Quarantine', 48; Kraut, *Silent Travellers*, 134; idem, 'Plagues and Prejudice', 66, 70–4; and Rodgers, 'A Disease of Cleanliness', 98. *Washington Times*, 11 July 1917, 3, blamed polio violence against doctors, nurses, and quarantine regulations on 'foreign parents'.

[95] Jones, *Influenza 1918*, 7.

women from volunteering in great numbers to assist the inflicted.[96] Her thesis that Winnipeg's general strike was the product of the pandemic might be questioned: the evidence rests on a chronological coincidence alone. Nonetheless, she sees the general strike not as dividing society but building bonds of empathy and trust paralleling the influenza experience of volunteers caring for the sick.[97]

These recent works have suggested a new departure in the history of epidemics since the spread of HIV/AIDS in the 1980s, by emphasizing the spread of volunteerism in such crises rather than hate and blame. Moreover, they signal a new dimension in volunteerism missed in the mid-1970s by Collier and Crosby: overwhelmingly the volunteers were women and mostly from educated, middle-class white families, many of whom crossed class, ethnic, and racial barriers for the first time in their lives.[98] Foley describes organizations, such as the Women's National Health Association, and women from the Citizen Army who, under the direction of the physician and Sinn Féin radical, Kathleen Lynn, cleared a house in Dublin and equipped it to care for influenza patients.[99] In Ireland's Great Influenza, middle-class and elite 'ladies' were instrumental in caring for the stricken, attending to menial tasks and supplying meals to the ill and dying. To explain this preponderance of 'ladies', Foley turns to local causes based on Ireland's particular nineteenth-century traditions of charity that had placed responsibility on women.[100] Yet their philanthropic response appears much the same as in Canada and the US: those risking their lives, entering neighbourhoods of the poor to care for the influenza-stricken were also predominantly middle- and upper-class ladies. Moreover, no equivalent trend can be seen elsewhere previously.

Similarly, Bristow interprets the 'distinctly female' volunteerism as 'distinctly American', explained by particular aspects of women's history in late nineteenth- and early twentieth-century America. By the time of the Great Influenza, 'women had gained new access to the American public sphere'. This platform enabled them to volunteer en masse in key positions to assist the afflicted.[101] Yet despite the strikingly different histories of women in Ireland, Foley has seen the same outcome. Moreover, Foley hypothesizes that Irish women's high levels of volunteerism could account for that country's low rate of casualties compared with other European countries.[102] But this challenging hypothesis needs testing: was Ireland atypical in the degree to which women risked their lives for the disease-stricken in 1918–19? Did volunteerism correlate with influenza casualty rates? Was volunteerism significantly higher in England, where casualty rates were among the lowest in Europe, or in Italy, where they were the highest?[103] Was this spirit of volunteerism lower in South Africa or New Zealand, where cases and mortalities were substantially higher?

---

[96] Ibid., 52.   [97] Ibid., 93.

[98] Also McGinnis, 'The Impact of Epidemic Influenza'; and Luckingham, *Epidemic in the Southwest*.

[99] Foley, *The Last Irish Plague*, 111–12.   [100] Ibid., 113.

[101] Bristow, *American Pandemic*, 59.   [102] Foley, *The Last Irish Plague*, 164.

[103] According to Tognotti, *La 'Spagnola'*, 18, and 'Scientific Triumphalism', 98: along with Portugal, Italy had the highest influenza mortality rates in Europe, around 600,000 in 1918–19. She does not, however, evaluate these problematic statistics from a time when physicians were not required to 'notify' deaths from influenza and pneumonic complications in most European countries and when these diagnoses were clouded in confusion. On these problems, see Witte, *Erlärungsnotstand*, 317–23 and 381.

If women's participation in the public sphere during the late nineteenth and early twentieth centuries was key to explaining the outpouring of volunteers in 1918–19, why was volunteerism so unremarkable, especially among women, in other late nineteenth- and early twentieth-century epidemics—smallpox, plague, typhus, poliomyelitis, and cholera? The only other epidemics to have spurred significant levels of volunteerism were cholera in Italy during the 1867 and 1884–7 epidemics and yellow fever in the Deep South from the last decades of the nineteenth century to its pandemic finale of 1905. But these were staffed almost exclusively by men and their organizations.

Only with the polio epidemic of 1916 had a female group formed an association to confront an affliction. However, these ladies' actions differed fundamentally from what occurred with influenza two years later. In August 1916 the Mothers' Militia to Fight Paralysis and Help Your Neighbors was founded. The one paper to report its doctrines—*The Evening World*—may have been behind the organization. Its founder was identified not by her own name but first by her fourteen-year-old prodigal son, then her husband, a federal health officer. This Mrs Stoner 'adopted' the *Evening World*'s 'Plan in Organizing the Women of the Afflicted Sections' of New York City and intervened first with a lecture tour. These lectures employed war metaphors to a heavier extent than ever heard from any woman volunteers two years later, despite the guilt the latter felt for not having served in combat or as battlefield nurses. Mrs Stoner's reliance on war metaphors, in fact, goes beyond anything Susan Sontag cites in her attack on metaphors utilized to describe cancer or AIDS.[104] Stoner's lectures began: 'When every mother in New York enlists for the war on polio the enemy will be conquered'. She then detailed her commands for invading homes of the poor to 'instruct' them on 'how to keep clean and healthy'. For each neighbourhood, she pledged to appoint 'the most intelligent and energetic woman as a general in my militia', with the task 'to guard a certain fixed area against disease and dirt.' Her 'generals' were to go on patrol and inspect houses to see if these impoverished women were 'keeping their rooms clean' and 'if their babies are bathed daily'. Mrs Stoner promised to start 'a soap and screen fund to aid the work' and reported that in Pittsburgh she had 'succeeded in stopping the filthy habit of expectorating on sidewalks, in public buildings, and street cars by 'escort[ing] the offenders to the nearest police station'.[105] Ironically, as discovered in 1949, polio was a disease of cleanliness. Cleansed of needed antibodies, children became vulnerable to this opportunistic virus. Polio in 1916, in fact, clustered in New York's wealthiest neighbourhoods, not in its Italian slums.[106]

In her study of the Great Influenza in Winnipeg, Jones questioned 'the discourse of heroism' that placed white middle-class women from old Scottish families (whom she contemptuously calls 'Mc' women) on a pedestal: they were 'clichéd descriptions of women's experiences as volunteers' that 'repeated stories of women...working for long hours or days to save one or two lives in working-class homes, and refusing

---

[104] Sontag, *Illness as Metaphor*.   [105] *The Evening World*, 19 August 1916, 6.
[106] Bollet, *Plagues*, 123–4.

to leave despite the risk to their own health'.[107] Yet she never denies that these 'Mc' women risked their lives performing menial tasks for the afflicted. Further, in her emphasis on rhetoric, neither she nor anyone else has brought to light from newspapers, personal diaries, or letters utterances akin to Mrs Stoner's class-ridden Mothers' Militia—top-down marching orders that blamed polio on the poor and threatened to punish them because of their alleged dirty habits, irresponsibility, and stupidity. By contrast with women risking their lives through hands-on care delivered to the contagious poor, newspapers fail to disclose a single Mrs Stoner in 1918, who from sanitized lecture halls preached against the poor.

* * *

The Great Influenza of 1918–20 can no longer justifiably be called the 'Forgotten Pandemic' and less so in America than anywhere else.[108] Except for AIDS and the Black Death, the social life of no other epidemic disease has received as much recent scholarly scrutiny. But even before the late twentieth century, bestsellers of imaginative literature from the 1920s to the 1980s, at least in America, centred on this pandemic, suggesting that it may never have been as forgotten as Crosby claimed. These include Willa Cather, *One of Ours*: book four, 'The Voyage of the Anchises' (1922); Virginia Woolf, 'On Being Ill', *The Criterion*, January 1926 and abridged as 'Illness: An Unexploited Mine', *Forum*, April 1926; and redrafted again as 'On Being Ill', in November 1930, as a Hogarth Press book; Thomas Wolfe, *Look Homeward, Angel: A Story of the Buried Life* (1929); John O'Hara, 'The Doctor's Son' (1935); William Maxwell, *They Came Like Swallows* (1937); Katherine Anne Porter, *Pale Horse, Pale Rider* (1939); Mary McCarthy, *Memories of a Catholic Girlhood* (1957); Katherine Fring's adaption of Wolfe's *Look Homeward Angel* for the stage in 1957, which appeared on Broadway for 564 performances, won six Tony awards and was awarded the Pulitzer Prize for drama in 1958; Sterling North's bestselling *Rascal: A Memoir of a Better Life* (1963); William Maxwell, *Ancestors: A Family History* (1972); and William Maxwell, *So Long, See You Tomorrow* (1980).[109] Nor was the pandemic forgotten in other arenas. In Britain, memory of the global devastation it wreaked was the driving force behind new research in virology with increased government expenditure, new research institutes, and pathology departments at Oxford and Cambridge. According to Michael Bresalier, 'The public and medical profile of influenza remained high throughout the 1920s' and prepared the groundwork for the identification of influenza and other viruses in the 1930s.[110]

Moreover, during the pandemic and to some extent afterwards, newspapers poured out daily directives on how to avoid it, reported cures and remedies,

---

[107] Jones, *Influenza 1918*, 82 and 89.

[108] On the surge in publications on the pandemic, especially during the first fourteen years of the twenty-first century, see Phillips, 'Second Opinion'.

[109] I know of no other national literary tradition to have produced notable works on the pandemic. The twenty-first century, however, has seen an upsurge in this literary production; for Spain, see Davis, *The Spanish Flu*, 4.

[110] Bresalier, 'Uses of a Pandemic', 409.

supposed medical breakthroughs and corresponding disappointments, daily counts of cases and deaths divided by numerous categories, closures of schools and other public places, and the public's reactions. These flooded small-town papers from Indian villages in the Dakotas to the bayous of Louisiana. 'Chronicling America' supplies 25,306 pages with 'influenza' for 1918 alone[111]—ten times more than for any wave of cholera covered by this database; in fact greater than any disease before 1922, when the database ended during my investigation. By early October, papers could contain more stories on influenza than on the war. They appear on front pages cast in large capital headlines, aided by the new photographic journalism that celebrated women's organizations and abnegation combating the pandemic.

US papers may have been more attentive to the progress of this pandemic than any other national press, but neither British nor Italian papers (where censorship was in effect) can be said to have reduced its reportage to 'brief tranquillizing paragraphs' on back pages in small print, as has been claimed.[112] For the *Scotsman*, for example, by the end of the summer of 1918 to 1919, articles on the pandemic appeared daily concerning trends and reactions in the UK along with places from West Samoa to Labrador. For the BNA, 29,449 pages on the pandemic have thus far appeared for 1918–19.[113] For Italy, articles on the pandemic were placed mostly in sections of regional news, but these appeared daily from 2 October 1918 to the end of the month, constituting the day's major story for a city. Their editorials included interviews with military doctors, directors of sanitary boards, and municipally employed physicians ('dottori condotti'). The following two chapters turn to these vast resources to sketch community reactions to the pandemic, one of the most contagious diseases known, and the one thus far to have scored the highest worldwide mortality in human history.

---

[111] Calculated on 16 April 2014, when 7,590,956 newspaper pages had been scanned, 1836 to 1922. Because often more than one article on influenza appeared on a single page and given 'Chronicling America's' poor OCR, the number of articles on the pandemic was much greater.

[112] Pierluigi, *Gli anni del colera*, 13 and 70: 'I grandi quotidiani nazionali...si limitavano a pubblicare brevi trafiletti tranquillizzanti sull'epidemia...'. Also, Alfani and Melegaro, *Pandemie d'Italia*, 124; and Cosmacini, *Medicina e sanità*, 1. According to Johnson, *Britain*, British newspapers and the medical press paid 'scant attention' to the pandemic (163). Bristow, *American Pandemic*, even claims US papers 'relegated [the pandemic] to back pages and small print' (10).

[113] Accessed on 10 June 2016. On West Samoa's mortalities, see Tomkins, 'The Influenza Epidemic'.

20

The Great Influenza
Quarantine and Blame

The previous chapter challenged an unexamined presumption, which has fascinated researchers of epidemics across time, that naming diseases after others was in and of itself to blame those people. Despite naming the Great Influenza 'the Spanish influenza', 'Spanish flu', 'La Spagnola', and 'La Grippe Espagnole', prejudicial laws, individual assaults, even verbal insults against Spaniards for causing the disease have yet to surface.[1] The same absence of blame holds for the previous pandemic, 1889–94, named after the Russians. As for the 'Spanish' one, neither the American press nor others believed it originated in Spain but concluded that troops brought it there, while others believed its origins lay as far afield as China.[2] Although some thought the pandemic originated in Germany because of the conditions suffered by soldiers in the trenches, few attributed the disease to Germans, named it after them, or blamed them for it, despite widespread nationalist propaganda stirred by war frenzy. As seen in Chapter 19, the few attempts to suggest that Germans spread it as a biological weapon held little sway; newspapers viewed the stories mostly with scepticism, ridicule, or silence.

CRIES OF PROFITEERING

Some have tried to place the Great Influenza in a wider historiographical frame: that of past pandemics' supposed propensity to spread hatred and blame. Yet evidence has yet to appear of this or any previous influenza epidemic stirring mobs to persecute Jews, women, homosexuals, foreigners, or other 'others'. The Great Influenza did result, however, in some pointing the finger of blame at others. Even if justifiable, governments and newspapers accused landlords and others of profiteering. Such charges were certainly more common than allegations over shooting dogs or brief notices of German U-boats allegedly disseminating 'the influenza germ'. Yet resentment against profiteering in 1918 has yet to be studied.

In the US, these accusations first targeted unscrupulous landlords. Based on stories of evictions of impoverished influenza victims or tenants with common

---

[1] Nor was 'Spanish Flu' universal outside Spain. In Australia, it was 'Pneumonic Influenza'.
[2] See Chapter 19, note 62.

colds suspected of carrying the virus, newspapers and government officials led the battles against the privileged perpetrators. Protests against the inhumanity may have originated with neighbours and relatives but never stirred vigilante action. The first campaigns against these landlords appeared in the nation's capital and gained the ear of President Woodrow Wilson. The *Washington Times* appears to have been the major catalyst; with the front-page headline 'PRESIDENT TO RECEIVE PLEA TO CURB D.C. RENT SHARKS', it began: 'Hunnish inhumanities and cruelties are being outdone right here in Washington in the treatment of tenants and room-renters—notably homeless and defenceless girl war-workers—by many greedy landlords'. Landlord greed was placed in the context of the pandemic: 'Side-by-side with the ravages of influenza stalks an unprecedented epidemic of piratical attempts to profit financially from humanity's fright, accompanied by wolfish neglect and mistreatment of the ill.' It then appealed to the President 'to step in . . . to assume charge of the rent situation' and 'suppress [the] human hyenas'.[3] Yet, despite its emotional appeal, no authoritarian controls followed.

With increased cases and deaths during the first half of October, the District Health Department took on the crusade, accusing landlords of 'directly contributing to the spread of the influenza epidemic' by refusing to heat apartments.[4] Two days later, District Health Commissioner, W. C. Fowler, used the *Washington Herald*'s front page to persuade landlords to furnish heat to their tenants,[5] and landlords themselves (the 'Real Estate Men') passed a resolution to improve tenant conditions, urging owners and agents to heat their buildings.[6] Still, stories of exploitation and appeals for reform continued. The *Washington Herald*'s social column, usually reserved for the capital's socialites, featured a story of a 'girl war worker', who left her lodging house for work feeling ill. On her return, her landlady refused her entry, 'calmly insisting that she didn't want to be bothered with sick people'.[7] Other papers took up the cause 'of sick girls and women', 'virtually penniless and far from home . . . put into the street', with influenza or early stages of pneumonia. In mid-October, the Food and Fuel Administration and the War Trade Department intervened:[8] no more is heard of the landlords' 'unpatriotic behaviour'.

Washington was not the only city to feel the effects of callous landlords, blamed for the pandemic's spread. Yet nowhere else did complaints focus so sharply on them. In New York City, cries came later than in Washington but, as in the capital, emanated from the highest echelons of government, in this case, Health Commissioner Copeland. As seen earlier, he resisted taking coercive measures against the pandemic's spread more than any health officer in America, refusing to close schools or theatres and only advising businesses to stagger opening hours to reduce crowding on public transportation. When influenza-related deaths soared in the second and third weeks of October, political opponents began calling his policies 'acts of negligence'.[9]

---

[3] *Washington Times*, 8 October 1918, front page and 15.
[4] *Washington Herald*, 10 October 1918, front page.   [5] Ibid., 11 October 1918, front page.
[6] Ibid., 2.   [7] Ibid., 13 October 1918, 11.   [8] *Sun*, 16 October 1918, 16.
[9] See Dr Stephen Wise's attack, *New-York Tribune*, 21 October 1918, 14, and responses to Copeland's criticisms of doctors by Dr Davin.

Copeland turned the blame on others. His first targets were landlords. On 10 October into the following week, with front-page headlines he threatened to prosecute landlords who refused to heat their apartments.[10] On 25 October, a landlord was taken to court for not heating his flats. This was, however, the only notice in the papers of any such prosecution.[11] Curiously, complaints against landlords do not arise from my searches in other cities, despite the pandemic peaking later and in colder climes in places such as Chicago and Minneapolis.[12]

Papers attacked other forms of influenza-related profiteering. In Philadelphia, complaints were raised against high grave fees. But again the protest came from government officers, not angry mobs. In mid-October, the city coroner threatened to seize burial grounds from private owners.[13] Several days later, the *Evening Public Ledger* commented that 'cumulative evidence' showed that 'some undertakers, druggists, and even corporations that control cemeteries, profiteered heartlessly at the expense of afflicted families'.[14] Unlike the outrage against landlords, however, either the threats were effective or the complaints subsided: only one further article raised the issue. The Washington papers attacked only one form of profiteering beyond landlords' greed[15]—coffin makers—and the district's health officer dealt with it swiftly by 'commandeering' all coffins to be distributed directly to undertakers.[16]

For other charges against profiteering, New York City was exceptional, and its Health Commissioner was again at the vanguard. After landlords, Copeland targeted physicians as profiteering at the sufferers' expense.[17] And in Brooklyn, druggists were coupled with them as 'Medical Vandals'. Here the evidence went beyond newspaper rhetoric. The District Attorney received 'numerous complaints'. Yet, the prosecutor testified that, although 'heartless, selfish, and unpatriotic', such practices pertained to only a few doctors in 'certain congested districts': 'The vast majority of the doctors here in Brooklyn are making sacrifices of time, money, and strength to end this plague. They are also gratuitously giving their time to the government...'.[18] Several days later, Copeland lambasted doctors again, this time for laxity in reporting influenza cases.[19] In their defence, doctors used newspapers to point to the numerous deaths in their ranks and a decline in their livelihood because of the pandemic.[20] The papers supported them, describing the adverse conditions in which medical professionals worked: severe shortages, bodies piled high in morgues, exhaustion, and death within their cadres. In Brooklyn, these conditions almost came to a boiling point. Six interns at the Greenpoint Hospital,

---

[10] *Evening World*, 10 October 1918, front page; 11 October 1918, front page; 17 October 1918, 11.

[11] Ibid., 25 October 1918, front page. *Sun*, 22 October 1918, 14, announced a planned 'Round-Up of Fuel Landlords'. Already *New-York Tribune*, 24 October 1918, 14, reported a decline in complaints against landlords, but the same day, *Evening World*, 24 October 1918, 18, reported receiving many letters 'about greedy landlords'.

[12] At present, no Chicago papers are in 'Chronicling America' for 1918–20.

[13] *Evening Public Ledger*, 18 October 1918, front page.   [14] Ibid., 21 October 1918, 8.

[15] Andrews, 'Epidemics and Public Health'; in Vancouver, druggists raised prices on influenza remedies 'to excessive heights', causing 'public outrage' (39).

[16] *Chicago Daily Tribune*, 16 October 1918, 13.

[17] *New-York Tribune*, 21 October 1918, 14; and *Sun*, 21 October 1918, 4.

[18] *Evening World*, 22 October 1918, 8.   [19] *New-York Tribune*, 27 October 1918, 20.

[20] See note 9.

overwhelmed by the number of patients with decreasing members of staff and constant strain from six weeks of the pandemic, threatened to strike.[21] However, their strike action appears not to have materialized. Moreover, despite these superhuman demands spreading across the US, not a single notice in thousands of newspaper pages points to a strike or another threat of one by any within the medical profession.[22]

In the same week as the attacks on doctors and druggists, complaints of profiteering arose against two other professions considered vital in combating influenza: first, vendors of lemons and oranges seen among the poor as preservatives;[23] and second, undertakers. For the first, the Federal Food Bureau joined the attack, and the second made news beyond New York's boroughs, as far away as Bisbee, Arizona. Its daily labelled New York's undertakers 'coffin ghouls', accusing them of 'reaping a rich harvest' from victims and their families. Despite its rhetoric, the article clarified that only 'several' undertakers were under investigation,[24] and stories could turn in the other direction: the same week, top-page headlines described a New York undertaker, who on hearing of a father too impoverished to bury his son killed by the pandemic, put his hearse gratis at the father's disposal.[25]

Finally, from the city's East Side, another form of profiteering arose. The health department investigated complaints of Jews peddling printed invocations in Yiddish that supposedly protected against influenza. Allegedly, 'many of the gullible poor' in Jewish neighbourhoods were purchasing these written amulets for a dollar a piece to guard their households.[26] Despite this variety of charges, attacks against profiteering lasted less than a week, the third one in October, when Commissioner Copeland's barrage of optimistic prognoses and unorthodox public health policies started to crumble. None of the attacks drew crowds or resulted in violence. As with the charges against landlords, few complaints of these sorts of profiteering appear beyond East Coast cities.[27] The only piece in the West to mention undertakers appeared in small-town Ogden City, Utah, and was entirely sympathetic to the profession, already overworked in the early weeks of the pandemic.[28]

MUNICIPAL ORDINANCES AND CLOSURES

Severe restrictions on public life with closures or regulations imposed on almost all forms of public entertainment and gatherings (schools, theatres, cinemas, saloons, dance halls, fraternal meetings, bowling alleys, pool rooms and billiard parlours,

---

[21] *Evening World*, 29 October 1918, 10.
[22] Three days later, Brooklyn druggists blamed their jobbers for the rise; ibid., 25 October 1918, 17.
[23] *New-York Tribune*, 24 October 1918, 14; *Sun*, 24 October 1918; 25 October 1918; and *New-York Tribune*, 26 October 1918, 8.
[24] *Bisbee Daily Review*, 23 October 1918, front page.
[25] *Evening World*, 28 October 1918, 3.   [26] *New-York Tribune*, 23 October 1918, 2.
[27] Maybe complaints of price gouging of lemons and oranges went westward; the Federal Food Bureau enacted national price controls on fruit by the fourth week of October, *Evening World*, 24 October 1918, 12.
[28] *Ogden Standard*, 26 October 1918, 12.

soda fountains, public meeting halls, and places of religious worship) occasionally provoked defiance. In Philadelphia two saloonkeepers were arrested for extending bar hours beyond those set by the city's quarantine.[29] But in the city of brotherly love, more chaos and arrests were caused by drinking legally outside the quarantine restrictions. On Friday nights, Philadelphians crossed the river to Camden, New Jersey, where no bans on bars were in place, and in a debauched state the 'armies of thirsties' 'brought their troubles back to Philadelphia'.[30] In the same city, its chief coroner, relying on medical lore prevalent during previous pandemics but roundly refuted in the US by 1918, ridiculed the quarantine closure of 'liquor establishments' as 'a fool order' that cost lives: 'liquor is a good remedy'.[31] No such defiance, however, followed in other cities, and in Philadelphia no collective protest arose or led to arrests other than the two saloonkeepers.

Nor did closures of public entertainment or schools spark significant protest. In late October, Philadelphia's theatrical managers questioned a municipal ban on places of amusement decreed on 3 October,[32] but their questions failed to end the ban, and no more is heard of the dispute. Instead, according to the *Evening Public Ledger*, the managers became fatalistic about recouping losses, which exceeded $200,000.[33] Nor were outcries by theatre owners or actors heard in other cities, where bans threatened livelihoods.[34] Instead, in Oregon, Missouri, when influenza cases began to rise, the owners of the Royal Theatre did not wait for closures but voluntarily shut their premises and announced it in a gigantic half-page advertisement.[35]

The only quarantine to provoke the slightest signs of defiance concerned churches. In almost every case, however, the papers showed at most a mixed reaction from clergymen or their flocks. For example, two of Nashville's many churches announced services on Sunday 13 October—the first Sunday after the Health Board ordered churches to close to avoid crowds.[36] No reports suggested that the two stuck to their defiant decision. The following Sunday in Newark, New Jersey, pastors' protests appeared more widespread with 'many churches' insisting on services. The pastors grumbled that an 'open church was no worse in spreading influenza than saloons that remained open'.[37] Yet, as in Nashville, no news reports showed Newark's pastors sticking to their guns. In Philadelphia, pastors must have protested too, but we hear of it not from their actions but from those within the church who opposed the protests. A minister published a letter to Philadelphia's health director, supporting the closures and beseeching colleagues to turn their attention to the sick.[38] A week

[29] *Evening Public Ledger*, 25 October 1918, front page.

[30] Ibid., 26 October 1918, 2. Differences in local ordinances also created weekend bashes of Baltimore's 'thirsties'; *Baltimore Sun*, 28 October 1918, 12.

[31] *Evening Public Ledger*, 12 October 1918, front page.

[32] On bans on public places of amusement, schools, and churches, see ibid., 3 October 1918, 2; on their plans to protest, ibid., 26 October 1918, 4.

[33] Ibid., 26 October 1918, 10.

[34] The most significant conflict was between theatre and cinema owners in Lombardy; *Corriere della Sera*, 3 October 1918, 3; and 10 October 1918, 3; 18 October 1918, 2.

[35] *Holt County Sentinel*, 11 October 1918, 7.   [36] *Washington Times*, 13 October 1918, 17.

[37] *Sun*, 21 October 1918, 4.

[38] *Evening Public Ledger*, 21 October 1918, 2. He concluded: 'those who protest may be preachers but [they] are not pastors'.

earlier, a call was made to ninety of Philadelphia's Episcopal clergymen, asking Health Director Dr Krusen to end the ban on church attendance. Only twenty-three attended the meeting.[39] On the same Sunday, the rector of St Patrick's in Washington issued an appeal to reopen the city's churches—asking that 'there be an universal protest against the prohibition'—but the protest never happened.[40]

Such signs of defiance were not confined to big cities. In Stanford, Maine, the municipal court fined the pastor of a local Catholic church $50 for violating the church closures.[41] In Sumter, South Carolina, the pastor wrote a letter to a local paper, criticizing the closures. He resolved not to defy the law, however, only to ask for space in the paper 'to remind the Christian community not to be idle in their religious devotion'.[42] The parish priest of Notre Dame in Springvale, Maine, went further. By keeping his church open for services, he strove to test the ban, claiming it was unconstitutional. He was arrested, but no more is heard of his protest.[43] None of these protests even in America's Bible Belt galvanized congregations to follow their pastors, either in tribunals or the streets as frequently occurred with resistance to cholera and plague quarantines. Such closures were unique in many places, as the *Boston Globe* noted: for the first time in the city's 300-year history 'religious services in duly ordained houses of worship have been curtailed'.[44] The same was true for El Paso, reaching back 200 years to its Spanish origins. On the first day, its paper noted, 'people were astonished and uneasy'.[45] But no protest resulted.[46] In other places, congregations supported the decisions as necessary. In Cumberland, Maryland, the Catholic church adhered to the restrictions by erecting a temporary altar in the church's portico to perform Sunday mass to those outside.[47] In Catonsville, Maryland, the pastor said masses on the front lawn of the church.[48] In Salt Lake City, home of the Mormons, the weekly papers greeted closures of all public places including churches, 'though seemingly drastic', as 'entirely justified'.[49] The Episcopalian bishop of San Francisco suggested that the closures gave incentives to 'greater devotion'.[50] In small-town Franklin, Louisiana, the local paper enjoined its Bible readers to abide by the ordinance as 'the only way to stop the spread of Spanish Influenza'.[51] In Birmingham, Alabama, the Pastors' Union complied unanimously, 'pledging wholehearted support'.[52] And Detroit's Temple Beth-El cancelled services before any closures were called.[53]

Instead of resisting, the clergy often donated their premises, staffs, and students to the cause, as on 8 October when the capital's pastors offered their churches rent-free

[39] Ibid., 17 October 1918, 22.   [40] *Washington Times*, 16 October 1918, front page.
[41] *Sun*, 24 October 1918, 12.
[42] *Watchman and Southron*, 16 October 1918. A similar case comes from Evanston, Illinois; *Evening Public Ledger*, 10 October 1918, front page.
[43] *Boston Globe*, 23 October 1918, 2.   [44] Ibid., 6 October 1918, 4.
[45] *El Paso Herald*, 23 October 1918, 10.
[46] Few letters to editors criticized orders for church closures. In one from the *Baltimore Sun*, 23 October 1918, 6, a Presbyterian pastor argued that the ordinance fanned the pandemic's ferocity but gave no hint of resistance.
[47] *Baltimore Sun*, 6 October 1918, 11.   [48] Ibid., 19 October 1918, 9.
[49] *Goodwin's Weekly*, 12 October 1918, 6.   [50] *San Francisco Chronicle*, 19 October 1918, 6.
[51] *Era-Leader*, 10 October 1918, front page.
[52] *Birmingham Age-Herald*, 9 October 1918, 5.   [53] *Detroit Free Press*, 22 October 1918, 7.

as temporary hospitals for influenza patients.[54] In Philadelphia, the Catholic arch-bishop volunteered seminary students to dig graves for the piles of unburied influenza victims,[55] and several weeks later converted church buildings into emergency influenza hospitals.[56] Such acts of kindness and sacrifice spread westward with similar cross-denominational zeal as seen in Philadelphia, where the pastor of the Union Tabernacle Church ministered to the sick of 'Hebrew' families.[57] San Francisco's archbishop donated equipment and resources to the Red Cross and later addressed the inadequacies of the Red Cross relief stations by 'commandeering' the Sisters of Mercy to work under the Red Cross until further notice, to 'treat every needy case immediately...without reference to race, sect, creed, or color'.[58] In summary, America's Great Pandemic may not have been entirely free from blame. The blame, however, differed markedly from the deadly accusations made against Jews or beggars during the Black Death or against the Chinese, blacks, and tramps with smallpox. Influenza complaints hardly spread beyond three big cities on the East Coast, and none galvanized mass murder or even individual acts of violence. Draconian impositions, instead, led to cooperation and offers of charity.

QUARANTINE

To understand socio-psychological reactions to the Great Influenza—the near absence of blame and total absence of mass violence in the face of the most conta-gious pandemic in world history—sociopolitical contexts, especially those sur-rounding the Great War will be discussed in the penultimate section of Chapter 21. Another context produced by the pandemic itself was, nevertheless, essential for our understanding of the reaction to it and is more perplexing. That context con-cerns the thicket of ordinances passed by municipalities, states, and the federal government to combat the disease and efforts to change behavioural norms imme-diately. Such advice appeared daily in large- and small-town newspapers across America, such as 'Uncle Sam's Advice' scripted by Surgeon General Rupert Blue.[59] These ordinances and guidelines intruded more deeply into daily routines of ordin-ary people than yellow fever or smallpox quarantines and arguably more so than with any other disease or national emergency in US history.

The decrees varied from one locale to another. Not all places closed all venues of public assembly, as we have seen with Philadelphia's 'thirsties' allowed to escape their city's alcohol restrictions by crossing the river to New Jersey or with New York

---

[54] *Washington Times*, 8 October 1918, 15. For similar altruistic acts, see *Sun*, 6 October 1918, 12; and *Evening Public Ledger*, 30 October 1918, 10.
[55] *Evening Public Ledger*, 9 October 1918, 2.　　[56] Ibid., 24 October 1918, 9.
[57] *Evening Public Ledger*, 30 October 1918, 10.
[58] *San Francisco Chronicle*, 24 October 1918, 9. For a similar hospital conversion, see *Ogden Standard*, 17 October 1918, 10.
[59] Another, entitled 'Official Health Bulletin on Influenza: Latest Word on Subject', appeared regularly in small-town newspapers such as *Pullman Herald*, 18 October 1918, 4; and *Monroe City Democrat*, 18 October 1918, 7.

City's more relaxed recommendations.[60] But overwhelmingly, across the country, closures of public places of entertainment and engagement from schools to soda parlors were the norm. Newspapers' social pages lamented cancellations of concerts and parties, while sports pages notified disruptions to college football and district baseball.[61] In Chester, Pennsylvania, the Public Health Department requested that all funerals be prohibited, 'especially of influenza victims', but of other deaths as well.[62] In Boston, all trials by jury were suspended.[63] In Corpus Christi, Texas, and other places, restrictions on public gatherings went further, disallowing men from congregating in barber shops or at shoe-shine stands.[64] In early October, the *Washington Times's* social pages reflected on 'living under what amounts to a city-wide quarantine', concluding that 'there was nothing left to do but eat and pray but not in groups'.[65] Colleges and universities such as Bryn Mawr,[66] Amherst,[67] Mount Holyoke,[68] and the Christian Girls' College of St Louis[69] not only closed classrooms but became virtual quarantine camps, imposing strict rules prohibiting students from leaving campuses for the disease's duration. At the University of Missouri (Columbia), fear of contracting influenza on trains led to ordinances preventing women students leaving town in September before the disease even hit the Midwest.[70]

With the pandemic sweeping south and west, communities adopted wholesale quarantine restrictions and closures more quickly than had happened in the northeast. On 7 October, 'as a precautionary measure' (with no influenza cases yet in town), the county sheriff closed all schools and other institutions of learning along with churches, picture shows, and 'all other places of public gathering' in Columbia, South Carolina.[71] Already, a week earlier, its military academy and university, the Citadel, had closed, 'furloughing' all students.[72] In Cloverport, Kentucky, before local physicians had diagnosed a case, the State Board of Health closed all public places.[73] Similarly, with only 'a few cases' reported in the entire county of Lancaster and Garrard, officials closed 'all public meeting places',[74] and the list goes on, with Warren, Minnesota,[75] Bisbee, Arizona,[76] Tombstone, Arizona,[77] and the entire state of Colorado[78] closing public places after a few isolated cases or none at all. Instead of resisting such measures, which newspapers often labelled 'drastic', organizations

---

[60] *Sun*, 10 October 1918, 8; and *New-York Tribune*, 29 September 1918, 18. While Copeland believed the subway was spreading the pandemic, he only 'advised against the overcrowding of cars'. The Navy took more vigorous steps, closing the subway to all sailors; *Evening World*, 18 October 1918, 16.

[61] See, for instance, *Washington Times*, 21 September 1918, 10.

[62] *Evening Public Ledger*, 5 October 1918, front page.

[63] *New-York Tribune*, 9 October 1918, 7.

[64] *Corpus Christi Caller*, 22 October 1918, 4.   [65] *Washington Times*, 6 October 1918, 14.

[66] *Sun*, 6 October 1918, 18.   [67] Ibid., 13 October 1918, section 6, 5.

[68] Ibid., 5 October 1918, 5.   [69] *Evening Missourian*, 7 October 1918, 4.

[70] Ibid., 26 September 1918, 4. The paper does not explain why the ban pertained to women only.

[71] *Keowee Courier*, 9 October 1918, front page.   [72] Ibid., 9 October 1918, 5.

[73] *Breckenridge News*, 9 October 1918, 5.   [74] *Central Record*, 10 October 1918, 4.

[75] *Warren Sheaf*, 16 October 1918, front page.

[76] *Bisbee Daily Review*, 6 October 1918, front page; also the University of Arizona (Tucson) was quarantined before influenza arrived; ibid., 5 October 1918, front page.

[77] *Tombstone Epitaph*, 6 October 1918, front page.

[78] *Bisbee Daily Review*, 8 October 1918, 2.

and businesses (like the owners of the Royal Theatre in Oregon, Missouri) and city councils (as in Lancaster, Kentucky) imposed or voluntarily extended quarantine on themselves before they were legislated. In Corpus Christi, the city's soda-fountain businesses agreed amongst themselves to close indefinitely.[79] Mount Vernon, Kentucky, called on the entire county to quarantine itself. Houses with suspected cases were to be placarded with rules recently established at Louisville, with every case 'rigidly' isolated for at least ten days or until 'the patriot' entirely recovered, and with family members agreeing to be isolated.[80]

As this last example illustrates, these quarantines were not restricted to public spaces; they entered the private sphere. The long list of closures in Perrysburg, Ohio, made these strictures clear: after listing 'all public, private, and parochial schools, the library, motion picture shows, churches, Sunday schools, billiard and pool tables, dance halls, soda water fountains, soft drink parlors', 'all gatherings public or private... either indoors and outdoors' were forbidden.[81] Such regulations penetrated the inner sanctum of the family. In Welsh, Calcasieu Parish, Louisiana, the mayor ordered that no gatherings were to take place, either of 'a public or private nature'. In addition, parents were responsible for keeping their children off the streets and from visiting friends' houses.[82] In Chicago, children were not allowed on the streets, and the police were ordered to disperse street-corner gatherings of any sort.[83] In Bismarck, North Dakota, the City Health Commissioner supplied greater detail on matters of parental control. 'A special police' was formed to patrol the streets, instructed to arrest children not kept at home. Parents were held responsible 'to which absolutely no exceptions will be made'. The Commissioner assured citizens that this notice was not simply a local ordinance; rather, Surgeon General Blue had endorsed it as 'a war measure'.[84] In Little Falls, Minnesota, the city council added another layer to the enforcement. Two members of the home guard were stationed in each ward to spy on children, seeing to it that those belonging to different families remained separated.[85]

Placarding houses, apartments, and hotels containing suspected cases became another general practice across the US and its territories.[86] In Corpus Christi, health authorities threatened violators of quarantine even within their own homes with deportation to pest houses.[87] Raising special forces to enforce influenza ordinances was not just a measure of small-town America. Despite Copeland's laissez-faire approach, as early as 30 September, he posted guards to patrol the city's

---

[79] *Corpus Christi Caller*, 22 October 1918, 4.

[80] *Mount Vernon Signal*, 18 October 1918, front page.

[81] *Perrysburg Journal*, 17 October 1918, 4.

[82] *Rice Belt Journal*, 11 October 1918, front page.

[83] *Bisbee Daily Review*, 19 October 1918, front page.

[84] *Bismarck Tribune*, 9 October 1918, 3.

[85] *Little Falls Herald*, 1 November 1918, front page; *Alliance Herald*, 24 October 1918, reported that they were 'doing the police work', enforcing quarantine 'night and day'.

[86] For instance, city and state departments in Salt Lake City placarded homes 'in large letters—INFLUENZA'; *Ogden Standard*, 30 October 1918; *Evening Missourian*, 15 October 1918, front page. For the Hawaiian Islands, *Mani News*, 25 October 1918, 2. For Norwood, Massachusetts, Fanning, *Influenza and Inequality*, 78.

[87] *Corpus Christi Caller*, 24 October 1918, front page.

railway stations for suspected cases. Physicians and nurses were ordered to 'round up' all influenza suspects,[88] and on 10 October he created a new 'Health Squad' of seventy-five policemen to enforce influenza regulations.[89]

With cases and deaths rising sharply through October, not only those with influenza or suspected of carrying it were isolated. At Klamath Falls, Oregon, children with common colds were turned away from schools.[90] Even with cases of influenza on the decline at the end of October, the capital's Health Board excluded all pupils with heavy colds from attending school,[91] and 'all employees with colds' were forced to quit work.[92] Here, the state intruded into people's lives in other ways. War workers were allowed to hail any car not already filled, and the driver was coerced to stop and transport them.[93] And at least in one town—Minersville, Pennsylvania, where the mortality rate had jumped to 3 per cent with victims' bodies left in houses for days—the military imposed martial law.[94] Quarantine control of military camps was more severe. Detailed regulations and permits were imposed on officers and enlisted men alike. At Fort Bliss, outside El Paso, no officer or enlisted man was permitted to leave his post or camp, and those in El Paso at the time of the order (16 October) seen 'loitering' were to be arrested immediately.[95]

A more in-depth study of special anti-influenza town ordinances would expose further examples of Draconian infringements on civil liberties and constitutional rights as Patricia Fanning has shown for Norwood, Massachusetts. During the pandemic, all wakes and informal visitations were banned; immigrants were removed from their neighbourhoods to quarantine centres; new statutes required disinfection of infected homes with $100 fines for any opposition or violation. Permission was granted to the town's Board of Heath to enter and inspect homes. Private citizens were required to notify officials of any outbreaks of the disease within their premises. Yet Fanning has found only three arrests for violations, all of which concerned doctors' failures to report cases of influenza.[96] Nonetheless, she speculates: 'Such measures could easily create a climate of conspiracy and suspicion within ethnic neighbourhoods.'[97] However, despite her scrupulous archival research and later interviews of survivors, she reports no conspiracies or resistance to these measures.

COUGHING, SPITTING, KISSING, AND BIG TALKERS

The advice of the press and tools of the state intruded still further into the minutiae of everyday intimacy. This preaching equalled or surpassed any degrees of surveillance into private lives that even seventeenth-century Puritans might have envisioned. They extended to ordinances patrolled by special police to arrest those coughing, sneezing, kissing, and even talking during the pandemic. First, across America, from

[88] *New-York Tribune*, 30 September 1918, 20.
[89] *Evening World*, 11 October 1918, front page.
[90] *Evening Herald*, 11 October 1918, front page.
[91] *Washington Times*, 31 October 1918, 2.   [92] Ibid., 21 October 1918, 3.
[93] Ibid.   [94] *Evening Public Ledger*, 12 October 1918, front page.
[95] *El Paso Herald*, 16 October 1918, 5.   [96] Fanning, *Influenza and Inequality*, 100–4.
[97] Ibid., 102.

September 1918 on, the Surgeon General's 'latest word on the subject' of influenza, published across newspapers, listed points of practical advice from physicians and biologists on how to avoid the epidemic. The first line of every notice set in bold type the command: 'avoid contact with other people so far as possible', and 'especially crowds', 'persons suffering from "cold", sore throats and coughs'. The articles put the public on watch for 'any person who coughs or sneezes without covering his mouth or nose'.[98] On occasion, such condemnation of careless coughers and sneezers was more emphatic as during the week of 11 October. A headline, 'Coughs and Sneezes Spread Diseases', was accompanied by a drawing of a man sneezing and not covering his nose, and a caption that read, 'As Dangerous as Poison Gas Shells'.[99] Other newspapers editorialized their own condemnations. On 20 September, weeks before declared cases had crossed state lines to infect the non-military population, the *Evening Missourian* preached:

> To cough or sneeze without holding a handkerchief...is rudely careless at any time, but to do so...with influenza is scarcely less than criminal.[100]

The same day, an article in the *New-York Tribune* under the headline 'War on the Sneezers and Coughers' praised Commissioner Copeland for his strategies, in particular calling on 'movie' picture men, theatre owners, and transport officials to engage in 'a campaign of placards...to warn the public against the dangers of sneezing and coughing'. It proclaimed that influenza was spread 'almost entirely through these two anti-social acts'. The paper then called for public action that, in effect, endorsed vigilante violence:

> The public might well adopt toward the sneezers and coughers the slogan of our pugnacious American Tank Corps: 'Treat 'Em Rough' [see Figure 20.1]. It would then not be very long before this pest was generally abolished.[101]

By October this war was not solely one of words. On the 6th, in what appeared to be an about-face in his laissez-faire policies, Copeland placed a notice in the *Sun*:

> Sneezers to be put out: I have had my inspectors visit these places, see the managers and direct them to instruct their waiters to watch the people and if they catch them sneezing to invite them to leave at once.

A week later, 'coughing or sneezing in a public place without covering the mouth or nose' was made a criminal offence, punishable by a fine up to $500 (almost a year's average wages[102]), one year in prison, or both.[103] In addition, the pandemic inaugurated 'crusades against spitting'. New York launched its campaign on 12 September,[104] and on 26 October, Copeland bragged that his 'crusade against

---

[98] For instance, *Pullman Herald*, 18 October 1918, 4.
[99] *Mount Vernon Signal*, 11 October 1918, 4; and *Monroe City Democrat*, 18 October 1918, 7.
[100] *Evening Missourian*, 20 September 1918, 4.
[101] *New-York Tribune*, 20 September 1918, 8. In October, moving picture shows broadcasted the 'Dangers of Sneeze and Kiss'; *Detroit Free Press*, 9 October 1918, 9.
[102] Douglas, 'Wages and Hours'.
[103] *Bisbee Daily Review*, 12 October 1918, 4: '$500 per sneeze'.
[104] *New-York Tribune*, 12 September 1918, 3; and *Sun*, 12 September 1918, 12.

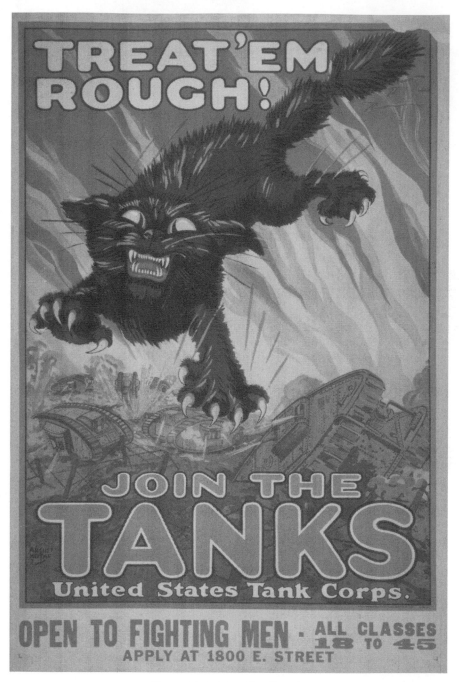

Figure 20.1. Treat 'Em Rough.

spitters' had arrested 500 and added it was still in progress.[105] In late September, Boston posted 'Big placards' throughout the city, announcing 'dire penalties to spitters'.[106] By 5 October, anti-spitting laws spread to Philadelphia and by the 6th to Washington.[107] At the end of October, Paris in Bourbon County, Kentucky, was imposing fines of $5 on anyone with a cold spitting on pavements or in any public place. The local paper claimed that a large number of cities were fining those failing to cover their mouths or noses with a handkerchief.[108] By the end of October, penalties for spitting increased from a maximum sentence of ten days in gaol and $25 to three months in the county prison.[109] News of America's coughing ordinances even made the Chinese press.[110]

With the resurgence of influenza in Boston in December, authorities condemned not only coughers and sneezers, but also 'talkers' as dangerous. The city health commissioner called 'forcibly talking in crowds' one of the 'most potent agencies of spreading influenza'; such acts were 'assaults upon assembled persons'. The perpetrators were 'dangerous at best' and were to be excluded from crowded places. The Health Department prepared placards to be displayed throughout the city prohibiting coughers, sneezers, and talkers from entering places of assembly.[111] In Lynchburg, Virginia, in mid-October, the mayor issued a proclamation forbidding people from stopping on the street to talk, and police were given special orders to break up public conversations.[112] Other countries also turned on spitters. In Adelaide, Australia, the city council promised 'to take stringent action' against persons spitting on city footpaths.[113] And Milan's *Corriere della Sera* blamed the spread of the disease on 'too many people, who with impunity spit in trams, railway cars, cafés, and inns'.[114] Even the air was patrolled. In Phoenix, Arizona, a special police force was hired to prevent groups from gathering, warning businesses 'that each customer must be allowed at least 1,200 cubic feet of air space'.[115]

Advice and ordinances entered further into intimate zones, one which had little, if anything, to do with public space—kissing. Well before the pandemic reached Missouri, the *Evening Missourian* demanded of its readers: 'Don't kiss'.[116] When influenza struck, the paper's admonitions became sterner, with the onus put on women. Citing a Dr Clarke, it charged, 'Kissing is criminal' and advised, 'Now is the time for University women to be unsociable'.[117] Eight days later, advising 'How to Avoid Influenza', a Kansas City physician asserted: 'I believe the epidemic had its start in Kansas City by girls kissing soldiers in the army, schools, and cantonments, who had become carriers of the disease.'[118] Also, in Salt Lake City, in September,

[105] *Birmingham Age-Herald*, 26 October 1918, front page.
[106] Ibid., 23 September 1918, 2.
[107] *Evening Public Ledger*, 5 October 1918, front page; and *Washington Times*, 6 October 1918, 22.
[108] *Bourbon News*, 29 October 1918, front page.
[109] *San Francisco Chronicle*, 24 October 1918, 9.
[110] *Millard's Review*, 14 December 1918, 62.   [111] *Boston Globe*, 19 December 1918, 2.
[112] *Baltimore Sun*, 15 October 1918, 8.   [113] *Barrier Miner*, 4 February 1919, 4.
[114] *Corriere della Sera*, 14 January 1919, 3; and *Il Messaggero*, 11 October 1918, 3.
[115] Luckingham, *Epidemic in the Southwest*, 45–6 and 51.
[116] *Evening Missourian*, 20 September 1918, 4.   [117] Ibid., 10 October 1918, 4.
[118] *Kansas City Star*, 18 October 1918, front page.

well before signs of flu appeared, the Health Commissioner warned that kissing was the most effective means to spread the disease and commanded: 'Hooverize on kissing'.[119] Phoenix, Arizona, true to form, had already gone further, passing an anti-influenza ordinance outlawing kissing on 2 October. As the *Tombstone Epitaph* clarified, 'It makes no difference whether people are engaged'.[120] A week later, the state's chief health officer called a conference of Arizona's 'prominent doctors' and agreed on seven 'rules and regulations to be enforced throughout the state'. Posters of the laws were placarded 'in all public places' and attached to homes with influenza. Its second rule instructed against coughing, sneezing, kissing, and shaking hands.[121] Even if other cities did not pass ordinances banning kissing, their advice was the same. Dr Max Starkloff, Health Commissioner of St Louis, regularly published his 'list of Don'ts', which included: 'Keep away from other people' and 'Do not kiss anyone', especially babies. His columns spread westward from Missouri to small towns as far as Oregon.[122]

The papers do not always reveal how the ordinances were enforced, but advice from papers, physicians, health officers, and the Surgeon General in weekly reports posed clear deterrents with a barrage of warnings to avoid crowds, to leave the ill to themselves, even to 'rough up' those contravening social norms. In this climate of fear and Draconian measures for disease prevention, what should have been expected from crowds when someone on a tram suddenly was seized by uncontrollable sneezing, coughing, or the need to expectorate? What is curious with this most devastating pandemic was that not a single paper recorded a single incident of violence against the afflicted, nothing like the multitude of assaults faced by the smallpox-afflicted across America during recent epidemics that were less contagious than the Great Influenza. Despite bold headlines demanding that the public shun crowds and especially those showing the slightest symptoms, kin, neighbours, priests, surgeons, nurses, and law enforcers are not reported abandoning loved ones or their responsibilities, as seen during the Black Death or smaller epidemics of cholera, plague, yellow fever, and smallpox. Out of thousands of news pages, I have found only one story in which fear led professionals to shirk service. In Somerville, outside of Boston, patrolmen 'balked' at driving the police ambulance to convey influenza patients to the hospital.[123]

THE MASK

Rather than fear, it was its absence that contributed to the most sustained opposition to state infringement on personal liberties during the Great Flu. This opposition focused on mostly municipal ordinances requiring citizens to wear

[119] *Salt Lake Telegram*, 20 September 1918, 13: 'Beware the Kiss!'; and *Montgomery Advertiser*, 28 October 4: 'Outlaw the Kiss'.
[120] *Tombstone Epitaph*, 6 October 1918, 5.
[121] Numerous papers published it, for instance, *Bisbee Daily Review*, 12 November 1918, 8.
[122] For instance, *Red Lake News*, 1 November 1918, 2; *Rogue River Courier*, 11 October 1918, 4; and *Deming Graphic*, 11 October 1918, 6.
[123] *Boston Globe*, 30 September 1918, 4.

masks in public, which in some cities included the great outdoors. However, thus far, significant resistance to these laws has emerged in only one city across the entire world—San Francisco.[124] Pushed by the city's Head of Public Health, Dr William Hassler, citizens on 24 October were forced to don specially designed gauze influenza masks anytime they ventured from home, except while eating in restaurants.[125] A week later, influenza cases declined, and Hassler and San Francisco were credited for the success. Nonetheless, citizens soon resented the impositions, which some considered a violation of constitutional liberties. Some wore masks drooped from chins, while others refused to wear them altogether. Hassler and the police retaliated, raiding hotel lobbies and arresting 'hundreds' with fines from $5 to thirty days in gaol.[126] With cases dropping, the city's Health Board rescinded the ordinance on 21 November.[127]

Within a week, cases climbed, and the mayor and city council made the mask compulsory on 7 December. Opposition now became more vocal and cut across class lines. Scepticism over its efficacy grew, and the press pointed to contradictions in its rationale—that it was required in wide-open spaces as in parks but not in crowded restaurants.[128] In mid-October, scientific news that influenza's agent was far too small to be blocked by any gauze reached headlines worldwide.[129] But the most important opposition came from merchants and shopkeepers, who feared the law would curtail Christmas sales.[130]

Unlike even the most respectable of anti-vaccine demonstrations in late nineteenth-century England,[131] mask opposition did not extend to mass rallies or organized demonstrations, and certainly was not reminiscent of events in San Francisco only eighteen years before, when the national public health authority placed Chinatown under quarantine, sparking legal battles and city-wide demonstrations that occasionally turned violent.[132] The only threat of public violence connected with the mask was an act by an unknown lone figure who planted a bomb probably intended for Dr Hassler. It never exploded and, if intended for the commissioner, was delivered to the wrong address.[133] Another act of violence, not reported by any secondary source I know, derived not from the public, but from a public health official, who shot a horseshoer in broad daylight for not wearing a mask.[134] No reported charges against the officer ensued; no riots, no complaints, not even city-wide coverage of the event.[135]

---

[124] Crosby, *America's Forgotten Pandemic*, ch. 7, 91–121, taken mostly from the *San Francisco Chronicler*. Also, Bristow, *American Pandemic*, 115–18.

[125] *New-York Tribune*, 25 October 1918, 14; and *Bourbon News*, 29 October 1918, 4, claimed that fines for violations as high as $1,000.

[126] Crosby, *America's Forgotten Pandemic*, 105.   [127] Ibid., 106.   [128] Ibid., 109.

[129] Several US papers reported the discovery less than three days after the news broke in Paris: for instance, *Oklahoma City Times*, 15 October 1918, 8.

[130] Crosby, *America's Forgotten Pandemic*, 109.   [131] See Chapter 10.

[132] See Chapter 14.

[133] Crosby, *America's Forgotten Pandemic*, 110; and *Hays Free Press*, 26 December 1918, 2, from an interview with Dr Hassler, who received threatening letters.

[134] *Rogue River Courier*, 29 October 1918, 4; and *Los Angeles Times*, 29 October 1918, 16.

[135] I found no reference to the incident in the CDNC.

Again, with the fall in influenza cases, the mask ordinance was rescinded on 19 December. When the pandemic returned in a third wave, the mask was imposed again on 17 January, and influenza cases fell. Emboldened by success, Hassler's men staged raids arresting 'hundreds' found without masks, prompting the 'Anti-Mask League' to form. Splintered by various conflicting political persuasions, its life was short, failing to survive even the first meeting. During shouting matches among attendees, the man renting the hall switched off the lights and all left.[136]

Instead of mass demonstrations or attacks aligned by class that challenged the latest scientific findings, the mask's controversy concerned convenience or at most individual liberties: 'the average man' wore the mask 'slung to the back of his neck' until he came in sight of a policeman, and most people 'had holes cut into them to stick their cigars and cigarettes through'.[137] The issues were also fought with sophisticated debates on medical breakthroughs and statistical correlations presented in newspapers. Hassler had the good fortune that moments of imposing the mask roughly matched falls in influenza cases. Yet other places, where no mask ordinances had been imposed, showed the same trends, such as San Mateo in the Bay area.[138] The head of California's State Board of Health presented statistics from San Francisco's best-run hospital: trained nurses had consistently worn masks but 78 per cent of them caught the disease.[139] Out-of-state papers entered the fray, highlighting cities such as Chicago, where there were no mask ordinances but the consequences were 'no worse'.[140]

*   *   *

No one has yet attempted to evaluate the extent of mask ordinances in the US or other countries: was San Francisco's experience the tip of the iceberg, or an exceptional case of civil disobedience? First, in the metropolitan regions and suburban towns of the north-east, in New England and the Mid-Atlantic states, no news of universal mask legislation appears. At most, masks remained a recommendation or compulsory only for certain professions. For the north-east, Washington receives the most headlines. On 12 October, its head of Public Health advised citizens to wear masks and placarded the city with his request, but it remained only a request.[141] The next day, he recommended that only barbers and dentists wear them,[142] and several days later, 'prescribed' it for any riding streetcars.[143] No opposition was reported. Instead, DC's residences seem to have embraced it enthusiastically with 'Washington's army of women war workers' appearing 'on crowded street cars and at their desks, muffled in gauze shields',[144] a '"Flu" harem of masks'.[145]

---

[136] Crosby, *America's Forgotten Pandemic*, 112.
[137] *Garland City Globe*, 28 November 1918, front page.
[138] Crosby, *America's Forgotten Pandemic*, 112.
[139] Ibid., 112–13. Also, *Sausalito News*, 1 February 1919, 6, charged that Hassler's statistics had been massaged.
[140] *Oklahoma City Times*, 14 December 1918, 10.
[141] *Washington Herald*, 12 October 1918, front page; and *Washington Times*, 12 October 1918, front page.
[142] *Washington Times*, 13 October 1918, 17.   [143] *Sun*, 16 October 1918, 16.
[144] *Oklahoma City Times*, 16 October 1918, 3.   [145] *Washington Times*, 20 October 1918, 3.

By mid-October, New York City's head of public health ordered barbers to wear them, but, according to the papers, the mask never became contentious.[146] Baltimore's health commissioner recommended that hospital attendants nursing influenza patients wear masks along with waiters and waitresses and others serving food in hotels and restaurants.[147] Little more is heard of mask recommendations or ordinances in these cities. Only at the end of December did Boston require doctors, nurses, dentists, and barbers to wear them, but only when 'in close proximity with influenza patients'. The city's Health Commission made it clear that mandatory wearing 'was not even contemplated' and that it regarded such orders as 'of little value'.[148] From Boston to Columbia, Missouri, I find only two further cities passing mask ordinances. In Jersey City, barbers were required to wear them while cutting hair and shaving,[149] and at the end of the year, Buffalo's policemen, but here it appears the law was not taken seriously: '[it] presented a loophole: policemen were allowed to cut holes in their masks in order to smoke'.[150]

In the Midwest, mask ordinances were slightly more in evidence. As the pandemic reached its peak, Chicago 'warned' citizens to wear masks,[151] but as a story later in this section suggests, the warning appears to have gone unheeded. In Detroit, unlike in neighbouring Chicago, the mask seems to have taken hold. With increased influenza cases in mid-November, health authorities in Indianapolis, Indiana, decreed that every resident 'must go about his business today wearing a mask'. The restriction does not appear to have included the outdoors, and the penalties fell on businesses or theatres, not individuals.[152] At the end of the month, the health board of Des Moines, Iowa, compelled 'everyone' to wear masks while in public.[153] In Cresco, Iowa, persons attending influenza patients were asked to wear them.[154]

In addition, special mask laws were imposed for special places. At the military base of Camp Gordon, south-west of Augusta, Georgia, servicemen were required to wear masks while attending performances.[155] At the University of Missouri, returning soldiers in late October were required to wear them in classrooms, before that rule was extended to all students.[156] In the cattle pens of Bourbon County, Kentucky, 'colored men and women' were forced to wear them.[157]

Urging the populace to wear influenza masks, or enacting legislation to make it compulsory, was far more pervasive in the Far West. Yet even here such ordinances appear in only fourteen municipalities from my searches, and several pertained to tiny places—Logan, Utah; Miami, Arizona; and Lynden, Washington. For some, the

---

[146] *Princeton Union*, 17 October 1918, 4, made it a joking matter.
[147] *Baltimore Sun*, 10 October 1918, 16.   [148] *Washington Herald*, 29 December 1918, 2.
[149] *Breckenridge News*, 23 October 1918, 7.
[150] *Daily Gate City*, 26 December 1918, 6. For ordinances in Americus and Macon, Georgia, see Chapter 22, note 36.
[151] *Chicago Daily Tribune*, 20 October 1918, A1.
[152] *Evening Missourian*, 19 November 1918, 2.
[153] *Daily Ardmoreite*, 30 November 1918, front page.
[154] *Cresco Plain Dealer*, 18 October 1918, front page.
[155] *Evening World*, 23 October 1918, 8.
[156] *Evening Missourian*, 26 October 1918, front page; 28 October 1918, front page.
[157] *Bourbon News*, 15 November 1918, 5.

law was brief as in Lynden: citizens 'wrestled' with the ordinance 'but for one day'.[158] California appears as the leader. Not only did San Francisco receive the widest attention, it was first to adopt city-wide enforcement. Moreover, California was one of the few states to enact the laws beyond a municipality. Before San Francisco's ordinance, the State Board of Health ordered barbers and hotel-room attendants to wear them,[159] and no opposition followed.

The next ordinance requiring masks to be worn appeared in Miami, Arizona, but pertained only to barbers, waiters, soda dispensers, and clerks.[160] Mask legislation and protests against it were more significant in Tucson and Phoenix. Tucson required everyone to wear one at all times outside the home, and twenty-five plain-clothes policemen were hired to patrol the city and enforce this law. After fifty-one days, with influenza on the decline, quarantines on a large range of public places and gatherings were rescinded but not the mask. Instead, the mayor of Tucson stepped up enforcement, sending a policeman into every church to ensure compliance. A prominent city banker defied the law, was arrested, challenged it in the courts, and won his case. Yet 'most citizens' cooperated with the law.[161] In Phoenix, a mask ordinance was passed later, on 26 November, with heavier penalties than elsewhere, reaching $100, thirty days in gaol, or both. Papers reckoned that 95 per cent of the population abided by the law, though some poked holes in their masks to smoke.[162]

In late October, the *Ogden Standard* reported with foreboding that Utah would compel 'every person in the state' to wear masks at work.[163] The ordinance was never enacted. Yet Ogden City already had a local ordinance compelling those with flu to wear one when leaving home. Not until the third week of November does another ordinance appear. Denver's commissioners demanded rigorous enforcement with 'drastic steps'.[164] At the outset, policemen were stationed on street corners to prevent anyone without a mask from boarding streetcars.[165] But Denver's experience did not replicate San Francisco's with surprise raids or arrests of 'hundreds'. Instead, health officials recognized the difficulties of enforcement and quickly annulled the law.[166]

Around the same time, debate on whether the mask should become mandatory in Utah intensified. First, the proposal was delayed for physicians to seek advice on its efficacy.[167] By early December, physicians had launched a campaign against it, arguing that the measures were not only ineffective but could be 'a positive menace'. Evidence came 'pouring in from all over the country' testifying to the mask's deficiencies.[168] Nonetheless, several communities in Utah enacted restrictions: one was Ogden City, despite its paper's strong opposition. But its Health Board

---

[158] *Lynden Tribune*, 14 November 1918, 3.   [159] *Ogden Standard*, 19 October 1918, 11.
[160] *El Paso Herald*, 26 October 1918, 5.   [161] Luckingham, *Epidemic in the Southwest*, ch. 4.
[162] Ibid., 53–4. San Diego also imposed heavy fines; *Los Angeles Times*, 12 December 1918, I, 17.
[163] *Ogden Standard*, 26 October 1918, 14.
[164] It was the only other city that Crosby, *America's Forgotten Pandemic*, 112, examined regarding the mask.
[165] *El Paso Herald*, 25 November 1918, 5.
[166] It lasted only a few days; *Ogden Standard*, 23 November 1918, 5.
[167] Ibid., 5.   [168] Ibid., 3 December 1918, 4.

refused to enforce the fines.[169] The final place found in 'Chronicling America' newspapers was another small town—Douglas, Arizona. Like Denver, it posted police on street corners. Their ordinance outlived Denver's but lasted little over a week until Christmas Eve with only four ever charged.[170] Other sources report further places where the ordinances were promulgated, as illustrated by a story in Manchester's *Guardian*. In March, a woman travelling from Chicago, where mask wearing was not compulsory and little practised,[171] stepped from her train at Pasadena, where the ordinance was in force. The sight of masses covered in white masks reduced her to delirium, not from fear of influenza but because she thought she had been besieged by the Klu Klux Klan.[172]

The California Digital Newspaper Collection (CDNC) provides further insights into the mask and its reception. Newspaper reports in this database for 1918–19 cluster in Marin County, north of San Francisco. Coverage of the flu from the two papers paying greatest attention to the pandemic (*Marin Journal* and *Sausalito News*) was more akin to archival documents than newspapers, detailing town meetings—who attended, what was said, what was decided. In addition, these papers reported news on mask laws in neighbouring towns. The *Sausalito News* proudly boasted that its town was among the first in the Bay Area to pass the legislation.[173] Two others—Mill Valley and the county seat, San Rafael—soon followed, and then criticized Sausalito's supposed slack enforcement.[174] Town meetings also relate how the legislation was received. On 2 November, a few days after the ordinance had passed but before it came into force, Sausalito's town councillors ('trustees') were indignant that the ordinance was not yet being enforced, even though the law had yet to take effect. The paper tarred the maskless as 'slackers...menacing public health and flaunting their criminal foolhardiness in the faces of the prudent people'.[175] But despite this seeming division between 'slackers' and the 'prudent', no physical hostilities flared up that day or afterwards.[176] With the return of influenza in December, Sausalito's trustees now refused to follow San Francisco's lead;[177] no more is heard on the mask from Sausalito.

Belief in the mask's effectiveness was much more pronounced in the US than elsewhere, except possibly in Australia, where initially the government of an entire state—New South Wales—imposed it on everyone on the streets or at public gatherings.[178] By contrast, papers in Italy, France, and Scotland hardly mention

---

[169] Ibid., 10 December 1918, 4.   [170] *Bisbee Daily Review*, 24 December 1918, 4.

[171] US papers such as *Oklahoma City Times*, 14 December 1918, 10, corroborated the *Guardian's* assertion.

[172] *Guardian*, 3 March 1919, 3. Some in Pasadena made a joke of the ordinances; see *Los Angeles Times*, 22 January 1919, I 16; and 24 January 1919, I 15. For Los Angeles' pride in keeping cases of influenza lower than San Francisco's without the mask, see ibid., 21 January 1919, II, front page. Portland, Washington, was another Western city where the mask was mooted but rejected; *Seattle Star*, 26 October 1918, 5.

[173] *Sausalito News*, 26 October 1918, front page; 2 November 1918, front page.

[174] Ibid., 2 November 1918, front page.   [175] Ibid.

[176] Along with Oakland and San Francisco, Sausalito discarded the mask on 23 November (ibid., 23 November 1918, 3).

[177] *Marin Journal*, 16 January 1911, 5; *Sausalito News*, 1 February 1919, 6.

[178] See, for instance, *Guardian*, 2 February 1919.

mask ordinances. For England, where coverage from online papers is more comprehensive than on the Continent, the mask was advised as a precautionary measure in large cities but only for certain groups—those nursing influenza patients in Manchester and Liverpool,[179] clerks in Bolton,[180] and theatre-goers in Liverpool.[181] None supported it with the zeal of San Francisco's Dr Hassler, and no opposition arose based on civil liberties. Questions over the mask became spirited only towards the end of the pandemic (early March 1919), six months after Nicolle's demonstration of the virus's filterability.[182] But those debating it appear restricted to the scientific community. Its supporters were few: Manchester's health officer, Dr Niven, several doctors in Liverpool,[183] some in Bolton.[184] By March, Britain's scientific community was united against it: the *Lancet* dubbed it 'a dubious remedy'.[185]

For Canada, no mask ordinances or recommendations arise, even for specific occupations, east of the Rockies. The single reported case of mandatory masking was in Alberta. Initially, it pertained to railway passengers only, and those without masks were only refused travel, not arrested, fined, or imprisoned.[186] Yet Alberta's legislation endured longer than San Francisco's, and later the penalties appear to have stiffened with 'scores' fined in police courts.[187] But by the end of November, the 'approved method of wearing a mask' was to keep it strapped beneath the chin 'until a policeman appears'.[188] As in Britain and most of the US, mask wearing in Canada failed to provoke conflict or civil disobedience.

*   *   *

Back to context, with those closest to the pandemic beset by the imposition of quarantines, ordinances against coughing, sneezing, spitting, kissing, talking, and mandated mask wearing, along with incessant advice to avoid crowds and shun the sick, certainly, no disease in American history imposed a net of restrictions as intrusive into private life as those produced during the Great Influenza. Given hypotheses by historians such as Sir Richard Evans that 'contagionism' and state policies such as quarantine that impinged on the rights of the public were key to understanding the power of epidemics to wreak violence,[189] the Great Influenza should have sparked conspiracies, rioting, hatred, and blame on a scale beyond the worst days of cholera violence. The following chapters on the Great Influenza instead illustrate the opposite. Despite these infringements and official encouragement to shun, even 'rough up', the ill and those in need, a contagion of volunteerism, compassion, and self-sacrifice stamped this pandemic.

*   *   *

---

[179] *Guardian*, 15 February 1919, 6; 20 February 1919, 7; and 28 February 1919, 7.
[180] Ibid., 1 March 1919, 7.   [181] Ibid., 25 February 1919, 4.
[182] Ibid., 2 March 1919, 5.   [183] Ibid., 20 February 1919, 7; and 28 February 1919, 7.
[184] Ibid., 1 March 1919, 7.
[185] Cited in Ibid., 1 March 1919, 6. It reported other physicians who condemned it.
[186] *New-York Tribune*, 22 October 1918, 12, from Calgary. The news appeared in numerous US papers; for instance, *Tulsa Daily World*, 22 October 1918, 4 and 6.
[187] *Bismarck Tribune*, 29 November 1918, 5.   [188] Ibid.
[189] Evans, 'Epidemics and Revolutions'; and Jones, *Influenza 1918*, 192.

Tangier's history of the Great Influenza poses a counterfactual case. Here, the pandemic created another micro-context, which might have sparked extreme violence against a traditional target—Jews. 'The epidemic found Tangier totally unprepared'. Because of its peculiar international status, governed by a council of the British, Spanish, and French, little was done to combat the disease or assist its victims. Death counts soared among the city's Moors and Europeans. The one group to protect themselves were Jews, who took 'rigorous measures' to guard their large, impoverished, and overcrowded population. While hundreds of Europeans and Moors died, 'not a single death' occurred within 'the Jewish colony'.[190] Yet no accusations of blame, conspiracies of poisoning, or pogroms against Jews stirred. Had a similarly striking religious disparity in death counts occurred during an attack of cholera, smallpox, or plague, would the consequences have been the same?

[190] *Guardian*, 12 October 1918, 5. Ten days later, death tolls of Moors and Europeans climbed rapidly; yet officials failed to act; ibid., 22 October 1918, 5. Finally, the French Protectorate intervened; the Sultan granted sums to clean the city and acquired additional doctors for the poor; ibid., 29 October 1918, 5.

21

The Great Influenza
A Pandemic of Compassion

Despite its rapid contagion, mysterious strain, and authorities' incessant campaigns to criminalize spitters, sneezers, and coughers, the Great Influenza across America failed to provoke social violence against victims of the disease or any 'others'. Admonitions from the press and health boards to avoid crowds and shun anyone showing the slightest signs of influenza certainly justified self-centred behaviour in the face of this deadly disease. Yet the medical profession and press were not all of one voice. On the same pages headlining 'Uncle Sam's Advice on Flu' and reporting resolutions of medical conferences warning the public to avoid the sick at all costs, health officers pleaded for nurses and teachers, now made idle by school closures, to dedicate their time to cleaning the houses of the afflicted, caring for the thousands orphaned, and nursing the dangerously ill.[1]

Given reactions to epidemics such as cholera, plague, and smallpox—less deadly (in terms of mortality rates), less contagious, and then less mysterious than the Great Influenza—the magnetic draw of this pandemic to mobilize volunteers to risk their lives for utter strangers is puzzling. In addition, those most eager and enthusiastic to do so were among the most susceptible to this influenza—young adults and especially young adult women in the prime of their lives.[2] It was also a rare moment in the history of the press, when praise of service and heroism overwhelmingly and disproportionately represented women. On occasion, the press may have even unfairly favoured women over men in acknowledging their volunteerism and martyrdom. A short article in Philadelphia's *Evening Public Ledger* commemorated together the lives of Dr Edwin Smith and Miss Rose Cummings, a student-nurse. Both worked and died the day before at St Joseph's Hospital in Philadelphia, 'martyrs to duty in ministering to influenza patients'. But the article placed the student nurse in the limelight. Only she received a full sentence praising her 'devotion assiduously to the task of attending the ill' for which she was stricken.[3] Similarly, an article in the *Baltimore Sun* announced that

---

[1] See Washington's desperate appeal for nurses; *Washington Times*, 6 October 1918, front page.

[2] Overall, women died in greater numbers than men from the Great Influenza, especially among young adults (Echeverri, 'Spanish Influenza'; Johnson, 'The Over-Shadowed Killer', 41; Ramanna, 'Coping with the Influenza', 89; *Le Matin*, 10 November 1918; *Le Figaro*, 31 December 1918 (for Paris). However, in Hartford, Connecticut, more men died than women, by as much as 58 per cent; Tuckel et al., 'The Diffusion of the Influenza', 170. According to Rice, 'Australia and New Zealand', 68, women and men died in equal numbers in Australia, New Zealand, and Europe.

[3] *Evening Public Ledger*, 9 October 1918, 2.

physicians from Johns Hopkins Hospital had volunteered for service against the pandemic. None was mentioned by name, but the article followed by reporting that seven professional nurses and twelve nurses' aides had registered the same day at the Red Cross, including three 'colored High School girls': all were named with their schools or addresses. The article's headline celebrated them, not Johns Hopkins' physicians.[4]

THE CHURCH

Nonetheless, men and gender-neutral institutions such as church congregations volunteered their services and facilities to combat the pandemic and were praised for doing so. Presumably, the thirty divinity students of the St Charles Seminary at Overbrook in Philadelphia who answered their archbishop's call to dig graves to relieve the city's piles of unburied influenza victims were mostly male.[5] As noted previously, Philadelphia's pastor, Dr Hunter, cared for influenza-stricken 'Hebrew families', when 'their ordinary devotional comfort could not be had'.[6] In early October, Philadelphia's *Evening Public Ledger* commemorated a Reverend Limmerick and unnamed priests at Gloucester and Camp Meade who sacrificed their lives, 'ministering to the sick and dying'.[7] In late October, the *Washington Times* praised one of the city's priests, who before his ordination had been a cabinetmaker; now he made caskets for his parishioners in his spare time.[8] On 7 October, the *Baltimore Sun* commemorated a priest and a male nurse, who died caring for soldiers at the camp: 'One does not have to go to the European battle fronts to learn stories of heroism.'[9]

To these few examples of male churchmen across denominations, contributions by Catholic nuns can be added. In fact, they appear as a more significant force in the US struggle against the pandemic. In its early stages in Baltimore, with cases still confined largely to nearby Camp Meade, the city's Cardinal Gibbons ordered the Sisters of Mercy to assist in caring for afflicted soldiers. In Philadelphia, 'one brave little nun' saved a family of seven, 'all stricken with influenza at once'. The paper made clear that this nun's sacrifice was not an isolated event. City officials and physicians gave her 'heroic sisters' 'unstinted praise', and a 'deluge of letters' sent to the archbishop celebrated their sacrifice.[10] Several days later, a sister of charity died of influenza 'nursing university boys' in Albuquerque, New Mexico, before which she had nursed men training for the army.[11] After the pandemic had peaked across the eastern seaboard, the *Baltimore Sun* reported that their city's 'nursing

---

[4] *Baltimore Sun*, 13 October 1918, 10.
[5] *Evening Public Ledger*, 9 October 1918. Three days later, more than 1000 bodies of influenza victims awaited burial, forcing the city to transfer hundreds of labourers from street, water, and sewer departments, and commandeering convicts for the task; ibid., 12 October 1918, front page.
[6] Ibid., 30 October 1918; and *Baltimore Sun*, 7 October 1918, 7.
[7] *Evening Public Ledger*, 7 October 1918, 2.   [8] *Washington Times*, 25 October 1918, 6.
[9] *Baltimore Sun*, 7 October 1918, 7.   [10] *Evening Public Ledger* 24 October 1918, 9.
[11] *Evening Herald*, 29 October 1918, 5.

nuns' had been praised by city, state, and federal officials, including the Surgeon General, for 'loyal self-sacrifice' caring for flu victims.[12] By the end of the pandemic, various after-effects became pressing. One was housing and caring for large numbers of orphans. Baltimore's Daughters of the Eucharist stepped in, providing for them at the nuns' nursery and kindergarten, raising funds for food and clothing, and organizing card parties.[13]

These examples of self-sacrifice by priests, pastors, and nuns, however, pale by comparison with the great outpouring of volunteerism from secular forces, especially secular women in 1918–19. Moreover, organizationally, the assistance offered by the religious differed: now the initiative came from the higher echelons of the hierarchy. Stories of pastors like Hoboken's Louis Schuyler, who on his own volition raced to Memphis to serve in 1878 and died for it, or of sisters like those of Saint Mary, who organized an emergency orphanage in the heat of that same yellow fever epidemic, fail to appear.[14] Only in Boston do the papers reflect on specific Jewish relief organizations for victims, which called the shots, procuring the services of seven physicians, organizing automobiles for an emergency service, and a Jewish women's canteen committee that distributed food to victims and their families, crossing denominational lines to answer calls regardless of religion and without compensation.[15]

CROSS-GENDER ORGANIZATIONS

Other organizations not tied to religion institutions flourished during the pandemic and increased in number as the disease reached its crisis in October. As early as mid-September, a neighbourhood club and the 'Women's Preparedness League' of Quincy, on Boston's outskirts, 'quickly' established an emergency hospital to care for the influenza-stricken in boarding houses. The club packed up its furniture and donated it to the new hospital: 'Men and women of independent means' prepared the premises for service.[16] In Washington and elsewhere the Red Cross formed special influenza committees collecting funds to establish temporary hospitals and 'diet kitchens', staffed by volunteers (presumably of both sexes), to treat and serve liquid meals to influenza sufferers.[17] In mid-October a wealthy couple loaned their 8-acre estate in Georgetown as a convalescent home for women war workers recovering from influenza with 'no place to go'.[18] The capital established a free taxi service 'run entirely by volunteers', staffed by 'over 150 chauffeurs and chauffeurettes' to transport the afflicted. By the end of October, it was answering over a thousand

[12] *Baltimore Sun*, 31 December 1918, 4.

[13] Ibid., 14 December 1918, 4; the Sisters at St Vincent's Infant Asylum did the same, ibid., 9 January 1919, 4.

[14] See Chapter 17.   [15] *Boston Globe*, 6 October 1918, 27.

[16] Ibid., 20 September 1918, 7.

[17] *Washington Herald*, 15 October 1918, front page. The committee also raised funds for the same in Alexandria, Virginia; ibid., 26 October 1918, 3.

[18] Ibid., 16 October 1918, 3; and *Washington Times*, 16 October 1918, front page.

calls a day.[19] The capital's Chamber of Commerce assisted in the care by appealing to the city's druggists to fill prescriptions up to $10 gratis for 'certified' cases of influenza. By 25 October, fifty-one druggists had joined the scheme.[20] In Philadelphia, students of the Pennsylvania School for Social Services (presumably male and female) 'volunteered as a body' as nurses' aides at the newly opened emergency influenza hospital.[21] The Bell Telephone Company of Pennsylvania ran a page-printed advert, thanking 'the people of Philadelphia' for their assistance in helping the company weather the crisis.[22] Private families opened their homes to children orphaned by the epidemic.[23]

Such fundraising and cross-gender volunteerism received praise beyond major cities of the East Coast. Citizens of small-town Coeburn, Virginia, raised $2,000 to establish an emergency influenza hospital with fifty beds, organized nurseries to care for orphans, and took others into their homes.[24] In Delaware, Ohio, Ohio Wesleyan University converted two fraternity houses into emergency hospitals 'with trained nurses and men of the students' army training corps' as assistants.[25] The Red Cross chapter at Mount Vernon, Ohio, received an urgent call from members of the Gambier branch appealing for sheets and other items for students at Kenyon College down with 'Spanish Influenza'. Immediately, citizens went to work and by evening had gathered sufficient articles for the students.[26] Aided by donations and labour from citizens, El Paso converted the Aoy High School for Mexican children into a hospital to accommodate a hundred flu-infected patients. According to the *El Paso Herald*, because of the generosity of men and women in the city, 'no influenza patients suffer for care or food'. Peyton's meat market donated the meat for the hospital, and women made sandwiches for the nurses, provided hot soup for patients, and opened their own kitchens to ensure the supply of nourishment.[27] With cases on the decline in the principal north-eastern cities by the third week of October,[28] Surgeon General Blue paid tribute to the 'flu fights', praising thousands for 'deeds of heroism' that had led 'to martyrdom not confined to the battlefield'.[29]

CROSS-BORDER CHARITY

As Mount Vernon's contribution to Garnier suggests, efforts to alleviate suffering were not limited to one's own neighbourhood or city. In addition to networks and governmental agencies,[30] individual volunteers crossed boundaries within the US and between the US, Canada, and Mexico. When Boston and other localities in Massachusetts succumbed to the pandemic in September, Canada and nearby

---

[19] *Washington Times*, 26 October 1918, 4.
[20] Ibid., 25 October 1918, 16; and *Washington Herald*, 29 October 1918, 3.
[21] *Evening Public Ledger*, 9 October 1918, 3.   [22] Ibid., 25 October 1918, 19.
[23] Ibid., 16 October 1918, 9.   [24] *Big Stone Gap Post*, 30 November 1918.
[25] *Democratic Banner*, 22 October 1918, 5.   [26] Ibid., 18 October 1918, 5.
[27] *El Paso Herald*, 22 October 1918, 8.   [28] *Sun*, 20 October 1918, front page.
[29] *Washington Herald*, 20 October 1918, 6.
[30] See examples in Collier, *The Plague of the Spanish Lady*.

states 'rushed' to their aid.[31] By the end of the month, eleven nurses from Hamilton, Ontario, and four recent graduate nurses from Woodstock, Southwestern Ontario, had answered Boston's calls.[32] In the first week in October, Canada sent 300 graduate nurses to Boston, twenty-five to Washington, DC, and more than 400 to places in the Midwest.[33]

At the same time, Arizona announced they were sending 'nurses and physicians in large numbers to hard-hit out-of-state military camps.[34] At the end of September, Maryland sent 'a special hospital-train' with forty beds for treating influenza patients to East Braintree, south of Boston.[35] A few days later, nurses from Hartford and Providence crossed state lines to volunteer in Quincy.[36] With influenza subsiding in Boston at the end of October, the city sent forty nurses and twelve physicians to Springfield,[37] and several days later with the crisis nearing its peak in central Pennsylvania sent eleven nurses to Harrisburg. Boston's head nurse explained: 'I am sure the people of Massachusetts will never forget the ready response of the Pennsylvania authorities, nor the sacrifices of the fifteen nurses sent to us from that state, four of whom succumbed to the disease.'[38] The Red Cross called out its defence nurses from across the country, assigning them to camps, hospitals, and shipbuilding plants on the eastern seaboard.[39] At the beginning of October, when the pandemic had infected 2000 in small-town Custer, Illinois, nurses 'rushed' from Kalamazoo, Battle Creek, and Ann Arbor, Michigan, to care for the afflicted.[40] Two days later, with cases doubling in Custer, nurses from other Michigan towns offered their services.[41] Later, a Wisconsin committee offered aid to women war workers in the nation's capital afflicted by the disease and expressed a desire to locate and befriend any in need of attention.[42] As late as the end of November, pleas were answered from other states when communities became overwhelmed with new cases, as in Sandusky, Ohio. From across Lake Erie, Michigan, answered its call.[43] Certainly, such eagerness to cross state and municipal borders to aid the afflicted was no universal sentiment, as seen with the internal quarantines constructed during smallpox epidemics and the last outbreaks of yellow fever, which hampered relief and divided states as though enemy territories.

MEN

One of the first acclaimed as 'a martyr' to the pandemic was the 'well-known physician' Dr Frederick Demling, who 'worked untiringly day and night over patients' at the City Hospital (Boston), before he contracted the disease and died.[44]

---

[31] *Sun*, 29 October 1918, 9.   [32] *Globe and Mail*, 30 September 1918, 2–3.
[33] *Baltimore Sun*, 6 October 1918, 7. Also, see *Washington Times*, 29 September 1918, 19.
[34] *Bisbee Daily Review*, 29 September 1918, 3.   [35] *Detriot Free Press*, 1 October 1918, 18.
[36] *Boston Globe*, 20 September 1918, 7; and 28 September 1918, 4.
[37] Ibid., 30 October 1918, 14.   [38] Ibid., 1 November 1918, 5.
[39] *Washington Times*, 29 September 1918, 4.   [40] *Detroit Free Press*, 2 October 1918, 18.
[41] Ibid., 4 October 1918, 3.   [42] *Washington Herald*, 27 October 1918, 5.
[43] *Detroit Free Press*, 30 November 1918, 14.
[44] *Washington Herald*, 23 September 1918, 2.

Early on, Philadelphia's *Evening Public Ledger* commemorated 'men of prominence in the city', who died of Spanish Influenza, 'many of them martyrs through devotion to families and friends'.[45] The following week, when recorded influenza deaths trebled, the paper proclaimed two more 'among the grip dead' as 'Physician Martyrs'.[46] Further male martyrs to flu can be found in smaller towns, such as Port Chester, New York, where thirty-six-year-old Dr Rittenberg died 'fighting the Grip' and was hailed for his sacrifice by a two-line notice in New York's *Sun*.[47]

Such recognition did not necessarily depend on dying. With the supply of nurses in crisis by mid-October, Health Commissioner Copeland appealed to businesses and professional men to volunteer for night shifts.[48] Since we hear no more of these desperate appeals, presumably these men served. In the capital, medical students (most, if not all, male) volunteered to treat influenza patients and were sent into private homes or wherever 'immediate relief was needed'.[49] A delegation from Howard University Medical College (a black institution) offered their services to the Public Health Commissioner, who assigned them 'to look after members of their own race'.[50] 'A number of physicians' from Johns Hopkins volunteered to relieve local physicians 'terribly overworked' because of the pandemic.[51] While medical students in New York City may not have solicited their health board to fight the pandemic, with a spurt of new cases on 10 October, the Health Department 'drafted' seniors in medical schools across the city to serve as nurses, and they accepted.[52] Yet, as we shall see, despite constituting a much smaller proportion of students, university women served far more readily, individually and collectively as members of departments and colleges, to combat the pandemic.

In Washington, men of the armed forces also donated free time to assist stricken civilian communities. In mid-October, ten Navy Yard men volunteered to drive ambulances, which papers celebrated with front-page headlines.[53] Days later, in a famous case, nine sailors stationed in the Boston naval district were lauded for '"flu" heroism', after volunteering to be inoculated 'with the disease scrum'.[54] The YMCA was another organization that encouraged men to volunteer. The *Washington Times* interviewed two, who had been working there between fourteen and eighteen hours a day. They explained: 'We get nothing out of it except knowing that we have done some good' and, according to the paper, this was 'typical of Washington's volunteer workers'.[55] At the same time, in Philadelphia, fourteen firemen, after their shifts, gave extra hours as nurses in the men's ward of the emergency hospital.[56] Similarly, men devoted their money, time, and often their lives in Winslow,

---

[45] *Evening Public Ledger*, 7 October 1918, 2; and praised its 'doctor martyrs to duty'; 8 October 1918, front page.
[46] Ibid., 12 October 1918, 2.   [47] *Sun*, 17 October 1918, 18.
[48] *Bisbee Daily Review*, 19 October 1918, front page.
[49] *Washington Herald*, 8 October 1918, front page.
[50] Ibid.; *Washington Times*, 8 October 1918, front page.
[51] *Baltimore Sun*, 13 October 1918, 10.   [52] *Sun*, 10 October 1918, 18.
[53] *Washington Herald*, 15 October 1918, front page.
[54] *Washington Times*, 20 October 1918, 4.   [55] Ibid., 23 October 1918, 3.
[56] *Evening Public Ledger*, 14 October 1918, front page.

Arizona, where the town's merchants organized an emergency ambulance service to carry influenza patients to two schoolhouse hospitals.[57] In Detroit, when schools shut in late October, not only did teachers (mainly women) volunteer to nurse the afflicted; school janitors offered care for the children.[58] In San Francisco, the Boy Scouts transformed their clubhouse into an influenza hospital, opened a soup kitchen, ran errands, carried soup to those too ill to send for it, and became volunteer nurses.[59]

Finally, businesses and men's clubs occasionally supported the anti-influenza struggle. The Western Maryland Railway Company converted the clubhouse of the Haggerstown Country Club into an influenza emergency hospital; and the Baltimore and Ohio Railroad converted one of its bunkhouses into a hospital at Brunswick, Maryland, supplied it with two nurses and two physicians, and placed a dining car on site to prepare meals for staff and patients and a sleeping car for nurses.[60] In the wealthy northern suburbs of Chicago, Exmoor Golf Club turned its clubhouse into an emergency hospital and by early October was caring for fifty-four influenza patients.[61] Another exclusive male country club in Chicago, this one at Indian Hill, converted its clubhouse into a 'flu hospital', staffed by 'society women'.[62] Yet such notices of men volunteers were rare among the thousands of pandemic-related pages in 'Chronicling America', even if the papers make clear that the daily strain of the pandemic on physicians (then mostly male) was great, as gleaned from such stories as 'Bad news from El Paso', when on 19 October, the city's Health Department abandoned any attempt to gather vital statistics, because of doctors' exhaustion.[63] However, men and their businesses rarely appear in the limelight as happened only thirteen years before with America's last yellow fever pandemic. A case in point of men's benign inaction comes from Birmingham, Alabama. Its lucrative State Fair coincided with the rise of influenza in October. The city health commissioner closed its gate, striking a 'serious financial blow' especially to the agricultural sector. Businesses, however, accepted the decree, and the local paper praised their cooperation as displaying a 'fine spirit' in 'Willingly Sacrificing Investment on Altar of Public Welfare'.[64]

WOMEN

Stories of men's volunteerism, heroism, and martyrdom illuminated by the press during a few months of the Great Influenza appear to have surpassed examples from both sexes over the whole course of cholera, plague, or smallpox across multiple epidemics in America. Yet the press's attention to the contributions of men and their fraternal organizations towards fighting the pandemic amounts to a tiny sliver of that offered by women. Moreover, the stories of martyrdom, courage,

---

[57] *El Paso Herald*, 16 October 1918, 5.   [58] *Detroit Free Press*, 23 October 1918, 6.
[59] *San Francisco Chronicle*, 25 January 1919, 11; also 16 February 1918, B6.
[60] *Baltimore Sun*, 19 October 1918, 5.   [61] *Chicago Daily Tribune*, 3 October 1918, 14.
[62] Ibid., 10 October 1918, 7.   [63] *Bisbee Daily Review*, 19 October 1918, front page.
[64] *Birmingham Age-Herald*, 9 October 1918, 5.

and abnegation that emerged during the Great Influenza contrast sharply with those surrounding yellow fever, in which men's organizations and their stories predominated and women hardly figured at all.

Was this volunteerism 'as a distinctly female activity' based on long-term trends from the late nineteenth century?[65] As mentioned earlier, other diseases—plague, yellow fever, poliomyelitis, typhus—continued to explode with epidemic force into the twentieth century with papers recording few, if any, stories of women's self-sacrifice. Rather than long-term trends in women's history, the historian might turn to the immediate circumstances of the Great War: the patriotic chest-thumping by the media with daily stories of heroism and an ever-present drumming-up of support for war from those left at home to organize and contribute to Liberty Bonds. Although these drives were organized predominantly by men,[66] the zeal, guilt, and competition they stirred up redounded upon women. Earlier, many had endeavoured to join the front as nurses, even when they did not possess the training. Linda Quiney has examined such women among Canadian teachers, who strove to join Voluntary Aid Detachments (VADs). In interviews conducted towards the end of their lives, she recorded their reasons for sacrificing careers as teachers to risk their lives on the front. One veteran VAD recalled the abundance of propaganda posters proclaiming, 'Your King and Country Need You'; another pointed to competition with her younger brother, fighting on the Western Front.[67]

The press certainly called on patriotism in its appeals for women to volunteer in the struggle against the pandemic. But given the near omnipresence of patriotic language in campaigns that advertised everything from Liberty Bonds to the most mundane household goods, the use of war rhetoric to attract women's assistance against the pandemic appears surprisingly rare. In a short article appealing for women volunteers—'Heroic Women Aid in "Flu" Fight'—the *Washington Times* said 'the appeal was put on a patriotic and humanitarian basis' but little was made of the 'patriotic': beneath a photograph of an unidentified young woman wearing an anti-influenza mask, the caption reads: 'She needs no name or identification. She is one of the volunteer workers. There are hundreds like her rising to this emergency.'[68] Several days later, the same paper reported that 'many patriotic women of Washington have interested themselves in the problem of convalescent girl war workers'. The paper did not dwell on patriotism, but instead reported how ladies at the top of society, such as Mrs Samuel A. Ellsworth, a director of the YWCA, and Mrs Herbert Hoover, wife of the Federal Food Administrator (later 31st President of the United States, 1929–33), were involved in the campaign.[69] Philadelphia celebrated more than fifty of its 'Unselfish Girl Scouts', serving in hospitals 'as patriotic duty'.[70] But the appeals to and praise of women played more on humanitarian strings than patriotic causes. At the same time, another Washington daily appealed to women, especially those owning automobiles, to bring food to

[65] Bristow, *American Pandemic*, 59.
[66] Men who had not gone to war seem to have been the mainstay, see Porter, *Pale Horse*, 183–8.
[67] Quiney, 'Borrowed Halos'. Also, idem, 'Rendering Valuable Service'.
[68] *Washington Times*, 9 October 1918, 3.   [69] Ibid., 12 October 1918, 2.
[70] *Evening Public Ledger*, 28 October 1918, 10.

those with pneumonia and influenza. It neither employed war metaphors nor made references to patriotism; it simply added that the food for these patients was already being prepared by other women.[71]

More than patriotism, appeals to women seen in editorials and interviews with volunteers turned on adventure, self-worth, respect, achievement, personal development, and liberation. Unlike short articles or brief obituaries that acclaimed male flu fighters as martyrs, those concerning women could stretch to full-page spreads studded with photographs of women ready for action and filled with personal touches. Many of these rested on new technologies and expertise that the pandemic opened for women, especially driving automobiles and joining new 'Women's Motor Corps'.

In a long editorial on Women's Motor Corps, New York City's *Evening World* recounted their perilous tasks during the munitions plant explosion in Morgan, New Jersey, when these women transported 'night and day' army influenza victims to the base hospital.[72] After the explosions, thirty women driving fifteen ambulances worked for two weeks transporting the soldiers suffering with influenza. Their captain, Katherine Richards, a Californian, was described as having 'a splendid simplicity, equally removed from blatant boasting, and in charge of between seventy-five and eighty-five volunteer workers'. During her service, she became afflicted with influenza, but returned to work after two days. Her interview lived up to her characterization:

> The influenza is nothing, though, unless you let it develop into pneumonia. We never think of trying to avoid it. Yesterday we had six calls to go to different addresses…in New York and take soldiers who had come down with the disease…we didn't wear masks…I don't think they do much good.[73]

The article ended by listing what the women cited as the job requirements: 'All must know how to drive unusually well and how to repair it. The task requires more knack than physical strength…two girls can lift the heaviest man…we have to lift the loaded litter over our heads'.[74]

Philadelphia and Washington also celebrated their 'Ambulance Girls' with full-length stories, interviews, and photography. One with Miss Marion Keating Johnson during a rest stop on her nightly ambulance run (Figure 21.1) chisels many of the same features seen with Richards. Johnson, an ambulance driver for the Bryn Mawr Emergency Hospital, was described as possessing 'a quiet gallantry' and 'an inspiration to countless others'. She said little about herself or the part she was playing, but she had organized a motor corps as an auxiliary to the Main Line Branch of the Red Cross. Her responses to questions were direct: 'You do see pretty

---

[71] *Washington Herald*, 20 October 1918, 6.

[72] On the multiple munitions explosions and their effect on influenza, see *Sun*, 6 October 1918, 12; *Evening World*, 8 October 1918, 5; and Galishoff, 'Newark', 250: over 500 were left homeless.

[73] Less than five days after the interview, one of Richards' co-workers died of influenza: *New-York Tribune*, 14 October 1918, 16.

[74] *Evening World*, 9 October 1918, 16, by Marguerite Mooers Marshall.

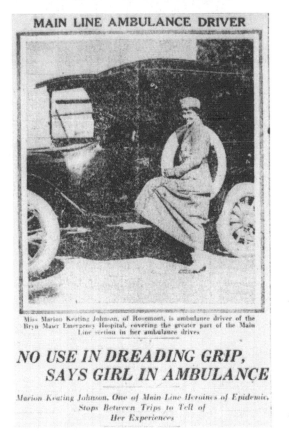

MAIN LINE AMBULANCE DRIVER

Miss Marion Keating Johnson, of Rosemont, is ambulance driver of the Bryn Mawr Emergency Hospital, covering the greater part of the Main Line section in her ambulance drives

NO USE IN DREADING GRIP, SAYS GIRL IN AMBULANCE

Marion Keating Johnson, One of Main Line Heroines of Epidemic, Stops Between Trips to Tell of Her Experiences

Figure 21.1. Marion Johnson, ambulance driver; *Evening Public Ledger*, 23 October 1918, 10.

dreadful things… I'm not afraid of getting it [influenza]… When we first opened, about a hundred girls from the college volunteered and worked like beavers'.[75]

In a multi-column story with photographs and interviews, the *Washington Herald* focused on one incident in a day's work of one woman driver of the Red Cross's Motor Corps, whose team was aiding infected women war workers. Yesterday, the driver related:

> a doctor found a girl suffering with Spanish influenza in a rooming house, three flights up—homeless, as war workers are in this city of magnificent distances and prices. He telephoned to the garage of the American Red Cross Motor Corps and in a few minutes an ambulance driven by one of us drove to the door. The driver [that is, the interviewee] ascended the stairs with a woman stretcher-bearer, and after the patient had been placed on a stretcher, an attempt was made to carry her down. The twisting winding stairway prevented this and so the driver took the sufferer on her back, carried her downstairs and into the ambulance.

[75] *Evening Public Ledger*, 23 October 1918, 10.

The article concluded: 'the Motor Corps has forty-five members and is looking for recruits. There are six ambulances.'[76]

Two weeks later, another Washington daily took another snapshot of the Motor Corps women. Accompanied by a large photograph of the women and their male orderlies (of whom nothing is said), it spread across five columns. It too emphasized the women's tough determination, the dangers they faced, and their understated courage. In addition, it gives a sense of how the influenza experience had rapidly transformed women's lives and character. I cite only a few sections from this lengthy exposé:

> In less than half an hour a uniformed girl ambulance driver stood on one side of the cot, her soldier orderly on the other [of a girl war worker, critically ill with pneumonia in a room with a cot, kitchen table, six empty milk bottles, and a typewriter]...the young girl ambulance driver, who a few months ago knew little about life except the fox trot and the smartest angle at which to wear a new hat, held up one end of the stretcher. A moment later the same girl was driving the clanging ambulance to the newly opened influenza hospital...That case and the girl is typical of the epidemic now raging in the city, typical of the shameful housing conditions of women war workers, typical of the heroic service being given by the Red Cross women ambulance drivers...
>
> Already this month the Women's Motor Corps have responded to more than 500 emergency calls...Some drivers have reported a total of more than a hundred hours a week. Several have worked thirty-six hours at a stretch. They have taken patients from mansions and hovels, from canal boats and hotels. They have not balked at a single condition from carrying patients weighing over 200 pounds to entering homes where a family of nine was prostrate with the disease.
>
> Maybe you have seen one of the women drivers at the wheel of an ambulance...and maybe you sniffed as I did a week ago: 'Oh, yes, society girls, with a new fad.' Yesterday, I saw the other side of the picture...I saw them carry helpless patients on their backs when flights of stairs were too numerous, too narrow, and too steep to accommodate a stretcher. I saw them entering where the filth and squalor were revolting even to accustomed eyes. I saw them render first aid, comfort bereaved children, even care for the dead. And these women, one the wife of a Western Congressman, a Boston society woman...one a daughter of the inventor of the telephone...one the wife of a well-known naval commander...pleaded with their superior officer for cases, and yet more cases...Four...have contracted the disease.[77]

No doubt, the article's language and class bias, or at least praise of society ladies, might provoke scepticism. Still, nothing revealed here or about other 'Motor Corps Girls' in any city smacks of the risk-free posturing or the preaching seen with women polio crusaders two years earlier and their undisguised contempt for the lower classes. Instead, this article and its interviewees were disgusted by 'the shameful conditions' in which they found isolated war workers and the

[76] *Washington Herald*, 6 October 1918, 12.
[77] *Washington Times*, 20 October 1918, 4.

impoverished dwellings of dying families of nine. Their tasks were not risk-free: four of the twenty contracted the deadly disease.[78]

The *Boston Globe* also ventured into the new photojournalism to praise its women volunteers, again concentrating on those who had donated automobiles, time, and organizational talents, like the Simons College administrators, who in one day alone requisitioned and put into service ninety-five ambulances from private motorists.[79] Praise of women and their automobiles was not limited to cities on the East Coast. With large photographs and stories of typical days in the life of volunteers, Detroit's major newspaper also celebrated its 'girl' ambulance drivers, claiming that in the 'fight' against influenza, 'no agency was more useful than its motor corps'. As with the East Coast, the paper described the 'girls' herculean shifts of fourteen to sixteen hours, their skill in driving, and endurance'.[80]

Nonetheless, this high-profile, well-publicized volunteer work of women combatting the pandemic was the tip of the iceberg in terms of social class and numbers volunteering. To qualify, the women had to have been experienced drivers before the epidemic, and already own their own automobiles, which in the early twentieth century constituted a restricted portion of the population even after Henry Ford's assembly line production in 1903.[81] However, the newspapers, perhaps surprisingly, could be almost as ebullient when praising less glamourous volunteer work by women in nursing, running diet kitchens, cleaning, and caring for rapidly rising populations of orphans, even if their stories were shorter and photographs more sparse. Here, women, principally of the lower middle classes, who held skilled jobs such as teaching, willingly rushed to fill these needs, and incurred many of the same risks confronting their better-heeled sisters behind the ambulance wheels. These stories of abnegation and courage were far more common. Before turning to their stories, we start with another group of women volunteers far more privileged than debutante ambulance drivers.

In October 1918 society pages of major East Coast cities fixed their glare on ladies contributing their time and wealth to arrest the pandemic, featuring women at the pinnacle of the political and economic elite, such as Mrs Samuel A. Ellsworth, Mrs Herbert Hoover, and Mrs Vanderbilt, who 'volunteered' their motor cars. Mrs Vanderbilt may have gone further than some. On 26 October, she spent her day transporting nurses 'to patients in the poorer homes of the city'.[82] Another large photograph showed her with seven other Washington grandees; its headline gushed: 'Washington Society Women Work Day and Night as Emergency Chauffeurs'. A long list of women followed, who had 'volunteered

---

[78] On the plight of women war workers, see *Baltimore Sun*, 22 October 1918, 2. Because of near starvation conditions and 'no one to look after their needs', the government on 21 October established an 'experimental kitchen' to provide them with 'three decent meals a day'. See *Birmingham Age-Herald*, 20 October 1918, B2, on their difficulties finding lodging: they were 'often homeless and sometimes foodless'.

[79] *Boston Globe*, 27 October 1918, 35.

[80] *Detroit Free Press*, 27 October 1918, 11, focused on ambulance driver Captain Marjorie Whitehead.

[81] See the low-paid gossip columnist in Porter's *Pale Horse*, who comments that 'at a pinch' she might drive an ambulance. 'I have driven a Ford for years' (209).

[82] *New-York Tribune*, 27 October 1918, 13.

their cars and services, transporting doctors and nurses, carrying hot food' and had demonstrated that 'they are afraid of nothing'. Among them were others of Vanderbilt's ilk: Mrs Cary T. Grayson, wife of the President's physician, and Mrs Thomas Gore, wife of Senator Gore.[83] Whether they actually did the chauffering is difficult to know. In Washington, papers also praised prominent women who aided influenza patients by making medicated gauze masks. Three were singled out: Mrs Fletcher, the wife of an admiral in the Navy, Mrs Lansing, wife of the Secretary of State, and Mrs McAdoo, wife of the Secretary of the Treasury. (The paper did not bother mentioning that she was also the President's daughter.[84]) But no matter how cynical we might be about these society ladies' risks or their assistance bathed in photo opportunities, one thing is certain: the contemporary press bestowed no comparable attention on men at the top of society for their sacrifices fighting the pandemic—even in stories of Surgeon General Blue, William Gorgas, Surgeon General of the Army, or other big-city health commissioners such as 'Director Doctor Krusen' of Philadelphia, and Brownlow, Fowler, and Mustard, directors of the health boards for DC and Washington, all of whom by the third week of October had succumbed to flu in the line of duty.[85]

Throughout October the social column of Philadelphia's *Evening Public Ledger*, 'Just Gossip about People', was stuffed with the details of city women volunteering; many were debutants or had recently completed university. The language of these strikes us today as flippant, but I think they must be read with dead seriousness. Below are a few, prefaced by 'Nancy Wynne discusses Influenza':

> Just Gossip 'Nancy Wynne Tells of Various Girls Who Are Nursing in the Hospitals'
> Do you know it's simply wonderful the way the women of this city have come to the fore and are working their hands and heads off in the hospitals and other places, helping the doctors and nurses to combat the influenza. Down at Pennsylvania Hospital, for instance, there are Estelle Sanders, Jean Bullitt,[86] Marian Wurts and six or eight others...[87]
> Bryn Mawr College girls are busy today scrubbing and painting the old Lancaster Inn...being equipped as an emergency hospital for...influenza victims...At the Emergency Hospital Mrs. Walter Chrystie of Bryn Mawr directed the cleaners yesterday...The Bryn Mawr Community Center will run the hospital kitchen and pantry with Mrs. Branson and Miss Hilda Smith in charge.
> A staff of nurses' aides, organized by Mrs. Richard E. Norton...will assist the regularly trained nurses...[88] Miss McDay has been doing her work too. Imagine in one case she went to a house and the woman called her in and begged her to help...five little children in one room all burning up with fever and very ill with the influenza and in the next tiny room a sixth child that had died that morning.[89]

---

[83] *Washington Times*, 25 October 1918, 5.   [84] *Evening World*, 26 September 1918, 12.
[85] *Washington Times*, 19 October 1918, 3; and 25 October 1918, 6.
[86] Later, she caught flu nursing at the Pennsylvania Hospital; *Evening Public Ledger*, 19 October 1918, 9.
[87] Ibid., 8 October 1918, 9.   [88] Ibid.   [89] Ibid., 11 October 1918, 13.

Isn't it wonderful, the amount of hard work women are doing now without saying anything about it. And there's so much going on that most people know nothing about it…[90]

Health Commissioner Copeland corroborates these 'gossips', that the work of these women (as opposed to donations alone) was essential. In praising the work of volunteer women nurses in New York City, he added: 'If you want to learn more about them look in the Social Registry.' The article was followed by an interview with one of the socialites behind an influenza gauze mask at a tenement, a Mrs Austin, who added: 'None of us mind being here. In fact, we consider it a privilege… important work for any woman in New York who can use a scrubbing brush, make up a bed or do plain cooking'.[91] In addition, women's elite clubs, such as the Civic Club of Philadelphia, were engaged in relief efforts that involved more than monetary contributions.

> They entered hospitals as nurses' aides, doing the more prosaic jobs to free more time for the urgently needed trained nurses… Unselfishly, they offered their services with all their zeal, whatever [was] assigned them. Some have been caring for children, who have been orphaned; others have undertaken the management of stricken households, where often as many as six or seven members have lain without help of any kind, unable even to cook their own food.[92]

Photojournalism and multi-column supplements did not, however, focus only on socialites, debutants, or college girls who owned automobiles. At the end of October, a *Boston Globe* supplement centred on the 'Fine Work Done By the Alston Canteen' in a working-class quarter west of Cambridge. It celebrated its closing after three weeks distributing soups and other foods 'among the needy sick'. Again, the initiative came from women, organized by the League of Catholic Women in cooperation with women from the Red Cross of St Anthony's parish and the St Vincent de Paul Society. The paper listed twenty-five volunteers, all of whom were women.[93] In the same issue with half-page photographs, the paper praised the District Nursing Association as 'one of influenza's worst enemies'. At one time, it had cared for as many as 3000 influenza patients: 'The spirit of the entire nursing force, trained and untrained, volunteer and regular… never flagged'.[94]

Photojournalism in praise of women could reach still further down the social ladder. In Kansas City, Missouri, one of its dailies featured an article on 'the ladies of the Auxiliary School of Nurse Assistants', housed in the city's general hospital in its 'colored division' accompanied by a photograph of its first graduating class, 'the first of its kind to be graduated in this country'. The paper lauded 'the ladies' as comprising 'of some of the best citizens of Kansas City, Missouri and Kansas City, Kansas'. Here, the paper's notion of 'best citizens' had nothing to do with status; rather it concerned character. The graduates had trained not as a necessity but to 'render assistance to the boys over there' and to those returning. The pandemic

---

[90] Ibid., 25 September 1918, 13.   [91] *New-York Tribune*, 14 October 1918, 16.
[92] *Evening Public Ledger*, 19 October 1918, 9.   [93] *Boston Globe*, 27 October 1918, 25.
[94] Ibid., 27 October 1918, 35.

interrupted those plans; now they 'voluntarily rendered most valuable service' to their civilian populations.[95]

Beyond East Coast cities, the newspapers' focus on socialites in the fight against flu was thin.[96] Elsewhere, whether in small towns or metropolitan centres, the women so praised tended to be hospital head matrons or head nurses, as in the community of Algiers on New Orleans' south side.[97] To be sure, these volunteers highlighted in the press were white and middle class. In the case of El Paso those praised were 'clean cut efficient women and girls from the best homes', who prepared 'steaming soup…in [their] most luxurious homes' and gave their automobiles and time running errands to facilitate the work of hospitals. Papers described them 'cheerfully and tenderly, in their tub frocks of gingham and their crisp white aprons…risking their lives that the less fortunate of the city's population may be cared for during the influenza epidemic'.[98] Not only class divided carers and patients; also ethnic and racial barriers stood between them. As the city's vital statistics show, the worst-hit neighbourhoods were in the poorest parts of town with the highest concentrations of Mexicans.[99] Yet, as Bradford Luckingham has shown, white elite women were not the only ones to volunteer. Care in El Paso's barrios depended on Spanish-speaking volunteers. Anglos and Mexicans joined forces, and within the Mexican community, charity also crossed class lines, as with a new social club of Mexican businessmen, who solicited contributions from Mexican residents, and businesses such as La Victoria bakery, which donated their products.[100]

'THE THOUSANDS OF DEEDS OF HEROISM'

Despite the gossip columnists' interest in high-profile women who were engaged in charity work, it was 'the thousands of deeds of heroism' in the words of Surgeon General Blue that played the more significant role combating flu, and newspapers in extraordinary numbers reported these stories across the country. Overwhelmingly, these concerned women. With influenza on the rise in New York City, 'thousands of volunteer nurses' went into the homes of sufferers to provide medical care and distribute food and supplies 'without recompense'.[101] These women became the nucleus of the 'Influenza Emergency Committee of the Mayor's Committee of

[95] *Kansas City Sun*, 19 October 1918, front page.

[96] An exception comes from *San Francisco Chronicle*, 25 October 1918, 9, praising socialite ladies in Belvedere, who commandeered a vacant suite of apartments to convert into hospital wards.

[97] *Herald*, 24 October 1918, front page.

[98] *El Paso Herald*, 22 October 1918, 8: The next day, the paper listed several society ladies who prepared broth in their kitchens and searched for needy infected Mexican families; ibid., 23 October 1918, 8.

[99] Ethnicity and class were determining factors in influenza mortality rates in 1918–19; see Tuckel et al., 'The Diffusion of the Influenza'; Fanning, *Influenza and Inequality*, 119; Noymer, 'Epidemics and Time', 148–9; and Swedlund, 'Everyday Mortality'.

[100] Luckingham, *Epidemic in the Southwest*, 10–15.

[101] *Evening World*, 11 October 1918, front page.

Women on National Defence', which recruited other women without nursing skills, who were assigned to other tasks aiding the afflicted and their families. By mid-October, forty-five centres staffed by women emergency workers had been organized across the city.[102] One was the Winifred Wheeler Nursery, 'converted by these women' into a home for babies and young children whose families were incapacitated by flu.[103] Other organizations, such as the Henry Street Settlement, supplied nurses and aides throughout the city: 'women and girls entered homes of all sorts and most worked without pay'. The Department of Health admitted that no provision existed for an emergency of the current scale. Only 'through the kindness of volunteers' and by galvanizing further women volunteers to make house calls and care for the afflicted could the crisis be confronted.[104] A woman in another New York City organization—one not known for feminine inclinations—also made inroads. Mrs Ellen A. O'Grady, acting commissioner of the Fifth Department of the New York City Police, organized an appeal for funds to aid families of policemen who were stricken or had died of influenza.[105]

Early on in the pandemic, Philadelphia formed its own women's corps of volunteer nurses to supplement the Red Cross. Unlike in New York, where the mayor and health commissioner organized emergency women's corps, here the impetus came from a woman (Miss Elizabeth Stites). According to the *Evening Public Ledger*, 'Women have come to the front in great numbers and the stories of their personal sacrifices in running the hazards of the disease have imbued everybody with a new courage'. The paper told their stories.[106] Another women's volunteer group, 'armed with mops, brooms, scrubbing brushes, soap and milk cans filled with hot water', directed by Miss Meta Jones, head of the social service department of the Woman's College Hospital, cleaned houses in the city's most congested southern districts, where influenza cases were highest.[107] A women's organization at the New York Ship Company, at Camden Docks, across the Delaware River from Philadelphia, volunteered for relief work at the homes of ship workers crippled by influenza and organized a nursery to relieve mothers too ill to care for their children.[108]

In Washington, volunteers came mainly from teachers freed from work by school closures. A call from the Nurses' Bureau of the American Red Cross on the morning of 7 October registered women, who began their duties the next morning. They aided nurses, scrubbed floors, and entertained the children of afflicted mothers.[109] Other women's committees ran diet kitchens, preparing liquid food that fed the 'hundreds' of the afflicted 'from every part of the city'.[110] The extent to which the volunteers cut through the capital's social layers is shown by the dedication of one of the most impoverished and exploited groups in the city, if not the

[102] *New-York Tribune*, 16 October 1918, 18.

[103] Ibid., 27 October 1918, 13. This committee assembled 'every women's committee of note in the city'; *Evening World*, 19 October 1918, 12.

[104] *Sun*, 22 October 1918, 14.   [105] *Evening World*, 26 October 1918, 4.

[106] *Evening Public Ledger*, 7 October 1918, 2.

[107] Ibid., 14 October 1918, 2; 24 October 1918, 11.   [108] Ibid., 18 October 1918, 9.

[109] *Washington Herald*, 8 October 1918, front page. For Boston, see *Boston Globe*, 6 October 1918, 9.

[110] *Washington Herald*, 21 October 1918, front page.

country—women war workers. After their daily government clerical jobs, they volunteered at night for emergency nursing. In at least one instance, one of them even received her photo opportunity. Featured in the *Washington Times*, the story of Mrs Eleanor Stanford, the first war worker to volunteer as a night nurse for the influenza-stricken, reported nightly at the Webster School, headquarters of the Public Health Service, for emergency calls. She worked there until midnight, completing seven-hour shifts during the day and eight at night.[111] As we have seen, women willingly left their homes, and crossed city and state lines to volunteer, like the nurses from Hartford and Providence who travelled to Quincy. 'Although tired out by the journey', they 'scorn[ed] a night's sleep' and asked to see patients at once. A nurse, Miss Helen Riley, was placed in charge.[112]

In contrast to the geographical distribution of socialite ladies, the efforts and sacrifices of women in general did not cluster in eastern metropoles but spanned America, running through large and small towns alike. The most important group supplying these volunteers was the teaching profession. In El Paso, they responded to appeals for nurses in mid-October, when influenza cases suddenly spiked. The Aoy School was converted into the city's main influenza emergency hospital, and its principal, Miss Katherine Gorbutt, played the leading role, organizing services and ministering to the ill in the city's worst-hit area,[113] the Mexican neighbourhood.[114] In Carlsbad, New Mexico, schoolteachers were reported as the ones 'unusually active during the epidemic', giving 'unselfish devotion' in caring for influenza sufferers.[115] With the closure of St Vincent's Academy at Albuquerque, all eight of its teachers, 'Sisters of the Church', volunteered to nurse sick students at the University of New Mexico, hit badly by the pandemic in October. In Ogden, Utah, schoolteachers responded to calls for nurses' aides, assisting with home care and staffing the emergency kitchen at the civic centre.[116] The school's superintendent organized boys and girls, made idle by school closures, to assist the afflicted.[117] In Sumter, South Carolina, the girls' high school became the nerve centre of their influenza relief programme,[118] and as in Ogden, teachers enrolled their students in the relief efforts. In Winslow, Arizona, girls from the domestic science class were the ones to volunteer; nothing was said about any boys.[119] In Bourbon County, Kentucky, women answered emergency calls to nurse in rural areas.[120] In Birmingham, Alabama, women's clubs delivered the services of their members—untrained nurses—to the 'stamp out' the flu, and twenty-five women graduates of the Hoover Kitchen (south of Birmingham) volunteered preparing the meals.[121]

Universities and colleges also produced women volunteers, who far outnumbered their male counterparts. Early on in the pandemic, the Women's Medical College

---

[111] *Washington Times*, 28 October 1918, 15.
[112] *Boston Globe*, 20 September 1918, 7. Also, see note 40.
[113] *El Paso Herald*, 17 October 1918, 6; and Luckingham, *Epidemic in the Southwest*, 10.
[114] See note 99.   [115] *El Paso Herald*, 24 October 1918, 5.
[116] Ibid., 24 October 1918, 7.   [117] *Ogden Standard*, 17 October 1918, 10.
[118] *Watchman and Southron*, 23 October 1918, 5.
[119] *Times-Herald*, 19 October 1918, front page; also, *El Paso Herald*, 16 October 1918, 5.
[120] *Bourbon News*, 15 October 1918, 4.   [121] *Birmingham Age-Herald*, 12 October 1918, 5.

in Philadelphia 'loaned' its third- and fourth-year students to hospitals to care for influenza patients.[122] Later, students in the social service department of the Women's College Hospital in Philadelphia volunteered to clean homes of the afflicted in the city's most destitute neighbourhoods.[123] Students of the Pennsylvania School for Social Services (mainly women) 'volunteered as a body' as nurses' aides in a newly opened emergency influenza hospital.[124] In Boston with its concentration of universities and medical schools, the paucity of students playing a significant role in the city's influenza relief is notable. The *Boston Globe* mentions none from Harvard, Boston College, or Boston University.[125] Instead, the one college to receive praise in its pages for students' assistance was a women's school, Smith College (Western Massachusetts). Freed from classes, they became 'farmerettes', devoting their energies not directly to the influenza-stricken or their families but to 'solving the farm labor scarcity' created by the war and more critically by the pandemic. Several hundred joined the work of haying, and in the autumn dug potatoes and husked corn.[126] The paper also signalled that individual students from the Boston area were volunteering and had risked their lives; these too were women. Towards the end of October, the paper reflected on the recent donation and conversion of private homes into emergency influenza hospitals. The volunteers did not come from one association or religious group but represented a broad coalition of:

> students, social workers, Sisters of Charity, one minister, women with Red Cross training, one dietician, and just women—women with common sense, who had nursed their own families or never nursed at all. They never flenched [sic] but went where they were sent.... The courage and self-sacrifice of these workers was remarkable.[127]

Moreover, college administrators and teachers joined these forces and assumed leadership roles: those named were women. Miss Anne Hervey Strong, director of Simmons College School of Public Health, headed an Emergency Committee and organized an ambulance motorcade of privately donated cars. Miss Evelyn Walker, a volunteer and ex-registrar of Simmons, organized the flow of 'enormous quantities of supplies', received calls, and directed the makeshift ambulances. Miss Mabel Anderson of the Teachers' Club worked with this organization daily for three weeks. And Boston's women schoolteachers comprised the rank and file.[128]

In New York State, 'more than four hundred' students from the women's college, Vassar—even though hard-hit by the pandemic—volunteered to help local authorities in their efforts to combat the disease, making hundreds of garments needed for the poorer patients. Many of these women had already been at work in Poughkeepsie and Arlington.[129] At the University of Missouri, 'university women played...an important and helpful part in handling the Spanish influenza'. Nothing was said about male students, and a woman (Mrs Guy L. Noyes) 'took

---

[122] *Evening Public Ledger*, 5 October 1918, front page.
[123] Ibid., 14 October 1918, 2.   [124] Ibid., 9 October 1918, 3.
[125] Yet it reports work by students from New York City's medical schools; *Boston Globe*, 10 October 1918, 4.
[126] Ibid., 20 October 1918, 49.   [127] Ibid., 27 October 1918, 35.
[128] Ibid.   [129] *Sun*, 22 October 1918, 14.

charge of the women'. Ninety-eight volunteered immediately as nurses; others ran errands, acted as 'telephone girls', gave their automobiles over to hospitals, and made sputum cups. According to their director, there was 'nothing they have refused to do'.[130]

Finally, as in the north-east, women in cities and towns across the Midwest and West assumed leadership roles and were involved in founding and organizing influenza relief efforts. El Paso's Miss A. Louise Dietrich organized a nurses' aid corps that quickly recruited over fifty volunteer nurses. Yet we only hear of her in the press when she came down with influenza in mid-October.[131] Women such as Mrs J. H. Nations, Mrs Mason Pollard, and her mother distributed soup to the stricken in the same city.[132] In Phoenix, Mrs Baron Goldwater (an Episcopalian, married to a practising Jew[133]) organized and supervised the city's Roman Catholic women, provisioning emergency hospitals with clothing, bedding, and other goods.[134] A Miss Esther Cummings was the General Secretary of the Warren District Relief Association in Bisbee, Arizona,[135] that organized relief 'to assist in any distress that might arise through the influenza throughout the city'.[136] In Corpus Christi, a dietician, Mrs Bessie Bellinger, took charge of the town's Red Cross soup kitchen and its volunteers.[137] At least one female-run organization responsible for influenza assistance extended beyond neighbourhood jurisdictions, cities, and counties. The Women's Benefit Association led by its 'supreme commander', Miss Bina M. West, with well-established hospital committees and 95,000 women members across the US, gave 'efficient aid to the government and civic authorities in checking the Spanish Influenza'.[138] In addition, women acted on their own without umbrella organizations but could still be celebrated in the papers: around the peak of the epidemic one 'thoughtful woman' from the small town of Whitman, Massachusetts, 'cooked up a great quantity of beans on Saturday night' and distributed them to families where the housewives were down with influenza.[139]

This extraordinary leadership, initiative, and self-sacrifice of women to assist strangers were unique in the history of American epidemics. Given the recent experiences with epidemics before 1918, yellow fever across southern and southwestern states until 1905, smallpox across America, and poliomyelitis in New York well into the twentieth century, it is difficult to pin women's dedication during the Great Influenza to any long-term nineteenth- or early twentieth-century trends in women's participation in the public sphere. Moreover, no epidemics crossing over into the twenty-first century in America or elsewhere—waves of flu, the re-emergence of tuberculosis, SARS, even HIV/AIDS—have shown anything akin to the massive

[130] *Evening Missourian*, 23 October 1918, 3.
[131] *El Paso Herald*, 17 October 1918, 6; and Luckingham, *Epidemic in the Southwest*, 10. Dietrich also worked at the emergency hospital and trained nurses.
[132] *El Paso Herald*, 24 October 1918, 8.   [133] Edward, *Goldwater*, ch. 1.
[134] Luckingham, *Epidemic in the Southwest*, 47.
[135] A mining district within Cochise County, which includes Bisbee.
[136] *Bisbee Daily Review*, 15 October 1918, 8. The organization originated in London, Ontario, in 1878; it also served as a fraternal society, providing low-cost life insurance.
[137] *Corpus Christi Caller*, 27 October 1918, 8.   [138] *Ogden Standard*, 15 October 1918, 6.
[139] *Boston Globe*, 3 October 1918, 12.

and disproportional contribution of women volunteers across American society that was seen in the Great Influenza, from Vanderbilts and McAdoos to black nurses and exploited 'girl' war workers.

THE GREAT WAR AND ITS SOCIAL CONSEQUENCES

Should this contagion of compassion and societal bonding against the odds, in the face of the horrific and deadly contagion of the Great Influenza, be attributed to the First World War? As can be seen in interviews and diaries, some women left behind unable to join the front as trained nurses or volunteer VADs regretted their lost opportunity to contribute.[140] Geoffrey Rice has argued that in New Zealand the war effort had already put in place the organizational structures for the 1918 response to the Great Influenza 'with numerous Red Cross societies and patriotic committees accustomed to fundraising projects'.[141] But in the US the volunteer relief relied heavily on neighbourhood and new grassroots organization, not top-down organizations emanating from energetic mayors, national civil servants, heads of churches, district leaders, or directors of local branches of the Red Cross, who in New Zealand happened to be men.[142] Besides, in the US, the heavy-handed fundraising campaigns of the Liberty Bond drives during the war may not have been as uplifting and unifying as newspapers portrayed them. The opening pages of Katherine Anne Porter's *Pale Horse, Pale Rider* illustrate instead the sarcastic, thuggish, bullying tactics of their 'inquisitors' as Porter dubbed them.[143]

More importantly, the First World War and the socio-economic contexts that immediately preceded it and contributed to its outbreak splintered civil society. Economic crises, civil unrest, anti-Semitic pogroms, and revolutions in Europe created a surge of East European and especially Jewish immigrants into over-crowded cities on the East Coast and the Midwest. Other cities in the American West had recently grown by even greater rates from cross-border Mexican migra-tion and internal movements within the US. El Paso's population jumped from 736 in 1880 to 77,560 in 1920 but was closer to 100,000 because of undercount-ing Mexicans.[144] As historians have shown, these demographic and ethnic changes in cities led to neighbourhood wars, pitting whites of Anglo-Saxon origins against newcomers as well as conflicts among the newly arrived—Italians against the Irish, Germans, or the Chinese. The same went for smaller industrial towns such as Norwood, Massachusetts, which had experienced waves of immigrant workers from Germany and Ireland since the mid-nineteenth century. Then, ethnic hostil-ities intensified during the first two decades of the twentieth century, with mass immigration from Southern and Eastern Europe. Jerry-built slum housing and linguistic isolation fuelled prejudice that worsened with the recession of 1913

---

[140] See note 67.   [141] Rice, *Black November*, 18, 71.
[142] Ibid., 71, 87, 95, 99, 104, 124, 140: James Henry Gunson, John Luke, Henry Holland, Dr Joseph Frengley, the Reverend Robertson-Orr, William Foster, and Bryan Canon King.
[143] Porter, *Pale Horse*, 183–8.   [144] García, *Desert Immigrants*, 31.

and loss of industrial jobs.[145] War frenzy and nationalist prejudices exacerbated these internecine conflicts. In Norwood, church services in German and even teaching the language were banned.[146] In Newark, all German street names were changed.[147] Beyond ethnicity and class, racial tensions during and shortly after the war further exacerbated this toxic mix. In 1917, one of the worst race riots in US history erupted in East St Louis that continued to 1919.[148] The same year another race riot lasting months spread through Chicago.[149] In 1921 whites destroyed an entire black town adjacent to Tulsa (Greenwood), burning nearly 4000 houses and murdering as many as 400 blacks, women and children included—an event largely hidden from US histories until as recently as 2011.[150]

Economic conditions continued to fan social divisions and hatred immediately before and during the pandemic. Because of a rise in streetcar fares to 6 cents a ride, riots continued for days in Detroit in August 1918 with streetcars turned over.[151] In February 1919, a general strike was called in Seattle, and in the autumn the famous Boston police strike sparked class hatred and violence, with Harvard athletes and Brahmin businessmen supplying the strike breakers. From 1918 to 1920 terrorist bombings, condemnation of Bolsheviks, and a hysterical red scare spread across America, along with the growth of the International Workers of the World, the imprisonment, trial, and ten-year sentence of Eugene Debs, and the trial and executions of Sacco and Vanzetti. In 1918–19, J. Edgar Hoover authorized the secret infiltration of labour unions and radical groups, compiling files on 200,000 alleged radicals. New laws were promulgated against anarchists, and after a spate of bombings in 1919 aimed against business leaders and government officials, including A. Mitchell Palmer, the US Attorney General, the government executed late night raids in eleven cities, arresting anarchists and deporting 249 'aliens'. In January 1920 these midnight raids expanded to twenty-three states with arrests of between 2000 and 3000 supposed radicals.[152] These years also witnessed the spread of Social Darwinism and eugenicist notions of racial and ethnic inferiority.[153]

VENEREAL DISEASE

Finally, as seen in Chapter 5, on the eve of the Great War and mounting through it, suspicions and social divisions cut along another axis—gender—with another epidemic that overlapped the Great Influenza but provoked far different reactions. Women and especially prostitutes bore the brunt of the blame for a rise in venereal diseases that threatened the country's war-readiness. Vice squads rounded up young girls, medical surveillance increased with intrusive and painful examinations,

[145] Fanning, *Influenza and Inequality*, 3–4, 49.
[146] Ibid., 60. [147] Galishoff, 'Newark', 247.
[148] Among other places, see Kraut, *Silent Travellers*. [149] Abu-Lughod, *Race, Space*, ch. 2.
[150] *New York Times*, 19 June 2011. [151] *Toronto Star*, 12 August 1918, 2.
[152] Fanning, *Influenza and Inequality*, 113–14. [153] Ibid., 48.

and organizations such as Michigan's Women's Committee on War Preparedness and the Sunday School Association of Battle Creek lobbied successfully for legislation requiring medical certificates to marry with hefty fines and jail sentences dealt to those carrying venereal diseases. On the eve of this epidemic (1917), six states had passed laws victimizing the victims of sexually transmitted diseases and throughout the influenza crisis eugenics societies pressured other states to pass these laws.[154] Big business supported state plans to eliminate 'vice contamination' by demanding that all factory employees be subject to periodic medical examinations.[155] Dr Olin, director of the Michigan Board of Health, declared that 60 per cent of all dishwashers in hotels and restaurants were unfit to work because of venereal disease and authorized the police to weed them out.[156] Arizona passed laws to dismiss and penalize anyone with venereal diseases 'handling food, acting as barbers, or engaging in occupations where they are likely to infect others'.[157] But as with campaigns against prostitution, the major force of these directives targeted women, even if these calls came predominantly from other women. Groups such as the Women's Committee on War Preparedness and Mothers of the Nation demanded that 'women of the streets do their bit in this terrible war and let the soldiers alone'. These women appealed to 'womanhood', 'kindness', and 'patriotism' not to infect soldiers.[158] With the Great Influenza rising, the health officer in Birmingham, Alabama, turned his attention to the 'curse' of venereal disease, utilizing the police department to rid the city of the disease by 'arresting all women of known questionable character', and, if found diseased, putting them 'in detention'.[159] To this end, they passed ordinances extending police powers to stamp out prostitution[160] and in November devised a programme 'to intern all affected persons...liable to spread the disease'.[161] In Arizona, health authorities blamed Mexicans as the ones especially harbouring venereal disease.[162] Such views about disease and blame appear worlds away from the Great Influenza's spread of compassion and abnegation, but the two were concurrent, appearing in the same cities and often authorized by the same boards of health and city commissioners.

This general milieu of division, distrust, and prejudice, coupled with political, social, and economic unrest was not limited to the US. Across its borders similar class tensions were rife. Winnipeg was 'on the brink of the largest labour confrontation in Canadian history',[163] and further strikes and riots cut across Canada during the Great Influenza. A riot in Toronto involving returning troops shows the tensions and prejudices that surfaced towards the war's end. With jobs scarce, soldiers railed against employing the supposed alien enemy and against aliens in

[154] *Detroit Free Press*, 16 August 1916, 2; 13 September 1917, 8; 23 August 1919, 8; *San Francisco Chronicle*, 14 January 1917, 7.
[155] Ibid., 10 February 1916, 8.   [156] Ibid.
[157] *Arizona Republican*, 15 February 1918, 7.
[158] *Detroit Free Press*, 13 September 1917, 8; also, 8 January 1918, 16.
[159] *Birmingham Age-Herald*, 5 October 1918, 9.
[160] *Birmingham News*, 4 October 1918, 19.   [161] Ibid., 3 November 1918, 4.
[162] *Arizona Republican*, 15 February 1918, 7.   [163] Jones, *Influenza 1918*, 8.

general who had not gone to war. In late September a crowd of 800 soldiers armed with sticks and cudgels attacked foreign shops, foreigners who happened to be nearby, and the police, who intervened to save a Greek. The following Saturday, a group of around 2000 soldiers and civilians attacked foreign citizens. Magistrates used the trials of the soldiers to turn on the national government, blaming the violence on its failure not to intern more aliens. In the same spirit, one of the city's aldermen raised a motion, compelling shopkeepers to display placards in their windows, declaring whether they were British subjects or aliens.[164]

At the end of 1918, the national government held an enquiry before the Industrial Relations Commission in London, Ontario, attended by employers and employees, to gain understanding of Canada's recent spate of unrest in industrial life. Numerous factors were found to be at play—the high cost of living, piecework, importation of strike breakers from the US, defiance of alien labour laws, and the lack of old-age, unemployment, and health insurance. Whatever the causes, one thing was clear: the social and economic setting of the Great Influenza was one of national strife and class division, hardly conducive to compassion and unity across neighbourhoods, class, ethnicity, and race. One of those interviewed was a retired conductor, who reflected on the divisions with pessimism: there was 'little hope; men would have to love their neighbors as themselves before labor troubles would cease'.[165]

In Mexico, the divisions were deeper and bloodier, especially along the border. The Mexican Revolution in 1910 amounted to a civil war that crossed borders with the American occupation of Veracruz in 1914, Pancho Villa's raid on Columbus, New Mexico, in 1916, and the massacre in Santa Ysabel on 10 January 1916, when sixteen Americans were killed.[166] Because of the Mexican threat of invasion, martial law was declared in El Paso. Police barricaded its major thoroughfare and the US sent in the National Guard and Pershing's troops.[167] Spurred on by the war, German efforts to ally with Mexico, the revelation of the Zimmerman Telegraph, rumours of German spies from Mexico sabotaging ranches across the American south-west, and raids across the border with savage reprisals by Texans against Mexicans, the Klu Klux Klan by 1915 found fertile soil in Texas and the south-west. By the time of the war, the Klan became triumphant in El Paso,[168] and the Santa Ysabel massacre ignited 'the city's first genuine race riot'.[169] Yet this general milieu of fear and hate failed to influence influenza. Instead, as we have seen, El Paso's white middle-class and elite women crossed neighbourhood borders, in many cases for the first time in their lives, to deliver care and aid to suffering Mexicans, risking their lives against the deadly contagion. Even with the recent rise of the KKK and anti-Mexican racism, the pandemic's spread from Mexico into El Paso and from impoverished Mexican neighbourhoods to those of middle-class whites did not spark blame against Mexicans or other minorities for causing the disease. Just as

[164] *Toronto Star*, 27 September 1918, 5.   [165] *Globe and Mail*, 25 December 1918, 2.
[166] Luckingham, *Epidemic in the Southwest*, 8; García, *Desert Immigrants*, 7, 188–9; and Lay, *War, Revolution*, ch. 2.
[167] García, *Desert Immigrants*, 189.   [168] Lay, *War, Revolution*, ch. 2.   [169] Ibid., 25.

the immediate context of the pandemic's health advice to avoid crowds and rough up spitters should have dampened people's desires to risk their lives for utter strangers, so too, the broader social and political conditions in North America immediately before and during the Great War should have borne ill for the flu's socio-psychological consequences. Instead, the disease prompted the greatest wave of volunteerism of any epidemic or pandemic in American history, overwhelmingly spearheaded and staffed by women. To what extent can the American experience be generalized?

22

The Great Influenza
(i) Comparative Vistas

To evaluate whether the socio-psychological reactions to the Great Influenza identified in previous chapters were broadly the same across radically different social, political, and ideological terrains, the historian must engage in comparative history. Did reactions in European countries where the war raged differ from those further removed from the battlefields, such as the US, Canada, Australia, New Zealand, South Africa, India, or even Great Britain and Spain, even if all these nations suffered considerable losses of lives and materiel in the war?[1] Before embarking on these transcontinental comparisons, let us look first at the US: were reactions across the country more or less the same?

PERSPECTIVES FROM THE DEEP SOUTH: NEW ORLEANS

Analysis of three major cities in the Deep South suggests regional differences. While papers in none of my three sample cities—New Orleans, Atlanta, and Birmingham—point to incidents where supposed perpetrators of the disease were blamed or the victims themselves were attacked, charity agencies and community responses in these southern cities differed from those sketched earlier. Instead of proudly celebrating a contagion of volunteerism, *the Times Picayune* sounded notes of desperation over the recruitment of health workers, rarely heard in cities examined in the previous chapter. As in other places, Louisiana's doctors and nurses began suffering serious loses less than a week after the first pandemic death was recorded in New Orleans on 29 September 1918.[2] By 5 October, the pandemic had taken from service fifty doctors and seventy-five nurses, and five ward-masters had died.[3] On 6 October, the paper called for nurses;[4] two days later the Red Cross repeated the call.[5] On the 11th, the Red Cross renewed its request. Several days later, the paper appealed for women to come forward to assist influenza nurses,[6] and the next day,

---

[1] To be sure, as Hew Strachan has emphasized, the First World War was a global war with battle-fields across parts of Africa, the Middle East, Central Asia, the Far East, and the seas, and not a solely a European one, but Europe was the central theatre; see Strachan, *The First World War*, chs 3 and 4.

[2] *Times Picayune*, 29 September 1918, 22.   [3] Ibid., 6 October 1918, 24.

[4] Ibid., 6 October 1918, 11.   [5] Ibid., 8 October 1918, 14.

[6] Ibid., 13 October 1918, 4.

for automobiles to transport nurses.[7] That day, the paper sounded a more desperate note. Beneath the headline, 'HOUSEHOLD HELP IMPOSSIBLE TO GET', it claimed that many 'alarmed by reports of the dreaded influenza' were refusing to work in any houses, where 'illness of any kind' was present. 'The panic' had spread to cooks, maids, washerwomen, and yardmen. The only ones willing to fill vital posts were 'negro women', who entered factories and lumberyards, 'taking up heavy labor to replace men'. Physicians, unable to find trained nurses, also turned to 'colored women adept in practical nursing'.[8]

Calls for qualified nurses in New Orleans continued through the worst weeks of the pandemic and in outlying areas of the city's coastal region until December.[9] Before the second half of October, few signs of volunteerism are seen: no stories of debutants sweeping floors, socialites donating automobiles, college girls assisting physicians, or other women working themselves to exhaustion. In mid-October, state officials and the *Times Picayune* in front-page headlines complained: 'Public Not Doing Share in Fighting Influenza'.[10] The same day, the acting director of Civilian Relief for the Gulf Division of the Red Cross elaborated: 'Our people do not seem to realize…what this situation is like.…We cannot supply sufficient nurses.' As it had done over the previous two weeks, the paper unleashed its desperate call for help:

> attendants…need not be trained…may be white or black, man or woman. Something must be done and done quickly, lest we face a hopeless situation…People are succumbing by the scores simply for the want of minor attention.[11]

The second half of the month, however, proved to be a turning point: the frequency of desperate appeals fell, replaced by an upsurge in articles attesting to acts of heroism and mass volunteerism. The first to answer the call were black women. Perhaps realizing (as the story above suggests) that they were more willing than whites to take the risks, the Red Cross 'scoured' the city to gather 'as many negro women for such service' as could be found to volunteer as 'assisting nurses', cleaning and caring for the influenza-afflicted.[12] Several stories followed with parallels seen in the previous chapters in other states. The captain in charge of the Red Cross auxiliary on St Charles Avenue paid tribute to 'business girls', who after work were making emergency masks.[13] The same day, an article gushed over citizens' sudden willingness to step forward 'to give aid in the present emergency'. That Wednesday, the nursing enrollment bureau was 'besieged all day' with men and women 'of all stations of life' offering their services, with the result that more than fifty volunteers were placed that day.[14] The next day, Claybourne Avenue Presbyterian Church donated its Sunday School classroom to a branch of the Red Cross.[15] By 20 October, women were responding to the calls for nurses and carers at a New Orleans asylum which held more than a hundred orphans under a year

---

[7] Ibid., 14 October 1918, 6.   [8] Ibid., 14.
[9] Ibid., 15 October 1918, 10; 19 December 1918, 13; 25 October 1918, 10.
[10] Ibid., 16 October 1918, front page.   [11] Ibid., 5.
[12] Ibid.   [13] Ibid., 17 October 1918, 8.
[14] Ibid., 6.   [15] Ibid., 18 October 1918, 8.

old.[16] On the 22nd, the Red Cross opened thirteen milk stations across New Orleans for the needy, sick, and convalescent. A woman was in charge.[17] By November accolades rolled in praising women volunteers, but the praise pertained almost exclusively to raising money for the war effort—the Liberty Bonds. Of twenty-one women singled out, only a Mrs Foxley had also 'found time' to nurse the sick infected by influenza.[18] Another exception appeared at the end of November: a college girl was remembered for her 'supreme sacrifice for patriotism'. She had contracted meningitis and died as a volunteer nurse at the Jackson Barracks, but she was the only college student mentioned sacrificing herself for the influenza-stricken.[19]

Not only does this meagre record of women's involvement in influenza relief pale by comparison with that seen in other regions, the way in which women participated in New Orleans was different. Here, the impetus came from the top down, with initiatives organized by established bodies, most prominently, the Red Cross; and, except for black women, in the beginning, men and women appear to have answered the calls to volunteer in equal measure. Reports of new organizations that could be seen as evidence of grassroots movements, such as neighbourhood soup kitchens, motorcades staffed by women, and groups of schoolteachers, school-age students, and university co-eds feeding, washing, and caring for the afflicted, do not appear.

The Male Response in New Orleans

New Orleans' turn from fear and panic to communitarian zeal had another side, one that differed from the patterns seen across much of the nation but was in line with its earlier yellow fever history.[20] This was to organize the charitable assistance through men's social clubs. On 15 October, members of the New Orleans Elks Club converted their organization into a free dispensary for drugs and medical services for influenza sufferers. By the 18th, three of its members—professional pharmacists—had filled a thousand prescriptions gratis, the club's physicians had made 498 house calls, and other members were loaning their automobiles to deliver medicines and transport doctors. In addition, the clubhouse had become a soup kitchen feeding the stricken. These middle- to upper-class men forfeited time from lucrative professions and promised to follow up all cases 'systematically' until the patients recovered. Enrolling a large corps of assistants, they worked night and day shifts. By the fourth day, news that physician members of the club were providing medicines and free medical attention spread through the city, and the dispensary became 'swamped'. Those at the desk worked from 7 a.m. late into the night. One of its 'expert' pharmacists had been on active duty not only 'every night but all night'. Other members donated money. In addition to providing poor patients

---

[16] Ibid., 20 October 1918, 10.   [17] Ibid., 22 October 1918, 6.
[18] Ibid., 3 November 1918, 5.   [19] Ibid., 30 November 1918, 8.
[20] See Chapters 17 and 18.

with medicine, milk, and food, the club made donations to other charities, such as St Vincent's Orphan Asylum, where the nurses and sisters caring for the children had been stricken by the pandemic.[21]

On 22 October, the Elks converted their 'home' on Canal Street into an emergency hospital.[22] Two days later, they equipped a banquet room of the St Charles Hotel to serve as sleeping quarters for physicians and interns, who treated patients round the clock.[23] By the 26th, they had recruited twenty-eight physicians and on that day alone treated 932 influenza patients free of charge.[24] The following day, the *Times Picayune* gave a statistical sketch of the club's contribution. In less than two weeks, its physicians had made 11,228 house calls; its pharmacists had filled 13,440 prescriptions; and 'thousands of eggs, crackers, oranges and hundreds of loaves of bread and gallons of milk' had been distributed to the poor, afflicted with influenza. By this time, fourth-year medical students at Tulane University had joined the Elks' physicians.[25] By 1 November, when the dispensary was discontinued because of the city's 'great improvement' in health, their house calls had exceeded 15,000.[26] On the 10th, the state Board of Health sent the Elks a letter of praise: 'no organization realized more keenly than yours the need of help during the influenza epidemic'.[27]

While the Elks Club was the first association in New Orleans to volunteer to fight the pandemic,[28] other male groups followed. In addition to Tulane's fourth-year medical students, New Orleans' dentists passed a unanimous decision to offer their services to the Health Board for the duration of the pandemic, 'wherever the board thought dentists could be most effective'.[29] A third group, travelling salesmen trapped in the city by the pandemic, assembled and called themselves the 'Knights of the Grip', discarding 'their badge of trade in favor of the Red Cross Brassard'. They volunteered as nurses, dispensed medicines under physicians' directions, waited on the sick, and posted adverts in newspapers, such as 'Will sit up with patients after midnight'; 'Will go on duty 10 pm to 2 am'.[30] The Southern Yacht Club at Lake Pontchartrain, north of New Orleans, formed a fourth group, donating equipment to the Red Cross Emergency Hospital and allowing anyone convalescing from influenza to stay in their clubhouse.[31] Finally, in November, yet another male group, the Negro Chauffeurs' Association, gave a vote of thanks to their employers for allowing them to have transported doctors, nurses, and other workers on emergency trips throughout the pandemic.[32]

Recently, historians have argued convincingly that the mysterious character of the Great Influenza might account for the peculiar fact that nurses received greater praise than physicians. The doctors' supposed discoveries, treatments, and cures had made little difference, whereas the simple care of nurses was in great demand and proved more efficacious. These divergent experiences account for differences in

---

[21] Ibid., 19 October 1918, 3.
[22] Ibid., 22 October 1918, 3.
[23] Ibid., 24 October 1918, 5.
[24] Ibid., 26 October 1918, 5.
[25] Ibid., 27 October 1918, 10.
[26] Ibid., 1 November 1918, 12.
[27] Ibid., 10 November 1918, 25.
[28] Ibid., 20 October 1918, 10.
[29] Ibid., 20 October 1918, 25.
[30] Ibid., 23.
[31] Ibid., 21 October 1918, 10.
[32] Ibid., 16 November 1918, 16.

outlook at the end of 1918: why nurses momentarily saw a bright future for their profession, while for doctors, the optimism that had steadily grown since the 1870s came to sudden, if temporary, halt.[33] While the character of this strange influenza was more or less the same across most of the globe, the perception of doctors and nurses appears not to have been everywhere the same. In New Orleans, parts of Louisiana, and I would speculate the Deep South more generally, this reversal in esteem did not happen. Here, the major praise, as with past epidemics of yellow fever, was showered on men and doctors. In December, at the end of the worst wave of the pandemic, Louisiana's Health Board celebrated physicians and surgeons for their 'fine and noteworthy part' in the Great War and during the influenza pandemic: 'no comprehensive history of the conflict can omit' these contributions that had cost the lives of 'as many as 35,000 doctors from America'.[34] No comment was made about nurses' sacrifices.

Atlanta

Even though keyword searches for 'influenza' and 'grippe' during the critical months from September to the end of 1918 produce more results from the pages of the *Atlanta Constitution* than the *Times Picayune*,[35] the coverage of local news in the former reveals much less about any rallying of volunteers to fight the flu— stories of self-sacrifice, organization of soup kitchens, and donations—or about issues such as price gouging, rent-raking, and protests against infringements of personal liberties. Instead, Georgians appear to have been cooperative, 'readily complied with' mask wearing (where it was imposed) along with closures of schools, theatres, and churches.[36]

Compared with cities of the north-east, as well as El Paso, San Francisco, and New Orleans, news of the pandemic in Atlanta was humdrum. At the beginning of October, before the pandemic touched civilians, cases at its nearby military installation, Camp Gordon, had reached a crisis: health authorities called for emergency nurses from Atlanta, and they responded.[37] But Atlanta's women were not the only ones or even the principal ones to answer the military's call. Two days earlier, 'a mob of registrants had besieged' the induction office at Camp Jessup for work in its transport corps, 'decimated by the epidemic': 'men, motorcycle men, and mechanical men of all ages' rallied to the call.[38] To meet the demand for nurses in hospitals and homes in mid-October, Atlanta's Red Cross opened a school to teach elementary home nursing so that 'every woman in Atlanta' could 'treat an influenza emergency' at home or meet the demand for volunteer nursing, which

[33] Bristow, 'You Can't Do Anything'; idem, *American Pandemic*, 13; Foley, *The Last Irish Plague*, 101; Witte, 'The Plague', 52 and 57; and idem, *Erklärungsnotstand*, 164–5.

[34] *Times Picayune*, 12 December 1918, 8.

[35] For the keyword 'influenza', 1 September 1918 to the end of December, the *Atlanta Constitution* produces 499 results, mostly in October (307 results).

[36] *Atlanta Constitution*, 22 October 1918, 4. It was imposed in Macon and Americus.

[37] Ibid., 3 October 1918, 4.   [38] Ibid., 1 October 1918, 5.

was 'becoming more urgent every day'.[39] No comment followed on whether Atlanta's women responded. But less than a week later, the Red Cross made 'an urgent appeal' for nurses, coaxing women 'to realize the great responsibility resting upon them', and defending their 'right to call for their patriotic co-operation'.[40]

Again, it is difficult to know how Atlanta's women responded. However, unlike in New Orleans, when the crisis intensified in the second half of October, the news did not encourage a sharp rally in volunteerism. The *Atlanta Constitution* hints only at a few positive signs. On 24 October, the Red Cross established canteens to aid the afflicted with Atlanta's women providing the services. In addition, they invented a new initiative—consoling 'heart-broken' soldiers infected with influenza. If they failed to recover, the women wrote letters of condolence to the soldiers' girlfriends, brides, or mothers, and provided fares for them to attend soldiers' funerals.[41] The paper divulges only traces of women's volunteer work in other Georgian towns, such as a notice in a column on Savannah's 'Social News': 'For the past two weeks the girls had been too involved with work for the Liberty Loan, the Red Cross, and the motor corps, leaving no time for other interests'.[42]

Perhaps women's volunteering and organizational initiatives were running apace with trends elsewhere, the difference depending instead on newspapers' sense of what was newsworthy. But this was not the case with women's involvement in the war effort, such as the care they provided in Georgia's military camps. During the war's closing stages, groups such as the Council of Jewish Women volunteered at nearby military camps mending garments for soldiers, and 'colored women of Atlanta' did the same 'for their men in the colored wards'.[43] By contrast, during the epidemic, there is an absence of reports on women joining motorcades, organizing soup kitchens, and running or staffing emergency hospitals, and for Atlanta and its region, less is heard of men's initiatives, nothing akin to New Orleans' Negro Chauffeurs, yachting elites, or the Elks Club pharmacists and physicians.

Birmingham, Alabama

The principal papers of Birmingham, Alabama, featured women, black and white, during the rise of the pandemic in October 1918, celebrating their organization and contributions to the Fourth Liberty Loan along with volunteer work at Birmingham's nearest military installation, Camp McClellan, in Anniston. The social pages reported their activities, such as the 'most excellent work' of Birmingham's Jewish women building a club room for their 'Jewish boys' at Camp McClellan.[44] But as with Atlanta and its region, almost nothing is mentioned about women or men volunteering as nurses, staffing diet kitchens, or organizing neighbourhood groups to assist the influenza-afflicted. Here, as elsewhere across the US, schools closed, creating 'enforced vacations' for teachers and students, and 'leaving women

---

[39] Ibid., 16 October 1918, 3.   [40] Ibid., 20 October 1918, B3.
[41] Ibid., 24 October 1918, 10.   [42] Ibid., 20 October 1918, B6.
[43] Ibid., 11 October 1918, 6. It also praised the city's 'Victory Girls', for collecting Liberty Bonds and donations for US forces; ibid., 31 October 1918, 4.
[44] *The Birmingham News*, 1 November 1918, 13.

teachers in an unsatisfactory frame of mind'.[45] But unlike developments in Boston, El Paso, Albuquerque, Carlsbad, Ogden, and many other cities, no news appears of teachers turning their pent-up energies to join or create organizations that entered homes to feed, clean, nurse, and care for the seriously stricken or their children.

* * *

Despite the possibility that newspaper reportage may have varied across the US, several conclusions can be drawn. Volunteerism in the Deep South differed from the form it took across much of the country, but despite the variation, nowhere did popular reactions lead to the ugly consequences that had flared up only several years before with smallpox and polio in America, or earlier with cholera across Europe. For no other disease in US history had women volunteered in such numbers and with such zeal, risking their lives, as in the autumn of 1918, even if places such as New Orleans may have proven outliers, where the traditions of yellow fever continued to form charitable habits with men providing the bulwark of relief.

THE VIEW FROM ITALY

Eugenia Tognotti supports Alfred Crosby's and others' claims that the Great Influenza was the Great Forgotten Pandemic. For Italy, she goes further, suggesting that even in its own time, news of it was largely snuffed from the Italian press. Notes on it appeared only occasionally and only within the columns on local city news (La Cronaca di Roma, di Milano, etc.).[46] She is correct in observing that the news of the pandemic appeared mainly as local news. Further, these papers commented on the international spread of the disease far less often than the US, Canadian, French, or Australian press. However, she is mistaken that Italian papers acted as though the disease was not among them. Milan's *Corriere della Sera*, *Il Secolo*, the socialist paper, *Avanti!*, Rome's *Idea Nazionale*, *Il Messaggero*, and provincial papers such as *Il Cittadino: Rivista di Monza e del Circondario* reported it regularly, some every day throughout October and into November, with articles occasionally spanning several columns and including more than statistics of supposed new cases and deaths.

Yet Italian papers, more than any others I have read, seem to have been engaged in a collective sense of denial. From their reports, it would be difficult to imagine that by October, Italy was experiencing among the highest mortality rates from the pandemic of any country in Europe.[47] The international press, however, reported that even in September, before the October upsurge, Italian cities such as Rome and Milan were suffering badly, with estimated deaths from influenza and pulmonary conditions reaching a hundred a day.[48]

Even Italy's questionable official statistics show a sharp climb in influenza cases and deaths in October. News coverage rose along with the rise in cases and then fell

[45] *Birmingham Age-Herald*, 21 October 1918, 5.   [46] Tognotti, *La 'Spagnola'*, 18.
[47] Ibid.   [48] *The Globe and Mail*, 27 September 1918, 5.

in November. Yet throughout October, papers insisted that the pandemic was in decline, stationary, or at most registering only slight increases. For instance, Rome's *Idea Nazionale* continued reporting into the second week of October that 'la Spagnola' was stationary or had appeared 'only in a mild form'.[49] With deaths reaching their peak in the third week, it claimed that 'the vast majority of cases' were 'not serious': less than 2 per cent, it maintained, resulted in death, and it was worse in other European countries.[50] This denial and seeming tranquillity in the face of mounting mortality is seen in a long interview with Colonel Mennella, director of the military's public health in Italy (Sanità Militare). He held that the public was calm. The problem lay with doctors raising alarms about bronchial/lung complications and requesting army medics to intervene. 'As always' the colonel reported, the army responded 'nobly' and sent civilians more than 8000 doctors, even though the alarm was unjustified. Mennella charged that they saw 'fever' deaths everywhere: if someone was run over by a tram, the death was called 'the Spanish Fever!' 'Such nonsense (*follia e di impressionabilità*) was spreading through all of Italy'. He reassured readers that 'in a few days influenza would be a vague memory'. The same day the municipal Office of Hygiene reported a sharp decline in cases for many Roman neighbourhoods but warned that 'alarmist voices' might spur on cases of other epidemic diseases.[51] On 25 October, it continued to claim that influenza was in steep decline.[52] Rome's widely circulating *Il Messaggero* was similarly reassuring, claiming as late as 11 October that the pandemic had reached only a few neighbourhoods and pneumonic complications were extremely rare.[53] When the disease reached its peak, the paper assured readers that the mortality remained low and was 'nearing its end'.[54]

Despite these assurances, concerns about the pandemic seep through local news items. By 5 October, in Rome 'without exception' relatives and friends were restricted from entering the wards of 'serious influenza cases'.[55] Two days later, *Idea Nazionale*, despite its cautions, reported that the numbers of sick and dying were climbing and better medical provisioning was necessary for the 'growing needs of the stricken, especially among the poor'. New sanitary legislation was enacted, requiring all doctors in Rome to be on call; and a crisis in the supply of milk had arisen, making it difficult to nourish infants.[56] Two days later, Rome's municipal government imposed restrictions on movie houses and other places of public entertainment.[57] *Il Messaggero* expressed concerns over sanitation in Rome's poorer quarters, calling on the population to help clean the streets and advising them not to approach the ill and to avoid crowded places.[58] By mid-October, *Idea Nazionale* admitted that 'no specific remedy' existed for the spread or cure of influenza, and

[49] *Idea Nazionale*, 8 October 1918, 2; 15 October 1918, 2.

[50] Ibid., 18 October 1918, 2; 19 October 1918, 2. *Il Cittadino: Rivista di Monza* presented a more realistic account; see 3 November 1918, 3; not until 7 November did it report the pandemic in decline.

[51] *Idea Nazionale*, 3 October 1918, 2.   [52] Ibid., 25 October 1918, 2.

[53] *Il Messaggero*, 11 October 1918, 3; see interview with Tivoli's deputy for public health; ibid., 12 October 1918, 2.

[54] Ibid., 15 October 1918, 2.   [55] *Idea Nazionale*, 5 October 1918, 3.

[56] Ibid., 7 October 1918, 2.   [57] Ibid., 9 October 1918, 2.

[58] *Il Messaggero*, 11 October 1918, 3; and 15 October 1918, 2.

medical supplies and personnel were not to be found in many of the province's communities. The municipality summoned doctors, pharmacists, and nurses to report to the Provincial Office of Medicine for service.[59] Two days later, *Idea Nazionale* admitted, shortages of doctors now affected not just the provinces but the city.[60] On the 18th, it reported that sanitary conditions were 'hardly normal' and military assistance for doctors, disinfectants, and medical supplies was needed.[61]

By the second half of October, the situation in the provinces had become more serious. The military had been summoned, but failed to solve the 'sanitary problems'. Military doctors were hard to find, and 'medical service along with guards and nurses is absolutely insufficient'. Forgetting its praise of and confidence in the military's intervention two weeks before, *Idea Nazionale* reported that 'military doctors now refused to obey orders and treat civilians'. It also accused those in the provinces of being hostile to any 'protective norms'; instead, 'all too often they relied on superstitious practices that worsened the epidemic'. Finally, it charged that pharmacists and 'occasionally the distrustful doctor' 'profited at the expense of the people, making the crisis terrible everywhere'.[62] However, unlike the violent incidents of cholera seven years before, neither this article nor others hinted at any individual or collective acts of hatred and violence.

Il Messaggero drew similar points on the same day, adding that the difficulty of finding pharmacists, especially at night, was worsening conditions in Rome, and in the South (Mezzogiorno) 'things were much worse'. On the 20th, it admitted that the epidemic had 'assumed exceptional proportions throughout the country' with only 'scarce medical resources' available to combat it.[63] By the 22nd, with influenza reaching its official peak mortality, the municipality took measures to close the city's theatres and passed an ordinance prohibiting the eight-day celebration of the dead, when cemeteries become overcrowded. It reduced opening hours of bars and restaurants (*osterie*) at weekends and required telephone operators to wear masks.[64] Two days later, the military's Health Works ordered that masks should be worn by its doctors and nurses in influenza wards.[65] In addition, new decrees threatened crooked pharmacists (*farmacisti ladri*) 'with grave consequences'; the city closed its largest cemetery (Verano), its 'variety' theatres,[66] and by the 27th, theatres of all sorts.[67] In November, with the pandemic in decline, *Il Messaggero* finally expressed some respect for this influenza: 'diseases such as cholera and smallpox were relatively easy to isolate and combat'. Influenza was different. 'Its cases continue to multiply by the hundreds'.[68]

As in so much of its past, post-unification Italy was not of one piece. Even in September, before influenza took off in October, Milan's *Corriere della Sera* reported the threat more realistically than seen in Rome. Unlike Colonel Mennella's opinion that to be concerned about Rome's influenza was no more than cowardly hypochondria, Milan's chief physician (*medico-capo municipale*) admitted as early as

[59] *Idea Nazionale*, 15 October 1918, 2.   [60] Ibid., 17 October 1918, 2.
[61] Ibid., 18 October 1918, 2.   [62] Ibid., 20 October 1918, 2.
[63] *Il Messaggero*, 20 October 1918, 2.   [64] *Idea Nazionale*, 22 October 1918, 2.
[65] Ibid., 24 October 1918, 2.   [66] *Il Messaggero*, 23 October 1918, 2.
[67] *Idea Nazionale*, 27 October 1918, 2.   [68] *Il Messaggero*, 10 October 1918, 3.

mid-September that 'the so-called Spanish Grip' had been serious since spring and that the public must confront it as a 'true and real influenza in epidemic form'. He then clarified that it was 'a pandemic, not the influenza in endemic form with which we are accustomed', and arresting it was 'humanly impossible'.[69] At the end of the month, against the central government's proclamation that the disease 'posed no cause for pessimism', the Milanese paper, relying on 'numerous scientists and doctors', revealed it to have been widespread for some time and presently 'unique in its rapid diffusion and virulence'.[70]

In early October, a month before Rome had enacted concrete measures other than disinfecting streets and houses in the worst-affected neighbourhoods, Milan began taking legislative action, and its chief paper, *Corriere della Sera*, pushed for further 'efficacious decrees'.[71] The municipality decreed that windows in trams be left open for better ventilation, believing that dust was one of the disease's vectors. By 3 October, the city's movie houses were closed and pharmacies' opening hours extended to ten at night;[72] military doctors were recruited, and sanitary assistance was offered free of charge. Schools remained open but with measures to avoid crowding. Several days later they were closed, and when reopened, examinations were postponed.[73] Milan's mayor decreed that doctors register all cases of influenza.[74] On the 13th, the city closed dives (*bettole*) and lower-class inns (*osterie*), prohibited funeral processions and the ringing of church bells, and integrated medical and pharmaceutical services with those of the military, placing both under the latter's command.[75] By the 19th, entry into city cemeteries to honour the dead was prohibited.[76] Trains and funerals were cancelled or suspended.[77] Throughout the month, because theatres were allowed to remain open, owners of movie houses protested the unfairness of theirs being closed. By the 21st, their protest had achieved some reforms: theatres now were allowed to remain open but only if rigorously disinfected and with admission limited to the galleries.[78] By contrast, in Rome only cinemas were closed and only for a few days.

Already by 2 October, Milan's municipal physicians (*medici condotti*) had been called repeatedly, often in vain, causing several to defect.[79] By the 17th, emergency services and 'Guardie Mediche', who addressed the most urgent cases, had reached a breaking point. The city faced a lack of doctors, and those who remained were worked to exhaustion—the city's health services grinding to a halt. The municipality appealed to private doctors (*liberi professionisti*), but the uptake was insufficient. The city decided to change tack, hospitalizing as many influenza cases as possible instead of sending doctors on thousands of house calls. The military offered Milan its hospital, the Fratelli Bandiera, with over a thousand beds. Yet 4000 to 5000 more were urgently needed.[80] Already by 2 October, the paper reported that an

---

[69] *Corriere della Sera*, 19 September 1918, 3.   [70] Ibid., 29 September 1918, 2.
[71] Ibid., 2 October 1918, 3.   [72] Ibid., 3 October 1918, 3.
[73] Ibid., 16 October 1918, 3.   [74] Ibid., 2 October 1918, 3.
[75] Ibid., 13 October 1918, 3.   [76] Ibid., 19 October 1918, 3.
[77] Ibid., 24 October 1918, 3.   [78] Ibid., 21 October 1918, 2.
[79] Ibid., 2 October 1918, 3.   [80] Ibid., 17 October 1918, 2.

absence of personnel had delayed funerals and burials.[81] Finally, as in Rome, people complained about the shortages and the excessive price of drugs.[82]

Yet, in contrast to papers in the US, Britain, and Canada, *Corriere della Sera* tried to convince its readers, perhaps under pressure from central government, that the pandemic was stationary or in decline, even as it raced toward peak mortalities in October.[83] It criticized 'alarmist' voices[84] and massaged the mortality figures, claiming throughout the first half of October that they were levelling off, and besides, the disease had been 'mainly benign'. No doubt, remembering Italy's cholera riots of seven years before, the paper speculated that anxieties could 'inseminate fantasies and terror among the less cultivated classes'. Even though admitting that the present influenza possessed greater lethality than normal, it consoled its readers that such 'developments are not new' and the disease's 'critical period' was about to pass.[85]

Turin's major paper, *La Stampa*, presents a third scenario. It best fits Tognotti's generalization of a near news blackout on the influenza.[86] During the worst month, when other papers were reporting influenza daily, its *Cronaca cittadina* remained mostly silent on the subject for Turin and its province but reported on trends in Rome and Milan. Before October, only two of its stories concerned the pandemic: one was a brief mention of the troubles it caused the German offensive;[87] the other an interview with Turin's director of medical services. Yet, unlike other major Italian newspapers, the article held that influenza had already risen sharply in September, had become a serious threat to public health, and had created disquiet among citizens. Unlike Rome's papers, and to a certain extent *Corriere della Sera*, the interview treated the disease seriously, commenting that it could strike a population 'as if it were lightning' and possessed all the markings of the 'la grande epidemia' of 1889–90.[88] It refrained from reporting the disease's daily tallies, reasoning that because doctors were not required to register them, the statistics were meaningless.[89] The paper's neglect of influenza news, however, did not reflect the city's or province's indifference to controlling it. By 6 October, Turin had passed ordinances regulating public spaces, which went beyond Rome's, Milan's, and (as *La Stampa* boasted) those of any major Italian city. Turin closed all theatres, movie houses, and 'caffè concerti' (bars with musical performances). Funeral cortèges were prohibited and pharmacies' night hours extended.[90] Priests were encouraged to register influenza cases and deaths and to restrict church services.[91] By mid-October, Turin doubled its core of physicians, by turning to the military for supplies and staff.[92] At the end of the month, *La Stampa* contended that influenza-related cases and deaths in Turin had been fewer than in other big cities and

[81] Ibid., 2 October 1918, 2; and 4 October 1918, 3.   [82] Ibid., 21 October 1918, 2.
[83] Ibid., 2 October 1918, 3; 5 October 1918, 2; 6 October 1918, 3; 17 October 1918, 2.
[84] Ibid., 3 October 1918, 3.   [85] Ibid., 21 October 1918, 2.
[86] Tognotti, *La 'Spagnola'*.   [87] *La Stampa*, 14 August 1918, 4.
[88] Ibid., 24 September 1918, 2.   [89] Ibid., 9 October 1918, 3.
[90] Ibid., 6 October 1918, 3.   [91] Ibid., 8 October 1918, 3.
[92] Ibid., 15 October 1918, 3.

attributed the difference to its enactment of numerous decrees that diminished crowding in public places and 'the discipline characteristic of our population'.[93]

Finally, the socialist paper, *Avanti!*, published in Milan, gives a fourth perspective, one critical of the government, more serious about the disease's threat, and more damning of the lack of scientific understanding of the disease. It was the only paper to attack the policies of government and the military to contain it. By the last week of September, it challenged the assurances given to the public that the disease was the usual influenza and questioned the discovery of its bacillus. 'A great deal of nonsense (*delle gran sciocchezze*) clouded the origins, development, and methods of treatment of the "grippe spagnuola"':[94] citizens had reason for alarm.[95] By early October, it recognized the plight of communal doctors: 'they had nowhere to turn. When they asked colleagues for help, they received no answers; when they sought help from "the famous military doctors", none was to be found!' Because of the deluge of patients and bureaucratic procedures, municipal physicians were forced to endure 'superhuman' hours. Hospitals turned away patients, because all the beds were full. Municipalities failed to enforce decrees to control the disease, and 'people were dying like dogs without assistance'. One of the *medici condotti* challenged readers: 'if you doubt these circumstances, then just walk the streets of working-class quarters in any major Italian city'.[96] The paper mocked 'the chatter' about cures and preventive measures announced at medical conferences. The disease was misunderstood and its medicine was 'the patrimony of charlatans'.[97]

Avanti! was even more critical of Milan's failure to act. No one, it alleged, dared to speak of the government's neglect of hygiene or implementation of decrees to inhibit overcrowding.[98] The city's sanitary state left much to be desired. Before the war it was poor; now the proletariat was forced to live in overcrowded conditions. Minimum standards of hygiene guaranteed by government had become a dead letter.[99] *Avanti!* stressed Rome's negligence: within days, the limited supplies of tobacco, thought to help prevent the disease, disappeared because speculators cornered the market, and pharmaceutical assistance remained insufficient.[100] The paper then turned to the military's contribution, so praised in other newspapers. With most civilians without medical assistance, it asked, 'where are the military doctors?'

Reactions in Italy

In Europe, criticism of profiteering from the pandemic's afflicted was even more muted than in the US. *Avanti!* pointed to the speculation of private enterprise but only with regard to one commodity—tobacco.[101] The Italian newspapers explored above show no evidence of landlords skimping on heat or expelling the afflicted.

---

[93] Ibid., 29 October 1918, 2.   [94] *Avanti!*, 26 September 1918, 3.
[95] See the reports by physicians Brunelli and Bruni in *Avanti!*, 27 September 1918, 3.
[96] Ibid., 3 October 1918, 3; also *Il Secolo*, 9 October 1918, 3.
[97] Ibid., 11 October 1918, 3; and 17 October 1918, 3.   [98] Ibid., 4 October 1918, 3.
[99] Ibid., 22 October 1918, 3.   [100] Ibid., 7 October 1918, 3.
[101] *Avanti!*, 7 October 1918, 3.

Nor do tales of profiteering by undertakers, gravediggers, or funeral directors appear, despite unburied bodies, overflowing cemeteries, and problems finding gravediggers.[102] Similarly, no hints arise that fruit sellers were charging excessive prices. Instead, the shortages that municipalities and papers saw as threatening were of bread and milk. Yet no charges of profiteering surfaced. The national government's ministry on provisioning (Il Ministero per gli Approvigionamenti ed i Consumi)[103] and municipalities[104] responded immediately by increasing supplies and ensuring milk was distributed directly to babies and the afflicted. The government also intervened to maintain supplies of medicine.[105] An alarm was sounded in Rome against profiteering by pharmacists, but only fleetingly since the city quickly passed an ordinance to control their prices.[106] Milan's Consiglio Sanitario warned of severe shortages of medicines and excessive prices, but neither the government nor the papers accused pharmacists of profiteering. Instead of punitive action, the municipality increased supply,[107] and the next day, *Corriere della Sera* singled out pharmacists for special praise: they had undertaken 'a veritable "tour de force"', keeping their dispensaries open until 11 at night to ensure medicines to fight the pandemic were not in short supply.[108] Their 'civic pride and humanity' had gained citizens' gratitude.[109] Milan was not alone in its praise. With the pandemic in decline by November, Turin's town council met to give thanks to its physicians (*medici condotti*), health officials, and pharmacists, particularly those in the provinces, 'for their abnegation and zeal in undertaking every request for assistance'.[110]

A second profession at times found wanting, especially when the pandemic was reaching its peak in October, were doctors. On 2 October, *Corriere della Sera* reported that five of the city's employed doctors (*condotte*) had defected,[111] and on the same day in Rome, Colonel Mennella chided civilian doctors as 'unjustifiable alarmists'. Even after the army's loan of doctors, the country kept making desperate pleas for doctors, pharmacists, and nurses, especially within the provinces.[112] On 18 October, the government again admitted the need for doctors in the province of Rome and appealed to the military for further medics.[113] They were 'making themselves scarce' and refused to treat civilians with influenza.[114] As we have seen, journalists were making similar charges against the military in Milan.[115] Yet these views were contested. The following day, a deputy from Rome's provinces charged that matters were not so atrocious as claimed: the military's medical intervention had been positive. Because of the distances between houses in the countryside, he argued, civilian medical corps had not been able to reach isolated places, but the military's health corps always arrived 'orderly and promptly...bringing comfort

[102] *Corriere della Sera*, 2 October 1918, 3; and 4 October 1918, 3.
[103] *La Stampa*, 22 October 1918, 3; *Il Messaggero*, 12 October 1918, 2.
[104] *La Stampa*, 6 November 1918, 3; *Idea Nazionale*, 7 October 1918, 2; 19 October 1918, 2; 30 October 1918, 2.
[105] *La Stampa*, 23 October 1918, 2.			[106] *Il Messaggero*, 23 October 1918, 2
[107] *Corriere della Sera*, 21 October 1918, 2.		[108] Ibid., 22 October 1918, 3.
[109] Ibid., 18 October .1918, 2.		[110] *La Stampa*, 2 November 1918, 3.
[111] *Corriere della Sera*, 2 October 1918, 3.
[112] Ibid., 15 October 1918, 2; and 17 October 1918, 2.		[113] Ibid., 18 October 1918, 2.
[114] Ibid., 20 October 1918, 2.		[115] *Avanti!*, 3 October 1918, 3.

and well-being everywhere'.[116] By November, as with the pharmacists, the press praised civilian doctors, both private practitioners and those employed by municipalities, for their long hours of work, sacrifices, and zeal, 'answering every call'. And despite trenchant criticisms against government authorities at every level and especially the military, *Avanti!* had only praise for the 'good will' of the overworked *medico condotto*.[117]

Except for *Avanti!*, Italian newspapers praised military doctors for contributing more than civilian doctors in protecting civilian populations. In Rome, Milan, and Turin their interventions were seen as essential. At the same time as the army's gift of 8000 medics to the civilian struggle against the pandemic, its local Milanese branch also answered calls from Milan's Ospedale Maggiore. With the numbers of afflicted soaring, the city was in desperate need of hospital beds. The military donated 1400 beds from its 'Fratelli Bandiera' and placed its military medical personnel 'at the complete disposal' of civil authorities. At the end of September, the army had already made similar provisions with other hospitals in the provinces, for instance, in Sesto San Giovanni and places near Como, where it had donated twenty-four of its doctors.[118] Three weeks later, it provided a hundred hospital beds for civilians afflicted in Monza.[119]

By the second week of October, for Milan's new strategy of hospitalizing influenza patients, the municipality depended on the resources of the military, which again responded, donating another 8000 beds to the city. The military answered further calls, supplying vans (*furgoni*) to the city to ease the growing problem of providing funerary services.[120] From *Corriere della Sera*, the military's contribution also appears extensive in southern and central Italy. In answering appeals for more doctors and pharmacists, the army sent 800 medics principally to southern Italy on 20 October.[121] And as seen from an interview with Tivoli's deputy, by the middle of October, the military had filled the breach in medical and health services in Lazio due to the lack of civilian personnel.[122]

In addition, government agencies assumed new charitable activities. National and local authorities engaged in providing provisions to the poor, the influenza-afflicted, and infants, especially bread, milk, and meat when they became dangerously scarce in early October. Even at the pandemic's peak, the Office of Hygiene guaranteed that anyone afflicted with influenza should be visited by a private doctor or one employed by the city.[123] Municipalities also intervened. Towards the end of October, Rome assumed extra emergency roles by providing housing and care for mounting numbers of orphans. In normal times these responsibilities fell to ecclesiastical bodies, such as the Congregazione di carità, but this influenza's peculiar mortality, killing off those in the prime of life, had drastically upset the balance. On 27 October, the Congregazione tried securing spaces for 300 babies

---

[116] *Idea Nazionale*, 21 October 1918, 2.
[117] *Avanti!*, 7 October 1918, 3; and 22 October 1918, 3.
[118] *Corriere della Sera*, 4 October 1918, 3; and *Il Secolo*, 2 October 1918, 3.
[119] *Il Cittadino*, 24 October 1918, 2.   [120] Ibid., 12 October 1918, 3.
[121] *Il Messaggero*, 20 October 1918, 3.   [122] *Idea Nazionale*, 21 October 1918, 2.
[123] Ibid., 19 October 1918, 2.

but found shelters for only seventy.[124] The following day, *Il Messaggero* reported that 250 orphaned infants still had nowhere to turn. The municipality (Il comitato di organizzazione civile) supplied another seventy.[125] Institutions caring for orphans in the province of Milan also became overburdened. The Milanese government had to suspend accepting further orphans into its homes. But one unit in the government, the Office of Assistance Because of the War, intervened, and 'gathered homeless orphans from the surrounding countryside, placing them in a house at Sordomuli donated by the Italian Red Cross. Milan's 'Comune' assumed responsibilities for running the new institute but encouraged others to assist by arranging parties and donating books and toys for the 'poveri piccini'.[126]

Volunteerism and Charity in Italy

Long-standing charity organizations, first the Church, then the Red and White Cross, played significant roles in addressing the crisis. On occasion, these went beyond the usual charitable acts. Not only do no protests surface from parish priests resisting restrictions on church services or the disinfection of sacred objects (as occurred seven years earlier during the cholera riots at Ostuni); in Milan, they volunteered to disinfect their buildings and homes around them.[127] The White Cross was also active in citizen relief efforts in Rome with special squads to disinfect the houses of anyone who asked.[128] Finally, the people of Rome thanked the American Red Cross, which from 1 November had intervened to provide assistance.[129]

On the other hand, Italian newspapers reveal little about grassroots organizations, individual initiatives, or collective acts of heroism, especially undertaken by women. Few stories, and certainly nothing akin to the US's in-depth interviews and photo supplements praising women's initiatives, appear in Italian papers. The absence of women might partly be explained by the relative lack of liberties and freedom of movement enjoyed by Italian women compared to their American or English counterparts, but in England (as we will see) women's involvement was equally lacking. A more compelling factor may have been the military's presence, which in Italy assumed responsibility for these vital tasks. Another reason may stem from Italian city-state traditions reaching back to the Middle Ages with the comunes employing the doctors, who provided medical services during emergencies often free of charge. But these bodies did not supply the urgent demand for nurses and nurses' aides, who tended to be women.

An exception may have come in November in Rome, where the soup kitchens ('le cucine economiche') of the Circolo San Pietro[130] and those 'of the family' in the Via Crescenzio and in the Piazza del Grillo[131] supplied 'entirely for free' 6000 rations for the needy every day. They were staffed by doctors employed by the city

---

[124] Ibid., 27 October 1918, 2.   [125] *Il Messaggero*, 28 October 1918, 2.
[126] *Corriere della Sera*, 23 October 1918, 3; also *Il Secolo*, 23 October 1918, 3.
[127] *Corriere della Sera*, 12 October 1918, 3.   [128] *Idea Nazionale*, 19 October 1918, 2.
[129] Ibid., 29 October 1918, 2.
[130] Founded by young noblemen in 1869 to sponsor Catholic solidarity and charitable activities.
[131] I find no information on these groups.

and the 'Committee of the Families of the Sick' ('Comitato alle familgie delle persone ammalate').[132] From their brief description, it is difficult to know whether municipal authorities with their employees (as with doctors) or the Catholic male youth of the Circolo San Pietro or volunteers from neighbourhoods were the prime movers and participants. Most probably, it was a combination of all three. However, the tradition of these 'cucine economiche', which reaches back at least to the early nineteenth century, appears to have been different from the grassroots voluntary neighbourhood organizations that were serving the afflicted in the US and Canada. The Circolo San Pietro originated with Pius IX (1792–1878) during the war between the Vatican and Garibaldi (1870). Originally, their pots were part of the war effort, distributed to the Pontifical army, the Zuavi.[133] Moreover, during Italy's previous epidemic of cholera, 1910–11, accompanied by economic crises in the South, the central government and local municipalities established and financed these bodies in places such as Barletta and Taranto in Puglia to quell crowds of outraged townsmen and peasants, who had stormed hospitals and attacked medical personnel.[134] Like the care of orphans and supply of hospitals beds, their initiative derived from the central organs of the Church and state, and their rank and file, at least in the case of the Circolo, historically had been composed of men. But in a second case, assistance came from outside the structures of Church and state. For Rome's orphanage crisis, ultimately the daily paper *Il Messaggero* intervened, using its paper to solicit private and corporative contributions to keep the children alive.[135]

The Italian news, however, occasionally singled out certain professions such as doctors and pharmacists for praise of their long hours of toil, skill, and self-sacrifice. In mid-October, the Council of Milan's hospitals (Il Consiglio degli Istituti Ospitalieri) used the Milanese papers to express their appreciation for the sacrifices of doctors, nurses, stretcher bearers, and morgue attendants, praising their 'admirable devotion' in caring for over 3900 cases of influenza. The institute then praised nurses for their sacrifices, over 700 of them, 236 of whom had succumbed to influenza. Eight were named, and all but one was a woman.[136] Monza's local weekly paper extolled the church's sisters and nurses, who cared for the flu-stricken in the town's hospitals. They had taken the largest losses: 'words could not express the importance of their arduous labour and self-sacrifice'.[137]

However, unlike the praise pouring from US newspapers on nurses and women volunteers performing a wide range of services, these are the only instances I have found of Italian papers recognizing women's contributions during the Great Influenza. The others celebrated by the press or by municipal governments were men—a Professore Devoto, director of the Clinica del Lavoro, who visited influenza

---

[132] *Idea Nazionale*, 29 October 1918, 2.   [133] Website of Vatican City.

[134] See Chapter 10.

[135] *Il Messaggero*, 27 October 1918, 2; 28 October 1918, 2; 29 October 1918, 2.

[136] *Corriere della Sera*, 17 October 1918, 2; *Avanti!*, 17 October 1918, 3; and *Il Secolo*, 16 October 1918, 3.

[137] *Il Cittadino*, 24 October 1918, 2.

victims in their homes free of charge;[138] Signore Bortelli, who in late October gave 5000 lire to help finance the new orphanage at Sordomuli;[139] and a municipal counsellor in Rome, Ausonlo Levi, praised for his vigilance over the city's health system throughout the pandemic and his efforts to enlist volunteers to keep the city clean.[140] The city council of Prati presented a Signore Chiappi Paolo with special thanks during the milk crisis; every morning he distributed from his estate 50 litres to influenza-stricken families.[141] Finally, early in the New Year 1919, first *Corriere della Sera*,[142] then Milan's counsellor for health (*assessore d'igene*) gave thanks to Professor Stefano Belfani for (supposedly) developing a vaccine against influenza.[143] Moreover, male-dominated professions were the ones singled out for praise—first doctors, then medical officials. As noted earlier, *L'Avanti!* extolled the 'superhuman' labour and abnegation of Milan's civilian doctors. Milan's *Il Secolo* praised military doctors and health workers 'who had already contributed in a superior measure to public health... forty-five medical officials and ten sergeants, students of medicine, had paid with their lives in the towns of Milan's Province'.[144]

As statistics from Milan's hospitals indicate, women and especially nurses may have given their lives more often than men in comforting the afflicted but were not recognized for it. Even the women's magazine, *La Madre Italiana: Rivista Mensile*, while praising Italian women's heroism nursing soldiers at the front,[145] stayed silent on their sacrifices during the Great Influenza. Nor did women's organizations such as the Società Cattolica Femminile relate any charitable deeds or sacrifices by its members to succour the afflicted. At its annual convention on 2 November, it praised services delivered to the poor but said nothing about 'la Spagnola'.[146] In contrast to America, evidence fails to point to Italian women gaining new, high-profile leadership roles in charitable organizations or initiating and staffing new organizations such as emergency hospitals or soup kitchens. To what extent did these differences in recognition reflect different social realities? To what extent might they be attributed to newspaper prejudices? As we have seen, Italian papers had not ignored Italian women's nursing and sacrifices on the battlefield. In addition, papers said little about the charitable roles of men or their initiatives beyond those organized by the military or national and municipal governments. The Great Influenza does not appear to have fired the enthusiasm and charitable vigour of young men with the spirit of unity of the new nation seen during the cholera epidemics in 1867, 1884, and 1887. Could it have been that not enough of them had been spared from war now to fight a second one against *la Spagnolo*? At any rate, the Italian case clearly differs from that in the US (and, as we shall see, in Canada, Australia, New Zealand, and South Africa). Nonetheless, in contrast

---

[138] *Il Secolo*, 3 October 1918, 3.   [139] See note 125.
[140] *Idea Nazionale*, 30 October 1918, 2.   [141] Ibid.
[142] *Corriere della Sera*, 11 January 1919, 3.   [143] Ibid., 14 January 1919, 3.
[144] *Il Secolo*, 21 October 1918, 2.
[145] Türr, 'Un'eroina della Guerra', recounts the 'virile courage' of an English nurse Hilda Wynne, who 'abandoned her life of splendours and wealth to enter battle camps at Dixmunde, Ypres, Furnes, Galizia', to treat troops on the front lines and organized transport of 4000 wounded.
[146] *Il Cittadino... di Lodi*, 2 November 1918, 2.

with nearly a century of cholera, the Great Influenza did not spawn conspiracies, blame, or hatred that had repeatedly ripped communities apart as late as 1911. In fact, with the near absence of blame directed at profiteers and lack of rancour over church closings, Italy's reactions to the Great Influenza appear more pacific than those in America.

FRANCE

As in Italy, the French reported the 'Great Influenza' less frequently than in the US, Canada, or Australia; in fact, various online newspapers in the Gallica collection show the French devoted fewer articles to this influenza than to much less serious waves before or after 1918–19.[147] Yet French reportage differed from the Italian. It did not present the influenza solely in sections of local news. Nor did it persistently try to convince readers that the pandemic was a bagatelle quickly to pass, even if early in the pandemic, it assured readers that their present 'grippe' was not as serious as the previous one in 1889–90.[148] As early as the summer wave, Paris's *Le Figaro* described it as abnormal, because of its fatal complications.[149] In early July and August, *Le Matin* reported that the pandemic spread rapidly through its region, infecting large numbers, and took a form often leading to death.[150] At the end of September, the paper reported it had inflicted 'cruel ravages' on French ports 'for some time', especially in Brittany.[151] By mid-October, Parisian headlines admitted the pandemic was failing to show signs of decline; the city had closed schools, and because of the 'great number of victims' insisted further measures were necessary.[152] In the same month, the grippe 'reigned' so severely in Lyon that the mayor had suspended funeral processions and curtailed the time the dead could be laid out with corpses carted immediately to the cemetery. In smaller towns such as Bourg and Molin, theatres, cinemas, lectures, and all meetings were prohibited.[153] And in various towns, church services were suspended.[154]

On other matters, the French press was more taciturn than the Italian. Complaints against profiteering landlords, undertakers, pharmacists, or lemon vendors fail to appear. One sign of discontent towards new ordinances came at the end of October from the diocese of Cherbourg but amounted only to regrets that all the churches of France had been closed (curiously, those in Cherbourg were not

---

[147] For instance, more results for 'grippe' arise in *Le Figaro* in 1907 (167), 1893 (145), and 1915 (151) than in 1918 (132). References to 'grippe' in *Le Matin* exceeded 1918 (128 results) even during a non-epidemic year, 1922 (163).

[148] *Le Matin*, 8 August 1918, 4; 24 October 1918; 9 November 1918; *La Presse* 8 August 1918, 4; *Le Petit Parisien*, 17 August 1918, 4; *Le Figaro*, 10 October 1918, 2.

[149] *Le Figaro*, 8 July 1918, 4.

[150] *Le Matin*, 7 July 1918, 2; 20 August 1918; and *La Presse*, 20 August 1918.

[151] *Le Matin*, 25 September 1918, front page; also 8 September 1918; and *La Presse*, 25 November 1918.

[152] *La Presse*, 17 October 1918, 2–3.

[153] *La Lanterne*, 17 October 1918, 2; and 19 October 1918, 2.

[154] Ibid., 11 November 1918, 2.

included in the ban).[155] France's National League Against Alcoholism voiced concern over an ordinance providing extra supplies of rum to aid sufferers. Unlike in the US where doctors since 1890 had changed their minds on alcohol's efficacy, the French stood by it and allocated pharmacies with quantities of rum to be distributed to the afflicted. The League did not, however, challenge the government's decision and the government would have agreed with the League's caution plastered on Parisian walls: 'Alcohol and rum in small doses does some good against the grippe but in large doses is injurious'.[156] Nonetheless, 'a scandalous traffic in rum' arose with some vendors selling it at 'truly excessive prices'.[157] This was the only instance of profiteering revealed by the press during the pandemic, and it appeared at the end.

In contrast to the US and even Italy, French papers reveal little about volunteerism in combating the pandemic—nothing appears about any new groups of men or women entering homes of the stricken, organizing soup kitchens, or donating automobiles. It is not as though the French state did not need assistance. When the pandemic was reaching its peak in the second half of October, the Under-Secretary of State appealed to the military for doctors to be released for emergency cases among civilians.[158] No later reports reveal whether the appeal was met. Several days later, Paris's municipal government requested any with a diploma as a midwife or nurse to care for influenza patients in Paris's hospitals. But this appeal was not exactly an example of voluntarism. The paper insisted that the applicants would be paid.[159] The Parisian papers pointed to terrible overcrowding in the hospitals,[160] but none of the papers I surveyed point to any organizations or individuals establishing emergency influenza wards or refurbishing buildings and supplying them with volunteer recruits as seen across the US. With the scourge near its peak in October, the municipal Office of Public Assistance suggested converting public schools into emergency hospitals, but the proposal was rejected, because the buildings lacked appropriate equipment.[161] The same, of course, was true of elementary and high schools in the US in 1918. What appears to be missing from Paris were initiatives from women such as Katherine Gorbutt, principal of El Paso's Aoy High School, along with throngs of young women volunteers. Even when advising their congregations on the proper behaviour to combat the pandemic, the Catholic Church recommended prayers, rosaries, and devotion to saints Roch and Sebastian, not self-sacrifice or voluntary work from their ranks or the laity to aid the afflicted.[162] As with Italy, one reason for the absence of voluntarism may have been the military's and governments' insistence on meeting the emergencies. In early October the military contributed six of its automobiles to the City of Paris to transport the stricken to Parisian hospitals.[163] Two weeks later, it 'donated' seventeen doctors

[155] Ibid., 28 October 1918, 2.   [156] *La Lanterne*, 24 November 1918.
[157] *Le Petit Parisien*, 19 December 1918, 2.   [158] *Le Figaro*, 20 October 1918, 3.
[159] Ibid., 23 October 1918, 2.   [160] *Le Petit Parisien*, 22 October 1918, 2.
[161] Ibid., 23 October 1918, 2.   [162] *La Lanterne*, 28 October 1918, 2.
[163] *Le Figaro*, 10 October 1918, 2.

to be stationed in Paris's fire department barracks, ready to receive calls from distressed patients.[164]

Similarly, the municipality of Paris made unusual donations to address the pandemic's demands, placing an automobile at every fire station in the city to transport anyone struck by grippe to the nearest hospital.[165] At every police station, it placed a cyclist on permanent alert to deliver medicines to the stricken.[166] No appeals or donations of automobiles from civilians fill newspapers. In addition, the national government intervened. In the last week of October, the Commissioner of Gasoline and Combustibles allocated 2.5 litres of fuel ('caburant') to every cab in Paris, if it transported medics to influenza patients.[167] To ensure drugs remained in adequate supplies without price gouging, the government (L'Office technique de pharmacie) provided 2500 kilos of sulphate of quinine, oil of ricin, and antiseptics to Paris's pharmacies and promised other chemical products.[168] In addition, the Under-Secretary of State mobilized pharmacists serving the military to extend services to civilians, as had already been ordered of military doctors.[169]

Finally, except for an appeal for women midwives and nurses (male and female) made only towards the end of October, none of the online newspapers in Gallica appealed for women to volunteer aiding nurses, delivering messages, preparing liquid diets, answering telephones, driving ambulances, or other tasks to stem the pandemic's advance. Moreover, the French press gave notice of only two cases of personal sacrifice in aid of influenza victims; both were brief and concerned young men. One, aged nineteen, died of influenza as a volunteer for the Société de Secours aux Blessés Militaires;[170] the other, seventeen, died while volunteering at the YMCA.[171] In addition, the municipality and the papers paid tribute to Mr Charles Gidden Osburne, transport director of the American Red Cross. 'Graciously', he made nine ambulances available to Paris, 'a precious addition to our sanitary services'. No doubt, women participated as Red Cross hospital workers ('many of whom had died...for their zeal and dedication'), thanked by the organization's director in the third week of October. Yet none was named or their deeds singled out.[172] Certainly, women were included in the tribute of Monsieur Godard, director of administrative services in Paris's town hall, when he praised nurses, male and female (*des infirmiers et des infirmières*) 'who paid the highest price with their lives'.[173] But, again, none was named.

The reasons for women's near absence may reflect biases by the French press, but were they any more sexist in 1918 than papers in the US or Italy? Certainly, indications of bias are easily found. *Le Matin* in November 1918, then *Le Figaro* in December, concluded that influenza mortality rates in Paris had been 'notably' higher among women than men, which may have been true (even if in places such as Hartford, Connecticut, women died in lower proportions). The papers' reasoning, however, was exceptional: women's higher rates depended on their greater

[164] Ibid., 24 October 1918, 2.   [165] Ibid., 3.
[166] Ibid., 25 October 1918, 2; and 27 October 1918, 4.   [167] Ibid., 25 October 1918, 2.
[168] Ibid., 24 October 1918, 3.   [169] *Le Petit Parisien*, 1 November 1918, 2.
[170] *Le Temps*, 25 October 1918.   [171] Ibid., 13 November 1918.
[172] *Le Figaro*, 24 October 1918, 3.   [173] *Le Petit Parisien*, 17 October 1918, 2.

'emotionalism (*cette émotivité*)', 'a fatal characteristic' that sprung from their 'phys-ical weakness and fear fixed by heredity'. Women, allegedly, had greater difficulties breathing and therefore 'were less resistant to infectious germs'.[174] But can such attitudes account for the stark differences observed between the US and France in the ranks of women volunteers? Like the American and Italian papers, the French were not reluctant to praise women heroines on the Western Front.

SWITZERLAND

With the spread of influenza in the summer of 1918, Switzerland received more attention from the international press than any country in Europe, except possibly Germany.[175] When influenza struck Swiss military camps and civilians in cities such as Berne with particular force, Swiss papers[176] did not attempt to convince readers that the present pandemic was without danger. Like the Italian, French, and British press, the *Journal de Genève* compared its present pandemic with the previous one of 1889–90, but came to the opposite conclusion: 'One thing is certain today…our present epidemic is more deadly than the one of 1889'. The paper pointed to two peculiar characteristics of the present one: it led more frequently to heart attacks and struck young adults most gravely.[177] At the end of the month, Lausanne's daily made no attempt to disguise the crisis: only three pharmacies remained open in the entire region, and waiting times for doctors even to examine the dead took at least two hours.[178] According to the paper, the war in part accounted for the medical crisis: most pharmacists had been drafted, leaving the public without sufficient assistance or medicines.[179] The paper did not, how-ever, see the crisis simply as one created by war or natural causes. Instead, it attrib-uted the extent of mortalities to the disarray among government authorities, each giving contradictory advice.[180]

By the third week of August, first in Berne, then other Swiss cities by early September, the pandemic was on the decline,[181] and criticisms of the government subsided. Papers now paid respect to their municipalities for having acted prudently. In fact, more than in Britain, France, and Italy, Swiss cities and their cantons had taken rigorous measures to control the disease with internal quarantines and closure of public spaces. Fribourg created a 'lazaret d'isolement' for its cases of influenza.[182] Berne closed its schools, refused to let churches hold Sunday services, and, while bars remained open, music and especially singing were banned. Church services were allowed to resume on 29 August but without singing, the assumption

---

[174] *Le Matin*, 10 November 1918; *Le Figaro*, 31 December 1918.
[175] See for instance *Evening World*, 24 June 1918; *New-York Tribune*, 22 August 1918; *Il Messaggero* 13 October 1918, front page; *Georgetown Herald*, 31 July 1918, 2; *Globe and Mail*, 25 July 1918, 2.
[176] Papers in Le Temps archives historiques.   [177] *Journal de Genève*, 18 July 1918.
[178] *Gazette de Lausanne*, 30 July 1918, 4.   [179] Ibid., 31 July 1918, 4.
[180] Ibid., 7 August 1918, front page.
[181] Ibid., 23 August 1918, front page; 10 September 1918, front page; 12 September 1918, 4 (Lausanne and Vevey).
[182] Ibid., 15 September 1918, 2.

being that the broadcasting spread the disease. On the same day, schools reopened but with health examinations to determine whether students should be admitted.[183] Because of the decline in influenza cases, Montreux in the Canton of Vaud rescinded its 'restrictive ordinances of July', with religious services to resume on 1 September.[184] Vevey ended all its restrictions two weeks later.[185] Finally, on 8 September, Zurich declared its city 'virtually grippe-free' and attributed its success first to the energetic response taken by its department of hygiene, and second, to the city's position with its 'open spaces and many gardens'.[186]

Switzerland's grippe did not, however, end in September. By early October, Lausanne recommended masks when caring for or in the presence of the ill; schools and cafés closed (with or without singing), and places of assembly were monitored with strict regulations.[187] In Neuchâtel classes at the university were closed.[188] In other towns, church services again were forbidden,[189] and isolation cars reserved for the sick were added to the train network.[190] This time, no complaints about government inaction or confusion arose, nor protests over the restrictions. Instead, Swiss papers give signs of volunteer work being undertaken and civilian sacrifices being appreciated.

Volunteerism in Switzerland

In early October, a society called the Good Samaritans (started during the Great War), comprised largely of health care workers, was officially praised for the sacrifices made by their doctors treating the influenza-stricken. In Lausanne, the medical corps of doctors was lauded as an 'intellectual elite', treating not only physical problems but moral ones 'with humanity and Christian zeal'.[191] At the same time, evidence of volunteers nursing influenza patients appears in Lausanne, with published precautionary instructions for their treatment, although none of the volunteers was named.[192] Much of the praise for sacrifice and volunteer work came from the military and concerned caring for soldiers. Even when volunteers visited homes of afflicted civilians, the carers were under military authority. Moreover, the volunteers were generally members of pre-existing societies. In the New Year, 1919, the *Journal de Lausanne* saluted the 'very precious' assistance of volunteers. The first to be mentioned were army doctors, followed by Red Cross workers, then the Society of the Good Samaritans, 'which worked for the public good in collaboration with the health services of the army'.[193] At the annual conference of Lausanne's Société des Samaritaines, the president of the society tallied up the group's services and accomplishments over that troubled year. These included repatriating captured soldiers, providing them with 50,366 litres of coffee, 800 cartoons of condensed milk, 9128 petits pains, and 1600 litres of hot

---

[183] Ibid., 23 August 1918, front page.   [184] Ibid., 31 August 1918, 4.
[185] Ibid., 12 September 1918, 4.   [186] Ibid., 10 September 1918, front page.
[187] Ibid., 8 October 1918, 2.   [188] Ibid., 19 October 1918, front page.
[189] Ibid., 11 November 1918, front page.   [190] Ibid., 21 November 1918, front page.
[191] Ibid., 5 October 1918, 2.   [192] Ibid., 8 October 1918, 2.
[193] Ibid., 19 January 1919, 2.

drinks. Their activities had concentrated on attending influenza-stricken soldiers. The Samaritans from Lausanne had been sent to the camps and battlefields. Only ninety-two of them had served at home ('garde-malades'). Yet these civilian initiatives differed from those in the US. Those of the Swiss happened under army supervision.[194] Another group praised at the end of the epidemic (August 1919) was the Swiss Red Cross: 742 of its 'sisters' had cared for the grippe-afflicted, soldiers and civilians, sixty-nine of them dying in service.[195]

One story, however, praised civilian volunteers who were not members of pre-existing organizations. Still, their self-sacrifice was for the armed forces and not their communities. In 1918, 'a great number' of French-speaking Swiss troops from the Vaudois were laid up, stricken with 'la grippe' at Zolingue (Zofingen), a German-speaking village in the Agrovienne (presently, the Canton of Aagau). At the end of the year the captain and chaplain of the regiment paid tribute to local doctors, soldiers of the health division of the Swiss German troops, and above all to 'a large cohort of local ladies and girls'. On their own initiative, they had converted their school into a hospital for the soldiers and had demonstrated 'exceptional zeal and perseverance' caring for them. Many of the locals paid the price with their lives. In addition, the captain praised them for 'their web of affection and confederation', which cut across linguistic barriers and more remarkably across the antipathies of war. The inhabitants of Zofingen had been allied with the Germans, and many of their families had been injured or killed by French Swiss soldiers. Yet on the grave of one of the Swiss French-speaking soldiers, who died of influenza and was buried in Zofingen's cemetery, the villagers erected a plaque expressing their condolences. The captain wished now to convey the gratitude of his soldiers. They thanked their 'dear confederates', the municipality, and the nurses, male and female, expressing 'the emotions, both of the sorrows and the charity, they had experienced together'. He wished to publish their sentiments 'so that this example should not be forgotten'.[196] Zofingen was not alone in bringing civilians to aid enemy soldiers stricken by flu. Less dramatically, individual civilians, professionals, and tradesmen such as pharmacists and the association of masons in the Vallée de Joux, Canton of Vaud, donated sums to comfort these soldiers and their families.[197]

More than the French papers, the Swiss singled out individuals who had lost their lives volunteering to succour the influenza-infected. As in North America and Canada (see Chapters 21 and 23), those celebrated were often women from the elites as well as from ordinary walks of life. A twenty-nine-year-old women, the concierge of Paudex College (Canton de Vaud) died while caring for 'les grippes' within the county, and on the eve of her passing, had continued her service 'at the bedside of her patients'.[198] In Bienne, another woman, aged twenty-eight, a volunteer of the Société des Samaritaines of her hometown, Yverdon, died in hospital caring for the soldiers afflicted with influenza.[199] A tribute was paid to a sister of the Red Cross, the daughter of a Swiss federal judge. For her treatment of afflicted

---

[194] Ibid., 24 March 1919, 2.   [195] Ibid., 29 August 1919, 6.
[196] Ibid., 28 December 1918, 2.   [197] Ibid., 24 November 1918, 2.
[198] Ibid., 21 October 1918, 2.   [199] Ibid., 3 January 1919, 2.

soldiers, the paper opined: 'just as medals were pinned on soldiers for their courage, so too this woman deserved hers'.[200] Women nurses were not alone in receiving praise, as we have seen with the recognition of the services rendered by doctors of the Good Samaritans in October. A month later, the *Journal de Lausanne* singled out two male doctors at the lazaret of la Broye in the Canton de Vaud for their sacrifices.[201]

One key difference between the emergency defences against the pandemic in North America and in places on or near Europe's battlefields appears to have been the centrality of the military. As in Italy, this presence may help explain the absence of grassroots movements and organizations to combat the pandemic and the comparative paucity of civilian volunteers, sacrificing their time, money, and ultimately their lives in this struggle. Nonetheless, despite the diversities across regions, one commonality appears. Instead of breaking societies asunder with accusations of blame and violence against the victims of the disease, the Great Influenza brought communities together: in the case of Zofingen, that union united bitter enemies in mutual respect for acts of abnegation.[202]

THE BRITISH ISLES

More than in Italy, France, or Switzerland, the British press reported developments of the pandemic at home and abroad, with weekly reports of cases and deaths in the major cities of England, Wales, and Scotland. More distinctive was its sustained attention to the pandemic's spread across the world, as it informed readers about the measures adopted by Portugal to combat the pandemic;[203] the pandemic's recrudescence in Swiss cantons;[204] misery in Hungary;[205] the need to mobilize military doctors to treat civilians in Paris;[206] and its spread through Ireland,[207] Denmark,[208] and Russia.[209] The British press cast its net far beyond Europe, reporting the disastrous mortalities in Mumbai at the end of September 1918,[210] high mortalities in Cape Town and citizens' responses;[211] extraordinary mortalities in Kimberley, South Africa;[212] the consequences for Tangier;[213] and the pandemic

---

[200] Ibid., 21 August 1919, 4.   [201] Ibid., 10 September 1918, 4.

[202] The Great Influenza united other antagonistic groups such as Protestants and Catholics in Temuka, New Zealand. While the Great War had intensified sectarian hatred, the Great Influenza brought volunteers from both religions to work together; Rice, *Black November*, 150.

[203] *Guardian*, 26 November 1918, 12.   [204] *The Times*, 10 October 1918, 5.

[205] *Scotsman*, 22 October 1918, 4.   [206] *Guardian*, 26 October 1918, 8.

[207] Ibid., 6 November 1918, 8; and 19 November 1919, 6.

[208] *Scotsman*, 2 November 1918, 4.   [209] *Guardian*, 19 November 1918, 12.

[210] Ibid., 27 September 1918, 5.

[211] Ibid., 10 October 1918, 5; 12 October 1918, 5; *Scotsman*, 15 October 1918, 4; 30 October 1918, 6; 25 December 1918, 7; *Guardian*, 18 September 1918, 8; 17 March 1919, 8.

[212] *Guardian*, 21 October 1918, 4; *The Times*, 31 October 1918, 5; 28 November 1918, 4. On Kimberley's experience, also see Phillips, '*Black October*'.

[213] *The Times*, 12 October 1918, 5; 22 October 1918, 5; and 29 October 1918, 5.

in Egypt,[214] Sierra Leone,[215] the Congo,[216] and Mauritius.[217] British papers charted the pandemic's progress through Canada[218] and noted policy decisions in the US down to the municipal level, as with Pasadena's mandatory masks.[219] It gathered details along the Yangtze and in Shanghai[220] and focused on regions where the mortality and lethality were greatest: in the Tonga Isles,[221] Upolu,[222] and other Pacific Islands,[223] with reports of expeditions into the Yukon[224] and villages along Labrador's coast, where populations had been extinguished almost entirely.[225] No other national press, the US included, comes close to Britain's global coverage. By contrast, readers of Italian papers may not have even known the Great Influenza was global.

On the other hand, British coverage of its own isles was less exciting than adventure stories thousands of miles from home—of dog sleighs, for instance, carrying doctors, nurses, and medicines from Dawson City to settlements in the Yukon, where the remnants of a community had barricaded themselves in their huts against their huskies, which had acquired a taste for human flesh.[226] Accounts of British experiences amounted mostly to dubious statistics. Yet in contrast to the Italian press, these made no effort to cover up the pandemic's advance. The *Scotsman* argued for the need to make influenza a notifiable disease and recorded Glasgow's high death rate in mid-October at 38 per 1000 inhabitants,[227] which climbed a week later to 41 per 1000.[228] Mortality in Kirkcaldy was even higher, at 65 per 1000.[229] At the end of September, with a second wave attacking Glasgow, six schools in the city were closed.[230] On 25 October, the Edinburgh Royal Infirmary closed its doors to all visitors,[231] and days later, Edinburgh shut its schools and barred children from movie houses.[232] At the same time, Parliament discussed the need to release military doctors for civilian purposes.[233] By the second week of November, the pandemic was on the decline in Scotland,[234] but 'serious increases' continued in England and Wales.[235] At the end of the month, the crisis appeared more serious in London and Birmingham than in any Scottish city.[236] The mortalities created shortages of gravediggers and undertakers. Dead bodies rotted in houses for as long as ten days. London's Lord Mayor summoned the military, and Birmingham's chief

[214] *Guardian*, 5 January 1919, 10.   [215] Ibid., 17 September 1918, 8.
[216] Ibid., 25 April 1919.   [217] Ibid., 1 June 1919, 15.
[218] *The Times*, 15 October 1918, 7; 4 December 1918, 7; and 5 December 1918, 9.
[219] Ibid., 30 October 1918, 7; *Guardian*, 3 March 1919, 3.
[220] *The Times*, 5 November 1918, 5.   [221] Ibid., 3 January 1919, 8.
[222] *Scotsman*, 25 December 1918, 4.   [223] *Guardian*, 26 January 1919, 6.
[224] *The Times*, 29 November 1918, 7.   [225] *Guardian*, 2 July 1919, 8.
[226] *The Times*, 29 November 1918, 7; and *Irish Times*, 7 December 1918, A5.
[227] *Scotsman*, 15 October 1918, 4.   [228] Ibid., 22 October 1918.
[229] Ibid., 6 November 1918, 2.   [230] *The Times*, 27 September 1918, 3.
[231] Ibid., 25 October 1918, 4.   [232] Ibid., 31 October 1918, 4.
[233] Ibid., 30 October 1918, 4.
[234] Ibid., 11 November 1918, 4; 13 November 1918, 4; and 15 November 1918, 4.
[235] Ibid., 7 November 1918, 4.
[236] *Le Figaro*, 1 July 1918, 3 and 3 July 1918, 3; and *Scotsman*, 27 November 1918, 4.

medical officer appealed for volunteer nurses.[237] But this was the *Scotman*'s sole mention of any requests for volunteers during the pandemic.

No complaints about profiteering, protests about church closures, or disputes over restrictions of personal liberties appear in the Scottish press. The clearest sign of discontent over policy came when influenza cases were on the wane. A deputation from theatre and cinematograph proprietors appeared before Edinburgh magistrates, asking that restrictions on theatres, music halls, and cinemas be rescinded. The magistrates refused, but no protest ensued.[238] A second possible scandal reported by the *Scotsman* concerned the military's inflexibility in meeting the need for doctors at the end of the war. A month after the Armistice, army doctors became 'miserably unemployed'. The situation was particularly irksome for those who had left lucrative practices in London for war service, made all the more annoying since doctors in London were 'worked off their feet' by the winter increase in cases.[239]

More surprising is the total absence of signs of volunteerism in Scotland or recognition of civilian self-sacrifice in combating the pandemic. Its absence cannot be attributed to editorial views that such information was without public interest. In late November, the *Scotsman* praised the Danish Red Cross for transporting 50,000 British war prisoners from Germany back to Britain, emphasizing the 'enormous number of Danish surgeons and nurses who had volunteered' to care for prisoners afflicted with 'Spanish influenza'.[240] The paper reported volunteers in Cape Town engaged against influenza, which by the end of November had killed 50,000.[241] At the end of the year, it reported in greater detail the nature of South African volunteerism in Kroonstad in the Orange Free State. Early in October, the public called a meeting to devise strategies for combating the epidemic, divided the town into districts, took a census, and organized patrols to find and assist the stricken. Volunteers with their own motor cars, soup, milk, and medicines entered homes to assist the afflicted. Influenza incapacitated two of the five volunteer doctors; when they recovered, the other three fell ill. Then their stocks of medicines ran out. Many of the nurses and VADs, who came from Durban, were laid low.[242] Perhaps the absence of news on Scotland's own volunteers was because they were not needed, despite the high death rates in Glasgow and Kirkcaldy. These certainly cannot compare with the mortality rates in Cape Town, Kroonstad, West Samoa, or among the Inuit, but they were on a par with other European cities as well as with North America, where the Great Influenza so forcefully spurred civilians, especially women, to risk their lives volunteering and organizing new associations.

* * *

Reportage of the Great Influenza in England runs along similar lines as for Scotland. First, restrictions were placed on public life—closing of schools, meetings, and places of amusement—but with much less rigour than in the US, Canada, New Zealand, Australia, Italy, or France, and this may explain why the disease

[237] Ibid., 27 November 1918, 4.
[239] Ibid., 7 December 1918, 7.
[241] Ibid., 30 November 1918, 6.

[238] Ibid., 15 November 1918, 4.
[240] Ibid., 20 November 1918, 3.
[242] Ibid., 25 December 1918, 7.

lingered longer in England and Scotland than in many wealthy countries in the Northern Hemisphere. As in continental Europe, the pandemic hit Britain with full force in the summer of 1918, well before striking civilian populations on America's East Coast. Yet it did not reach peak mortalities in Manchester,[243] London,[244] and other English cities until mid-February 1919,[245] when medical and other essential services were nearing collapse.[246]

Not until September 1918 were any restrictions placed on public gatherings in Greater London, and these were limited to cinemas, prohibiting admission to children under fourteen. Other forms of public entertainment could stay open so long as they closed every three hours for forty-five-minute breaks to clean the premises.[247] On 14 November, children's peace demonstrations were prohibited, and 'many' but not all schools and cinemas closed.[248] At the beginning of November, Manchester shut two of its elementary schools,[249] and with influenza raging as ferociously, if not more so, during the third wave at the end of February, the city's health board debated school closures but left them open.[250] In late October 1918, Leeds went further, closing of all its elementary and secondary schools and excluding children under thirteen from picture houses and other places of licensed amusement.[251] But few cities followed Leeds's example. During the third wave of influenza, the Isle of Man appears from papers to have been the only region to have closed schools or curtailed the hours of public entertainment.[252] Manchester's head of health, Dr Niven, warned that 'all dances and private entertainments should be avoided', but they continued unrestricted.[253]

In contrast to the US, especially west of the Mississippi, no British city at any moment of the pandemic imposed a complete shutdown of all public engagements from shoe-shine stands to public meetings. No notice comes of church services being prohibited or of churches deciding to hold services outdoors. Thus, unsurprisingly, little is heard of protests against anti-influenza policies. With the partial closure of cinemas in London, the Cinematograph Proprietors' Association criticized the regulation, but the health board held its ground and, as in Edinburgh, no more was heard of the complaint.[254] In Huddersfield, a town meeting was called to register that influenza sufferers could not obtain sufficient coal supplies and that whisky had run dry, but there were no accusations of corruption or profiteering.[255] Inadequacies in the British health service became apparent during the pandemic's later stages, but the papers and public framed their complaints as opportunities for future improvements, which received a positive response from government. In the last week of February 1919, the Ministry of Health confessed that little was known about influenza and 'the only thing to be done about it, is nursing'. It admitted

---

[243] Ibid., 22 February 1919, 6.   [244] Ibid., 20 February 1919, 7.
[245] *Guardian*, 16 February 1919, 10.   [246] Ibid., 10 March 1919, 7.
[247] *The Times*, 8 November 1918, 3. According to Tomkins, 'The Failure of Expertise', 454, cinema managers claimed they were victims of 'differential treatment' and threatened to disregard the regulations.
[248] *The Times*, 14 November 1918, 5.   [249] *Guardian*, 1 November 1918, 10.
[250] Ibid., 28 February 1919, 7.   [251] Ibid., 1 November 1918, 10.
[252] Ibid., 14 January 1919, 4.   [253] Ibid., 20 February 1919, 7.
[254] Ibid., 8 November 1918, 3.   [255] Ibid., 20 February 1918, 7.

that no organization for influenza research or mechanisms to extend nursing existed in the United Kingdom. Now, the Ministry promised to organize nursing 'and put it at the service of all'.[256]

Evidence of volunteer work and of neighbourhood organizations to combat the pandemic is even harder to find in England than in Scotland. When mortalities approached their apex with shortages of gravediggers and undertakers in London, the city's medical officer appealed to partially trained nurses 'and others' to offer their services; the *Guardian* reported that the campaign had drawn 'a number of volunteers'.[257] During the pandemic's second wave in early November, citizens in Manchester, led by Lady Leigh, mounted a public appeal and organized a bazaar to raise funds for a College of Nursing. According to Leigh, nurses had few friends and when they fell ill often had no one to care for them; some, she claimed, were even shunned because of suffering from influenza caught on duty.[258] But the bazaar was a one-off event, not an ongoing organization with resources or the will to support existing nurses or recruit new ones to assist their depleted ranks.

Appeals for volunteers were made, but the results differed from the US where women eagerly volunteered. The English papers make clear that these appeals often failed. During the crisis weeks of early November, London's Local Government Board announced that numerous districts had difficulty obtaining 'sufficient nursing assistance'. The Board eventually had to turn to their own members to persuade 'health visitors and other members of the female sanitary staff of the Council' to assist in the task of nursing influenza patients. They also turned to partially trained nurses, VADs, and untrained women to act as 'home helpers', but the papers give no indication of whether the calls were answered. Finally, to stretch depleted resources, the Board had to revive the Public Health Act of 1875 that authorized nurses and assistants to dispense prescriptions.[259] Over the same days, local boards advertised for 'Home Help for Influenza Patients', admitting that patients often confined to their homes and 'too weak to make their beds' received no attention. Papers beseeched women not occupied with war work to offer help to district nursing associations: many women with children were stricken and could not receive help because district nurses and doctors were overworked, their ranks in desperate need of replenishing. The *Guardian* pointed to what was missing—'some sort of organization'[260]—and from reports on influenza in Britain through its third wave to April 1919, none seems to have evolved.

As in Italy, France, and Switzerland, British towns turned to the military for help. When Birmingham needed undertakers and labourers to dig graves in late November 1918, the Lord Mayor asked for soldiers.[261] At the same time and for the same reasons, the town of Mansfield pleaded for military assistance.[262] The number of unburied bodies in Manchester may have been the worst: 'all the mortuaries' were full. Undertakers were working day and night but could not keep up with the

---

[256] Ibid., 22 February 1919, 6.   [257] Ibid., 27 November 1918, 3.
[258] Ibid., 7 November 1918, 3.
[259] Ibid., 8 November 1918, 8; and *The Times*, 8 November 1918, 3.
[260] *Guardian*, 7 November 1918, 4.   [261] *Scotsman*, 27 November 1918, 4.
[262] *The Times*, 29 November 1918, 3.

demand. Because of the lack of gravediggers, the dead waited eight to ten days for burial. At the end of November, Manchester's health commissioner pleaded with the War Office for skilled coffin-makers and gravediggers.[263]

The shortages of medical services and personnel persisted with the pandemic's recrudescence in 1919. Local health boards again appealed to the military. In late February, Manchester's board asked military authorities to release twenty doctors to serve in the city's heavily hit industrial zones;[264] a week later, the board appealed to the military for VAD nurses.[265] Even into March, civilian needs brought about by the pandemic remained acute in many regions of England, and central government sent 'a most urgent call for nurses'. No simple transfer from military to civilian service was, however, now possible. Army nurses either had been or were about to be released and had been granted paid vacations for 'their strenuous labours during the war'. The government pleaded with the nurses to defer their 'well-earned holiday' to attend the needs of influenza victims.[266]

As seen earlier, the civilian authorities turned to the military to resolve the problems of supplying doctors to meet the influenza crisis once the war ended. But at least a month before the Armistice, the military had been releasing large numbers of doctors and now had fewer to meet the growing influenza crisis.[267] In March 1919, influenza continued to rage throughout Britain. The availability of doctors and nurses became critical, but too few came forward even to provide 'casual attention to patients'. Following the Armistice, medical staff in armed services remained idle, while doctors at home were 'pressed to their wits' end', even after two million men had been released from the army. In Manchester and Salford, fears arose that those in general practice would collapse under the strain.[268]

Certainly, British journalists were well aware of other countries' methods of facing the influenza crisis that involved citizens' voluntary organizations and acts of abnegation. They turned not to North America but to New Zealand, South Africa, and India. In November 1918, soon after the pandemic had broken New Zealand's maritime defences, the *Guardian* described their rigorous restrictions—closing of schools, colleges, hairdressers, hotels after 4 p.m., religious services after 5 p.m., and prohibition of public meetings. In addition, New Zealanders formed 'vigilance committees' organized and comprised of ordinary citizens to assist influenza sufferers and their families.[269] In Cape Town, large numbers of voluntary workers organized soup kitchens and free medical depots spread across South Africa.[270]

Finally, one the longest articles on the Great Influenza to appear in British papers concerned India and an organization of women in the Presidency of Bombay, 'Sava Sadan' (the Royal Service Society), comprised mostly of lower-caste, impoverished, and illiterate women. It focused on their work in Pune going door-to-door

---

[263] *Guardian*, 30 November 1918, 6. To address the scarcity of gravediggers in Leeds, they turned to its engineers' department; 1 November 1918, 10.

[264] *Guardian*, 20 February 1918, 7.   [265] Ibid., 27 February 1919, 7.

[266] Ibid., 10 March 1919, 7.   [267] Ibid., 30 October 1918, 6.

[268] Ibid., 5 March 1919, 7.

[269] Ibid., 21 November 1918, 5; and 22 September 1918, 10.

[270] Ibid., 30 November 1918, 6; and 12 October 1918, 5.

through the most impoverished neighbourhoods nursing the sick. Other women replaced nurses incapacitated by flu at the Sassoon Hospital; still others travelled to villages visiting influenza victims. By the correspondent's account, these women 'stuck to their posts irrespective of personal danger', showed 'skill and cheerfulness' in the care of their patients, and saved 'many lives'.[271]

Even across the Irish Sea, English papers highlighted the self-sacrifice and devotion of volunteers who helped flu victims. *The Times* of London praised Reverend Thomas Murray of the Mater Misericordiae Hospital, Dublin, who died from a severe attack of influenza while visiting patients.[272] Two days later, the *Guardian* eulogized two further Dublin priests who had died attending 'to the spiritual needs of the many patients in the hospital stricken with influenza'.[273] By contrast, my searches through British papers have produced only one such instance of praise of a man or woman from England, Scotland, or Wales. But even this exception occurred beyond British shores and was in military service. Probationer nurse Michael of Glasgow died of influenza while nursing patients at Edmonton's military hospital and was buried in the town's Heroes' Corner with full military honours.[274]

Ireland

So did Ireland's reaction to the Great Influenza or the representation of that reaction differ categorically from England's or Scotland's? Here, I focus briefly on one of Dublin's dailies, the *Irish Times*, which produces as many results from keyword searches of influenza in 1918–19 as any English and Scottish paper.[275] Only by the second half of October did influenza bring about strains in Ireland's health service and a need to solicit volunteers. On 16 October, Lady Molony sought to revive the earlier work of Dublin's 'Cooked Food Depots' that originated at the time of the Great Famine. She advised creating a new 'scheme of communal kitchens or some kindred institution', arguing that better nourishment would decrease the number of influenza cases, especially among schoolchildren.[276] A week later, owing to the critical shortage of nurses, the Local Government Board in Rathdown, County Dublin, tried recruiting volunteers to visit the homes of the afflicted.[277] But throughout the pandemic's worse days, the *Irish Times* provides no evidence of volunteers, men or women, answering the call, and two days after the Rathdown plea, the signs were negative. Dublin City Corporation called for doctors and nurses, but local authorities in various districts reported that the response had not been sufficient. A Dublin alderman described the 'absolute helplessness of influenza sufferers', because of the 'appalling want of medical assistance'. At the same time, he pointed to three Dublin physicians languishing in English

[271] Nihal Singh, 'The Work of "Seva Sadan"', *Guardian*, 30 March 1919, 16.
[272] *The Times*, 26 October 1918, 7.
[273] *Guardian*, 28 October 1918, 4. When I conducted this research (18 October 2014), BNA contained no Irish newspapers for the years of the Great Influenza.
[274] *The Times*, 21 October 1918, 5.
[275] Accessed during October 2014; I found 404 results from 1 June 1918 to 30 June 1919.
[276] *Irish Times*, 16 October 1918, 4.   [277] Ibid., 24 October 1918, 4.

gaols because of political opposition and one on the run, Dr Kathleen Lynn.[278] The corporation asked for their release to combat the flu and won their appeal.[279]

It was not until the second week of November when the pandemic reached its 'worst phase' in Dublin[280] that the paper suggests a turning point in the response to these desperate pleas. The first signs came from small-town Dundalk on the Irish Sea, where 'a number of ladies' answered their parish priest's pleas to aid the town's poor who were suffering from influenza. The women established commit-tees for relief; one housed at the town's technical school provided beef tea and 'other nourishing foods'. Similar movements emerged elsewhere during the week. In Athy, south-west of Dublin, a communal kitchen opened at another local tech-nical school, and the town's Guardians provided meat at the homes of the afflicted. The town solicited the services of a nurse to visit the afflicted poor and supply them with hot meals. In Trim, north-west of Dublin, the picture was not as pretty: nurses, an assistant doctor, and several clergymen were stricken, and attempts to meet the demands of flu sufferers pushed the remainder of the medical staff to exhaustion.[281]

By the end of the third week, 'a number' of VADs in Dublin volunteered to nurse the afflicted in hospitals and in private homes.[282] Yet supply fell behind the demand triggered by the pandemic. On 7 December, with the city's nursing staff overstretched, Dublin appealed to the War Office to send nurses to Dublin's hos-pitals, but the War Department refused, despite the Armistice having been signed almost a month earlier.[283] By February 1919, conditions had improved, and those at St Patrick's Nurses' Home reflected on Dublin's influenza experience. Dr Ella Webb had offered the services of the VADs and patients had shown their appreci-ation by contributing small funds to the home.[284] The public also continued its charity. The Irish Auto Club offered the Public Health Commission a motor ambulance to transport influenza patients (the first such contribution reported by the *Irish Times*), and the St John Ambulance Brigade supplied stretcher-bearers.[285] The next week, Rathfarnham and Whitechurch Nursing Association in South Dublin praised its district nurse, who in a month made over 600 house visitations to influenza victims.[286]

This small harvest of charitable and volunteer work largely from one city, Dublin and its environs, and from a single paper presents considerably more than what I gathered from the three principal national papers of Scotland and England over the same period, covering more or less the entire United Kingdom. The Irish examples, moreover, show some similarities with the US: predominantly women served on these front lines, used their organizational talents, and were praised for it. The Irish volunteer contribution, however, even if taken from a single paper (yet a major one of the capital), was meagre compared to the pages of praise of women's initiatives and self-sacrifice seen in the US in one month alone, October 1918. The praise was not simply a matter of American jingoistic journalism; foreign

[278] See later in this section.
[279] *Irish Times*, 26 October 1918, 4; *Guardian*, 1 November 1918, 10.
[280] *Irish Times*, 8 November 1918, 2.   [281] Ibid.   [282] Ibid., 20 November 1918, 7.
[283] Ibid., 7 December 1918, 5.   [284] Ibid., 24 February 1919, 7.
[285] Ibid., 8 March 1919, 8.   [286] Ibid., 11 March 1919, 6.

presses observed it as well, and, as we shall shortly see, it became a model of volunteerism, organizational zeal, and charity for Australians when their pandemic battle finally commenced in 1919.

More on these charitable initiatives and especially women's predominance in this Irish struggle can be taken from Caitriona Foley's extensive research based on diaries, medical reports, and government archives. Her analysis reveals that doctors and civil society were at the centre of the pandemic's relief, aided by various 'Volunteer Aid Associations'. Her emphasis falls on the remarkable radical Sinn Féin freedom fighter and physician Kathleen Lynn, who directed the Women's National Health Association.[287] In addition, Foley points to the role of more traditional Catholic societies: branches of St Vincent de Paul provided aid to the poor and afflicted across Ireland and 'galvanized others to do so'. The same came from female religious orders,[288] and middle- and upper-class 'ladies' caring for flu victims in various towns, mobilizing aid and supplying daily meals.[289] Still, we see far fewer such initiatives in Ireland, whether at the neighbourhood or national level, and fewer women with commanding positions in these charitable endeavours than in single US cities or national organizations, such as the 'supreme commander' of the Women's Benefit Association, Miss Bina West. Foley's in-depth research and my searches through the *Irish Times* and newspapers in England and Scotland uncover only one woman whose initiatives were on the same remarkable plane as many cited in the US—Kathleen Lynn. Was the US then the odd one out in stimulating such exceptional levels of charitable sacrifice mainly from women? We now turn to the experiences of three other nations removed from the Great War's immediate battlefields.

---

[287] Foley, *The Last Irish Plague*, 63 and 111–12.　　[288] Ibid., 112.　　[289] Ibid., 113.

23

The Great Influenza

(ii) Comparative Vistas—Beyond the Battlefields

CANADA

How did countries further from the battlefields of Europe compare? As a Dominion of the United Kingdom, did Canada follow the lines of the British Isles or of France in its French-speaking states? Did it fit a North American pattern in its reactions to the Great Influenza, with a great number of volunteer initiatives, staffed principally by women? Or did it hew its own distinctive niche? A word of caution: our view of Canada relies heavily on the availability of searchable online newspapers, which concentrate on Ontario (OurOntario.ca Community Newspapers) and within Ontario on Toronto, with its two major newspapers, the *Toronto Star* and *Globe and Mail*. These, however, had a much wider remit than the city of Toronto. They reported daily from other towns in Ontario such as Brantford, Kingston, and Windsor, but also across Canada: Edmonton, Winnipeg, towns in the Rockies, on the west coast, Yukon and Northwest Territories, as well as Ottawa, Montreal, Quebec City, and their regions.

In contrast to Italy and to a certain extent other countries investigated in Chapter 22, these papers made few attempts to persuade readers that the flu of 1918–19 was nothing new and without any cause for alarm.[1] Tracing the disease that was spreading across Canada and the US at an alarming rate, *Kingsville Reporter* informed its readers that physicians recognized it as 'much more serious than they had believed' and advised them to stay at home.[2] Three weeks later, *Newmarket Era* reported 'thousands of cases of the strange malady'.[3] At the end of Canada's first wave of influenza, it concluded: 'Never since the Black Death has such a plague swept over the world'.[4] Another Ontario paper made it clear that 'La Grippe' was no laughing matter of sniffles and sneezes and described its symptoms as gruesome as those of plague or cholera.[5] Months before the disease became epidemic in Canada, an Ontario paper's front-page headline warned: 'A Mysterious Disease is Sweeping Spain; Forty Per Cent of Population Affected'.[6] Certainly, Italy's reaction to the

---

[1] Initially McCullough, director of Public Health, Province of Ontario, preached against raising alarm about the flu outbreak (*Toronto Star*, 24 September 1918, 2) but changed his mind quickly once deaths mounted in mid-October.

[2] *Kingsville Reporter*, 17 October 1918, 8.   [3] *Newmarket Era*, 17 October 1918, 5.

[4] Ibid., 27 December 1918, 4.   [5] *Leamington Post*, 21 November 1918, 2.

[6] *Windsor Evening Record*, 28 May 1918, front page.

Great Influenza illustrates Charles Rosenberg's Act I of epidemics' 'dramaturgic events': 'the slow acceptance, failure to acknowledge the presence of an epidemic disease, or even the frank denial of its existence'.[7] But across Ontario, that model fails to hold.

Quarantines and Closures

Canadian cities and towns were not slow to react as had been seen with some US cities of the north-east. By the beginning of October, schools were closed across Quebec.[8] In some places, movies were allowed to stay open but for a limited time only,[9] and early on, the Board of Health in Toronto demanded that churches close or limit their services, and the clergy complied.[10] By mid-October, with influenza deaths increasing, Toronto enacted more stringent measures; new regulations appeared daily. On the 16th, the city's Medical Officer, Dr Hastings, closed schools and prohibited public gatherings but allowed theatres and places of public amusement to stay open, as long as managers evicted anyone coughing or sneezing and barred school children from attendance.[11] A day later, several colleges were shut; all lodge meetings were cancelled; and most theatres voluntarily closed.[12] On the 18th, the policy tightened: theatres, movie houses, and billiard rooms shut.[13]

Further east, closures were more comprehensive from the start and imposed by fiat rather than agreement. By 8 October, Canada's then largest city, Montreal, closed 'all theatres, schools, picture shows, dance halls, and other places where the public congregate'.[14] The city's Health Board also asked the military to keep their soldiers confined to barracks and requested closures of large retailers at 4 p.m. to avoid congestion.[15] In the first week of October, Quebec mandated much the same,[16] as did various Ontario towns—Kitchener,[17] Brantford,[18] and London—a week later[19] along with other towns as far west as British Columbia by mid-October, even before the pandemic arrived.[20] Moreover, train passengers from the infected cities of Boston and New York were inspected, and by the 17th, the checks extended to 'every passenger train in Canada, whatever its origin'.[21] Not only do these perhaps overzealous actions contradict the dramaturgy of denial; they run against the assumption that such Draconian measures should stir unrest and distrust: nowhere in Canada did they provoke violent protest.

---

[7] Rosenberg, 'What Is an Epidemic?'.   [8] *Mail and Globe*, 2 October 1918, 5.
[9] Ibid., 5 October 1918, 7.   [10] Ibid., 7 October 1918, 14.
[11] Ibid., 16 October 1918, 8.   [12] Ibid., 17 October 1918, 6.
[13] Ibid., 18 October 1918, 8.   [14] Ibid., 8 October 1918, 3.
[15] *Gazette*, 8 October 1918, front page.   [16] *Globe and Mail*, 9 October 1918, 14.
[17] Ibid., 8 October 1918, 5; and 14 October 1918, 3.   [18] Ibid., 12 October 1918, 13.
[19] Ibid., 15 October 1918, 2; 18 October 1918, 2; for Saskatoon, Saskatchewan, 19 October 1918, 4; Fort William and Port Arthur (Ontario), 180 km north-west of Ottawa, 19 October 1918, 4; North Bay, Ontario, 350 km north-west of Ottawa, 23 October 1918, 3; Sault Ste. Marie, 13 December 1918, 12.
[20] Ibid., 17 October 1918, 3.   [21] Ibid., 18 October 1918, 2.

Controversies

As in the US, the pandemic sparked controversies in Canada but as elsewhere did not lead to attacks against victims of the disease or anyone else. Canada's conflicts differed from those south of the border. The papers reveal no outcries against profiteering or the closure of churches. Instead, in one of the most thoroughly regulated cities, Montreal, where all the churches were closed, the archbishop endorsed the Health Board's anti-influenza policies.[22] The following day, Cardinal Bégin went beyond Quebec's regulations, issuing a circular to the clergy, 'requesting pastors of every parish where influenza exists to suppress all religious services'.[23] And a pastor in Toronto publicly praised the city's director of health after the churches had been closed.[24] Only one protest by any church appears. Canada's Methodists passed a resolution against allowing the sale of alcohol. Unlike in the US, many doctors and health boards in Canada believed spirits were effective against influenza, and proposed that they be sold openly.[25] The Church was not the only constituency that opposed lifting the ban. In Acton, Ontario, 'many physicians of high renown' questioned the efficacy of alcohol and alleged that liquor dealers were behind the plan; it was 'the whiskeymen's Prussian trick'.[26] Only after the pandemic had passed did the Church express its regrets about church closures. In June 1919, the Anglican Bishop of Toronto complained that civilian authorities had closed churches, while allowing big department stores to remain open.[27]

Instead, the controversy that made headlines and endured over much of the course of the Great Influenza centred on Toronto and involved squabbles over jurisdictional authority, first between the mayor of Toronto and the medical health officers of Ontario, then between the mayor and the national government in Ottawa, and finally between the mayor and the military. Ad hominem recriminations on policies, procedures, and conditions of hospitals were acrimoniously exchanged. Much of the conflict stemmed from the personality of Toronto's mercurial mayor, Mr Church. These controversies, however, concerned professional rivalries, jurisdictions, and egos of political and military elites, and they raged in editorials, not in the streets. It is not clear the public were engaged at all, except for one soldier's father, who lodged a complaint about the overcrowding of a military hospital that tested the boundaries between the military's and Toronto's jurisdiction.[28]

Volunteerism and Women

To combat the Great Influenza, volunteerism from men and women in Canada was a greater force than anything experienced in Britain or the Continent. As in the US, the military, instead of being the principal resource aiding civilian society during this crisis, was on the receiving end, dependent on civilian volunteers,

[22] Ibid., 18 October 1918, 2.   [23] Ibid., 19 October 1918, 4.
[24] Ibid., 4 November 1918, 8.   [25] Ibid., 12 October 1918, 5.
[26] *Acton Free Press*, 17 October 1918, 2.   [27] Ibid., 4 June 1918, 8.
[28] *Globe and Mail*, 2 November 1918, 8; 8 November 1918, 8; and *Toronto Star*, 27 September 1918, 5.

usually women, caring for its influenza-stricken soldiers based in military camps at home. As in the US, Canada's pandemic began with the military. By 10 October, a hundred civilian nurses from Toronto were treating infected soldiers. Three University College men's residences had been converted into influenza hospitals staffed by nursing sisters and VADs.[29] At the start, women manned these front lines.

In contrast to the British Isles, continental Europe, and to some extent the US, Canadian health boards from small municipalities to the national one in Ottawa urgently appealed for voluntary assistance from civilians as soon as cases and deaths began to mount in the middle of October, and these appeals were directed at women. Initially, notes of desperation were sounded, suggesting the calls were not readily heeded. On 14 October, Ottawa's mayor 'again' issued an 'urgent appeal' for voluntary nurses: 'people are dying in our midst... but we have nobody to send... Knitting socks for soldiers is a very useful work, but we are now asking the women of Ottawa to get in the trenches themselves.'[30] On the 15th, Toronto's Health Board directed by Dr Hastings and the regional board under Colonel McCullough created a new volunteer organization, the 'Sisters of Service'. Meeting at Toronto's Parliament Building, they sought volunteers, principally women, to be quickly trained as nurses, and to spread the word for the 'Great Need of Helpers'.[31] The following day, their plea hit newspapers: 'Young woman, you can serve your country by helping fight the influenza'.[32] The same day, Toronto's director of nursing appealed to motorists to lend their services to the Victoria Order of Nurses.[33]

Shortly thereafter, articles made clear that these calls were being answered, but the pleas persisted. On the 18th, the board of the emergency hospital in Brantford went to the clergy asking for help recruiting volunteer nurses and others to treat growing numbers of influenza patients and to form a local branch of the Sisters of Service.[34] The next day, with cases increasing 'throughout the whole of Ontario', provincial health boards followed Brantford's example, appealing to the clergy through Toronto's province to solicit voluntary nurses.[35] A day later, the province turned to all teachers off-duty because of school closures to volunteer as nurses' aides or attend the crash courses on influenza nursing at Toronto's Parliament Building.[36] On the 21st, the province's Chief Health Officer appealed for an additional 500 volunteers to attend the lectures.[37]

Recruitment in other cities of Ontario was not as positive. Windsor's Health Board announced: 'competent nurses are so scarce here that returned soldiers with overseas hospital experience are being pressed into service'.[38] Despite the downturn in cases by the last week of October, pleas for volunteers continued with the headlines 'NEED FOR WOMEN TO FIGHT INFLUENZA'.[39] Cries for assistance edged into November with Colonel McCullough, Dr Hastings, and others using newspapers to broadcast the 'great need' for new nurses: 'NEW ARMY TO

---

[29] *Globe and Mail*, 10 October 1918, 6.   [30] Ibid., 15 October 1918, 2.
[31] Ibid., 10.   [32] Ibid., 16 October 1918, 6.   [33] Ibid., 8.
[34] Ibid., 18 October 1918, 2.   [35] Ibid., 19 October 1918, 9.
[36] Ibid., 4; and ibid., 'An Appeal'.   [37] Ibid., 21 October 1918, 7.
[38] Ibid., 28 October 1918, 14.   [39] Ibid., 29 October 1918, 10.

FIGHT "FLU" ... CONSCRIPT EVERYBODY'.[40] In addition, volunteer groups that had formed over the past two weeks became starved of funds, like the 'Neighborhood Workers', whose daily expenditures were costing $200.00 (Canadian) with only $60.00 coming in.[41] These continuous appeals for assistance by health authorities and newspapers separated Canada's fight from that of the US, where volunteers appeared to have sprouted organically from neighbourhood groups and the individual initiatives of women, such as at El Paso's Aoy High School. But even more distinctive were Canada's strenuous efforts to 'conscript everybody' in contrast to the European approach, which relied on long-established organizational forces—the Red Cross, VADs, and especially the military.

Canada's volunteerism differed from the US's in another respect. Initiatives came largely from above, at the level of the province and its Health Board, and were directed mostly by men. But, here, unlike in Europe, the pandemic created a new institution dedicated to resolving the problem of inadequate care for the colossal number of casualties. After convening a meeting at Toronto's Parliament Building, the Honourable W. D. Paterson, the Provincial Secretary, was elected president of the new organization, and Colonel McCullough, director of the provincial Board of Health, was clearly a prime mover as seen at this meeting and with later calls for volunteers. Other medical doctors from other organizations formed the board. Dr C. J. Copp, head of the St John Ambulance Brigade, offered his facilities and was elected Vice President. Despite its name—the Sisters of Service—and mission to recruit 'young lady volunteers',[42] only one women sat on the board, head nurse and the organization's principal lecturer, Dr Helen MacMurphy.[43]

The 'Sisters' were founded to supply urgently needed influenza nurses to enter the houses of the afflicted as quickly as possible. Its strategy was to train women, most with little, if any, experience in nursing, through public lectures alone. After three or four days of lectures, the volunteers were sent into homes. By 17 October, 120 'Sisters' were seeing patients in Toronto and beyond.[44] Within a week, the organization had requisitioned offices in towns throughout Ontario, and had converted the quarters of the Army and Navy Veterans into an emergency hospital.[45]

In the second half of October, women's organizations active during the war joined the movement. The most prominent was the IODE (Imperial Order Daughters of the Empire), created in 1900 to promote patriotism. At its St George's chapter in Toronto, women converted the Central Technical School into a kitchen providing food 'for the hundreds' down with flu.[46] The Daughters of the Empire (later to become a branch of the IODE) did the same in Hamilton.[47] In other rooms of the Technical School, they formed 'sewing bees', making towels and

---

[40] Ibid., 2 November 1918, 10.   [41] Ibid., 29 October 1918, 10.
[42] Ibid., 16 October 1918, 9.   [43] Ibid., 4.
[44] Ibid., 17 October 1918, 6. After five days, the pace slowed with only 175 volunteers placed (19 October 1918, 9). A week later, however, they increased to between 700 and 800 (24 October 1918, 9).
[45] Ibid., 18 October 1918, 2; 21 October 1918, 3; 22 October 1918, 2.
[46] Ibid., 21 October 1918, 8.   [47] Ibid., 22 October 1918, 2.

pneumonia jackets.[48] In Kitchener, along with the Victoria Order of Nurses 'and kindred organizations', the Daughters aided with transportation.[49] Other organizations comprised principally or even exclusively of women without connections to the war also volunteered. One was the Ontario Voluntary Health Auxiliary, a new branch of which began on 21 October in Collingwood, Ontario.[50] A Miss Pressley of the Toronto branch lectured to women on influenza treatment, organized a branch of the Sisters of Service, and converted rooms of the Elks Lodge into an emergency hospital, where three women nurses officiated.[51] Another group to become active in the second half of October was the Women's Patriotic League, which supplied soup, other foods, bed linen, and pneumonia jackets to the flu-infected in Toronto neighbourhoods and surrounding towns, with its headquarters as a collection centre for contributions.[52]

Other women's groups aiding influenza victims were attached to political parties or the Church. The Women's Liberal Association, headquartered in Toronto, produced pneumonia jackets and collected bedding, which they sent to the Red Cross and the Neighbourhood Workers' Association (hereafter NWA, to be discussed in the next section).[53] 'Ladies' of Toronto's St James' Presbyterian Church established a committee to 'work hand in hand' with the city's nurses, making soups and jellies. When the nurses discovered a family with influenza they called the committee and the pastor of their church to distribute the food. The inspiration for the service came from the pastor, who first consulted the Ministry of Health 'and then got the ladies working'.[54] In Woodstock, 'ladies' organized a committee to provide 'food and comforts' to influenza victims.[55] In late autumn, similar groups, which had been working throughout October, appeared in the press for the first time. The Ladies' Auxiliary of War Veterans distributed bedding and clothing to afflicted families but was forced to close at the end of October: all of its workers had caught the flu. Toronto's Jewish women and another group called the Montefiore Patriotic Society, under the presidency of Mrs Goldstein, supplied pyjamas and pneumonia jackets. The Ladies' Section of the High Park Bowling Club distributed aid in Toronto's worst-hit neighbourhoods of Mimico and Long Branch.[56] An unnamed women's club in Toronto ran 'a sort of motor corps', delivering soups and other meals to victims and transporting nurses and volunteers from one afflicted household to the next.[57] At the end of October, 390 women in Woodstock formed a new organization to provide relief, and when the Great Influenza ended decided to maintain their organization to provide services for any future epidemic.[58]

During the last influenza wave, from March to mid-May 1919, further women's organizations sprang into action but can be grasped only in the notes of annual meetings, expressing gratitude for members' sacrifices. They include the Women's

[48] Ibid., 21 October 1918, 8.   [49] Ibid., 14 October 1918, 3.
[50] Ibid., 21 October 1918, 3.   [51] Ibid., 22 October 1918, 3.
[52] Ibid., 26 October 1981, 10.   [53] Ibid., 25 October 1918, 8.
[54] Ibid., 21 October 1918, 6.   [55] Ibid., 24 October 1918, 8.
[56] Ibid., 29 October 1918, 10.   [57] Ibid., 15 November 1918, 10.
[58] Ibid., 31 October 1918, 10.

Patriotic League of North Toronto, the Jewish Council of Women, Toronto's Public and High School Teachers (comprised mostly, if not entirely, of women), and the High Park Soldiers' Comforts' Club.[59] At its annual meeting in June 1919, the YWCA noted that its domestic science room had been converted into a diet kitchen, distributing soup, custard, and jelly.[60] At the annual meeting of the Board of Home Missions and Social Services of the Presbyterian Church in Winnipeg, a Miss Goldie, was singled out for 'High praise': she and her team had fed 4362 families with 65,430 meals.[61]

Other problems and needs arose towards the end of the pandemic. As elsewhere, given this influenza's peculiar mortality rates which clustered among young adults, orphan numbers swelled. Again, women came to the fore as in Brantford, where the Social Service League formed to care for the pandemic's orphans.[62] At the end of the year, three Hamilton women led a deputation to create a new institution in Toronto 'for soldiers' orphans and those left parentless by the epidemic'.[63] By November, the economic consequences of the pandemic were being felt: problems such as loss of property ownership because families had been splintered and breadwinners made unemployed. Moreover, other diseases were believed to have emerged from it, such as infantile paralysis (poliomyelitis) and encephalitis. Women spearheaded local Samaritan clubs to provide groceries and pay the rents of those left bereft by the pandemic.[64]

At times, individual volunteers appeared who were unattached to established women's groups, churches, or patriotic associations, yet created new organizations or acted on their own, such as Miss Kay, a domestic science teacher at the Normal School in Toronto, who organized teachers to run a diet kitchen.[65] In Edmonton, a woman from New York City established and operated an electric laundry in the basement of a Methodist church to wash and disinfect clothes from homes where no one was capable of doing the chores.[66] Yet, in contrast to the US, these individual and small-group initiatives appear exceptional in Canada's Great Influenza response.

Cross-Gender and Men's Work in Fighting the Pandemic

The wide range of women's organizations and initiatives during the pandemic is impressive, especially when viewed from across the Atlantic, where such zeal, organization, and self-sacrifice—beyond the international and national branches of the Red Cross and in the British Isles, the VADs—were meagre. However, in contrast to the US, the inspiration and organizational direction for these women volunteers often appear to have derived from men, as was the case with the largest group in Toronto (and probably Canada), the Sisters of Service. Other women's groups also took their lead from men, such as the ladies of St James Presbyterian

59 Ibid., 14 May 1919, 8.   60 Ibid., 23 June 1919, 10.   61 Ibid., 22 March 1919, 12.
62 Ibid., 30 October 1918, 3.   63 Ibid., 25 December 1918, 2.
64 Ibid., 6 November 1918, 10.   65 Ibid., 22 October 1918, 3.
66 Ibid., 22 March 1918, 12.

Church, whose idea to organize a diet kitchen came from their pastor. More strik-ing, the Canadian volunteers did not draw such a stark contrast between sexes as in the US. First, a number of these Canadian organizations were neither clearly feminine nor masculine but comprised of both sexes probably in near-equal numbers. In Toronto the group after the Sisters of Service to receive the widest publicity was the NWA, whose social origins reached further down the social ladder than the Sisters'. Quickly, it became a vast operation with twenty-four stations for relief and diet kitchens across Toronto, caring for over 500 families daily.[67] By the end of October, it had established twenty-seven 'relief-work food and supply depots', aiding 1876 families.[68] Like the Daughters, its headquarters were in the Technical High School.[69] Like the Sisters, it soon spread to other towns in Ontario.[70] The organization had a multifaceted approach to relief. For one, it served as a credit union for working-class men, seeing this support as of direct importance in fighting the flu. Perhaps the physician's soundest advice to the flu-ridden was to stay in bed, but for workers that was a 'prescription for financial suicide'. In addition, the organization distributed bed linen to sufferers and their families, made pneumonia jackets,[71] and established diet kitchens, for which vari-ous women's organizations volunteered.[72] Furthermore, it organized Toronto's charitable landscape. On 26 October, it asked the Women's Patriotic League to assume responsibility for the neighbourhoods west of Younge to Bloor Street, while it supervised other areas.[73] Unlike women's organizations funded by the provincial government, the NWA depended on contributions from the public and throughout the pandemic was in debt.[74]

Other volunteer groups cut across the sexes. The YMCA provided another 'army of community service workers'. Like the NWA, it coordinated its efforts with other groups including the NWA, recruited 'large numbers of workers from various churches', and used Boy Scouts and Girl Guides to run messages and deliver food to influenza victims.[75] In mid-October, the Archbishop of Montreal gave consent for nuns and friars in his dioceses to be placed at the disposal of the health author-ities to nurse the stricken.[76] Like the Sisters, the Salvation Army trained and deployed its 'cadets' to serve flu sufferers throughout the city. The 'cadets', however, were not entirely men. One story of a 'cadet' treating a 'poor man' was, in fact, a woman, who afterwards fell critically ill for a month.[77] Other groups comprising men and women included the Social Service League in Brantford, which at Christmas sent cheques and supplies to the families of influenza victims.[78] The congregation of the Trinity Church in Toronto organized volunteers to carry food baskets to seventy afflicted families in the parish.[79] A club called the Parkdale Society in Toronto, composed of men and women, looked after 'needy cases' throughout the

[67] Ibid., 29 October 1918, 10. [68] Ibid., 14 May 1919, 8.
[69] Ibid., 2 November 1918, 10. [70] Ibid., 24 October 1918, 6.
[71] Ibid., 25 October 1918, 8. [72] Ibid., 4. [73] Ibid., 26 October 1918, 10.
[74] See note 53. [75] Ibid., 26 October 1918, 10. [76] Ibid., 18 October 1918, 2.
[77] Ibid., 31 October 1918, 10. [78] Ibid., 25 December 1918, 3. [79] Ibid., 6.

pandemic.[80] Finally, by mid-November, the epidemic had spread to Canada's most frigid and remote places. Volunteer doctors and nurses on dog sledges drove thousand-mile treks over snow from outposts such as Dawson City (Yukon) and Fort MacPherson (Northwest Territories) where the flu had had a devastating impact. While all the participants named on these missions were men, some of the nurses may have been women.[81]

Other groups clearly had a male component although the balance between the sexes is not always clear. With the upsurge in cases in Ontario, medical students volunteered to serve 'in the war against influenza'. Fifty-five from the fifth year were already assisting before the Board of Health called for volunteers in mid-October. Third- and fourth-year students now joined their ranks.[82] As in the US, overwhelmingly, they would have been male students. However, in contrast to the US, this was the only college or university group highlighted by the press to have volunteered. In Canada, waves of co-ed volunteers do not appear, even though in both countries, colleges remained closed for most of the pandemic. Early on, Boy Scouts came forward to assist nurses. On 17 October, eight appeared in Toronto's Arlington Hotel ready for action, and soon two hundred appeared, prepared 'for any kind of service'.[83] A week later the *Globe and Mail* praised them for their 'splendid work', carrying soup to 'helpless victims', distributing literature to businesses, and advising on influenza prevention and care.[84] In annual reports the following year, the Boy Scouts were recognized for their services during the pandemic. On the other hand, Girl Guides were mentioned only once.[85]

As in New Orleans, businesses and men's clubs in Ontario contributed with donations, their buildings, automobiles, and time. On 17 October Dr Hastings praised the innovation of Mr George Wright, proprietor of two Toronto luxury hotels, for engaging qualified nurses at his own expense to care for any guests down with flu.[86] On 22 October, Brantford's merchants and manufacturers called a meeting to discuss 'further means for fighting the epidemic' and how to stem the shortage of drugs, principally quinine.[87] During the second half of October, Toronto's postmen and the Rotary Club joined forces to provide doctors and health boards with better statistics on those afflicted with influenza and pneumonia. The Rotarians printed 10,000 survey forms; the postmen distributed them.[88] Foresters across Canada were another male group to contribute. First, they volunteered for hospital work, dedicated to their members, and then deducted 1 per cent of their salaries to help families of the afflicted. Along with a concert after the pandemic, they raised nationwide $4,000,000.[89] In Brantford, the Rotary Club

[80] Ibid., 7 March 1918, 4.
[81] Ibid., 14 November 1918, 9; 15 November 1918, 2; and 27 November 1919, 14.
[82] Ibid., 16 October 1918, 9.   [83] Ibid., 17 October 1918, 6.
[84] Ibid., 22 October 1918, 9.   [85] Ibid., 14 May 1918, 8.
[86] Ibid., 17 October 1918, 6: Walker House and the Carls-Rite Hotel.
[87] Ibid., 21 October 1918, 3.   [88] Ibid., 24 October 1918, 6.
[89] Ibid., 13 November 1919, 8.

delivered a Christmas tree to a children's shelter housing recent orphans of influenza victims and gifts to 142 further influenza orphans across the city.[90]

Perhaps these businesses and men's clubs may not have been on the front line, sacrificing their lives and working to exhaustion, as seen with New Orleans' doctors and pharmacists, and certainly they had not made as significant a contribution as the Sisters of Service, women's patriotic clubs, or the NWA. Some of their sacrifices and contributions might even be questioned, such as the Toronto hotelier, who assisted his wealthy clients alone, which may have drawn scarce medical services from needy neighbourhoods. Another group, predominantly of men, however, did risk their lives in Canada and across much of the globe and paid a heavy price—doctors. As Nancy Bristow, Caitriona Foley, Esyllt Jones, and others have described, nurses, not doctors, were the victors of the Great Influenza, and perhaps for the first time in medical history were praised more than their much better-remunerated male bosses.

Evidence from Ontario, but reaching places as far west as Winnipeg, may have been different, as it was in the American South. From the *Globe and Mail* I have found thirteen obituaries or stories in praise of those who sacrificed their lives during the Great Pandemic. Ten of the eulogized were men and only three women. Of the men, all but one was a physician who died attending influenza-stricken patients. These stories often recounted the number of cases a physician had been attending the day before or even on the day of his death; for a Dr Faulds of Elmira, it was 160 patients.[91] On 2 November, a longer story appeared about a physician in his eighties, who came out of retirement to treat the pandemic's victims. Before succumbing, he had visited ninety-four patients and on the day before his illness, eighty.[92] Of the three women who were eulogized, one was a teacher.[93] Even if the newspaper stories of women, who risked their lives or made noteworthy contributions but did not die, are added, the women's numbers increase by only two, both described in the previous section—the laundress who went to Edmonton[94] and Winnipeg's superintendent.[95] In these stories, nine were physicians and two were nurses. As we have seen, the gender differences for most of the US swung in the opposite direction. Yet, despite these differences, Canada and the US appear similar in their outpouring of and dependence on volunteers, certainly more so than any two countries yet compared. How do other nations far from Europe's battlefields compare?

[90] Ibid., 25 December 1918, 3. Another men's club, the Gunaikes, with only twenty members, volunteered, but the paper did not specify what they did (4 October 1918, 10).

[91] Ibid., 29 October 1918, 16.

[92] Ibid. 2 November 1918, 10. The other obituaries are from ibid., 25 October 1918, 2; 30 October 1918, 2–3 (eulogies of three physicians); 4 November 1918, 3 (two physicians); 7 November 1918, 9. The only male so eulogized, who was not a physician, was a seventeen-year-old 'lad', who died in London, England, as an orderly in an influenza hospital; 31 October 1918, 5.

[93] Ibid., 4 November 1918, 14, for the obituaries of the two nurses: 9 November 1918, 11; and 25 November 1918, 2.

[94] See note 66.   [95] Ibid., 22 March 1919, 12.

AUSTRALIA

Other chapters have addressed aspects of Australia's response to the Great Influenza. As historians have remarked, no other nation or continent was better prepared for it than Australia. By their surveillance, they managed to postpone the scourge by nearly seven months after it ravaged Europe in the summer of 1918 and by four months from its spread across the US and Canada. A survey of newspapers in the Trove database shows Australians, even in isolated towns of the interior, well informed. Their newspapers cited medical journals, well-known scientists, and reported developments across the globe before the disease breached defences in New South Wales (NSW) and Victoria at the end of January 1919.[96] Perhaps in part as a consequence, Australia was less severely battered by the pandemic than any inhabited continent of the globe. It was not, however, free of controversy or conflict.

Quarantine Battles

Across its federalist structure bequeathing individual states extensive powers, especially over public health, levels of surveillance and closure of public places was as widespread throughout Australia as for any country facing the pandemic. With the earliest cases—only four in Sydney on 28 January—theatres and schools immediately closed,[97] and a special committee was called to prohibit churches, music halls, and picture shows from opening.[98] On the same day with the first cases in Melbourne, the government of Victoria closed all places of amusement, churches, and schools.[99] As influenza penetrated regional quarantines and spread to the other Australian states, closures and precautions rolled into place. There was not the varied patchwork of preventive measures seen in the US, Canada, and Italy, depending on the philosophies of individual directors of health boards as in New York City and Vancouver. Despite these rapid measures, even before any deaths from 'pneumonic influenza' occurred,[100] little was heard of any protest. Churches, Protestant and Catholic, abided by state prohibition of services 'indoors or outside' without signs of pastors breaking the law or protesting against secular decisions as seen in the US. On the first Sunday after the church closures, Sydney's Protestant ministers devised means of instructing their congregations without exposing them to contagion. The following Monday, they published weekly sermons in a local newspaper with each denomination given a column.[101] Even if they thought the state and federal governments' decisions were 'drastic', as Australia's Catholic

---

[96] *Cootamundra Herald*, 15 July 1918, 2; *The Register*, 26 October 1918, 12, which discussed medical notions of 'infecting principles'; and *Brisbane Courier*, 30 October 1918, 6, which cited the *Deutsche Medizinche Wochenscritt* on the 'influenza bacillus of Pfeiffer'.

[97] *Wyalong Advocate*, 28 January 1918, 2.   [98] *Molong Angus*, 31 January 1919, 3.

[99] *Bunbury Herald*, 29 January 1919, 3.

[100] For closures in Brisbane with the first cases in May, see *Townsville Daily Bulletin*, 6 May 1919, 5.

[101] *Leader*, 3 February 1919, 2; and *Watchman*, 6 February 1919, 5.

hierarchy believed, they kept it to themselves in their publications.[102] Furthermore, Australian newspapers reveal no accusations against profiteers, such as Washington's 'cruel' landlords or New York's 'coffin ghouls'. Australian states felt no need to intervene as happened in New Zealand in November 1918, when, because of 'scandalous profiteering', the government 'commandeered all oranges and lemons, fixed their prices', and considered regulating pharmacists.[103]

Australia's struggles over quarantine, however, filled more newsprint than any controversy linked to the pandemic in any country. These matters went beyond questions of prevention and turned on Australia's ideology of federalism—the rights of states. With the official declaration at the end of January 1919 of the first civilian cases of influenza in its two most populous states—NSW with Sydney and Victoria with Melbourne—controversy over internal quarantine borders exploded in volleys of accusations by one state against another and by states against the Commonwealth and its Federal Director of Quarantine, Dr John Cumpston.[104] First, several states accused Victoria of alleged carelessness in allowing influenza to breach the nation's quarantine.[105] Second, NSW was accused of wresting control from the Commonwealth, violating an agreement of November 1918, which placed interstate traffic in the Commonwealth's hands. Other states also began violating the agreement almost immediately with the first declared cases of influenza. At the end of January, Western Australia arrested a transcontinental train and placed the passengers in quarantine. Many were citizens of Victoria, who lodged grievances with the Commonwealth.[106] At the same time, border patrols sprouted up on the frontiers as in Albury and Tocumwal in NSW to prevent influenza entering from Victoria.[107]

The delays and blockages at harbours and internal border controls of Australian troops returning from Europe caused further disputes. A steamer transporting several hundred troops, who had been given a clean bill of health by Commonwealth doctors, was nevertheless blocked by Sydney's quarantine authorities.[108] Another clash between state and Commonwealth flared up at Lynton quarantine hospital, where the State of Queensland feared soldiers might escape and spread 'pneumonic influenza' through the state.[109] A few days later, soldiers, anxious to return home after long voyages and delays, broke the quarantine. Some were arrested; others, however, were not found.[110] The quarantining of returning troops in various states against the wishes of local populations made headlines throughout February[111]

[102] *The Catholic Press*, 6 February 1919, 27.   [103] *The Advertiser*, 16 November 1918, 11.

[104] See Roe, 'Cumpston'. During the pandemic, Cumpston strove to broaden his department's remit into a wider training unit in general health and in March 1921 achieved it with himself as the first director.

[105] *Forbes Times*, 31 January 1919, 4; and *Richmond River Herald*, 31 January 1919, 2.

[106] *Argus*, 31 January 1919, 5.   [107] *Albury Banner*, 31 January 1919, 44.

[108] *Cairns Post*, 3 February 1919, 5.   [109] *Brisbane Courier*, 5 February 1919, 9.

[110] *Queensland Times*, 6 February 1919, 5.

[111] *Daily Observer*, 10 February 1919, 2; *Morning Bulletin*, 10 February 1919, 9; *Kalgoorlie Miner*, 12 February 1919, 3.

and continued until July 1920.[112] Because of one cold, sore throat, or mild fever on board, entire shiploads containing a thousand soldiers could be quarantined for seven days, even after medical officers had declared no cases after ocean voyages from Europe.[113]

Soldiers were not alone in being harassed by internal quarantines, competing jurisdictions, or general confusion over intercontinental travel. Citizens were subjected to the same seven-day quarantines, unjustifiably long given influenza's short incubation. The central government strove to shorten the period, but Queensland and Western Australia vetoed the reform. Passengers' journeys were blocked by internal quarantines and often ended in detention in quarantine camps.[114] Stories were told of travellers stranded at border posts, thrown into quarantine when they longed to return to their families,[115] and fined up to £20 or imprisoned as long as three months if they broke quarantine.[116]

On first impression, these impositions might recall plague protests in India in the early twentieth century, illegal municipal quarantines in the US sparked by smallpox, or legal 'shotgun' quarantines that divided southern states during their last yellow fever epidemics. But complaints over the quarantine's 'greasy utensils'[117] were not quite the equal of conditions faced by Indians—strip searches, sexual humiliation, and refusal to supply infants milk, which went on for months, not seven days. Nor did the Australian restrictions replicate the quarantines of vigilante farmers taking the law into their own hands, preventing passengers entering or leaving their own towns. In the vast number of Australian papers, no collective or individual acts of violence are detected, not even peaceful demonstrations. These wrangles instead occurred at the highest political levels, with one Acting Premier of a state complaining against another Acting Prime Minister, or against the indefatigable Dr Cumpston, Director of the Commonwealth's Quarantine Service, and vice versa. They filled long, convoluted columns of newsprint but did not cause unrest in the streets.[118] Another set of state decrees, however, had a greater impact on public opinion.

The Mask

Australia's zeal for enforcing mask ordinances comes closest to the US. But its legislation concentrated at least initially on one state alone, NSW. On 30 January 1919, an ordinance required all Sydney's citizens to wear masks along with towns or settlements within the state as soon as influenza was declared.[119] On 4 February,

---

[112] Also, in China, the pandemic recurred in 1920, reaching peak mortalities in Hong Kong; Langford, 'Did the 1918–19 Influenza?', 479.
[113] *Mercury*, 8 July 1919, 6.
[114] *Border Watch*, 4 March 1919, 2; for further inconveniences, see *Northern Star*, 31 May 1919, 3.
[115] *Maryborough Chronicle*, 7 February 1919, 3.
[116] *Western Australian Times*, 23 April 1919, 8. [117] *Daily Observer*, 1 March 1919, 2.
[118] See for instance *Daily News*, 4 February 1919, 6.
[119] Numerous Australian papers reported the decision; for instance, *Northern Star*, 30 January 1919, 2. The Canadian and British press covered it: *Globe and Mail*, 7 February 1919, 11 and

a bylaw required everyone travelling on trains or trams or waiting on station platforms to wear masks, with steep fines of £10 per violation.[120] Immediately there were reports of slackness in heeding the legislation: not even stretcher-bearers, who carried influenza victims, bothered donning the mask.[121] Papers pointed at judges, who deliberated their judgments without obeying the law.[122] Yet others celebrated Sydney's embracing of the mask with a full-page issue, picturing theatre-goers, society ladies, policemen, and tramway men proudly sporting them.[123] Papers give no sign of collective opposition to masks, only that many did not wear them or 'slung theirs around the neck walking down streets, smoking their pipes'.[124] Papers reported occasional arrests and fines,[125] but these were not in the hundreds as in San Francisco.[126] The only hint of ideological opposition to them came from the acting Prime Minister of Australia in a telegram to the Premier of NSW, claiming the new regional ordinance was unconstitutional.[127] And only one case of individual resistance appears. A Sydney physician was brought to trial for refusing to wear the mask, went to gaol, and refused bail.[128]

By early March with cases on the decline, the law was rescinded but within two weeks with influenza mounting again was reinstated.[129] The second time round, the strictures were less onerous and pertained mainly to travel: passengers in trains, trams, motor buses, cabins on ferries, while waiting on wharves, and in lifts were compelled to wear them.[130] Otherwise, the public was 'advised' to wear them where travellers congregated. In small towns, that was the post office.[131] In early February 1919, Victoria and its capital, Melbourne, mooted following NSW's example. Following physicians' advice, the authorities initially refused to make the mask mandatory. Later, however, they imposed a law.[132] In Brisbane and Queensland mask legislation was not passed until August 1919, modelled on NSW's later modified laws pertaining to travel, but it was also imposed on public spaces, targeting one profession—deliverers of foodstuffs.[133] Unlike those of NSW, neither foreign nor Australian papers gave them much attention. Finally, when the pandemic infected Tasmania, eight months after it entered mainland Australia, the question of compulsory masks surfaced but they were imposed by one municipality alone: by then, late August 1919, the tide had turned against the mask.[134]

Guardian, 2 February 1919, 6, respectively; on border towns, see *Border Morning Mail*, 22 February 1919, 2.

[120] *Riverine Grazier*, 4 February 1919, front page; *Daily Observer*, 3 February 1919, front page; and *Daily Telegraph*, 4 February 1918, 6.
[121] *Sunday Times*, 9 February 1919, 11.   [122] *Daily Telegraph*, 18 February 1919, 6.
[123] *Mirror*, 7 February 1919, front page; and *Cairns Post*, 3 February 1919, 5.
[124] *Daily Telegraph*, 4 February 1919, 6. Also, *Northern Herald*, 26 June 1919, 52.
[125] *Daily Observer*, 1 March 1919, 2.
[126] Crosby, *America's Forgotten Pandemic*, 105 and 112.
[127] *Northern Star*, 4 February 1919, 2.   [128] *Irish Times*, 19 February 1919, 4.
[129] *Border Morning Mail*, 27 March 1919, 2.
[130] Ibid.; *Western Champion*, 27 March 1919, 11; *Riverine Grazier*, 15 April 1919, 2.
[131] *Riverine Grazier*, 15 April 1919, 2.   [132] *Maitland Daily Mercury*, 1 February 1919, 6.
[133] *Daily News*, 24 May 1919, 8.
[134] *Daily Telegraph*, 18 August 1919, 5, from *Medical Journal of Australia*.

Controversy over the mask in Australia was largely limited to discussion of its scientific value. Interventions came from physicians with references to medical journals. Immediately following NSW's decision, the press supported the mask's advantages, alleging that San Francisco had recovered from the pandemic more quickly than any city in the US and concluding that 'credit must be given to masks'.[135] Five days later, another paper comparing influenza-related deaths in San Francisco and Los Angeles, which did not have the legislation, concluded the opposite: adjusted for population, San Francisco's casualties doubled Los Angeles'.[136] As early as 30 January, Dr Cumpston remarked that the mask was 'of as little practical value as powdering the face'.[137] Citing the *Medical Journal of Australia*, another paper questioned the mask's utility: 'at best' it covered 'only a very small surface of the body'.[138] As elsewhere, by May 1919, Nicolle's findings had weakened mask arguments.[139] Australian headlines boldly announced his findings: 'Anti-Influenza Masks: Like Using Barbed Wire Fences to Shut Out Flies'.[140] Yet, despite this negative near-consensus, mask-wearing ordinances persisted longer in Australia than anywhere else, from late January 1920 to the end of August.

Abnegation

Before the advent of the pandemic in Australia, the Australian press surveyed socio-psychological reactions to the scourge, reporting stories of neighbourhood organization, charity, volunteerism, and abnegation as they emerged, first from the US, then from less privileged places, such as Tonga and parts of South Africa where death rates mounted as high as 10 per cent, and finally from New Zealand. Australian journalists reflected on 'object lessons' for themselves, if the disease were ever to penetrate their maritime defences. Sydney's *Freeman's Journal* looked to the Catholic community in Boston and compared its organization and courage to Carlo Borromeo's during the plague of 1575–7 and to the seventeenth-century St Vincent de Paul and his care of the poor.[141] Another paper extolled the heroic deeds of nuns at hospitals in Philadelphia, citing a physician who proclaimed that in thirty-three years of practice he had never witnessed 'such heroic devotion to duty', adding, 'And I am a Methodist'.[142]

Australian papers described volunteers in Tonga burying the dead and starting soup kitchens,[143] and providing relief in Cape Town, such as a hundred students of the South African College, who made house calls to thousands of the afflicted.[144]

[135] *Queensland Times*, 1 February 1919, 8.
[136] *Daily News*, 5 February 1919, 7, from *Christian Science Monitor*.
[137] *Geraldton Guardian*, 1 February 1919, 3.
[138] *Maryborough Chronicle*, 6 February 1919, 3.   [139] *World's News*, 10 May 1919, 2.
[140] *Albury Banner*, 6 June 1919, 33, and papers in NSW, Western Australia, South Australia, and Tasmania, and raised other objections, such as Tasmania's *Daily Telegraph*, citing the *Medical Journal of Australia*, 18 August 1919, 5.
[141] *Freeman's Journal*, 5 December 1918, 13 and *The Catholic Press*, 19 December 1918, 19.
[142] *The Catholic Press*, 9 January 1919, 6.   [143] *Adovocate*, 27 February 1918, 4.
[144] *Zeehan and Dundas Herald*, 11 October 1918, 3.

Once the pandemic struck Australian cities, another article elaborated on South Africa's relief programmes: depots opened to distribute soup, bread, and medicine; voluntary workers 'of both sexes' visited the stricken. Medical students took temperatures in homes across the city. 'Boy Scouts were everywhere, and as is always the case in emergencies, women rose to the occasion'.[145] Cape Town was not the only South African guide. In a letter from a friend at the heavily hit mining town of Kimberley,[146] a man from Boolaroo, NSW, praised their commitment: 'from the highest to the lowest', they 'threw themselves into' voluntary relief work:

> The Mayoress could be seen anytime during the day washing dishes at the City Hall Soup Kitchen, while staid city men took on all and sundry jobs from district nursing to burials....In addition to house-to-house work, the general hospital and the three additional hospitals...were mainly staffed by city men, their wives, and daughters— all free voluntary service.[147]

The examples most often cited by the Australian press, however, came from New Zealand. The *Catholic Press* described New Zealand's Catholic schools being converted into emergency hospitals, nuns serving as nurses in 'houses of the dead and dying'; priests 'working day and night'; and the charitable tasks of numerous other Catholic organizations.[148] In bracing for the pandemic's arrival in Brisbane, a local woman gave 'practical suggestions' taken from her recent visit to New Zealand on forming soup kitchens, posting SOS notices in shops, and directing women to houses where services were needed. She even advised Australia's 'medical men' on a system developed in New Zealand, whereby every doctor divided his district into squares and delegated sections to volunteer nurses and those supplying food.[149] In May 1919, when the pandemic struck Brisbane, the paper republished the lady's advice.[150] A day later, 2000 km across the continent, one of Adelaide's papers cited examples from Christchurch during its blackest days in mid-November, extolling the charitable deeds and organization of groups such as the Plunkett Society, the Society for the Protection of Women and Children, the city's churches, nuns, sisters, the Marist Brothers, VADs, and Boy Scouts. They cared for children, offered aid, drove ambulances, and carried messages, medicine, and food to the poorest, most crowded areas of the city. A voluntary staff established a convalescent home for sick children, ran playgrounds, established soup kitchens, and prepared two meals daily for 500 children (see Figure 23.1).[151] A Tasmanian paper published a letter from Christchurch to a friend in Hobart, describing not only 'the very drastic precautions' but the *esprit de corps* and altruism of the citizens:

> Every district has its kitchens for making beef tea and jellies, etc, and a depot for the issue of free medicines....Patrols were organized, and every house in each street was visited and all cases reported. The Automobile Association got all the motor cars and

---

[145] *Brisbane Courier*, 29 January 1919, 9.   [146] See Chapter 22, note 211.
[147] *Newcastle Morning Herald*, 1 February 1919, 2.
[148] *Catholic Press*, 19 December 1918, 19.
[149] *Brisbane Courier*, 29 January 1918, 9.   [150] Ibid., 3 May 1919, 5.
[151] Ibid.; *The Register*, 30 January 1919, 8.

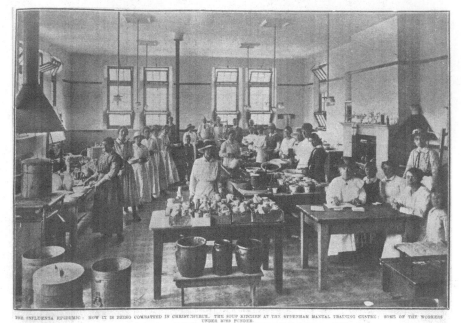

THE INFLUENZA EPIDEMIC: HOW IT IS BEING COMBATTED IN CHRISTCHURCH. THE SOUP KITCHEN AT THE SYDENHAM MANUAL TRAINING CENTRE: SOME OF THE WORKERS UNDER MISS PONDER.
The staff of the soup kitchen have done very fine work in providing useful foods for the many patients in the Sydenham and Waltham districts.　　　C. Behm

Figure 23.1. Epidemic soup kitchen at the Sydenham Manual Training Centre, Christchurch, 1918.

cycles; the boy scouts are always on duty, and girls and nurses are at the Central Depot, being sent out night and day to any place they are required.[152]

In Australia, volunteers were called and they came forth even before cases had developed beyond the nation's quarantine centres. On the eve of its press claiming that the country would soon be declared the only continent on earth to escape the pandemic,[153] small-town Narrandera, NSW, asked Sydney for assistance dealing with an influenza outbreak 'in the event that it ever gained a foothold'. Sydney's municipal council appealed for nurses who would treat influenza patients; 'several women' came forward, 'fully knowing the risk involved', and willingly were inoculated.[154] As soon as the pandemic struck Australia's two major cities in January 1919, the municipalities began soliciting volunteer nurses and others to assist.[155] By the end of January, women volunteers of the VAD patrolled each of Sydney's eighteen wards, searching for cases and those needing assistance.[156] After a respite in March, influenza rebounded in April; Sydney again relied on and praised its 'relief organizations ready to work'. The city was also blessed with 'a very large

[152] *Examiner,* 3 January 1919, 6. For further 'object lessons' from New Zealand, see *The Advertiser,* 4 November 1918, 5; 14 November 1918, 6; 16 November 1918, 11; 10 December 1918, 5; *Land,* 27 December 1918, 6.

[153] *Camperdown Chronicle,* 9 January 1918, 4.　　　[154] *Land,* 20 December 1918, 6.

[155] *Age,* 27 January 1919, 6.　　　[156] *Molong Angus,* 31 January 1919, 3.

number' of volunteers who belonged to no established organization, yet who were 'only too anxious to serve in any capacity'. A Sunday paper claimed that over the past few days, offers to help had 'besieged' Sydney's Red Cross influenza headquarters. Its soup supply depots were 'entirely filled with volunteers at work' and others were 'doing a thousand odd jobs'.[157] Independent volunteers were busy in Sydney's suburbs: women used their homes to establish soup kitchens and served 'the needy sick in their neighbourhood'.[158] At Broken Hill, NSW, the head doctor and nurse matron of the town's hospital addressed a meeting of the Red Cross: 'many' citizens offered to volunteer as aid workers, and VADs took over establishing soup kitchens.[159] Upper-middle-class women, unattached to established charities, arrived in force in Brisbane, led by the Mayoress and the wives of council chairmen.[160] With this second wave, women without clear organizational ties became the backbone of relief programmes in medium-sized and small towns, founding and staffing soup kitchens in Blackall and Ipswich (Queensland);[161] Ballarat (Victoria), where a Jewish woman with fifteen 'young ladies' began a soup kitchen at City Hall;[162] Launceston (Tasmania);[163] Newcastle (NSW);[164] Cessnock (NSW);[165] Singleton (NSW);[166] Tenterfield (NSW);[167] Cobar (NSW); New Norfolk (Tasmania);[168] multiple ones at Hobart;[169] and many more. These women also joined 'patrols' visiting the neediest, supplying medicines and nourishment, and, when possible, calling doctors or nurses.[170] Other women supplied automobiles or drove them.[171] Still others gave literature and flowers. Men also contributed: butchers donated meat; farmers, eggs and milk; others drove automobiles, delivering meals.[172] In one Tasmanian town, the Town Council refused to open a soup kitchen, which sparked protest. After two weeks, the Council conceded, turning its Town Hall into the town's soup kitchen.[173]

Towards the end of the pandemic, papers congratulated towns and cities on their heroic unity to battle the disaster. Ipswich's paper boasted:

> the hearts of folks of Ipswich are in the right place when it becomes a matter of assisting comrades in distress...The authorities of the Ipswich General Hospital only required to tell the good people of the city how badly they were in need of assistance

[157] *Sunday Times*, 13 April 1919, 3.   [158] Ibid., 20 April 1919, 14.
[159] *Barrier Miner*, 31 January 1919, 4.   [160] *Brisbane Courier*, 3 May 1919, 5.
[161] *Morning Bulletin*, 2 June 1919, 8; and *Queenslander*, 7 June 1919, 10.
[162] *Jewish Herald*, 27 June 1919, 10.   [163] *Examiner*, 30 May 1919, 8.
[164] *Cessnock Eagle*, 4 July 1919, 3.
[165] Ibid., 4 July 1919, 2; 11 July 1919, 2; and *Maitland Daily Mercury*, 8 July 1919, 7; 1 August 1919, 2.
[166] *Singleton Argus*, 28 August 1919, front page.   [167] *Northern Star*, 25 July 1919, 7.
[168] *Mercury*, 29 August 1919, 5; 18 September 1919, 5; 23 September 1919, 5.
[169] Ibid., 29 August 1919, 5; 13 September 1919, 5; 20 September 1919, 7.
[170] *Cessnock Eagle*, 11 July 1919, 2; and *Maitland Daily Mercury*, 8 July 1919, 7.
[171] For instance *Cessnock Eagle*, 11 July 1919, 2; and *Maitland Daily Mercury*, 8 July 1919, 7; in the second case, husband and wife conveyed food and medicine from a soup kitchen: the husband provided the automobile; his wife drove it.
[172] *Mercury*, 26 August 1919, 5.
[173] *Advocate*, 27 October 1919, 3; *Examiner*, 10 November 1919, 5; *Advocate*, 10 November 1919, 2.

when it was made available.... Whilst knowing full well the dangers...there was always a band of workers willing to help.[174]

Similarly, at Chelmsford, NSW, the local paper congratulated themselves:

> Most clouds are said to have silver linings, and the silver lining in this matter has been the abnegation and self-sacrifice exhibited by uninfected neighbours. Household duties have been attended to, day and night nursing undertaken, and milking and corn husking and shelling seen to, so that the wheels of industry have been kept going and the invalids and children have received adequate attention.[175]

On community organization and cooperation, all was not, however, sweetness and light. From the beginning, desperate pleas for volunteers occasionally slip through.[176] In Wynyard, Tasmania, the Red Cross asked for volunteers in case the pandemic broke out: only one lady came forward.[177] In Forbes, a small town in NSW, a public meeting was called at the end of April to coordinate programmes for combating the pandemic, 'but of all the VADs only one volunteered', and no help came from the hospital nursing staff. Only a husband and wife arrived to help a single nurse. The mayor appealed to its sister town, Parkes, but only one lady agreed to come. A lone doctor was treating twenty-eight to thirty patients with 'pneumonic influenza' at a temporary hospital in the old gaol with only one nurse and a VAD assisting. Finally, a lady from the country volunteered, but because of poor health, had to be rejected.[178] Two months later, shortages of nurses and a 'heavy strain on the medical staff' caused Goulburn, a small town 200 km south-west of Sydney, to close its federal quarantine station to further cases.[179] Following a long article celebrating the response to the pandemic in Sydney, which was 'besieged' with offers of help, an article in the same issue reflected on the 'troubles' facing volunteers. Occasionally, women were asked to do extraordinary services for families, when women boarders without children—'among the best to offer their services'—were present. But their landlords prevented them from volunteering, and those who already had were given an ultimatum: 'Leave this establishment, or leave the influenza service.'[180]

*   *   *

Despite Australia's federalist constitutional wrangles and the voices of some landlords, its experience with the Great Influenza may have been the most positive of any nation. Few signs surface of profiteering by undertakers, druggists, or doctors, or protests against impositions to control the disease. Instead, newspapers overflow with stories of volunteerism and self-sacrifice across the continent. Australians had time not only to improve on regulatory practices seen in other parts of the globe but to study modes of behaviour and organization of community assistance.

---

[174] *Queensland Times*, 14 June 1919, 6.   [175] *Northern Star*, 16 July 1919, 3.
[176] *Age*, 27 January 1919, 6: 'Volunteer Help Needed'.
[177] *Daily Telegraph*, 14 February 1919, 4.   [178] *Forbes Advocate*, 29 April 1919, 2.
[179] *Goulburn Evening Penny Post*, 17 June 1919, 2.   [180] *Sunday Times*, 13 April 1919.

Because volunteers in Canada and the US were predominantly of middle-class, even elite families, it might be assumed that levels of volunteerism depended on a region's socio-economic status. Yet in Australia these acts and organization spread across small farming communities in the interior, and Australian models of altruism derived from some of the most impoverished places on earth, such as the inhabitants of Tonga and black miners in Kimberley. Finally, the rise of disproportionate numbers of women risking their lives to answer calls for charitable action needs explanation. Why was it so pronounced in the US, Canada, Australia, and South Africa but not in Britain, France, Switzerland, or Italy? The relative importance of women's emancipation, at least if the right to vote or their coming into the public sphere are key, cannot explain it, especially given the sacrifice and altruism of black women in South Africa, where universal suffrage was not introduced until 1993. One variable that distinguishes whether volunteers—men or women—rushed to aid the dangerously ill was a country's geographical position: whether it was enmeshed in the Great War's European battlefields. Countries further afield, despite involvement in the war and even if armed struggles touched their shores, appear to be the regions where volunteerism was more likely. As we have seen, relief in the countries where the principal battlefields lay or countries adjacent to them (Britain and Switzerland) was top-down, organized by national governments and especially dependent on the military. Unlike in New Zealand, Australia, Canada, and South Africa, volunteers here did not 'besiege' health boards to assist the afflicted. Instead, military and governmental agencies largely assumed the responsibilities. We turn now to a final case—India—another country far from Europe's battlefields.

INDIA

Newspapers in the US, Canada, Australia, and Britain kept their readers abreast of soaring mortalities caused by the pandemic in Mumbai during October, the worst month of the scourge in the Presidency. The international press, however, reported little from the worst-affected areas, which were far removed from the services of major cities, and which native Indian newspapers claimed had been completely neglected. Unlike the coverage of Tonga, Samoa, Pretoria, and especially Cape Town, the foreign press did not describe voluntary relief organizations, college students assisting nurses, or soup kitchens in India, that is, except for one article in Manchester's *Guardian*, detailing a mission of poor women, who went door-to-door nursing the afflicted in the most impoverished neighbourhoods of Pune and Mumbai.[181] Did the pandemic spark waves of abnegation and altruism through the subcontinent similar to the initiatives in the US, Canada, Australia, New Zealand, South Africa, and Tonga?

---

[181] See Chapter 22, note 271.

Complaints from India's Newspapers

Weekly reports from hundreds of native Indian newspapers translated and excerpted for surveillance by the colonial government in the Presidency of Bombay reveal little about any voluntary organizations to fight flu, whether initiated by men or women during the pandemic's worse months, mid-September to mid-November. Given the colonial criteria on what to extract, it may not be surprising that such details failed to register on the government's radar. The extracts, however, are laden with comments on the pandemic in the Presidency as well as outside it in Kolkata,[182] Ahmedabad,[183] Broach City,[184] and Hubli Taluka.[185] Throughout the pandemic, these papers repeated complaints that differ radically from the problems that had troubled Indian populations two decades earlier regarding the British approach to plague, which produced the most widespread and violent demonstrations connected with any epidemic disease in Indian history. Now, the complaints turned in the opposite direction. Instead, of attacking heavy-handed, humiliating, and abusive intervention with severe quarantine, segregation camps, and strip searches, indigenous papers accused the Crown and municipalities of abrogating their responsibilities.

When influenza deaths mounted at the end of September, these papers appealed to the Presidency's governor, demanding public meetings, consultation of native leaders, price controls on basic foodstuffs, and relief funds to ensure the poor were fed and had access to medicines and care.[186] In October, with casualties reaching their peaks, the papers protested against the absence of basic supplies and remedies such as quinine, while the government sat 'with folded hands'.[187] Papers demanded organized measures 'in cooperation with charitable and philanthropic agencies'. Still, by 20 October, the *Sunday Chronicle* claimed that the municipal government had so far left 'everything' to 'philanthropy': 'laissez-faire is most dangerous and reprehensible at this crisis...a gross dereliction of duty'. It demanded facilities to treat the poor, the building of temporary, open-air hospitals, and use of 'up-to-date' treatment.[188] The *Jam-e-Jamshed* was more stentorian: 'What has the Government done?...the mass of poor and fever-stricken humanity lies helpless in the different nooks and corners of the town'.[189] Neither voluntary organizations nor zeal on the part of the populace were lacking; rather it was the Crown's refusal to assume responsibility.[190]

By the second week of November with the pandemic on the wane, the *Bombay Chronicle* demanded that the municipal government explain why it had not closed

[182] L/R/5/174, week ending 28 September 1919, no. 40, *Praja Mitra and Pdrisi*, no. 27; and week ending 9 November 1918, no. 49, *Bombay Chronicle*.
[183] Week ending 12 October 1918, no. 46, *Times of India*.
[184] Week ending 12 October 1918, no. 47.
[185] Week ending 2 November 1918, no. 46, *Bombay Chronicle*.
[186] Week ending 28 September 1918, no. 39, *Praja Mitra and Pdrisi*.
[187] Week ending 12 October 1918, no. 46, *Gujaráti*.
[188] Week ending 19 October 1918, no. 26; also no. 27, *Gujardti*.
[189] Ibid., no. 28, *Jam-e-Jamshed*.
[190] Numerous papers made similar complaints: ibid. nn. 25, 47; week ending 19 October 1918, no. 25; week ending 26 October 1918, nn. 52, 53; also, Ramanna, 'Coping with the Influenza', 88.

schools as Kolkata had done and contrasted Kolkata's diligence with Mumbai's 'policy of masterful inactivity'.[191] Other papers claimed that in villages, 'doctors, volunteers and hospital arrangements' cannot be had, and called on the government to maintain travelling dispensaries and appoint itinerant doctors immediately.[192] For villages outside Hubli, central government and the Board of Health had distributed 'absolutely' no medicines.[193]

Early on, native papers called on the governments of Mumbai and Kolkata to employ well-known bacteriologists presently in the subcontinent, such as Major Glen Liston at Parel and Dr Fowler at Bangalore.[194] They advised circulating leaflets in indigenous languages outlining 'simple directions about precautions' against 'the influenza epidemic'.[195] In early October, the *Sdnj Vartaman* asked government to sponsor a special medical conference bringing medical men to Mumbai to investigate the disease and discover remedies and appealed to the Municipal Corporation to employ a bacteriologist from England.[196] Others petitioned for investment in 'large scientific Pharmacological Institutions' to supply India with drugs, thereby lessening its dependence on medicines from 'far off Europe and America, which were costly and unreliable'.[197] By the end of the month, the Corporation appointed a committee of scientists and medical men, which the papers applauded.[198] As with plague, now influenza, the native press's hostility was not against Western medicine but against colonial inefficiencies and neglect. As these complaints suggest, voluntary groups were the country's only salvation.[199] Yet the extracts mention little about appeals for volunteers, their organizations, and whether they depended on established societies such as the Red Cross or had created new grassroots movements.[200] The extracts fail to reveal who comprised the volunteers: schoolteachers, middle-class women, or whether, as in America, they included some from the highest social echelons. Were they in the main women? The one organization mentioned in the British press—Sava Sadan—does not even appear in these extracts connected with the pandemic.

Volunteerism

To answer these questions, I turn to one native paper recently made available online, Mumbai's *Times of India*. More than a local paper, it reported the pandemic

[191] Week ending 9 November 1918, no. 49, *Bombay Chronicle*.   [192] Ibid., no. 46, *Kesari*.
[193] Week ending 2 November 1918, no. 46, *Bombay Chronicle*; also, see Ramanna, 'Coping with the Influenza', 87.
[194] Week ending 28 September 1918, no. 40, *Praja Mitra and Pdrisi*; also week ending 16 November 1918, no. 62.
[195] Week ending 28 September 1918, no. 40; and ibid., no. 45, *Akhbar-e-Islam*.
[196] Week ending 12 October 1918, no. 47, *Sdnj Vartaman*.
[197] Week ending 2 November 1918, no. 47, *Deccan Ryot*.
[198] Week ending 26 October 1918, no. 45, *Bombay Samachar*. Also, *Times of India*, 8 November 1918, 8.
[199] Week ending, 12 October 1918, no. 47, *Hindusthan*; no. 46, *Gujaratti*; week ending 20 October 1918, no. 26, *Sunday Chronicle*.
[200] Pune voiced a rare expression of gratitude, praising volunteers for their 'good and commendable work'; week ending, 16 November 1918, no. 63, *Kesari*.

in South Africa,[201] London, and Indian cities and regions such as Simla,[202] Delhi,[203] Bhávnagar,[204] Hubli, Karnataka,[205] Surat,[206] Lahore, villages in the Punjab,[207] and Rangoon (Myanmar, then part of British India).[208] In contrast to the extractions, the *Times* lodged no criticisms against the Crown or municipal governments. However, it treated the two levels of government differently with the Crown receiving little notice or praise, while municipal governments were portrayed as engaged with charitable organizations, endeavouring to control the pandemic and provide medicines, food, and care. It reported Delhi's municipality opening city dispensaries and distributing medicine and disinfectants;[209] Hubli's, distributing medicines to the poor free of charge and opening 'a Spanish influenza hospital' at a local high school;[210] Lucknow's, implementing new relief measures and providing free medical relief to sufferers, supplies of firewood at cremation ghats, and shrouds for the dead;[211] and Rangoon's, opening ten dispensaries to supply medicines and advise the infected.[212] Yet Mumbai's daily had little positive to say about the municipality. The best it could report was that it had hired thirteen doctors and three medical students when influenza mortalities suddenly soared in early October.[213]

Nonetheless, the *Times* corroborates an impression suggested by the government's extracts. The Presidency of Bombay and other Indian cities were forced to confront the crisis with a strong volunteer movement. Unlike the extracts, however, the full texts reveal much more—names of charitable organizations, their directors, and praise of individual acts of self-sacrifice, which, as the examples below show, united groups across class, castes, and creeds. Yet given expectations raised by the *Guardian*'s article on the women's organization, Seva Sadan, the view from the *Times* is surprising: overwhelmingly, the charitable response in Mumbai, as well as in other places, was driven predominantly by men.[214]

First, a number of groups to succour the infected give no notion of the volunteers' gender. Early on in the pandemic, the pre-existing Social Service League formed 'a band of volunteers' to afford relief.[215] Further articles specified the organization's tasks: volunteers advised on treatments and organized other volunteer agencies to work with the poor afflicted with influenza.[216] These articles did

---

[201] *Times of India*, 28 October 1918, 11.   [202] Ibid., 28 October 1918, 7.
[203] Ibid.   [204] Ibid., 29 October 1918, 5; *c.*90 km west of Rajkot in Gujarat.
[205] Ibid., 29 October 1918, 8.   [206] Ibid.
[207] Ibid., 28 October 1918, 7.   [208] Ibid., 12 October 1918, 10.
[209] Ibid., 28 October 1918, 7.   [210] Ibid.; and 7 November 1918, 5.
[211] Ibid., 13 November 1918, 9.   [212] Ibid., 12 October 1918, 10.
[213] Ibid., 9 October 1918, 12.

[214] See Chapter 22, note 271. Of numerous voluntary organizations listed in Ramanna, 'Coping with the Influenza', Seva Sedan is never mentioned; instead, they were male-led and male-dominated organizations. Moreover, she mentions only one woman by name—Lady Chinubhaim, 'the pioneer of public health in Ahmedabad', who lent automobiles to neighbouring villages. Hardiman, 'The 1918 Influenza', 659, mentions a few voluntary organizations in the villages of South Gujarat like the Patidar Youth Association, comprised of young men, but mentions no women.

[215] *Times of India*, 1 October 1918, 8.

[216] Ibid., 2 October 1918, 9; and 3 October 1918, 8, praises it 'as the labouring heart and soul among the poor, teaching, preaching, persuading'.

not identify volunteers by class, caste, religion, or sex. But the organizers were men. When the League took its mission to the stricken villages of Wadhwan and Rajkot,[217] the four directors were men,[218] and in Mumbai, when it opened a new centre in Grant Road, it requested that only men who knew the locality need apply.[219]

Various religious groups donated funds and space in their hospitals to treat influenza patients, such as the Hindu Medical Association's ward and the Jain Hospital. At the end of October, Mumbai's Hindu citizens met to devise anti-influenza measures and collected 'considerable funds' on the spot.[220] In December, the association presented their volunteers with silver medals for their sacrifices. No women were mentioned.[221] The Prabhu community donated a ward at their hospital. Wilson College organized its students to assist and offered a building for hospitals. But by 9 October, more hospitals were needed. Unlike the anti-plague controls which had struck fear into the native population, 'the people' now sought out hospital care without any suspicions reported.[222] The Parsis asked for a hospital where they could offer their assistance. Their graduates made house-to-house visitations, supplying medicine, milk, and jackets. The beneficiaries, however, were not restricted to Parsis; rather they visited 'every house in a given locality, regardless of caste and creed.'[223] Another established organization, in this case an international one, the St John Ambulance Brigade, also served sufferers across caste and religious divides.[224] Similarly, the Liberty Club's relief efforts crossed India's dominant social barriers, distributing medicines to any without the means to purchase them, 'to all castes and creeds'.[225] In Lucknow, the pandemic brought Hindus and Muslims together to discuss anti-influenza policies, and together they donated materials for a large number of burials.[226] In Mumbai, the Israelite Brotherhood assisted influenza sufferers, who presumably were not exclusively, or even mostly, Jews.[227]

This cooperation, uniting rival religious groups in common action, occurred against a backdrop of violent conflict between Hindus and Muslims. From 8 to 13 September 1918, major riots erupted between the two at Kolkata, after the Bengal government cancelled a Muslim 'monster meeting' aimed at defending themselves against Hindu agitation and insults against Islam.[228] Numerous demonstrators were shot; the numbers were not even known until weeks later. The government's firing on the Nakhoda Mosque in Kolkata led to further death, with riots continuing for at least a month afterwards, that is, throughout the height of the pandemic.[229] Even according to a Hindu newspaper, the violence and the government's gross

---

[217] In Gujarat, 109 km north-east of Rajkot.   [218] *Times of India*, 15 November 1918, 8.
[219] Ibid., 10 October 1918, 5.   [220] Ibid., 28 October 1918, 7.
[221] Ibid., 2 December 1918, 6.   [222] Ibid., 2 October 1918, 9.
[223] Ibid., 10 October 1918, 5.   [224] Ibid., 19 November 1918, 8.
[225] Ibid., 17 October 1918, 8.   [226] Ibid., 13 November 1918, 9.
[227] Ibid., 11 October 1918, 5.

[228] Even before the Kolkata riot, *Political Bhomiyo* on 6 September (L/R/5/174, week ending 14 September 1918, no. 20) decried the helplessness of Muslims in Hindu–Muslim riots, alleging that Hindus generally instigated the disturbances. It pointed to massacres of Muslims during their festivals of Bakr-Id at Arrah and Shababad the previous year and called on Muslims to arm.

[229] Ibid., week ending 14 September 1918, nos 21–2, *Sdnj Vartaman, Hindusthan, Praja Mitra, and Parsi*; and *Shri Venkatshwar*; week ending 21 September 1918, no. 23, *Young India*; week ending 28 September 1918, nos 16–19: *Gujardti; Sudhaka*; and week ending 12 October 1918, no. 17, *Kesari*.

mismanagement 'spread discontentment fast' throughout India.[230] A month later, the Hindu massacre of Muslims during their festival of Bakr-Id at Katarpur (United Provinces) suggests the extent of animosity: twenty-three Muslims were killed and to add to the humiliation, their enemies burnt their bodies, 'regarded as a great sin by Islam'.[231] The paper called for a 'defence' from the Muslim community, which, in effect, was a call for violence.[232] No women were mentioned.

Another group not defined by gender, the Salvation Army, aided influenza sufferers in hard-hit villages. It was directed, however, by a man, Colonel Spooner, and its rank-and-file probably also consisted principally of men,[233] like the Telugu Volunteers, comprised of doctors and medical student volunteers, who treated 7000 patients and prescribed medicines gratis 'to all communities without distinction of caste or creed'. Of the six individuals named for extraordinary sacrifice at its annual meeting in December, five were doctors and one a senior medical student: all were men.[234] The following day another group of similar composition, the Daivadnya Association of Mumbai, congratulated its doctors and volunteers.[235] At Ahmedabad, the political party, Gujrat Sabha (which played a leading role in a peasant revolt in Kheda in 1918 and was later famous for its freedom fighters) opened a hospital for influenza patients and collected funds to supply medicines to flu-infected villagers.[236] The paper listed no female volunteers.

In villages such as Balasore voluntary associations formed to nurse the sick, but it is unclear whether they were staffed by men or women.[237] At the end of October, the Depressed Classes Mission (DCM) initiated relief work in Hubli, severely hit by influenza just as it was lifting from Mumbai. With the closure of Hubli's schools, the Mission employed teachers to distribute medicines house-to-house in the city's most depressed areas.[238] By mid-November, its Bangalore branch was providing medical assistance to 1070 influenza patients in the city and surrounding villages.[239] Another group in Hubli, the Karnataka branch of the DCM, organized three medical depots, made house calls, inspected and advised 500 householders daily, and distributed medicines gratis to 1000 influenza victims. From its dispensary, they supplied meals and arranged doctors' visits free of charge.[240] The gender composition of its volunteers, however, was unspecified.

As in the US, Canada, Australia, and New Zealand, schoolteachers and students volunteered in India, delivering messages, medicine, and food, and caring for afflicted families and orphans. The big difference, however, was that while women dominated these organizations in other countries, in India schoolmistresses (as opposed to schoolmasters) are mentioned only three times and schoolgirls, never. At the annual meeting of the Gokhale Education Society, only the boys at the

---

[230] Ibid., week ending 14 September 1918, no. 22, *Hindusthan*.

[231] Ibid., week ending 12 October 1918, no. 16, *Political Bhomiyo* claimed the assaults 'wounded the religious feelings of the Muslims of the whole world'.

[232] Ibid.   [233] *Times of India*, 23 December 1918, 11.

[234] Ibid., 6 December 1918, 7.   [235] Ibid., 7 December 1918, 9; and 13 December 1918, 7.

[236] Ibid., 19 November 1918, 7.   [237] Ibid., 14 October 1918, 12.

[238] Ibid., 29 October 1918, 8.   [239] Ibid., 22 November 1918, 7.

[240] Ibid., 7 November 1918, 5.

schools of this society were awarded.[241] In Baroda, schools and teachers appear to have been the strongest charitable body. Their buildings were converted into dispensaries, from which teachers distributed medicines with a Mr Pendse in charge. Later, the high school's headmaster organized a corps of young volunteers, who gained support from the public and a 'munificent gift' from one man. Two hundred teachers volunteered for the Medical Department, started relief work in the region's infected towns and villages, and deputed officers to organize relief in other districts.[242] In October and November, 200 teachers volunteered in the capital and 4000 in the districts, tending dispensaries, making house calls, and distributing food and medicines 'to about 275,000 sufferers'. They participated in local committees, collected funds, and organized distributions of milk and other essential commodities free of charge 'to thousands of patients' and helped with the funerals of the needy. The schoolmasters 'managed' the nursing in the temporary hospitals, which they established in school buildings, 'and even in the Mofussil, schoolmistresses volunteered as nurses and did excellent work', suggesting that women were the exception, even if, finally, they were recognized. At their annual meeting, schoolmasters and several schoolmistresses were awarded medals and certificates. The women had opened a crèche and an orphanage in Baroda City for those left isolated by the pandemic.[243]

In November, the paper published a map showing over 200 influenza relief centres with names of the charities that had organized them. Not one was identified as a women's group, and the one student organization was a 'Brotherhood'.[244] In addition to established and newly founded charities to combat the pandemic, businesses (no doubt, directed by men) provided resources for the needy, and 'numbers of cattle owners' gave milk free of charge.[245] In Delhi, Hindu and Muslim merchants paid funeral expenses for the poor.[246] In Mumbai, the Japanese and Shanghai Silk Piece-Goods Association opened two relief stations, paid a doctor to treat poor patients, and provided food and supplies.[247]

The *Times* also honoured individuals for their organizational skills, care, and sacrifices. Early on in the pandemic in Mumbai, a Dr Turner applied to the military for a hospital to treat impoverished victims. With applications to the municipality and private agencies, he established a 500-bed facility, attracted volunteer workers, and distributed milk and stock medicines for the poor.[248] In early November, Dr Ratilal Bakshi was praised for his house calls, advice, and medicines gratis in Jamnagar.[249] A Dr Ghia founded the Social League Service in the district of Wadhwan and Rajkot, and was praised for supplying milk, ice, cologne water, and 'even food' to his patients. In twenty days, he made 550 house calls.[250] At the same

---

[241] Ibid., 17 April 1919, 9.   [242] Ibid., 2 November 1918, 9.
[243] Ibid., 24 December 1918, 7. The only other mention of women combatting the pandemic I have found was in Simla: 'a number of ladies' volunteered as nurses; ibid., 28 October 1918, 7.
[244] Ibid., 8 November 1918, 9.   [245] Ibid., 9 October 1918, 12.
[246] Ibid., 28 October 1918, 7.   [247] Ibid., 19 November 1918, 7.
[248] Ibid., 2 October 1918, 9.
[249] Ibid., 5 November 1918, 8. Jamnagar, 90 km west of Rajkot.
[250] Ibid., 15 November 1918, 8.

time, a Raj Saheb, who opened an emergency hospital and donated milk, medicines, and pneumonia jackets, and made rounds with a Dr Thakkar in the worst-afflicted areas, was celebrated for contributing to the pandemic's decline in Vankaner.[251] Because of the high mortality in Bhávnagar, the poor suffered from acute shortages of firewood needed for burials; Parmar Hirji Zina opened a fuel shop and fund to provide the wood to the needy.[252] In mid-November, Mr Shivabhoy Motibhoy Patel, a High Court pleader, died of influenza and was honoured for providing milk to poor sufferers.[253] In Ahmedabad, Dr Tankartwalla was recognized for his 'hard work at the influenza hospital founded by Gujurat Sabha'.[254] In December, Reverend W. A. Thomas had worked with numerous patients in a village in the Ninnar and died attending afflicted families. 'Christians and non-Christians' in the village paid him tribute.[255] This collection of pandemic honours is striking: not a single nurse or woman appears.

Was this absence of women simply a matter of the *Times*'s selection? As seen above, the listing of charities, organizations, businesses, and notable individuals recognized for their contributions came not only or primarily from the newspaper but from prior recognition given in reports by distant correspondents in other parts of India, awards granted at annual meetings of charities, and other organizations such as schools and businesses, and from a government map and surveys. Besides, the *Times* often mentioned women's charitable organizations but for deeds unrelated to the Great Influenza. The Women's Branch of the Bombay Presidency War Fund and the Bombay Council of the Women's Famine Relief appear in the news in 1918 and 1919, praised for their good works and recognized at end-of-year ceremonies. Stories of the organizational skill, determination, and self-sacrifice of these women did not, however, concern the Great Influenza.[256] And what about Sava Sadan? During the pandemic, they also appear, celebrated by the *Times* in two articles: one reporting the activities of its Mumbai branch; the other about its work in Pune, praising its principles and contributions to female education and emancipation, its benefits to poor women and children, and its homes for homeless women.[257] In February 1919, the paper covered the society's annual meeting marking these women's achievements in 1917 and 1918: no sacrifices were mentioned concerning influenza.[258] Only in an article on 'Enlightened Indian ladies', did the paper mention, but only in passing, that 'several members of Sava Sadan...had helped as volunteers in the recent influenza epidemic in the Hindu and Parsi Fever hospitals'.[259]

Similar to the US, Canada, Australia, New Zealand, and South Africa, involved in the Great War but removed from Europe's battlefields, India shows its dependence on philanthropy and the lively response of individuals and community groups

---

[251] Ibid., 14 November 1918, 8. Vankaner (now Wankaner), 50 km north-east of Rajkot.
[252] Ibid., 15 November 1918, 8.   [253] Ibid., 18 November 1918, 11.
[254] Ibid., 19 November 1918, 7.   [255] Ibid., 21 December 1918, 6.
[256] Ibid., 8 November 1918, 8.   [257] Ibid., 12 July 1918, 9 and 17 August 1918, 13.
[258] Ibid., 28 February 1919, 9. Later, it recorded that *The Times* (31 March 1919, 8) had drawn attention to this group.
[259] Ibid., 12 July 1919, 12.

to assist victims of the pandemic. In the Preliminary Government Report of India in 1919, the Crown expressed its appreciation: 'Never before, perhaps, in the history of India, have the educated and more fortunately placed members of the community come forward in such large numbers to help their brethren in time of distress.'[260] The Indian case, in fact, highlights the need to rely on such groups because of government indifference and neglect or, unlike in France, Switzerland, and especially Italy, the absence of a military ready to intervene with medical and charitable assistance to civilians crippled by the pandemic in the last days of the war and during the peace. But in contrast to most other regions beyond European borders, India's response relied overwhelmingly on men and their institutions. Nonetheless, along with other nations in and outside Europe, India experienced the Great Influenza, like the epidemics in Livy's ancient Rome, as a force for unity. Like the plague at the turn of the century, this pandemic brought classes, castes, even the warring religious communities together throughout the subcontinent.

Of epidemics and pandemics, none can compare with the Great Influenza. As far as current research goes, most remarkable was its global reach and the absolute numbers felled. The preceding chapters illustrate another dimension equally remarkable, especially given current expectations that epidemics across time and space have 'spawned sinister connotations', resulting in violence and scapegoating of 'others'. Worldwide, this pandemic unleashed waves of compassion, volunteerism, and self-sacrifice. To be sure, these chapters show a wide spectrum of governmental, community, and individual reactions. In Italy, France, and Britain the sources shed little light on the formation of grassroots organizations to assist the afflicted or of individuals heroically battling the dangerous contagion for utter strangers, at least in comparison to the outpouring of altruism that besieged local health boards, municipalities, and international organizations across the US, Canada, Australia, and India. Switzerland and Ireland fit an intermediate position perhaps also reflecting their roles in the war, the first as a neutral country, the second as a defector after the Easter Rising of 1916, especially around Dublin, where my samples have been taken. Yet, even in places where levels of volunteerism were little in evidence, suspicion, hatred, or violence towards governments, elites, physicians, or victims of the disease is not found. The worst story of cruel indifference comes from 'the fashionable residential district' of San Rafael, north of San Francisco. Nocturnal ramblings of an influenza sufferer 'delirious with fever' enraged some citizens enough to sign a petition demanding that those suspected of influenza be interned at a county farm. Yet only fifty signed, and the petition failed miserably.[261]

Of the few to have recognized the Great Influenza's failure to spark hatred and violence, some have reasoned this resulted because the disease was a normal seasonal ailment that people joked about. This influenza, however, quickly became no joking matter. Instead, from small-town papers to scientists as exalted as America's leading pathologist, it was seen as new and mysterious. In fact, diseases that continued to produce hate and violence into the twentieth century—smallpox,

---

[260] Cited in Ramanna, 'Coping with the Influenza', 86.
[261] *San Francisco Chronicle*, 29 October 1918, 7.

poliomyelitis, occasionally typhus, and most dramatically, cholera—had by then become medically understood and familiar. One might hypothesize that the Great War's galvanizing patriotic pull had created a milieu of community-inspired cooperation. But instead, the war had fragmented communities across class, ethnicity, race, and ideology. However, against this backdrop, the pandemic brought white debutants into El Paso's barrios; Jews and Catholics together in support of hospitals; blacks and whites together in the Deep South; Muslims and Hindus together in Lucknow; and even enemies at war to assist each other in mutual respect, like the French soldiers and German-speaking peasants in the Swiss mountain village of Zofingen.

24

Conclusion

This book challenges a dominant hypothesis in the study of epidemics across time: that mysterious diseases with no preventive measures or cures to hand were the ones to provoke 'sinister connotations', spurring hatred and blame towards 'the other' and victims of disease. If this were true, then why were such incidents so rare before the spread of cholera through Europe in the 1830s? As we have shown, these violent reactions hardly appeared in antiquity, and for the Middle Ages the Black Death has cast a long shadow that needs contesting. Recurrences of plague after 1348 into the sixteenth century did not rekindle the horrors of the Black Death, which pervaded social relations and brought about not only the burning of Jews but also the more diffused cruelty of abandoning loved ones in their moment of need. Even with resurging fears of plague spreaders in the sixteenth century, neither Jews nor other minorities were then the butts of prejudice and persecution; rather, insiders from solid artisans to bankers were the usual suspects. Moreover, those tried, tortured, and executed did not amount to thousands; nor were entire communities exterminated as in 1348–50. In the most studied case, the torture and execution of alleged plague carriers in Milan in 1630, only ten executions are recorded. The Black Death was a colossal exception, not the rule for a pre-'laboratory-revolution' past when almost all diseases were without cures to hand.

Should we then suppose that a socio-psychological immunity developed, with epidemics losing their capacity to terrorize and spark widespread violence after their first mysterious appearances? The answer was usually no. Sometimes we forget that cholera first struck parts of Europe in the early 1820s, not the 1830s, and first spread through Russia's Volga basin without traces of social violence.[1] But it returned there for the next five cholera waves with deadly socio-psychological effects, as in the 1890s, when crowds of 10,000 killed a governor, physicians, and soldiers and destroyed an important industrial town, present-day Donetsk. Such recurrences were not limited to authoritarian regimes that brutally enforced sanitary controls. In Italy, cholera's social violence, instead of declining or disappearing with successive bouts of the disease, expanded geographically. With its first attack in 1836–7, riots were confined almost exclusively to Sicily. By its last major wave, 1910–11, riots had advanced through Puglia, Calabria, and Abruzzi, invading towns in the centre-north, such as seaside resorts north of Rome, and by some accounts, Venice. With the same fantasies and fears of the 1830s, crowds attacked town halls and

---

[1] I know of only one riot during cholera's first wave. In Manila, 9 October 1820, thirty to forty Europeans and eighty Chinese were massacred; Peckham, 'Symptoms of Empire', 192.

hospitals, killed doctors and mayors, and 'liberated' afflicted neighbours, whom they triumphantly carried on their shoulders back to their homes.

Cholera was not the only epidemic disease that failed to acquire immunity to attacks of blame and violence. While rioting accompanied the first spread of plague in Mumbai in 1896, social violence mounted with successive strikes of the disease and peaked with its largest, most deadly revolt in March 1898, joined by shopkeepers who closed their businesses and workers who went on strike. The same holds for plague in the Middle East, where social violence was not triggered by the first appearance of the disease but after four plague seasons had passed.

Smallpox's trajectory of violence was more striking. If the Antonine pandemic of the 160s CE was smallpox, as historians now believe, it provoked no known cases of blame, persecution, or violence. Quite the opposite: tensions along Rome's bellicose borders eased. Nor did the Middle Ages record any smallpox riots or persecution, and the same appears to have been the case when it arrived in the New World and later in colonial Latin America. Instead, sustained smallpox violence that blamed outsiders—the tramp, 'Negro', 'Chinaman', and 'Bohemian'—came late in the day with the pandemic of 1881–2 in the US and mounted in frequency and cruelty into the twentieth century, that is, after it had become a familiar disease both epidemically and endemically, and after an effective means of prevention had been discovered.

AGGRESSORS AND TARGETS

Smallpox highlights a second theme running through this book. The violence spawned by various epidemic diseases was not all alike, nor was it what historians have supposed. People perceived as the 'other'—ethnic and racial minorities, the outsider, the foreigner, the Jew—were not predominantly the victims. Rather, aggressors and their targets assumed different sides, depending on the epidemic. Although officials, intellectuals, and physicians may have decried the ignorance and filth of the labouring classes, seeing them as cholera's cause, elites were the victims of this disease's rage. As René Baehrel claimed sixty-six years ago, these were matters of class struggle, but one to which neither Marx nor Engels paid any heed. Across a wide range of political regimes from Czarist Russia to liberal Manchester, the poor and marginal—recent Irish Catholic immigrants in English, Scottish, and North American cities; Asiatic Sarts in Tashkent, impoverished women and children in Glasgow and Edinburgh, fig-growers and fishermen in Sicily and southern Italy—produced similar fantasies that accused elites of plotting to cull populations of the poor. Here, the 'others', instead of being the butts of blame, were the perpetrators, who attacked physicians, pharmacists, mayors, and police.

On first impression, plague riots, mostly in India in the years 1896 to 1902, may appear to have followed cholera's suit. These riots, however, rarely divided communities. Instead, they unified castes and classes, bridging differences even between Hindus and Muslims in common cause against colonial and municipal abuses, military searches, destruction to temples and homes, and disrespect for local customs. In contrast to the bulk of cholera riots, which show few signs of prior organization, planning, or leadership, plague riots usually began with open meetings, resolutions, newspaper editorials, and letters to colonial commissioners. Despite initial criticisms of violence or lower-class 'superstitions', intellectuals and indigenous elites often ended up supporting the demands of the lower classes against abuses, incompetence, and notions of plague control that dated back to the Middle Ages, but by 1898 had been discovered to be counterproductive.

Plague protest as a force for unity was not exclusive to the subcontinent. The national Public Health Service's discriminatory quarantine on San Francisco's Chinatown and coercive vaccination of the Chinese alone not only united the city's Chinese community across class, it moved white merchants to support their Chinese neighbours with demonstrations, business closures, and legal actions in marked contrast to their earlier attitudes and actions during outbreaks of smallpox, tuberculosis, and syphilis. Similarly, Honolulu's plague experience ultimately was a force for unity, despite white citizens' initial fears and armed quarantine entrapment of Chinese, Japanese, and native Hawaiians, while their homes and businesses burnt to the ground. No class or ethnic massacre ensued. Instead, white elites succoured the afflicted: charity and compassion were the upshots.

The epidemic disease that best fits the present view that diseases inspired hatred with the victims of the disease often being victimized was smallpox in America, which historians have yet to realize. This disease's social violence was also one of class struggle, but the perpetrators and victims of violence now switched sides. Smallpox 'mobs' were mostly comprised of small-town white citizens, businessmen, or propertied farmers and were led (unlike cholera protesters) by adult males. In such cases, the victims were doubly victimized, first by the disease, then by elite violence. Smallpox violence differed in another respect. Although these crowds could number in the thousands, more characteristically, gangs or small vigilante groups greeted those seeking help with double-barrel shotguns, or worse, burnt their pesthouses to the ground, sometimes with the incumbents cremated inside. Other epidemics showed more complex alignments, as in Milan in 1630. Those who perpetuated myths of plague spreaders and persecuted those who were accused by means of brutal legal procedures participated in an unspoken alliance between the poor—often women—and elites, comprised of physicians, senators, and the Cardinal-Archbishop. The alleged *untori* on the other hand were not outsiders or the lowest of plague cleaners, as historians now assume, but insiders, native Milanese, who proudly announced it when summoned before the authorities who interrogated and tortured them.

UNITY

Across the wide sweep of recorded epidemics, blame and persecution were not the usual outcomes. As Livy and authors in antiquity highlight, epidemics often interrupted the course of human events, ending, at least temporarily, conflict between tribes and nations, such as between Rome and Velitrae or the Volscians during the fifth century BCE, or internal battles, such as the ongoing strife between senatorial classes and plebeians. When epidemics were particularly mysterious, oracles or sacred books were consulted. Instead of casting out beggars or persecuting 'others', ancients heeded oracles' calls by opening their doors to strangers, breaking the manacles binding prisoners, granting work-free holidays, providing grain for the poor, and inventing new forms of hospitality. Similarly, with the two great pandemics of late antiquity, the Antonine Plague of 165–180 CE and the Justinianic Plague beginning in 541, unity and charity, not division and hatred, were the outcome. Emperor Marcus Aurelius was praised for his charitable offerings to the afflicted, and despite war with the Germanic tribes, his previous persecution of Christians, and the fact that this pestilence was new, mysterious, and originated beyond the Empire's borders, no blame or persecution ensued. Instead, new opportunities and privileges were extended to 'barbarian' outsiders.

The depiction of the Justinianic Plague once it reached Constantinople was more extraordinary, especially given the disposition of its principal historian, Procopius, towards Emperor Justinian. Before the pandemic, Procopius depicted Justinian's greed, corruption, and cruelty that divided the city through factional strife, sponsoring the circus of the Blues and murdering their rivals. Yet with the coming of the plague, Procopius heaps praise on Justinian's charity, which through his minister, Theodorus, rallied public assistance to the poor and afflicted, and buried the mounds of plague corpses threatening the city's survival. The circuses' perennial divisions temporarily ended. Those who before the plague despised one another now united to honour the dead.

The late Middle Ages also experienced these moments of unity in the midst of pestilence. Not only was the Black Death unique in its horrific socially inflicted carnage, half a century later, a flagellant movement was born from a plague that was the polar opposite of the previous movement in 1349. Instead of re-enacting Black-Death division and hate, the Bianchi was a peace movement that united elites and commoners, crossed city walls into the countryside, and brought men, women, and children together to end social conflict from everyday litigation to factional strife among aristocratic clans and war between territorial states.

Even if the Black Death was not a turning point in epidemics' power to fuel hatred, it awakened a new awareness of the transmission of diseases, inspiring new regulations and organizations to protect communities in plague time by evicting suspected carriers and undesirables. Yet it was the birth of a new disease in Europe at the end of the fifteenth century—the Great Pox—that launched endeavours to track the movement of disease, as physicians turned from their reliance on antique and Arabic sources, to chart Columbus's voyages and the possible routes by which the new disease progressed to Naples, then across Europe and beyond. With this disease, however, tracking of contacts did not lead to blaming and certainly not to persecution. Instead, the leading edge of hate-fuelled disease in early modernity was Europe's old companion, known now for two centuries—plague. The sixteenth- and early seventeenth-century accusations, tortures, and executions did not hinge on ignorance or a sudden unleashing of folkloric superstition previously locked in mountain hollows. Instead, those at the forefront of medicine and science were the ones to justify the state's onslaught on innocents. Yet these injustices did not amount to massacres, certainly not on a scale comparable to the Black Death slaughter or to cholera and plague riots in the nineteenth and twentieth centuries.

COMPASSION

Even with modernity and new notions that diseases were carried by people (although miasmas continued to figure), few epidemic diseases ignited collective violence against victims of disease, outsiders, insiders, or elites. Instead, some of the most feared and deadly diseases, whose causative agents remained mysterious into the twentieth century, provoked waves of compassion and volunteerism rather than division and hate. Like Livy's ancient plagues, yellow fever in America and the Great Influenza of 1918–20 globally eased class, ethnic, sectional, and racial tensions and extended care and charity through the donation of resources and relief provided by priests, nuns, doctors, nurses, and others who often journeyed from distant places and died as a consequence of their charity. The mass evacuation of Philadelphia in 1793, New Orleans in 1853, Memphis in 1878, and many smaller towns across the Deep South throughout the nineteenth century suggests that yellow fever sparked greater fear and panic than any disease in US history. Fear and panic did not, however, spell blame and violence. Instead, it cut in the opposite direction, spurring clubs and business to assist the afflicted, with people from the North volunteering in the South and blacks sacrificing their lives for the white afflicted. These waves of abnegation, moreover, sprouted in historical contexts not conducive to such sentiments, such as the South's epidemic of 1853, when sectional tensions between North and South were on the rise, or in 1878, during a racist backlash against the advances of post-Civil War reconstruction.

Charitable outpouring and self-sacrifice were more widespread during the Great Influenza and differed from earlier waves of disease-inspired volunteerism. Women now played the principal role, at least across much of Canada, the US, and Australia. No doubt, the war played its part in the shift. But here too the general contexts—war-spun xenophobia, worldwide industrial strife, red-scare hysteria, the longest, most violent race riots in US history, and rising anti-Mexican hatred, even warfare, along the Texan–Mexican border—ran counter to humanitarian urges. But in El Paso, middle-class women and debutant girls crossed into the city's most impoverished and afflicted Mexican neighbourhoods to sweep floors, make meals, care for children, and nurse the dangerously ill. Such sentiments flourished across the country against advice from government bulletins and municipal decrees pillorying spitters, sneezers, coughers, and big talkers, and urging 'patriots' to blame them for flu's fatal spread. No collective violence, however, ensued against sufferers or any other 'others'.

THE IMPORTANCE OF DISEASE

This book has argued that local and national contexts are insufficient to explain how a disease such as cholera could have produced such similar and distinctive fantasies of blame and patterns of collective violence across radically different political and cultural regimes from Asiatic Russia to New York City. Moreover, other epidemic diseases struck some of these places at the same moments without stirring blame or igniting mass violence, such as an influenza pandemic in Paris, other places in France, and Europe in 1831 that caused more deaths than cholera did a year later. Similarly, a wave of typhus raged through Britain and Ireland in 1826, felling 20,000 in London alone, and again in the 1830s with no ramifications of social violence, and attacks of plague and typhus spread through the Volga in 1892, when cholera and the riots associated with it were rife, but here neither plague nor typhus spawned a single disturbance. In addition, many disastrous epidemics fill modern European history, such as typhus which accompanied the 'Great Hunger' in Ireland in the 1840s or that spread from Siberia in 1920–2 through parts of Russia and into Eastern Europe, but did not stir up violence.

Of course, neither cholera nor smallpox spread hate and blame everywhere. As we have seen, smallpox's social violence was situated mostly in the US and before 1881–2 had been extremely rare. Cholera also showed peculiar patterns. So far, only one major cholera riot has appeared in its birthplace, India, although cholera was rife at moments when plague protest neared its peak in May 1897 on the eve of the 'Tragedy of Poona' and with mass plague violence in Kolkata, Mumbai, and elsewhere. On the other side of the hate–compassion divide, an epidemic of poliomyelitis erupted in New York City in 1916. However, unlike influenza two years later, elite ladies, instead of risking their lives to clean, feed, and nurse the poor, blamed the poor for the disease and patrolled impoverished neighbourhoods to report habits they judged unsavoury to the police.

As shown in the chapter on smallpox and collective violence, pundits in the nineteenth century thought cholera was the disease most likely to provoke social violence in America. International news, however, and not their own history, fixed their views. In places such as Ireland, Britain, America, and to a large extent France, waves of cholera after the 1830s failed to spark mass social violence; whereas in Russia, Spain, Portugal, Persia, and places in the Middle East, the riots persisted throughout the nineteenth century, and, in Italy, may have reached their zenith during its last major wave in 1910–11. Moreover, in North America, cholera crowds in the thousands appeared only once. Even in the 1830s, when cholera pushed westward, devastating cities such as New Orleans and St Louis, no rioting or fantasies of doctors culling populations arose.

Certainly, such differences depended on multiple factors, which can be uncovered only through new comparative research, investigating attitudes and practices of ruling elites and medical authorities along with those of the poor, especially on sensitive matters of ritual and religion, such as the burial and handling the dead. In places, authorities appear to have learnt lessons, such as the reforms made by the

British for the provisioning of cadavers to anatomy colleges. In other places, such as Russia from the 1830s to at least the 1890s, elites instead stood fast to the same accusations, blaming the disease on the poor, castigating their supposed 'ignorance' and 'superstitions', and creating their own mythologies that labelled any cholera disturbance the work of outside agitators, while the state imposed heavier controls and harsher repression.

Similar measures by local and national authorities continued to provoke distrust and cholera unrest in Italy. From the first cholera wave in Italy in 1836–7 to the last major one in 1910–11, local authorities prohibited non-elites from performing their traditional burial rites, visiting afflicted friends and relations, and viewing the bodies of loved ones before burial, while elites were allowed to bury theirs in traditional church grounds. Such class-based impositions supported fears that doctors and the state were murdering the poor. Seeing their relatives unceremoniously 'thrown into ditches' of newly created cholera grounds, the *popolo* of Ostuni rioted in 1837. In 1910, the state's class-based burial restrictions remained in place, and fears of poisoning and burials alive resurfaced. In mid-November, Ostuni's collective violence exploded beyond any of its previous incidents: 3000 in a town of 18,500 wrecked the cholera hospital, 'liberated the patients', burnt down the town hall and health department, took possession of the town square, attacking health workers, stoning *carabinieri*, and destroying doctors' homes.

On the other hand, other places succeeded in quelling fears and distrust, which could have sparked social violence among populations unaccustomed to hospital care and where mythologies of doctors plotting to poison the poor already existed. Such was the experience during yellow fever's 1905 finale in Louisiana's bayous. Recently arrived Sicilian peasants, working the sugar plantations and imbued with cholera fantasies from their homeland of little more than a decade earlier, initially resisted doctors and fumigators entering their homes. In Old World fashion, they accused them of spreading the disease to cull their numbers. Through door-to-door canvassing by Italian-speaking neighbours and priests, and letters and lectures from trusted community leaders, their fears, however, faded: threats of collective violence turned to disease prevention.

A MODEL FOR EPIDEMIC DISEASES?

Few scholars have pointed to which diseases in the past or which of their characteristics were likely to spark social violence. Margaret Humphreys has delved deeper than others, arguing that childhood diseases and those that were endemic, despite being big killers—diphtheria, scarlatina, whooping cough, dysentery, typhoid, tuberculosis, and influenza—were not prone to ignite blame or hatred. Instead, those that struck suddenly and disappeared quickly were the socially dangerous ones. At times, this was certainly the case. However, America's socially most toxic disease—smallpox—was an endemic disease with epidemic outbreaks, and children more than adults were the victims. The same goes for poliomyelitis, which in 1916 was blamed on the poor, ethnic minorities, and victims of the disease, or their mothers. As for diseases that struck fast and vanished rapidly, this theory only partially works with cholera and plague: plague after 1348 and into the sixteenth century provoked no riots and rarely social loathing. Moreover, with modern plague, collective violence was confined mostly to India and the years 1896 to 1902, well before the disease reached its heights in the subcontinent. Other epidemic diseases also rose and disappeared quickly, such as yellow fever and the Great Influenza, which in many places wreaked its havoc within a month. Yet, these failed to spark mass violence or social victimization of the diseased victim.

Three further characteristics may have influenced epidemics' potential for hate and social violence. First, diseases that kill quickly such as cholera (in a day or two), plague in medieval and early modern Europe (in two to three days), and modern plague (around a week in bubonic form, twenty-four hours in pneumonic form, and less with septicaemia) could all provoke hatred, blame, and rioting. Yet fast killers, such as yellow fever (within a week) or influenza in 1918–20 (often within forty-eight hours) did not rouse violent recriminations. By contrast, smallpox, whose record of hatred and violence arose only in the late nineteenth century, was usually a slow killer. Second, diseases with signs and symptoms that produced reactions of disgust also could spread hate and blame. Here, the prime candidates were smallpox, leprosy, and syphilis and other venereal diseases that engulfed early modern Europe. But as we have observed, leprosy during the Middle Ages until the mid-nineteenth century rarely ignited hatred and sparked mass slaughter only once, in 1321, when no epidemic of it raged. Similarly, neither syphilis nor other venereal diseases spread blame or persecution of their victims until late into the sixteenth century and then it was limited mostly to England. Of the diseases renowned for disgust, only smallpox engendered popular hatred or rioting and this occurred principally in the US and only by the late nineteenth century.

Finally, lethality (and certainly not mortality) was a key variable. Lethality rates of medieval and early modern plague were high. As calculated from lazaretti records, they could range between 50 and 90 per cent and remained as high with modern plague until the diffusion of antibiotics. Cholera's rates were also high, usually over 50 per cent into the twentieth century, as were Ebola's in West Africa in 2014–15.[2] With both diseases, this lethality sparked repeated claims by victims' friends and families: 'Here, if the people come into the hospital, they don't leave alive.' And for both, these suspicions led to deadly consequences for doctors, health workers, and police. In addition, with cholera and Ebola, as well as plague in India, anger arose when health workers tried to disrupt traditional rituals of dressing and burying the afflicted. Yet as the recent history of Ebola in West Africa has shown, along with examples in this book stretching from Mumbai's slums to Louisiana's bayous, relations between governors and health

---

[2] By contrast, lethality rates of yellow fever and especially influenza, even the Great One, were much lower. In places with repeated strikes of yellow fever, mild cases arise that often go undetected. Even in severe epidemics like Philadelphia's in 1793, estimates of lethality are less than 20 per cent.

boards and the communities of victims were crucial. When the latter were permitted to negotiate and participate in measures such as search parties, the rioting and assassinations ended. While this book knows no easy answers, it has uncovered parallels and stark differences over the long history of epidemics. Just as different diseases affect our bodies differently, so too they have affected differently our collective mentalities.

25

Epilogue: HIV/AIDS
A Pandemic of Hate, Compassion, and Politics

The HIV/AIDS pandemic stimulated scholarly interest in the socio-psychological effects of epidemics in the past.[1] A wide range of commentators across academic disciplines and the press searched for historical parallels and readily found them. The message was univocal, one-dimensional, and transhistorical, resisting attempts to detect change over time or discover significant differences among diseases. Across time, space, and disease, epidemics, especially ones that were 'new', lacking tested cures or effective prevention, were seen as the triggers for all 'sorts of irrational hatreds and prejudice'.[2] This irrationality supposedly targeted the victims of disease or 'others'—the poor, the outcast, the Jew, the foreigner. Some added that AIDS was particularly virulent in sparking hate, because it was sexually transmitted, and as a consequence, parallels between syphilis and other sexually transmitted diseases in early modern Europe and during the nineteenth and twentieth centuries, were seized upon.[3] Finally, those perceived as susceptible to AIDS and accused of spreading it further fuelled the pandemic's social toxins, because, as supposedly in epidemics of the past, they came from marginal communities, already subjected to suspicion and prejudice: in the case of HIV/AIDS, homosexuals, IV drug users, prostitutes, and Haitians. This chapter differs from previous ones in that I rely on a vast secondary literature rather than mining original sources.

HATE AND VIOLENCE

Although difficult to measure, what were the manifestations of HIV/AIDS-related collective violence aroused within communities or from governments? Despite over 10,000 books and articles on HIV/AIDS published by 1986,[4] I know of none to catalogue the acts of violence, especially collective ones, sparked by AIDS globally

---

[1] For its early history, see Grmek, *Histoire di sida*; for more recent discoveries, Pepin, *The Origins of AIDS*; and Harden, *AIDS at 30: A History*.

[2] Tomes, *The Gospel of Germs*, 13, citing Burnham, *How Superstition Won*, comparing AIDS and tuberculosis a hundred years earlier in America. For other authors, see Introduction and Grmek, *Histoire di sida*, 82.

[3] Grmek, *Histoire di sida*, 179; Baldwin, *Disease and Democracy*, 203; McGough, *Gender, Sexuality, and Syphilis*, 150; Farmer, *AIDS and Accusation*, 237; Gilman, 'AIDS and Syphilis'; Eamon, 'Cannibalism and Contagion', 1–2; Brandt, 'Aids and Metaphor', 103; and Altman, *AIDS in the Mind of America*, 140–1.

[4] Feldman, *Plague Doctors*, 3.

or within any nation or region. Yet authors have readily characterized AIDS violence 'as depressingly reminiscent of medieval Europe's response to Black Death, when Jews...were rounded up and exterminated'.[5] Outside of Africa, no journalist or scholar has repeated more than a handful of stories of physical violence against the AIDS-afflicted, their families, or imagined carriers. As for mass protest, no one has reported any violence. Below are the instances I have gathered from the literature. I begin with the most-repeated examples.

On the night of 28 August 1987, after a week of bomb and death threats against Clifford and Louise Ray, their three sons, and a daughter, and with parents boycotting the children's school in Arcadia, Florida, a fire mysteriously destroyed the Rays' home. No one, however, was injured. The three boys were haemophiliacs 'known to have been exposed' to AIDS, and had been banned from school. Their parents sued and after physicians testified that the boys' condition posed no health risks, they were readmitted, igniting the boycott by the school's parents' committee. Yet two days after the Rays' house had been torched, the committee offered the family food and clothing. The Rays declined the gift, asking instead that their charity go towards educating the community about AIDS.[6] It is still not known who or how many were involved in the arson.

An earlier incident of slightly longer duration involved greater numbers and has received scholarly attention. During September and October 1985, parents protested against a seven-year-old AIDS patient attending school in Queens, New York, first by bringing a lawsuit against the Board of Education, the Department of Health, and New York City's Commissioner of Health. The court decision allowed the unnamed child to attend class at an unspecified school within New York City's 622 elementary schools. On the first day of classes, parents of 10,000 children of the city's 960,000 elementary pupils boycotted classes. Marches with placards and chanting ensued but without violence to any AIDS victim, suspected carrier, or anyone else. A decision on 11 February 1986 ruled in favour of the School Board, declaring AIDS not 'a communicable disease' and allowing the anonymous AIDS victim to remain in school. The decision fuelled no backlash.[7]

Another case of discrimination but not of physical violence became a cause célèbre: Ryan White, diagnosed with AIDS at thirteen, was barred from attending school in Kokomo, Indiana, in January 1985.[8] Afterwards, with his mother, he founded an organization to educate the nation on AIDS. A few months after his death (8 April 1990), Congress passed the AIDS bill (CARE, Comprehensive AIDS Resources Emergency Act) named after him. A fourth case of what might be considered collective physical violence (although, as with the three above, the victims amounted to less than a handful) has been mentioned in the literature far less often. On 12 November 1987, the *Wall Street Journal* reported three men in Texas brutally beating a man diagnosed with AIDS. When asked what they were doing,

---

[5] Eamon, 'Cannibalism and Contagion', 1.   [6] 'AIDS Panic'; Foege, 'Plague', 14.

[7] Nelkin and Hilgartner, 'Disputed Dimensions of Risk'; Bayer, 'The Dependent Center', 138; Brandt, 'Aids and Metaphor', 105. For a dramatization of the story, see Black, *The Plague Years*, 174–6.

[8] Brandt, 'AIDS'; idem, 'Plagues and Peoples', 192.

an assailant responded, 'Killing AIDS'. But nothing was said about or against homosexuals. The victim returned to his hometown, Williamson, West Virginia, where after he swam in a local pool, mothers fled with their children. Townspeople (the number is unrecorded) then circulated a petition to ban his younger sister and her boyfriend from school, because they were believed to be infected. Unlike in Texas, no violence occurred. Clearly, their phobia did not hinge on homosexuality or prejudices against non-whites, foreigners, or outsiders; the sister and boyfriend were white, heterosexual, and from town.[9] I have found a fifth case in one source alone and whether its violence was collective or committed by a single miscreant is not revealed. Here, the victim was not a victim of AIDS but probably a gay rights advocate. The house of a student director of a production of Larry Kramer's *The Normal Heart* at the University of Missouri was firebombed. The culprit(s) appear not to have been apprehended; their number went unreported.[10] A sixth incident (which also comes from a single source) was reported in the *San Francisco Chronicle* on 1 October 1984, but occurred at an unspecified time in the previous summer. On a Sunday afternoon in San Francisco's 'bucolic Sigmund Stern Grove', 'a gang' of about twenty drunk teenagers with sticks and stones attacked and chased 'gay men and lesbian women' at a picnic sponsored by 'the gay Catholic group Dignity'. The teenagers shouted, 'Unclean' and 'Faggots got AIDS', and one 'big hulk of a kid…threw rocks at a lesbian'.[11] There is no evidence that any of the victims were HIV-positive, or that the 'kids' inflicted injuries.

Finally, according to anthropologist-physician Paul Farmer, citing Renée Sabatier, the decision of the Center for Disease Control at Atlanta (CDC) in 1982 (and not rescinded until 1985), which defined Haitians as an AIDS risk-group, sparked attacks on Haitian schoolchildren and led to families being evicted from their homes.[12] The evidence comes from an uncited and undated reference to a report by an unnamed 'New York City Commission'.[13] The number of incidents it recorded and the nature of the violence, whether it consisted of playground bullying or collective violence involving adults, is not specified. Reflecting on the same legislation, Alan Kraut is slightly more concrete: in Miami, children were 'ostracized even on the school playground', phrased as if this were the worst of the violence.[14] To be sure, stigmatization of Haitians at home and within the US increased sharply in 1982–3, and they paid for it psychologically and economically. Yet the literature describes no 'mobs' or riots against any Haitian AIDS scapegoats.

Other collective actions against AIDS sufferers, presumed carriers, or their families certainly occurred in the US. *Time* magazine reported that in New York City attacks against homosexuals increased from 176 in 1984 to 517 in 1987.[15] A special congressional hearing in late 1986 concluded that violence against homosexuals had increased, 'much of it linked to AIDS'.[16] But I know of no studies to analyse these figures for New York or elsewhere. Were they all physical assaults?

---

[9] Rushing, *The AIDS Epidemic*, 155. [10] Goldstein, 'The Implicated and the Immune', 39.
[11] Cited in Altman, *AIDS in the Mind of America*, 69. [12] Sabatier, *Blaming Others*, 86.
[13] Farmer, *AIDS and Accusation*, 214; and Sabatier, *Blaming Others*, 86.
[14] Kraut, *Silent Travellers*, 3. [15] Rushing, *The AIDS Epidemic*, 155.
[16] Altman, 'Legitimation through Disaster', 313; and idem, 'Gays Testify'.

How many involved multiple assailants? Were the targets predominantly Haitian or foreigners? Could any of them be described as riots? To be sure, some physicians refused to treat AIDS patients,[17] and some were 'even denied transportation to the grave'.[18] Yet, despite claims in the literature of physical beatings, stigmatization, and discrimination with the loss of jobs, homes, and friends, the six cases above are the only specific ones that I have found in the US which hint at collective violence. These, moreover, clustered into just over three years, from the summer of 1984 to December 1987.[19]

For Europe, even less appears in the secondary literature, and there are no reports comparable to the US incidents. This meagre harvest of HIV/AIDS-fuelled violence in the West stands in striking contrast to the hatred and suspicion spawned during the nineteenth and early twentieth century by cholera, smallpox, and plague. These epidemics led to occasions when protesters in the US, Canada, India, Britain, Italy, Russia, and other countries assembled in streets and burnt municipal buildings, clinics, and hospitals, often maiming or murdering health workers and government officials and, in the case of smallpox, the afflicted. As seen in earlier chapters, the riots they sparked could involve thousands of people, last for months, and take over or destroy entire towns. By contrast, HIV/AIDS, for all its fear and prejudice, failed to produce a single reported riot in the West (unless 'kids' in a San Francisco park, attacking a gay Catholic picnic with sticks and stones is so labelled).

In Africa, where the number of cases of HIV as of 2014 became the highest in any continent,[20] the story is different. Incidents of physical violence (or at least the recognition and publicizing of them) against AIDS victims came to light later but became more widespread and extreme. Since the dominant African strain of HIV-2 has led to relatively fewer cases among homosexuals or IV drug users than seen in the West, the social violence in Africa has targeted principally heterosexuals. According to John Iliffe, '[S]uspicion focused [at first] especially on infected men alleged to spread the disease deliberately, "so as not to die alone." ' However, he cites only one case where such suspicion led to collective violence: a mob in western Uganda (its numbers unreported) beat to death a man suspected of being infected with AIDS, who boasted of having sex with over thirty women.[21] Nonetheless, Iliffe cites more cases of physical and collective violence to AIDS victims than any I have found for Africa or elsewhere. In KwaZulu-Natal, a province in South Africa, papers in 2001 reported that houses of AIDS sufferers were burnt to the ground; some 'barely able to walk [were] chased by mobs into the bush', and teachers

---

[17] Brandt, 'Plagues and Peoples', 192; and Harden, *AIDS at 30: A History*, 79.

[18] In addition to the above, see Fineberg, 'The Social Dimension of AIDS', 106; Altman, *AIDS in the Mind of America*, 63; Patton, *Sex and Germs*, 70; and Weeks, 'AIDS', 26. On federal law not protecting the civil rights of AIDS victims in the 1980s and threats to previous anti-discrimination legislation, Brandt, 'Plagues and Peoples', 194.

[19] Farmer, *AIDS and Accusation*, 247; and Harden, 'AIDS in the U.S.', 7–13.

[20] Sub-Saharan Africa comprises nearly 71 per cent of people living with HIV, and South Africa, 25 per cent of these (2013); on the other hand, AIDS-related deaths have decreased by 48 per cent in South Africa since 2005; *UNAIDS Gap Report*, 26 and 28.

[21] Iliffe, *The African AIDS Epidemic*, 80. He does not date the case.

and pupils hunted down children infected with HIV because they were 'unclean'.[22] AIDS patients returning home after counselling at centres in Dodoma Region in Tanzania were rejected by their families with some locked up and treated as lepers.[23] In Sierra Leone, a man suspected of having AIDS had his house ransacked.[24]

Along with other authors,[25] Iliffe has argued that in place of homosexuals, haemophiliacs, and drug users, women in Africa soon bore the brunt of blame for spreading HIV/AIDS.[26] Certainly, much of the blaming took the form of domestic violence (most cases of which were unreported)[27] or collective stigmatization for which an increasingly large social science literature has produced evidence from interviews and questionnaires.[28] But as in the West, reports of large-scale riots against the victims have not surfaced. Cases of stigmatization leading to violence against individuals are, however, easily found. At Dar es Salaam, Tanzania, a local newspaper reported on 8 January 2004 that AIDS patients, 'who are mainly women', are refused food, and not even greeted by their families. In public, their families instead shout insults, calling them adulterous and prostitutes.[29] In 2004/5, vigilantes called Karavinas (from 'carbine') killed 'numerous' suspected witches alleged to be responsible for AIDS in Kaoma on Zambia's western border.[30] The number of attacks, those killed, and whether the attacks were acts of collective violence have not been established. The 'most atrocious case', and most often cited, concerned one victim alone. In 1998, in a Durban township (South Africa, the province of KwaZulu-Natal), Gigu Dlamini was stoned, kicked, and beaten to death after announcing on local radio she had tested positively for HIV. She was judged as 'dishonouring the neighbourhood'.[31] Scholars have claimed that 'many similar cases have been recorded',[32] but few have cited any others. Furthermore, Iliffe concludes that such AIDS-related acts of violence were short-lived in Africa, as in the West; with a better understanding of the disease's transmission, these incidents were on the wane in many regions of Africa by 2003.[33] But even so, in Africa they have persisted. In December 2003, Lorna Mlofana, a twenty-one-year-old Treatment Action Campaign (TAC) activist, was gang-raped in a public toilet in

---

[22] Ibid., 88.　　　[23] Ibid.　　　[24] Ibid.

[25] Pepin, *The Origins of AIDS*, 82–3 and ch. 6; the same can be said for parts of Asia; for China, see Hyde, *Eating Spring Rice*, 31, 103, 129, 173; for Burma, Altman, *Power and Community*, 55: Burmese girls forced into prostitution in Thailand became infected and were killed when they returned home.

[26] Women have accounted for 58 per cent of those with HIV in sub-Saharan Africa. The highest proportion of new cases is now among women between 15 and 24; *UNAIDS, Gap Report*, 26 and 32.

[27] Ibid., 31.

[28] See Schoepf, 'Culture, Sex Research'. Moreover, women and especially prostitutes have increasingly become targets of blame in the West; see Hart, 'Men Who Buy Heterosexual Sex'.

[29] Iliffe, *The African AIDS Epidemic*, 88.　　　[30] Ibid.

[31] Ibid., 89. Also, Phillips, 'HIV/AIDS', 35–6; Deacon, Uys, and Mohlahlane, 'HIV and Stigma', 105; for the consequences of AIDS on women's activism, Mbali, *South African AIDS*, 6, 7, 77, 79.

[32] Deacon, Uys, and Mohlahlane, 'HIV and Stigma', 105. Mbali, *South African AIDS*, 236, cites a similar case and others of 'corrective rape' against lesbians that led to death, but these were not necessarily tied to AIDS.

[33] Iliffe, *The African AIDS Epidemic*, 89. The June 2011 issue of *American Journal of Public Health* (Gruskin, 'Tackling Violence'), was supposed to launch a special issue on HIV/AIDS and violence, but only two articles, both on Africa, addressed the question and neither cited examples of collective violence.

Cape Town, then beaten to death when she told her attackers she was HIV-positive. Her horrific death became a cause célèbre, with the TAC staging a mass protest in front of Khayelitsha Magistrates' Court where the murderers were on trial. Educational 'blitzes' followed with door-to-door canvassing in Town Two, where Mlofana was killed.[34] In 2007, another highly publicized murder of an AIDS activist occurred. Sizakele Sigasa, a lesbian, active in the Positive Women's Network, was killed 'in a homophobic hate crime'.[35] In addition, wars, especially in Sierra Leone, the Democratic Republic of the Congo, Burundi, Rwanda, and Uganda, led to systematic violence against women, including rape, mutilation, sexual slavery, forced pregnancy, forced marriages, abduction, and torture, which in turn increased the spread of HIV. During the genocide in Rwanda, 60 to 80 per cent of rape victims were estimated to be seropositive, compared to 13.5 per cent of the population at large.[36] Yet, it is difficult to ascribe this violence to HIV/AIDS. Either it was a conscious strategy of war and terror, or an enduring practice of warfare that those in command tolerated but did not order. Finally, in the last years of the twentieth century, especially in rural parts of South Africa, the belief spread that sex with a virgin was a cure for HIV, which contributed to the rocketing of rape cases by 80 per cent between 1998 and 1999, with rape carried out against girls as young as six months.[37] Instead of the victims of the disease being the ones abused, this was a rare instance in the history of disease, when the perpetrators of violence were the diseased victims themselves.[38] Another violent incident occurred when police fired rubber bullets on TAC demonstrators who occupied a hospital in Queenstown, injuring thirty-five—the 'first ever police shooting of AIDS protesters anywhere in the world'. Yet, as Alex de Waal has argued, 'people living with AIDS' did not riot in the streets, bands of orphans did not rip societies asunder, and AIDS did not threaten the political and social fabric of sub-Saharan Africa.[39]

As horrific as individual acts of violence and abuse in Africa have been, more pernicious and with graver consequences have been the effects of governments' denial of the disease and their production of conspiracy theories to explain it. Most infamously, South Africa's Thabo Mbeki argued that AIDS, if it existed, was solely a matter of poverty or the product of Western capitalist imperialism, concocted in Western laboratories, and introduced by white homosexuals. The impact of these theories reached its apex in June 1999, when Mbeki claimed AZT was a toxic drug promoted by Western pharmaceutical companies to kill Africans and profit at the same time. The African National Congress (ANC) government, led by the newly elected Mbeki, banned aid to provide anti-retroviral drugs even to infected pregnant women. After four years of concerted protests, demonstrations, civil

---

[34] Robins, *From Revolution to Rights*, 120.   [35] Mbali, *South African AIDS*, 236.
[36] John-Langba, 'HIV, Sexual Violence'; and El-Bushra, 'How Should We Understand Sexual Violence', 245, on Rwanda.
[37] Flanagan, 'South African Men'.
[38] Even with the infamous case of Typhoid Mary, her desire to preserve her economic stability at the expense of her employers was exceptional; see Leavitt, *Typhoid Mary*.
[39] De Waal, *AIDS and Power*.

disobedience, and legal actions taken by the TAC, supported by Nelson Mandela and the international community, the ANC finally changed its policies.[40]

Other myths and conspiracies raced across Africa. Despite the disease being overwhelmingly transmitted heterosexually, it was initially considered a disease of 'white European homosexuals'. In Kinshasa in the Democratic Republic of Congo people believed AIDS was transmitted by foreign canned food. In Burkina Faso, villagers claimed it originated when a white man paid a woman to have sex with a chimpanzee.[41] In South Africa, rumours circulated that it was 'an Apartheid device' spread by teargas 'to decimate the black population'.[42] In addition, townspeople and villagers accused immigrants and refugees from other African countries of bringing the pandemic. Villagers blamed townsmen; elders, the young; men, women; and vice versa; and 'everyone blamed sex workers'.[43] The first major AIDS research programme in Rakai, Uganda, had to be suspended because people suspected research teams 'of draining their blood'. On World AIDS Day 1988, the District Medical Office in Masaka, Uganda, had to announce publicly that doctors were not lethally injecting patients with AIDS.[44]

Along with these, other stories circulated. In 1991, the South African magazine *Drum* published an article, 'Is AIDS a conspiracy against Blacks?' Its answer was a resounding 'yes', claiming the apartheid government had deliberately introduced the disease in its final days to combat African liberation movements, and in the early 1990s AIDS had been 'a plot devised by the government... to convince black people to have less sex'.[45] Disastrously, this myth-making seriously delayed mobilizing government and medical attention to confront the crisis, not only in Mbeki's South Africa, but in countries such as the Congo, where President Mobutu Sésé Seko, military dictator from 1965 to 1997, silenced the press following the first declared case of AIDS.[46] Yet, unlike cholera, smallpox, or plague a century or less earlier, the conspiracies failed to arouse armed crowds to assemble, attack, and murder the afflicted, health workers, government officials, or foreigners.[47]

Africa was not alone in inventing HIV/AIDS conspiracy theories. Paul Farmer has argued that conspiracy theories 'constituted a sort of Haitian reply to North American discrimination'.[48] Similar to those produced in sub-Saharan Africa, the Haitian beliefs held that 'AIDS had been created in a US military laboratory'.[49] Yet, Farmer maintains that these conspiracies served as a 'counterattack' to the US's false accusations against Haiti as the nucleus of the new disease, which destroyed its tourist industry, turning an already impoverished economy into one of the

---

[40] Iliffe, *The African AIDS Epidemic*, 145; Mbali, *South African AIDS*, 8, 11, 108, 120–31, 148; and Robins, *From Revolution to Rights*, ch. 5. While the rate of HIV/AIDS has slowed in Africa generally in the twenty-first century, the same cannot be said of Zimbabwe; see Echenberg, *Africa in the Time of Cholera*, 164.

[41] Iliffe, *The African AIDS Epidemic*, 80.   [42] Ibid.   [43] Ibid.

[44] Ibid., 91.   [45] Phillips, 'HIV/AIDS', 34.

[46] Iliffe, *The African AIDS Epidemic*, 66–7.

[47] However, as Gruskin, 'Tackling Violence', comments: 'Studies linking violence and HIV are heavily skewed toward examining violence as a risk factor for acquiring HIV, with few analysing HIV as a risk factor for experiencing violence.'

[48] Farmer, *AIDS and Accusation*, 192.   [49] Ibid., 228.

poorest on earth.[50] By contrast, the Haitian AIDS myths, according to Farmer, were simply the 'rhetorical defences' of powerless victims.[51]

In the mid-1980s, other conspiracy theories appeared in the media that were not pinned on the poor. In September 1986, three East German scientists produced a paper supposedly linking US military laboratories working in virology in 1979 with AIDS erupting thereafter. Papers and popular magazines in Russia (including *Pravda*), Nigeria, Costa Rica, Zimbabwe, India, and other countries polished the story, linking the spread of AIDS to its supposed laboratory invention in the US.[52] The myth also found its propagators within the US, though with different twists. At the Third International AIDS Conference in Washington in June 1987, a group called 'United Front Against Racism and Capitalism-Imperialism' published a broadsheet, claiming that research based on more than 300 scientific and medical papers proved the US Government created AIDS as germ warfare against gays and blacks.[53] Higher-profile figures such as black activist Dick Gregory repeated the story, adding that Haitian refugees served as the guinea pigs.[54]

Despite the fears, inhumanity, and bitterness aroused by HIV/AIDS in the 1980s, assertions that these reactions were comparable to Europe's during the Black Death or to cholera's in the nineteenth century show little reckoning with the recent or distant past. Plague scholar Robert Swenson pronounced: 'In the fourteenth century we burned Jews at the stake; today we burn hemophiliacs' houses for fear that they will transmit HIV infection...This is precious little progress in five hundred years.'[55] So the annihilation of hundreds of communities down the Rhine in 1348–9 with men, women, and children burnt alive on islands or in their synagogues, ending medieval Jewish civilization in its heartland,[56] was the equivalent of burning one house in Arcadia, Florida, where no one was injured? William Rushing (professor and chair of the Department of Sociology and Anthropology at Vanderbilt, 1975–9) claimed the hate and violence stirred by the Black Death and cholera formed the same sociological patterns as AIDS in the US: 'such forces emerge and lead people to act as their ancestors did in previous epidemics', blaming others and inflicting violence against the outcast, the poor, and afflicted.[57] The sociologist Irwin Sherman saw the Black Death and AIDS as 'History repeating itself': 'a cry goes out: find the source of infection. We may hear: "Let's get rid of the poor, the homosexuals, the drug users, the unwed mothers, the prostitutes, and so on."'[58]

* * *

[50] Ibid., 229. For the collapse of the Haitian tourist industry, see Sabatier, *Blaming Others*, 45–6.

[51] Farmer, *AIDS and Accusation*, 247.

[52] On these, see Grmek, *Histoire di sida*, 251; Farmer, *AIDS and Accusation*, 233; Gibbs, 'Poison Libels', 546; and Sabatier, *Blaming Others*, 62–4.

[53] Ibid., 64. For similar stories, see Altman, *AIDS in the Mind of America*, 43.

[54] Rushing, *The AIDS Epidemic*, 157. Also, Altman, *AIDS in the Mind of America*, 43, on a Trotskyist group spreading the same story.

[55] Swenson, 'Plagues, History, and AIDS', 198.   [56] Cohn, 'The Black Death'.

[57] Rushing, *The AIDS Epidemic*, xi, xii, and 129–80.

[58] *The Power of Plagues*, 112–13. For similar pronouncements, see Ruffie, 'SIDA et civilisations', 86–7; Strong, 'Epidemic Psychology', 255; Doka, *AIDS, Fear, and Society*, 117–18; Silverman, 'The Plague of Our Time'; Cogan and Herek, 'Stigma' 466–7; and Alcamo, *AIDS in the Modern World*, 77.

In place of mass violence, however, journalists, scholars, and activists have pointed more often to alarmist headlines and homophobic slurs made by religious fundamentalists and right-wing pundits, such as Pat Robertson, Pat Buchanan, Jerry Falwell, and William F. Buckley, but also heard from prominent members of Congress and religious leaders such as Pope John Paul II and Cardinal John O'Connor, Archbishop of New York (1984–2000).[59] Inflammatory homophobic statements, such as Buchanan's cry of 'homosexuals have declared war upon nature', Norman Podhoretz's 'gays get what they deserve', and Buckley's 'all asymptomatic persons infected with HIV should be identified and inscribed with a tattoo on forehead, genitals, and anal areas', have been more often repeated and are better remembered than examples of physical violence, like the burning of the Rays' home or a man beaten in Texas.[60] Such high-profile verbal attacks could inflict a meaner economic bite. In the US, insurance companies attempted to gain permission from regulatory agencies to deny coverage to persons at risk of AIDS, and several states proposed bills to quarantine AIDS patients, identify children or employees with AIDS to school officials, and extend techniques of venereal disease control by tracing the sexual contacts of persons with HIV/AIDS.[61] Such proposals also went to Congress. Incensed by the educational work of the Gay Men's Health Crisis of New York City (GMHC), North Carolina's Senator Jesse Helms introduced an amendment in 1988 to cut federal funds to this volunteer organization, the first of its kind in the struggle against AIDS, and any others providing AIDS education, because allegedly they promoted 'homosexual activities'.[62]

This verbal violence against AIDS victims found echoes in other industrialized democracies. Parts of the British press attacked homosexuals and targeted groups thought to be AIDS carriers, and these slurs could come from prominent public figures such as Greater Manchester's chief constable, James Anderton.[63] Carlo Donat-Cattin, Health Minister in Bettino Craxi's government in 1986, refused to control blood supplies for transfusions to combat AIDS, arguing that such interference would give 'publicity for anal intercourse and condoms': 'L'AIDS ce l'ha chi se la va a cercare' ('AIDS is acquired by those who go looking for it')—some message from a state's Minister of Health![64] As in America, seropositive children were not admitted to nurseries and primary schools in some Italian towns. Others testing positive were refused employment; workers were dismissed; drug addicts

---

[59] For these and others, see Poirier, 'AIDS and Traditions of Homophobia'; and Rushing, *The AIDS Epidemic*, 171 and 177.

[60] Among many citations to fundamentalist and homophobic rhetoric, see Irwin, 'Scapegoats', 619; Shilts, *And the Band Played On*, 311–12, 335, and 32, 244, 45, 311, 347–8. Altman, 'Legitimation through Disaster', 314; Poirier, 'AIDS and Traditions of Homophobia', 139–67; Brandt, 'AIDS and Metaphor'; idem, 'AIDS'; and Fox, 'AIDS', 18; for the first citation, Brandt, 'AIDS and Metaphor', 107; the second, Brandt, 'AIDS', 156; and the third, Poirier, 'AIDS and Traditions of Homophobia', 142–3.

[61] Fox, 'AIDS', 20–2.

[62] Altman, *Power and Community*, 50, and on the GMHC: ibid., 2–3; idem, *AIDS in the Mind of America*, 84–9; Kobasa, 'AIDS Volunteering', 174–84. On the Helms amendment, Patton, *Globalizing AIDS*, 13.

[63] Dorothy and Roy Porter, 'The Enforcement of Health', 114.

[64] Altman, 'Legitimation through Disaster', 313; and D'Amico, 'AIDS', 13.

were refused treatment at dental clinics.[65] In Germany, the president of the Federal Court of Justice proposed tattooing or quarantining those testing HIV-positive.[66] The Anglican Dean of Sydney, Australia, held that gays were responsible for AIDS, charging them with having 'blood on their hands', and the Premier of Queensland accused them of deliberately contaminating others with 'bad blood'.[67] In other countries with poorer human rights records, such as Mexico and Guatemala, imprisonment, deportation, bashings, isolation, burning houses, and murder of AIDS workers and gay activists were reported.[68] But in the literature beyond Africa, I have not found specific descriptions of 'mobs' or collective actions by vigilante groups against AIDS victims or supposed carriers of the disease.

Instead, mass demonstrations connected with AIDS in the 1980s were organized by those protecting the civil rights of AIDS victims and other targeted groups. Most spectacular of these was the 20 April 1990 rally organized by Haitian Americans and their supporters, who marched over the Brooklyn Bridge to protest against the Food and Drug Administration (FDA) and a federal regulation on blood donations stigmatizing Haitians and Africans. The police expected several thousand; instead, 50,000 by police estimates, and 100,000 according to the organizers, joined the march, making it the city's largest demonstration since the anti-war rallies of the 1960s.[69] Yet neither at this 'mammoth' demonstration nor others, such as one held in Washington, or candlelight rallies earlier,[70] did counter-demonstrations and violence staged by religious fundamentalists, anti-gays, anti-Haitians, or other groups erupt against the demonstrators. In this respect, these occasions differed markedly from anti-war protests and demonstrations for racial equality, women's rights, or pro-choice from the 1960s to the present. Moreover, the pro-Haitian demonstration was successful: in December 1990, the FDA withdrew its prohibitions against Haitians donating blood.[71]

As suggested above, attacks on AIDS victims and targeted groups may have been more subtle, more matters of stigmatization, discrimination, and measures prejudicially affecting the welfare of the victims. The effects of such 'structural violence' could inflict greater consequences with longer-term injury to individuals and communities than acts of direct physical violence, as Farmer has shown convincingly.[72] Many authors have pointed to the myriad prejudices raised against individual AIDS victims.[73] Few, however, have delineated trends, or compared quantitatively

---

[65] Altman, *Power and Community*, 54. [66] Piot, *No Time to Lose*, 151.

[67] Altman, *AIDS in the Mind of America*, 25 and 185.

[68] Altman, *Power and Community*, 54–5. For Cuba and the ex-Soviet Union, see Piot, *No Time to Lose*, 151.

[69] Kraut, 'Plagues and Prejudice', 65; Farmer, *AIDS and Accusation*, 219.

[70] Farmer, *AIDS and Accusation*, 218. In May 1983, candlelight rallies of around 8000 occurred in New York and San Francisco; Altman, *AIDS in the Mind of America*, 104.

[71] Farmer, *AIDS and Accusation*, 219. US persecution of Haitians suspected of having HIV continued when those fleeing the military coup that deposed Jean-Bertrand Aristide's democratically elected government on 30 September 1991 were detained at Guantánamo; Farmer, *Pathologies of Power*, ch. 2.

[72] Farmer, *Pathologies of Power*, for his definition, see 8–9.

[73] Following Michel Foucault, Antonio Gramsci, and others, Parker and Aggleton, 'HIV and AIDS-Related Stigma', argue that 'physical violence or coercion increasingly gave way to what

AIDS stigmatization and discrimination with the negative public attitudes experienced by those suffering from other diseases or disabilities.[74] One early study to unearth specific cases of unfair discrimination against AIDS victims was Larry Gostin's, based on cases adjudicated by the courts and the Human Rights Commission after George H. W. Bush signed into law the American Disabilities Act on 26 July 1990, the most sweeping civil rights act since 1964. It protected those living with HIV as a disability against discrimination in housing, employment, health care, and education.[75] As Gostin states, 'no studies' had revealed the scope and kinds of HIV-related discrimination since HIV began.[76] In fact, before the law's promulgation, it is difficult to know how such a systematic study of discrimination might be conducted.

For over a year (his exact dates are not stated), Gostin found 149 cases of discrimination against those presumed to be infected with HIV/AIDS brought before the courts and the Human Rights Commission. From these, he described a wide variety of offences—refusals to hire or promote; demotions and dismissals from jobs; exclusion of children from schools and other unjust impositions placed on them, such as requiring them to use separate, AIDS-only bathrooms; restrictions on those handling food; discrimination in nursing homes and housing. Yet Gostin never reflects on the significance of the number: were 149 cases surprisingly many or few? How does it compare with discrimination cases concerning other disabilities? The number might, in fact, be read as a success story of AIDS activism, correlating with trends such as increases in federal funding for AIDS research, post-AIDS gains in gay rights, improvements in public understanding of HIV/AIDS, and recognition of discrimination against HIV/AIDS victims as actionable in federal courts.[77]

COMPASSION

As late as 1987, scholars and activists were convinced that AIDS threatened 'to undo a generation of progress toward gay rights'[78] with the worst excesses of homophobia yet to come.[79] The literature emphasized the successes of the 'New Right' during the 1980s which used the AIDS crisis to reverse a wide range of progressive

[Foucault] described as "subjectification", or social control exercised not through physical force, but through the production of conforming subjects and docile bodies'. However, with other forms of discrimination and stigmatization, such as 'stop and search' procedures against blacks, collective physical violence and protest continue to arise in the US, Britain, and other countries. For others who have emphasized stigmatization with AIDS, especially in Africa, see notes 28 and 29.

[74] For these statements, see Nelkin and Hilgartner, 'Disputed Dimensions of Risk', 118; Brandt, 'AIDS', 153–4; Farmer, *AIDS and Accusation*, 214 and 247; and Bayer, 'The Dependent Center', 138.
[75] Gostin, 'The AIDS Litigation Project'.   [76] Ibid., 144.
[77] In the UK, laws against discriminating against those with AIDS in the workplace came into force only in 1996 and provided much less protection than the US legislation. In Britain, the law did not protect those with asymptomatic HIV; Adam-Smith and Goss, 'Opportunity Lost', 37.
[78] See Brandt, *No Magic Bullet*, 194, cited by Altman, 'Legitimation through Disaster', 313; Black, *The Plague Years*, 208. Some saw AIDS posing major social violence to gays in the US as late as 1997; Doka, *AIDS, Fear, and Society*, 49, 115, 120–30; and Shah, *Pandemic*, 129–30.
[79] Goldstein, 'The Implicated and the Immune', 37–8.

political achievements over the past decade, especially regarding lesbian and gay rights.[80] In the early 1990s, however, publications such as the essays in Dorothy Nelkin et al., *A Disease of Society*, Dennis Altman's *Power and Community*, and Jeffrey Weeks' work on Britain marked a turning point in perceptions. As with previous works, they pointed to governments' initial denial of the disease with disastrous consequences for medical research and care for the AIDS-afflicted and to the stigmatization of groups already stigmatized. Yet, with AIDS shifting in the US from a disease previously labelled 'GRID' (Gay-Related Immune Deficiency) and 'gay cancer' to one increasingly of IV drug users, blacks, and the poor, and transmitted heterosexually, these assessments of the long-term effects on gay and lesbian communities became points of departure.[81] Now studies stressed the mass volunteerism coming from within and outside the gay community to assist AIDS victims.[82] To be sure, volunteerism and its organizations began with the earliest publicized cases in 1981.[83] As Cindy Patton remarked in 2002, 'even before AIDS had a name...everywhere that someone was sick, individuals and networks banded together for mutual aid.'[84] By the mid-1980s in New York City, a formal task force comprised of volunteers and AIDS activists, representing twenty community-based organizations and twelve hospital-based volunteer programmes, met regularly at the Mayor's office, and each of the city's boroughs had 'its own volunteer and self-help HIV/AIDS organization'.[85] In San Francisco, grassroots, community-based organizations of volunteers (CBOs) expanded just as rapidly, achieving even closer relations with city government. The crisis here became 'a catalyst for organizational change and innovations in the delivery of AIDS care', with volunteers and nurses assuming new managerial roles, designing new systems of patient services and home care.[86]

Yet the first book to examine in any detail these waves of altruism in the US or elsewhere[87] was not published until 1994. Instead of stigmatism and violence, its history of AIDS focused on communities of volunteers, their services in

---

[80] See Patton, *Sex and Germs*, 80 and 145, and ch. 7; and Altman, *AIDS in the Mind of America*, 99–100, 109, who examined the AIDS crisis against the backdrop of right-wing governments in Britain, Europe, and Australia. Britain showed a mixed picture of public attitudes towards AIDS and homosexuality. On the one hand, public opinion in 1987 became less discriminatory on whether gays and lesbians should be barred from certain professions (compared with 1983); on the other, the public was less accepting of homosexual relationships; Weeks, 'AIDS', 28–9.

[81] Patton, *Sex and Germs*, 17; and idem, *Inventing AIDS*, 22–3; Black, *The Plague Years*, citations from an interview with Larry Kramer, 143; and on the divisions within the gay community on whether to close bath houses in San Francisco and New York in 1984–5, 161–3 and 171. On the significance of changes in naming this disease in common parlance and medical discourse, see Treichler, *How to Have Theory*, 26–34.

[82] Fineberg, 'The Social Dimension of AIDS', recognized community grassroots organizations as 'one of the most remarkable and heartening by-products of HIV' (110), but the future social and political course of the disease for him in 1988 stood on a knife's edge, as his rhetorical questions at the end of the essay illustrate (112). Even as late as 1997, Doka, *AIDS, Fear, and Society*, continued seeing the social significance of AIDS for the human and civil rights as more gloomy than hopeful (130) and as 'the great Divider' (134).

[83] Kobasa, 'AIDS Volunteering', 172.   [84] Patton, *Globalizing AIDS*, xvii.

[85] Ibid., 173.   [86] Fox et al., 'The Culture of Caring', 142–3.

[87] Aggleton, 'Series Editor's Preface', vii.

education, counselling, nursing, establishing emergency hotlines, opening and staffing new hospitals and hostels, providing meals and therapies, bridging communication between gay and 'straight' communities, and above all, manifesting an outpouring of disinterested compassion. Groups of experts in nursing, finance, and law clustered around new community centres with systems of 'buddies' providing emotional support for AIDS sufferers.[88] The GMHC, founded in September 1981, was the earliest of these organizations, but shortly afterwards Shanti in San Francisco,[89] the AIDS Action Committee in Boston, Toronto AIDS Action Committee, AIDS Project/LA, AIDS Atlanta, the Terrence Higgins Trust, which later opened the London Lighthouse in Ladbroke Grove, and others in smaller cities followed.[90]

While Altman concentrated on the countries he knew from first-hand experience— Australia and the US—he surveyed a similar growth in volunteerism for AIDS victims in Canada, Western Europe, the Caribbean, Uganda, South Africa, Tanzania, Eastern Europe, Latin America, Russia, and parts of Asia. Certainly, the trends were not all of one piece. Even in the West, some countries such as Germany, France, and especially those in Southern Europe lagged behind the US, Canada, Australia, and other countries in Northern Europe.[91] Most surprising was France. Although it was at the forefront of AIDS research[92] and possessed the highest number of cases in Europe, absolutely and per capita,[93] France had produced few AIDS volunteers and organizations compared with the Anglophone world. As late as the end of 1984, Paris did not have a single CBO assisting HIV/AIDS victims.[94] By the early 1990s, the largest AIDS organization in France, AIDES, comprised only 1500 volunteers across thirty-one cities.[95] In countries such as India, Argentina, and Russia, where volunteers faced greater obstacles and the afflicted, greater persecution, unsurprisingly, fewer of these organizations formed.[96] But across the globe volunteers from communities beyond those immediately affected supported such organizations. During the 1980s and 1990s, heterosexuals, especially middle-aged married women in North America and Australia, joined these groups, despite

[88] Altman, *Power and Community*, 39–40; for the US, Fox et al., 'The Culture of Caring', 136; Kobasa, 'AIDS Volunteering'; on 'buddies', Casper, 'AIDS', 206–7.

[89] Founded in 1974, as early as November 1981, it began an AIDS support group with only thirty recognized cases in San Francisco; Black, *The Plague Years*, 157–8. It became exclusively dedicated to work around AIDS in 1984; Altman, *AIDS in the Mind of America*, 85.

[90] Altman, *Power and Community*, 2–3, and 39–40; idem, 'Legitimation through Disaster', 303; idem, *AIDS in the Mind of America*, 89–91; Fineberg, 'The Social Dimension of AIDS', 110; and Berridge, 'AIDS: History', 53. By contrast, Patton, *Inventing AIDS*, ch. 1, saw these organizations aiding Reagan's cost-cutting measures and dividing lesbian and gay communities, with volunteers and paid experts, on one side and 'deserving' and 'undeserving recipients' on the other, 'sucking from the movement its radical politics' (22). On the increase in altruism and importance of the Terrence Higgins Trust, see Weeks, 'AIDS', 27.

[91] Altman, *Community and Power*, 22–3.

[92] Many have described the race to discover the virus between the French and Americans, led by Luc Montagnier at the Institut Pasteur and Robert Gallo at the National Cancer Institute; see, for example, Gallo and Montagnier, 'AIDS in 1988'; and idem, 'The Chronology of AIDS Research'.

[93] Sabatier, *Blaming Others*, 12.   [94] Altman, *AIDS in the Mind of America*, 91.

[95] Altman, *Power and Community*, 23.   [96] Ibid., 3–4.

many coming from traditional backgrounds, opposed to drug use or the sexual practices of the afflicted.[97]

In Africa, the issues and constituencies of the CBOs differed from those in the US and Europe. The most stigmatized, persecuted, and economically affected were women, followed by homeless orphans. Correspondingly, CBOs such as Ugandan Women's Efforts to Save Orphans, the AIDS Widow, Orphan and Family Support,[98] and organizations that combated violence against women with AIDS, such as Tanzania's Gender Networking Programme and Harare's Musasa Project, were the initiatives to arise in Africa.[99] But the most widespread and successful of these grassroots volunteer organizations were in South Africa, partially as protest groups against Mbeki's politics of denial, but also campaigning against the same 'Big Pharma' attacked by the ANC. The discoveries of cocktails of various anti-retroviral treatments in 1994–5, soon to transform HIV from a fatal disease to a chronic condition, were for Africa not a reality given its poverty. In 1998, the TAC, a broad-based activist group rooted in the anti-apartheid movement, was staffed by men and women across social classes and with international connections. The majority of its volunteers, however, were poor, unemployed African women, many of whom were 'HIV-positive mothers desperate to gain access to life-saving drugs for themselves and their children'.[100] Through international contacts, mass demonstrations, neighbourhood support groups, cafés, and the courts they overturned Mbeki's policies and ended multinational prohibitions against generic drugs from India entering Africa. The TAC's success fundamentally altered the trajectory of HIV/AIDS in the world's worst-hit continent.[101]

Similarly, in North America, Europe, and Australasia, these community-based organizations followed changes in the disease's epidemiology. With infection rates dropping sharply among homosexuals in the late 1980s but rising among drug users and heterosexuals, AIDS stimulated the rise of new CBOs, especially groups defending sex workers.[102] In 1987 'only a handful of Western countries' had organizations for sex workers; by the early 1990s, they increased rapidly in the West and appeared for the first time in African countries.[103] Less successful were AIDS

---

[97] Ibid., 40. The only work I know to anticipate these trends was Altman, *AIDS in the Mind of America*. His tone then was, however, tentative, claiming that volunteers came almost exclusively from the targeted groups (179). Further, he explained the rise of CBOs negatively, as 'a necessity', because of the government's failure to provide basic services (181) and argued that through the 1980s AIDS sharpened divisions between gay men and lesbians (94).

[98] Altman, *Power and Community*, 41.

[99] Baylies, 'Community-Based Research', 236–7. For women's groups in Tanzania and Zambia, Bujra and Baylies, 'Solidarity and Stress', 45–8. Also, Mbali, *South African AIDS*, for women activists in the TAC, ch. 3; and South Africa's Positive Women's Network, run by and for women living with HIV (97). For grassroots organizations supporting HIV/AIDS victims in the Ivory Coast and Burkina Faso, which were cross-gender or comprised principally of gay and bisexual men, such as Jeunes sans frontières, see Nguyen, *The Republic of Therapy*.

[100] Robins, *From Revolution to Rights*, 118.

[101] Ibid., ch. 5; Mbali, *South African AIDS*; Harden, *AIDS at 30: A History*, 222–7; Piot, *No Time to Lose*, 280–5, 311–12; and de Waal, *AIDS and Power*, ch. 3, arguing that the TAC never constituted a revolutionary movement.

[102] Altman et al., 'Men Who Have Sex with Men'.

[103] Altman, *Power and Community*, 157–8. On the political significance of these organizations; see Parker and Aggleton, 'HIV and AIDS-Related Stigma', 21–2.

awareness, education, and organization among drug users, constituting the most pressing challenge for AIDS control in the twenty-first century, especially in Eastern Europe and Russia, where the virus continues to be on the rise.[104]

These changes in perception were not limited in seeing the impact on AIDS-related organizations alone. During the 1990s, studies began to recognize how AIDS had altered notions of the family, kinship, and commitment more broadly. HIV/AIDS had forced the infected and their biological families to broaden notions of 'the family' for emotional and economic support, linking together traditional family members and friends with health workers and volunteer supporters, who increasingly assumed family functions. In May 1989, San Francisco passed the first law allowing unmarried homosexual and heterosexual couples 'to register publicly as "domestic partners", paving the way for them to obtain health benefits, hospital visitation rights, and bereavement leave'.[105]

The threats and tragedies of AIDS also caused gays and heterosexuals to reassess notions of friendship, expanding networks of 'love, support, and care for many people'. While the disease heightened what might be considered traditional values—'recognition of couple relationships',[106] marriage, and parenting—it forced governments to enact reforms granting legal recognition and rights to relationships previously not included within traditional notions of marriage or parenting. In large part because of the AIDS crisis, kinship is no longer restricted to blood and has become more a matter of choice. These changes have gone beyond family law to influence policies of hospitals and hospices on residence and visitation.[107]

POLITICS

Dennis Altman has called HIV/AIDS 'the most political of diseases'; and the American physician and founding director of the World Health Organization's (WHO) former global programme on AIDS, Jonathan Mann, declared, 'No other disease has so revolutionized attitudes to the meaning and provision of health care.'[108] Such claims come without comparative research in the history of diseases. For instance, an immediate after-effect of the Great Influenza of 1918–20 was to encourage the formation of national health programmes in Canada, New Zealand, South Africa, and Britain, and the revolution in the control of sewage and public water systems in cities which followed cholera outbreaks at various times and

---

[104] Small, 'Suffering in Silence?', 12–13. Controlling the spread of HIV/AIDS among prisoners has been another area where progress continues to be stymied; Stöver and Lines, 'Silence Still = Death'; and Clark, 'Gaps Remain in Russia's Response'.

[105] Levine, 'AIDS and Changing Concepts of Family', 50–1.

[106] Cited in Heaphy et al., 'Narratives of Care', 79. For a negative assessment of these trends, see Patton, *Sex and Germs*, ch. 8 and 133.

[107] Heaphy et al., 'Narratives of Care', 67–82.

[108] Altman, *Power and Community*, 136 and 17.

places, might call Mann's claim into question. For Altman, plague in India in the late nineteenth and early twentieth centuries could be a contender. As seen in Chapter 16, it forged alliances between diverse social groups, castes, and classes, that unified Muslims and Hindus in opposition to Britain's heavy-handed and culturally insensitive controls, and elites and intellectuals found common cause with impoverished sufferers and their families.

Nonetheless, perceptions began to change in the 1990s, running counter to the disquiet of the 1980s. HIV/AIDS invigorated gay communities politically with homosexuality gaining greater legitimacy in many parts of the world.[109] In the following decade (2000–10), the AIDS crisis sparked similar political gains for sex workers' and women's groups in Africa, despite AIDS simultaneously leading to increased violence towards women. Since the early 1980s, a mutually supportive relationship had arisen between the growth of community organizations assisting AIDS sufferers and often the same organizations as advocacy groups gaining political power and building worldwide networks.[110] As a result of these unforeseen developments, activists and scholars in the 1990s began to stress the positive aspects of the AIDS crisis.[111]

The beginnings of this change resulted in a shift in relations between the gay movement and national governments (even Conservative ones, such as Reagan's and Thatcher's administrations[112]) from an adversarial orientation to cooperation. Organizations such as GMHC, Shanti, and the Terrence Higgins Trust secured funding and implemented services and policies previously under government departments or that had not existed. It was a two-way street: gay activists began to participate in government, and governments were forced to recognize and fund gay organizations which they had earlier shunned.[113] By the mid-1980s, as in California, 'owing to AIDS', the tables turned from abuse, violence, and stigmatization to the increased visibility of gay communities, whose demands for civil rights were felt to deserve support. In 1986, New York City passed an anti-discrimination ordinance, protecting homosexuals, and in the same year, New Zealand finally decriminalized homosexuality.[114] The virus created the conditions for Australia's 'exceptional' success in empowering societal groups earlier marginalized.[115] By the end of the 1980s, AIDS had 'mobilized more gay men into political and community organizations . . . than any other event in the short history of the gay movement'.[116]

---

[109] Altman, *Power and Community*, 33; For Spain, Fouz-Hernández, 'Queer in Spain'.

[110] At the same time, the global effects of AIDS have produced 'increases in inequality within countries and between them'; Altman, *Power and Community*, 168.

[111] Ibid., 6. According to Goldstein, 'The Implicated and the Immune': 'Not even tuberculosis, that most "aesthetic" of epidemics, produced a comparable outpouring in so short a time' (17).

[112] For Britain, Weeks, 'AIDS', esp. 31: By the end of the 1980s, 'prosecutions for consensual homosexual offences had reached a new high (comparable with the previous high total in 1954, before the establishment of the Wolfenden Committee)', and new government initiatives in 1990/1, 'threaten[ed] to increase penalties for homosexual offences through the Criminal Justice Bill'.

[113] Altman, 'Legitimation through Disaster', 302–3.   [114] Ibid., 307.

[115] Edwards, 'AIDS Policy Communities', esp. 55.

[116] Altman, 'Legitimation through Disaster', 309.

Another aspect of AIDS-inspired creativity and compassion was reshaping the patient–physician relationship, first in AIDS clinics, later for medical practice in general. Given the long antipathy between the medical profession and homosexuals[117]—the former's conceptualization of the latter as a pathological condition with some nurses, doctors, and ambulance and emergency-room attendants turning to union representatives to escape treating those with AIDS[118]—such a development was not predictable. However, mutual respect developed with AIDS patients becoming involved in decision making, designing clinical trials and determining medical priorities to a greater extent than ever achieved with any other disease.[119]

The mystery of the disease with physicians unable to provide effective cures gave power to AIDS patients, who in the early stages in the West and Australasia tended to be educated middle-class males. Given the medical uncertainties, these patients felt obliged to remain abreast of the latest research developments and thus gained the confidence to challenge physicians' authority. The mystery of the disease and its threat to well-established hierarchies, instead of poisoning patient–physician relationships, achieved the opposite.[120] Because of physicians' inability to cure the disease, AIDS altered other medical hierarchies. Especially before AZT became widely available in the late 1980s (at least in the West), HIV/AIDS was 'essentially a nursing disease' with treatment centred on 'caring rather than curing'. As with the Great Influenza, nurses in the last decades of the twentieth century gained greater respect from patients, the media, and physicians.[121] Since HIV/AIDS was a disease of long duration, this effect was not as short-lived as it had been in 1918–20. The disease's long incubation period of eight years or more also meant that able-bodied HIV victims became active in charitable and political endeavours, and with the disease's transformation to a manageable condition, the time patients spent 'fit, keen, and able to organize' increased.[122] As seen above, the patients were not the only actors transforming HIV/AIDS from a disease initially perceived to have threatened to tear societies asunder to one of compassion and creativity, redefining traditional notions of the family, patient–physician relations, roles of nurses, women, sex workers, and marginalized groups.

[117] Patton, *Sex and Germs*, 8–9; and Casper, 'AIDS', 202–4. In Italy, the relationship from the 1960s to the 1980s had become violent; Wanrooij, ' "The Thorns of Love" ', 153.

[118] Patton, *Sex and Germs*, 71–8.

[119] Feldman, *Plague Doctors*, 144. On AIDS patients becoming 'collaborators and colleagues rather than constituents and subjects', also Engelmann, 'Photographing AIDS'.

[120] Feldman, *Plague Doctors*, 237. For confirmation of these trends into the twenty-first century, see Guarinieri and Hollander, 'From Denver to Dublin', 88. Moreover, as Brandt, 'How AIDS Invented Global Health', has argued, AIDS activism went beyond the patient–physician relationship; it changed the relationship of patients and the public to medical science and research more generally, creating a 'revolution' in public health, eroding the sharp distinction between curing and prevention, and inventing a new 'global health'. Also, Mbali, *South African AIDS*.

[121] See Chapter 21 and Fox et al., 'The Culture of Caring', 132, 141–2.

[122] On these factors enhancing possibilities for organization, see Iliffe, *The African AIDS Epidemic*, 144; Feldman, *Plague Doctors*, 90; Fee and Fox, 'Introduction', 4; Berridge, 'AIDS: History', 43; Phillips, 'HIV/AIDS', 41 (citation).

As this book began, the AIDS pandemic of the 1980s was a stimulus for scholars across a wide spectrum of disciplines to reflect on the history of epidemics and prise lessons from the past to confront the globe's new pandemic. Scholars' responses, however, have reduced the rich and changing variety of epidemics and their mentalities overwhelmingly to a single set of negative consequences. By these accounts, epidemics across time and space, especially when 'mysterious', without preventive measures or cures, have spawned moral panic, abandonment of the sick, stigmatization of the afflicted, blaming of 'the other', and deadly collective violence.[123] With this picture of disease-fuelled hate, little attention was paid to how different social classes might align as the targets or perpetrators of violence. More astoundingly, these views have reflected little, if at all, on the power of past plagues to ignite compassion, bringing volunteers to make sacrifices for complete strangers across class, ethnic, and racial divides. Nor do these accounts recognize epidemics' political effects that mobilized citizens to combat governmental neglect in medical and social services, dilapidated hygienic infrastructures, and unjust, abusive, and ineffectual controls that stigmatized and persecuted sectors of the population. Yet from the 1990s, writing on AIDS began to shift from a view darkly centred on blame to one forged by compassion and political activism. This transition has yet to inspire historians to revisit the long history of epidemics. This second, more nuanced, more positive (though hardly rosy[124]) view forms a new template through which to rewind the movie reel—'de rérouler à reculons',[125] as the medievalist Marc Bloch once put it—to analyse the past from perspectives of the present.

---

[123] Even skilled historians of epidemics such as Phillips ('HIV/AIDS') continue to project this fixed, ahistorical, and negative trope across time. However, Phillips sees some difference between HIV/AIDS and previous epidemics. Because of the long period of latency and managed care, those with HIV/AIDS have had time to organize, becoming politically active (41) and thus gaining new rights (43). Others using the past have made wild allegations such as the supposed massacres of witches during the Black Death; Sabatier, *Blaming Others*, 3.

[124] See, for instance, Mayer et al., 'AIDS 2016'.   [125] Bloch, *Les caractères originaux*, xiv.

Bibliography

ARCHIVES

Archivio di Stato di Firenze, Inventario delle pergame.
Archivio di Stato di Mantova, Archvio Gonzaga, busta 1693.

Biblioteca Ambrosiana Milano, ms G 127 Sussidio, *Elenco cronologico delle persone state giustitiate nella Città e Stato di Milano dall'anno 1471 al 1783.*

Biblioteca Apostolica Vaticana:
  Avvisi, Urbanato. Latino, 1100.
  Avvisi, fondo Vaticani Latini, no. 12948.

British Library: Indian Office Records and Private Papers:
  Report of Native Papers Published by the Bombay Presidency, IOR: L/R/5/150–158 (1895–1903) and 174 (1918).
  Selections from the Native Newspapers published in the Punjab, IOR: L/R/5/188 (1905–6).
  Native-Owned English Newspapers in Bengal, IOR: L/R/5/25–28 (1899–1902).
  Native Papers Examined by the Translators to the Government of Madras, L/R/5/109–110 (1899–1902).
  Selections from the Vernacular Newspapers published in the North-Western Provinces and Oudh, L/R/5/77–80 (1900–4).
  Native Papers Examined by the Translators to the Government of Madras, L/R/5/109–110 (1899–1902).

ONLINE ARCHIVES, BIBLIOGRAPHIES, LIBRARIES, JOURNALS, NEWSPAPERS

Acta Sanctorum, the Full Database (Proquest).
Brepols Library of Latin Texts (A).
'British Newspaper Archive' [BNA], from the British Library's holdings previously held at Colindale.
California Digital Newspaper Collection, 1846 to the present.
'Chronicling America: Historic American Newspapers' from the Library of Congress, 1789–1922.
Digital Kingston Historical Newspapers.
Edit 16: Il *Censimento nazionale delle edizioni italiane del XVI secolo.*
Emeroteca, online collection, Braidense Library, Milan.
Gallica, Bibliothèque nationale de France: les principaux quotidiens numérisés.
The Guardian, 1821–2003, and *The Observer*, 1792–2003, ProQuest Historical Newspapers.
Medical Heritage Library of Nineteenth-Century Sources, funded by JISC and the Wellcome Library.
Hong Kong's English-language papers—*The Hong Kong Telegraph, The China Mail, The Hong Kong Weekly Press.*
Loeb Classical Library, Harvard University Press.
The *New York Times* Archive, 1851–.
Newspaper SG: National Library Board of Singapore.

'The Nineteenth Century British Newspapers'.
OurOntario.ca Community Newspapers Collection.
Perseus 4.0, Tufts University.
ProQuest Historical Newspapers:
  Atlanta Constitution, 1868–1984.
  The Baltimore Sun, 1837–1991.
  The Boston Globe, 1872–1984.
  Chicago Tribune, 1847–1963.
  Chinese Newspaper Collections, 1832–1953.
  Detroit Free Press, 1831–1922.
  The Globe and Mail (Toronto), 1844–2012.
  Irish Times, 1859–2015, and *The Weekly Irish Times* (Dublin), 1876–1958.
  Los Angeles Times, 1881–1922.
  San Francisco Chronicle, 1865–1922.
  The Scotsman, 1817–1950.
  The Times of India, 1838–2007.
  The Toronto Star, 1894–2013.
  The Washington Post, 1877–1999.
Readex World Newspaper Archive:
  African American Newspapers, 1827–1998.
  America's Early Historical Newspapers, 1690–1922.
  Caribbean Newspapers, 1718–1876.
  Ethnic American Newspapers from the Balch Collection, 1799–1971.
  Latin American Newspapers, 1805–1922.
  South Asian Newspapers: India, Pakistan, and Sri Lanka, 1864–1922.
Le Temps archives historiques—Quotidiens numérisés (Switzerland).
The Times Digital Archive, 1785–2007.
Trove Digital Newspapers, from the National Library of Australia, 1803–2011.
Universal Short Title Catalogue (USTC, St Andrews).
Welsh Newspapers Online, National Library of Wales, 1804–1910.

PRIMARY SOURCES: NEWSPAPERS

Australia
The Advertiser (Adelaide, SA)
The Advocate (Burnie, Tas.)
The Age (Melbourne, Vic.)
Albury Banner and Wodonga Express (NSW)
The Argus and *The Argus Supplement* (Melbourne, Vic.)
Bairnsdale Advertiser and Tambo and Omeo Chronicle (Vic.)
Barrier Miner (Broken Hill, NSW)
Bendigo Advertiser (Vic.)
The Border Morning Mail (Albury, NSW)
Border Watch (Mount Gambier, SA)
The Brisbane Courier (Qld)
Bunbury Herald (WA)
Bunyip (Gawler, SA)
The Burrowa News (NSW)
Cairns Post (Qld)

Camperdown Chronicle (Vic.)
The Catholic Press (Sydney, NSW)
The Cessnock Eagle (NSW)
Clarence and Richmond Examiner (Grafton, NSW)
Cootamundra Herald (NSW)
Daily Herald (Adelaide, SA)
The Daily News (Perth, WA)
Daily Telegraph (Launceston, Tas.)
Daily Observer (Tamworth, NSW)
Empire (Sydney, NSW)
The Evening Statesman (Walla Walla, WA)
Examiner (Launceston, Tas.)
Freeman's Journal (Sydney, NSW)
Forbes Advocate (NSW)
Forbes Times (NSW)
Geraldton Guardian (WA)
Goulburn Evening Penny Post (NSW)
The Goulburn Herald and Chronicle (NSW)
Jewish Herald (Vic.)
Kalgoorlie Miner (WA)
Kapunda Herald (SA)
The Kiama Independent, and Shoalhaven Advertiser (NSW)
The Land (Sydney, NSW)
Launceston Examiner (Tas.)
Leader (Orange, NSW)
The Maitland Daily Mercury (NSW)
The Maitland Mercury & Hunter River General Advertiser (NSW)
Maryborough Chronicle (Qld)
The Mercury (Hobart, Tas.)
Molong Angus (NSW)
Morning Bulletin (Rockhampton, Qld)
Myrtleford Mail and Whorouly Witness (Vic.)
Newcastle Morning Herald and Miners Advocate (NSW)
The North Eastern Ensign (Benalla, Vic.)
Northern Star (Lismore, NSW)
Northern Territory Times and Gazette (Darwin, NT)
Port Pirie Recorder (SA)
Queensland Times (Ipswich, Qld)
The Queenslander (Brisbane, Qld)
The Register (Adelaide, SA)
The Richmond River Herald (NSW)
The Riverine Grazier (Hay, NSW)
Singleton Argus (NSW)
South Australian Register (Adelaide, SA)
South Australian Weekly Chronicle (Adelaide, SA)
Sunday Times (Sydney, NSW)
The Sydney Morning Herald (NSW)
Times and Liverpool Plains Gazette (NSW)
Townsville Daily Bulletin (Qld)

Wagga Wagga Advertiser (NSW)
Watchman (Sydney, NSW)
The West Australian (Perth, WA)
West Gippsland Gazette (Warragul, Vic.)
The Western Australian Times (Perth, WA)
The Western Champion and General Advertiser for the Central-Western Districts (Barcaldine, Qld)
Western Star and Roma Advertiser (Toowoomba, Qld)
The World's News (Sydney, NSW)
The Wyalong Advocate (NSW)
Zeehan and Dundas Herald (Tas.)

British Isles
Aberdeen Journal
The Aberdeen Weekly
The Belfast News-Letter
Birmingham Daily Post
Blackburn Standard (Lancashire)
Bucks Herald (Aylesbury, Buckinghamshire)
The Burley News
Burney Collection of 17th and 18th Century Newspapers
Bury and Norwich Post
The Caledonian Mercury (Edinburgh)
Chelmsford Chronicle
Cheltenham Chronicle
Corbett's Weekly Political Register (London)
Coventry Evening Telegraph
Daily Gazette for Middlesbrough
Derby Daily Telegraph
Dublin Morning Register
Dundee Courier
Edinburgh Evening News
The Edinburgh Evening Post
Elgin Courier (Elgin, Scotland)
The Era (London)
The Essex Standard (Colchester, Essex)
Evening Telegraph (Dundee, Scotland)
The Examiner (London)
Exeter and Plymouth Gazette and Daily Telegraph
Fife Herald (Cupar, Scotland)
Freeman's Journal and Daily Commercial Advertiser (Dublin)
Glasgow Herald
Gloucester Citizen
Gloucester Echo
The Guardian (Manchester)
The Hampshire Advertiser
Hertford Mercury and Reformer
The Hull Packet and Humber Mercury (Hull)
Inverness Courier

The Irish Times (Dublin)
Irish World
Jackson's Oxford Journal
The Lancaster Gazette and General Advertiser (Lancaster)
Leeds Intelligencer
The Leeds Mercury
Leicester Chronicle and the Leicestershire Mercury
The Liverpool Mercury
Lloyd's Weekly (London)
London Daily News
London Standard
Manchester Courier and Lancaster General Advertiser
The Manchester Times and Gazette
The Morning Chronicle (London)
The Morning Post (London)
Newcastle Courant (Newcastle upon Tyne)
Northern Echo (Darlington)
Nottingham Evening Post
The Observer (London)
Pall Mall Gazette (London)
The Preston Guardian
Preston Chronicle
Reynold's Newsletter (London)
Royal Cornwall Gazette
Saunders's News-Letter (Dublin)
Sheffield Daily Telegraph
Sheffield Independent
The Sheffield & Rotherham Independent
Shields Daily Gazette
The Standard (London)
Tamworth Herald (Staffordshire)
The Times (London)
Westmorland Gazette
Western Times (Devon)
Worcester Journal
Yorkshire Evening Post
Yorkshire Post and Leeds Intelligencer

Canada
The Acton Free Press (Acton, Ont.)
The Gazette (Montreal)
The Georgetown Herald (Ont.)
Globe and Mail (Toronto)
Kingston Chronicle (Kingston, Ont.)
The Kingsville Reporter (Kingsville, Ont.)
The Leamington Post (Leamington, Ont.)
The Newmarket Era (Newmarket, Ont.)
Toronto Star
The Windsor Evening Record (Windsor, Ont.)

China

The China Mail
The Chinese Recorder and Missionary Journal (Shanghai)
The Hong Kong Telegraph
The Hong Kong Weekly Press
Millard's Review of the Far East
The North-China Herald
The Shanghai Times

Europe

Le Figaro (Paris)
La Lanterne (Paris)
Le Matin (Paris)
Le Petit Parisien (Paris)
La Presse (Paris)
Gazzetta Piemontese (Turin)
Gazette de Lausanne (Switzerland)
Journal de Genève (Switzerland)
La Stampa (Turin)
Le Temps (Paris)

Italy from Microfilm

L'Avanti! (Milan)
Il Cittadino di Monza
Il Cittadino: Rivista di Monza e del Circondario
Il Cittadino; Settimanale di Lodi e circondario
Corriere della Sera (Milan)
Corriere di Roma
Corriere italiano (Rome)
Il Giornale di Roma
Giornale di Sicilia: Politico Quotidiano (Palermo)
Idea Nazionale (Rome)
La Lombardia: Giornale Politcio Quotidiano (Milan)
La Madre Italiana: Rivista Mensile (Florence and Milan)
Il Messaggero (Rome)
La Nazione (Florence)
La Perseveranza (Milan)
La Perseveranza (Naples)
Il Pungolo (Naples)
Il Pungolo: Corriere di Milano (Milan)
La Riforma (Florence)
Il Secolo (Milan)

Indian Subcontinent

Amrita Bazar Patrika (Kolkata)
Indian People (Allahabad)
The Leader (Allahabad)
Pioneer (Allahabad)
The Times of India (Mumbai)

Tribune (Lahore)
(In addition to these newspapers, searchable in their entirety, several hundred Indian newspapers are cited in the notes taken from the selections, extractions, and translations made
by colonial governments across the subcontinent.)

Latin America and the Caribbean
El Comerciò (Lima, Peru)
El Dictamen (Veracruz Llave, Mexico)
El Imparcial (Mexico City)
Estrella de Panama (Panama City, Panama)
Excelsior (Mexico City)
Mexican Herald
Panama Star & Herald (Panama City, Panama)
Royal Gazette (Bermuda)
La Voz de Mexico (Mexico City)

Singapore
Malaya Tribune
Mid-Day Herald and Daily
Singapore Chronicle and Commercial Register
The Singapore Free Press and Mercantile Advertiser
The Straits Times
Weekly Sun

United States and its Territories
Aberdeen Herald (Washington Territory)
Aberdeen Daily News (Aberdeen, SD)
The Abilene Reflector (Abilene, KA)
Adams County News Ritzville (Washington Territory)
Akron Daily Democrat (Akron, OH)
Albuquerque Evening Citizen
The Alexandria Gazette (Alexandria, VA)
Alliance Herald (Alliance, NE)
Anaconda Standard (Anaconda, MT)
The Anderson Intelligencer (Anderson, SC)
The Appeal (St Paul, MN)
Arizona Republican (Phoenix, AZ)
Daily Ardmoreite (Ardmore, OK)
Arizona Weekly (Prescott, AZ)
The Atlanta Constitution
The Augusta Chronicle (Augusta, GE)
The Austin Weekly Statesman (Austin, TX)
The Baltimore Gazette and Daily Advertizer (Baltimore, MD)
The Baltimore Sun
Barton County Democrat (Great Bend, KA)
Belmont Chronicle (St Clairsville, Ohio)
The Big Stone Gap Post (Wise Co., VA)
The Biloxi Daily Herald (Biloxi, MS)
The Birmingham Age-Herald (Birmingham, AL) [microfilm]

Birmingham State Herald [microfilm]
The Birmingham News [microfilm]
Bisbee Daily Review (Bisbee, AZ)
The Bismarck Tribune (Bismarck, ND)
Bismarck Weekly Tribune (Bismarck, ND)
The Border Vidette (Nogales, AZ)
The Boston Globe
The Boston Journal
Boston Evening Transcript
The Bourbon News (Paris, KY)
The Breckenridge News (Cloverport, KY)
The Brownsville Daily Herald (Brownsville, TX)
The Burlington Free Press (Burlington, VT)
The Cambria Freeman (Ebensburg, PA)
The Cape Grardeau Democrat (Cape Grardeau, MO)
The Capital Journal (Salem, OR)
The Central Record (Lancaster, KY)
The Charlotte Observer (Charlotte, NC)
Cheyenne Transporter (Darlington Indian Territory)
Chicago Daily Tribune and *Chicago Tribune*
The Citizen (Berea, KY)
Cleveland Daily Leader
The Coconino Sun (Flagstaff, AZ)
The Columbian (Bloomsburg, PA)
The Columbus Courier (Columbus, NM)
The Columbus Journal (Columbus, NE)
Commercial Advertiser (NYC)
Commercial Gazette and Daily Advertizer
Corpus Christi Caller (Corpus Christi, TX)
Cresco Plain Dealer (Cresco, IO)
The Daily Astorian (Astoria, OR)
The Daily Capital Journal (Salem, OR)
Daily Dispatch (Richmond, VA)
The Daily Gate City and Constitution-Democrat (Keokuk, IO)
Daily Globe (Canton, IL)
Daily Globe (St Paul, MN)
Daily Inter Ocean (Chicago)
The Daily Journal (Salem, OR)
The Daily Ohio Statesman (Columbus, OH)
The Daily Phoenix (Columba, SC)
Daily People (NYC)
Daily Press (Newport News, VA)
Daily Union and American (Nashville, TN)
Dallas Morning News
Deming Graphic (Deming, NM)
The Democratic Banner (Mount Vernon, OH)
Democratic Free Press & Michigan Intelligencer (Detroit, MI)
Desert Evening News (Great Salt Lake City, Utah)
Detroit Free Press

Donaldsonville Chief (Donaldsonville, LA)
The Edgefield Advertiser (Edgefield, SC)
El Paso Herald (El Paso, TX)
Evening Bulletin (Honolulu)
Evening Bulletin (Mayville, KY)
The Evening Critic (Washington, DC)
Evening Herald (Shenandoah, PA)
Evening Missourian (Columbia, MO)
The Evening News (Sault Ste. Marie, MI)
Evening Post (NYC)
The Evening Press (Grand Rapids, MI)
Evening Public Ledger (Philadelphia, PA)
Evening Star (Washington, DC)
Evening Star (Washington, DC)
The Evening Telegraph (Philadelphia, PA)
The Evening World (Brooklyn, NYC)
Fair Play (Ste. Genevieve, MO)
The Forest Republican (Tionesta, PA)
The Fort Worth Register
Gainsville Daily Sun (Gainsville, FL)
Gainsville Sun
The Garland City Globe (Garland, UT)
Gazette (Raleigh, NC)
Goodwin's Weekly (Salt Lake City, UT)
Graham Guardian (Safford, AZ)
Grand Forks Daily Herald (Grand Forks, ND)
Gulf Coast Breeze (Crawfordville, FL)
Harrisburg Telegraph (Harrisburg, PA)
Hawaiian Gazette (Honolulu)
The Hawaiian Star (Honolulu)
The Hays Free Press (Hays, KA)
The Herald (New Orleans, LA)
The Hickman Courier (Hickman, KY)
The Highland Weekly (Hillsborough, OH)
The Holt County Sentinel (Oregon, MO)
The Idaho Daily Statesman (Boise, ID)
Idaho Statesman (Boise, ID)
The Indianapolis Journal (Indianapolis IN)
The Intermountain Catholic (Salt Lake City)
The Iola Register (Iola, KA)
Iowa State Bystander (Des Moines, IO)
Iron County Register (Ironton, MO)
The Jackson Citizen Patriot (Jackson, MI)
Jackson Daily Citizen (Jackson, OH)
The Jasper Weekly Courier (Jasper, IN)
Kalamazoo Gazette (Kalamazoo, MI)
Kansas City Star (Kansas City, MO)
The Kansas City Sun (Kansas City, MO)
The Kansas City Times (Kansas City, MO)

Keowee Courier (Pickens Court House, SC)
The Kinsley Graphic (Kinsley, KA)
Lancaster Daily (Lancaster, PA)
Little Falls Herald (Little Falls, MN)
Little Falls Weekly Transcript (Little Falls, MN)
The Logan Republican (Logan, UT)
Los Angeles Daily Herald
Los Angeles Herald
The Lynden Tribune (Lynden, WA)
The McCook Tribune (McCook, NE)
The Mahoning Dispatch (Canfield, OH)
Manchester Democrat (Manchester, IO)
The Mani News (Wailuku, Maui, HI)
The Manning Times (Manning, SC)
Marion Daily Mirror (Marion, OH)
Marin Journal (San Rafael, CA)
Marshall County Independent (Plymouth, IN)
Memphis Daily Appeal
The Middlebury Register and Addison County Journal (Middlebury, VT)
The Milan Exchange (Milan, TN)
The Minneapolis Journal
Monroe City Democrat (Monroe City, MO)
Morgan County Democrat (Versailles, MO)
The Morning Call (San Francisco)
Morning Herald (Lexington, KY)
The Morning Star and Catholic Messenger (New Orleans, LA)
Mount Vernon Signal (Mount Vernon, KY)
Nashville Patriot (Nashville, TN)
National Republican (Washington, DC)
The Nebraska Advertiser (Nemaha City, NE)
The New Bloomfield, Pa. Times (New Bloomfield, PA)
The Newport Miner (Newport, OR)
New-York Daily Tribune
New York Herald
The New York Times
New York Times Magazine
The New-York Tribune
The News-Record (Enterprise, OR)
The Norfolk Virginian
The Ogden Standard (Ogden City, UT)
The Oklahoma City Times (Oklahoma City)
Omaha Daily Bee (Omaha, NE)
Omaha World Herald (Omaha, NE)
Palestine Daily Herald (Palestine, TX)
Patriot (Harrisburg, PA)
The Pensacola Journal (Pensacola, FL)
Perrysberg Journal (Perrysburg, OH)
Philadelphia Inquirer
Phillipsburg Herald (Phillipsburg, KA)

Pittsburgh Dispatch
Pittsburgh Gazette
Portsmouth Journal of Literature and Politics (Portsmouth, NH)
The Princeton Union (Princeton, MN)
Public Ledger (Memphis, TN)
Pullman Herald (Pullman, WA)
Raftsman's Journal (Clearfield, PA)
The Record-Union (Sacramento, CA)
The Red Cloud Chief (Red Cloud, Webster County, NE)
Red Lake News (Red Lake, MN)
The Rice Belt Journal (Welsh, LA)
The Roanoke Times (Roanoke, VA)
The Rockford Daily Register and Gazette (Rockford, IL)
Rogue River Courier (Grants Pass, OR)
Sacramento Daily Record-Union
The Salt Lake Herald (Salt Lake City, UT)
The Salt Lake Tribune (Salt Lake City, UT)
The St. Albans Daily Messenger (St Albans, VT)
St. Louis Republican
The St. Lucie County Tribune (Fort Pierce, FL)
St. Paul Daily Globe (St Paul, MN)
St. Tammany Farmer (Covington, LA)
San Antonio Express (San Antonio, TX)
The San Antonio Light (San Antonio, TX)
San Francisco Chronicle
The San Juan Islander (Friday Harbor, WA)
Santa Fe New Mexican
Saratoga Sentinel (Saratoga Springs, NY)
Saturday Press (Honolulu)
Sausalito News (Sausalito, CA)
The Scranton Tribune (Scranton, PA)
The Seattle Star
Sedalia Weekly Bazoo (Sedalia, MO)
Semi-Weekly Interior Journal (Stanford, KY)
Shenandoah Herald (Woodstock, VA)
Sioux City Journal (Sioux City, IO)
The Somerset Herald (Somerset, PA)
Springfield Globe-Republic (Springfield, OH)
The Star (Reynoldsville, PA)
The Stark County Democrat (Canton, OH)
The State (Columbia, SC)
The State Republican (Jefferson City, MO)
The Sun (NYC)
The Times (Richmond, VA)
The Times (Washington, DC)
The Times and Democrat (Orangeburg, SC)
The Times Dispatch (Richmond, VA)
The Times-Herald (Burns, OR)
The Times Picayune; The Daily Picayune (New Orleans, LA)

Tombstone Epitaph (Tombstone, AZ)
The Trenton Evening Times (Trenton, NJ)
Trenton State Gazette (Trenton, NJ)
The True Democrat (Bayou Sara, LA)
Tulsa Daily World (Tulsa, Indian Territory, OK)
The New Ulm Weekly Review (New Ulm, MN)
Vermont Phoenix (Brattleboro, VT)
Virginian-Pilot (Norfolk, VA)
Waco Examiner (Waco, TX)
Warren Sheaf (Warren, MN)
Washington Bee (Washington, DC)
Washington Herald (Washington, DC)
The Washington Times (Washington, DC)
The Ward County Independent (Minot, ND)
The Watchman and Southron (Sumter, SC)
Weekly Kansas Chief (Troy, KA)
The Wenatchee Daily World (Wenatchee, WA)
Wheeling Daily Intelligencer (Wheeling, WV)
Williams News (Williams, AZ)
The Witchita Daily Eagle (Witchita, KA)
Worcester Daily Spy (Worcester, MA)

OTHER PRINTED PRIMARY SOURCES

Acland, Henry Wentworth. *Memoir on the Cholera at Oxford in the Year 1854* (London, 1856).

Acta Sanctorum, ed. Société des Bollandistes, 68 vols (Antwerp and Brussels, 1643–1940).

'AIDS Panic Rocks Florida Town', <www.fact.com>, 4 September 1987.

Albertus de Bezanis Abbatis. *Cronaca Pontificum et Imperatorum*, ed. Oswald Holder-Egger, MGH: Scriptores rerum Germanicarum in usum scholarum (Hanover, 1908).

Alessandri, Francesco. *Trattato della peste et febri pestilenti, tradotto di latino in volgare* (Turin: per Antonio de' Bianchi, 1586).

Allen, Richard and Absalom Jones. *A Narrative of the Proceedings of the Black People, during the Late Awful Calamity in Philadelphia, in the Year 1793* (Philadelphia, 1794).

[Almenar, Joannes]. *Libellus ad evitandum et expellendum Morbus Gallicum ut nunquam revertatur noviter inventus ac impressus* (Venice, 1502).

Amari, Michele. *Descrizione del cholera di Sicilia*, ed. Carmela Castiglione Trovato (Naples, 1990).

Amato Lusitano [João Rodrigues de Castelo Branco]. *De Morbo Gallico et Gallica scabie*, in Luisini, I, 560.

Amato Lusitano. *Epistola ii*, 'De Gallica Scabie', in Luisini, I, 560.

Ammianus Marcellinus. *Rerum Gestarum Libri*, trans. John C. Rolfe, LCL 300, 3 vols (London, 1935–40).

Anche il colera: gli untori di Napoli, ed. Gennaro Esposito (Milan, 1973).

Annales Mechovienses a. 947–1434, in *Monumenta Germaniae Historica*—Scriptores (in folgio, SS) XIX, ed. G. H. Pertz (Hanover, 1866), 666–77.

Annales Ragusini Anonymi: item Nicolai de Ragnina, ed. Speratus Nodilo (Zagrabe, 1883).

Annales seu Cronicae incliti Regni Poloniae opera venerabilis domini Joannis Dlugossii canonici Cracoviensis, ed. I. Dabrowski, 10 vols (Warsaw, 1964–85).

Annali a Pietro Aliosio Doninio, in Corradi, 'Nuovi documenti', 361–2.

Annali delle Città dell'Aquila...Rome, 1570, in Corradi, 'Nuovi documenti', 365–6.

Annalium Hiberniae Chronicon ad annum MCCCXLIX, ed. Richard Butler, in *The Miscellany of the Irish Archaeological Society* (Dublin, 1849), 1–39.

'"Antagonism" to Smallpox, by Prophylaxis and by Riot', *Lancet*, 147 (22 February 1896): 501.

Apollodorus. *The Library*, trans. James C. Frazer, LCL 121–2, 2 vols (Cambridge, MA, 1921).

'Appearance of Human Plague at Shanghai', *Lancet*, 176 (17 December 1910): 1804.

Appian. *Roman History*, 8.1: *The Punic Wars*, trans. Horace White, LCL 2 (Cambridge, MA 1912).

Appian. *Roman History*, 10: *The Illyrian Wars*, trans. Horace White, LCL 3 (Cambridge, MA, 1912).

Appian. *Roman History*, 12: *The Mithridatic Wars*, trans. Horace White, LCL 3 (Cambridge, MA, 1912).

The Apostolic Fathers, I: *I Clement, II Clement, Ignatius Polycarp, Didache*, trans. Bart D. Ehrman, LCL 24 (Cambridge, MA, 2003).

'Armed Resistance in Georgia', *Lancet*, 142 (23 September 1893): 754.

Arreste du Parlement de Paris portant reglement sur le fait des malades de la Grosse Verole, and *Ordonnance du prevost de Paris pour les malades de la Grosse Verole*, in *Aphrodisiacus*, 69–71.

Arrests notables du Parlement de Tolose donnez & prononcez sur diverses matieres, civiles, criminelles, beneficiales, & feudales, ed. Bernard de La Roche-Flavin (Toulouse, 1617).

Arrests notable du Parlement de Tolose donnés et prononcés sur diverses matières civiles, criminelles..., ed. Bernard de la Roche-Flavin; nouvelle édition: Augmentée des Observation de Me François Graverol, Avocat de la ville de Nîmes (Toulouse, 1720).

Astruc, Jean. *Dissertation sur la contagion de la peste* (Toulouse, 1724).

Astruc, Jean. *De Morbis Venereis, Libri Sex. In quibus disseritur tum de origine, propagatione & contagione...* (Paris, 1736).

Augustine. *The City of God against the Pagans*, I: *Books 1–3*, trans. George E. McCracken, LCL 411 (Cambridge, MA, 1957).

Baldinucci, Giovanni. *Quaderno: peste, guerra e carestia nell'Italia del seicento*, ed. Brendan Dooley (Florence, 2001).

Bando di Filippo IV Re di Spagna relativo agli untori in Milano, Cremona e Lodi (Milan: Eredi di Pandolfo e Marco Tullio Malatesti, 1630).

Bannerman, W. B. 'The Spread of Plague in India', *Journal of Hygiene*, 6 (1906): 179–211.

Barbacciani, Prof. (Cesenatico). *Storia sul Cholera-Morbus Indiano sviluppatosi nella terra e circondario del Cesenatico nell'estate dell'anno MDCCCXXXVI* (Pesaro, 1836).

Basil. *Letters*, I: *Letters 1–58*, trans. Roy J. Deferrari, LCL 190 (Cambridge, MA, 1926).

Bell, Benjamin. *A Treatise on Gonorrhoea Virulenta and Lues Venerea*, 2 vols, 2nd edn (Edinburgh, 1797).

Beniveni, Antonio. *De Morbo Gallico*, excerpted from *Tractatus, ex libro eius de abditis morborum causis*, in Luisini, I, 345–6; and in *Aphrodisiacus*, 85.

Benzonus, Hieronymus. *Novae novi orbis historiae*, published in 1600; he made his observations in the New World between 1541 and 1556, in *Aphrodisiacus*, 141.

Berlerus. *Chronicon* (1510), in *Aphrodisiacus*, 124–5.

Biggs, J. T. *Leicester: Sanitation versus Vaccination* (London, 1912).

Bisciola, Paolo. *Relatione verissima del progresso della peste di Milano* (Ancona, 1577).

The Black Death, ed. and trans. Rosemary Horrox, Manchester Medieval Source Series (Manchester, 1994).

Blane, Sir Gilbert. *Warning to the British Public* ([S.L.], October 1831).

Blondus, Michael Angelis. *De origine morbi Gallici deque ligni Indici ancipiter proprietate* (Venice, 1542).

Boccaccio, Giovanni. *Decameron*, trans. G. H. McWilliam, Penguin Classics (Harmondsworth, 1972).

Boccaccio, Giovanni. *Tutte le opere di Giovanni Boccaccio, IV: Decameron*, ed. Vittore Branca (Milan, 1976).

Boismont, Alexandre Brierre de. *Hallucinations or, the rational history of apparitions...* (Philadelphia, 1853).

Bononia Manifesta: Catalogo dei bandi, editti, costituzioni e provvedimenti diversi, stampati nel XVI secolo per Bologna e il suo territorio, ed. Zita Zanardi, Biblioteca di Bibliografia italiana CXLII (Florence, 1996).

Borgarutius, Prosperus. *Methodus*, in Luisini, II, 151–85.

Borromeo, Federigo. *De Pestilentia (La Peste di Milano del 1630)*, ed. Giancarlo Mazzoli (Pavia, 1964).

Borsani, Luigi and Francesco Freschi. 'Osservazioni intorno al Cholera Asiatico fatte in Bergamo nei mesi di maggio e giugno del 1836', *AUM*, 79 (1836), f. 235.

Bower, Walter. *Scotichronicon*, ed. D. E. R. Watt, 9 vols (Aberdeen, 1989–98).

Bowring, Edgar Alfred. *Abstracts of Returns of Information on the Laws of Quarantine which Have Been Obtained by the Board of Trade* (London, 1860).

Brant, Sebastianus. *De pestilentiali scorra*. In *Aphrodisiacus*, 54.

Brasavola, Antonio Musa. *Examen omnium Loch,...ubi de morbo Gallico diligentissime copioseque tractatur* (Venice: apud Iantus, 1553).

Brasavola, Antonio Musa. *De Morbo Gallico*, in Luisini, I, 564–610.

Brasavola, Antonio Musa. *De radicis Chynae usu, tractatus*, in Luisini, I, 616–35.

Breve Chronicon Clerici Anonymi, in *Recueil des Chroniques de Flandre publié sous la direction de la Commission Royale d'histoire*, ed. J.-J. de Smet, t. 3 (Brussels, 1856), 5–30.

Brevi annali della Città di Perugia dal 1194 al 1352 da uno della famiglia Oddi, ed. Ariodante Fabretti, *ASI*, 16 (1850).

Brewer, Thomas. *The Weeping Lady, or London like Ninivie in Sackcloth* (London, 1625).

Briet, Guillaume. *Discours sur les causes de la peste survenve á Bordeaux...* (Bordeaux, 1599).

Briet, Guillaume. *Explication de deux questions politique touchant la Peste...* (Bordelais: Par S. Millanges Imprimeur ordinaire du Roy, 1599).

Briet, Guillaume. *Remede tres salutaire contre le Mal François* (Nîmes, 1591).

Brighetti, Antonio. *Bologna e la peste del 1630* (Bologna, 1968).

Bruni, Leonardo. *Historiarum Florentini populi, Libri XII [Dalle origini all'anno 1404]*, ed. Emilio Santini, in RIS, XIX/3 (Città di Castello, 1914).

Burton, Lady Isabel. *The Life of Sir Richard F. Burton* (London, 1898).

Caesar, C. Iulius. *Civil War*, trans. Cynthia Damon, LCL 39 (Cambridge, MA, 2016).

Calderini, Carlo. 'Cenno istorico del Cholera-morbus che ha regnato in Nizza, Cuneo, Genova, Torino e altri luoghi dello Stato Sardo, dal suo primo apparire fino al 18 settembre 1835', *AUM*, 81, f. 242 and 243 (1837): 401–75.

Campani, Niccolò. *Lamento di quel tribulato di Strascino Campana senese sopra il mal francioso* (Venice, 1523).

Carey, Matthew. *A Short Account of the Malignant Fever, Lately Prevalent in Philadelphia*, 4th edn (Philadelphia, 1794).

Casteen, Elizabeth. 'John of Rupescissa's Letter *Reverendissime pater* (1350) in the Aftermath of the Black Death', *Franciscana: Bollettino della Società internazionale di studi francescani*, 6 (2004): 139–84.

Chaumette. *Enchiridion, ou Livret portatif pour les chirurgiens, …* (Lyon: L. Cloquemin, 1571).

Chicoyneau, François. *Traité des causes, des accidens, et de la cure de la peste: avec un recueil…* (Paris: Chez Pierre-Jean Mariette, 1744).

'Cholera at Leghorn and in the Abruzzi', *Lancet*, 142 (14 October 1893): 948.

'Cholera in Europe', *Lancet*, 178 (30 December 1911): 1856–62.

Chronica Olivensis auctore Stanislao, abbate Olivensi, in *Monumenta Poloniae Historica* I, ser. VI (Lvov, 1893).

City of Aberdeen and its Vicinity (Aberdeen, 1831).

Clementius Clementius. In *Aphrodisiacus*, 120.

Clemow, Frank. 'The Cholera Epidemic in Russia', *Lancet*, 141 (6 May 1893): 1053–9.

Clemow, Frank. *The Cholera Epidemic of 1892 in the Russian Empire* (London, 1893).

Clemow, Frank. 'The Plague at Calcutta', *Lancet*, 152 (17 September 1898): 738–42.

Clowes, William. *A briefe and necessarie treatise, touching the cure of the disease called morbus Gallicus, or lues venerea…* (enlarged edition) (London: Thomas Cadman, 1585).

Consilium breve contra malas pustulas, in *Aphrodisiacus*, 41–6.

Cronaca Fermana di Antonio di Niccolò Notaro e Cancelliere della Città di Fermo dall'anno 1176 sino all'anno 1447, ed. Marco Tabbarini, in *Documenti di Storia Italiana* IV (Florence, 1870), 1–98.

Cronache anteriori al secolo XVII concernenti la storia di Cuneo, ed. Domenico Promis, Miscellanea di Storia Italiana 12 (Turin, 1871), 225–324.

Cronache di Ser Luca Dominici, I: *Cronaca della venuta dei Bianchi e della Moria 1399–1400*, ed. Giovan Carlo Gigliotti (Pistoia, 1933).

The Chronicle of Jean de Venette, trans. Jean Birdsall (New York, 1953).

The Chronicle of Pseudo-Zachariah, Rhetor: Church and War in Late Antiquity, ed. Geoffrey Greatrex, trans. Robert R. Phenix and Cornelia B. Horn, Translated Texts for Historians 55 (Liverpool, 2011).

Chronicon Galfridi le Baker de Swynebroke, ed. Edward Maunde Thompson (Oxford, 1889).

Chronicon Moguntinum 1347–1406 und Fortsetzung bis 1478 in *Die Chroniken der niedersächsischen Städte: Mainz*, ed. J. Hegel (Leipzig, 1882), 147–250.

Chronicon Monasterii Mellicensis, in *Aphrodisiacus*, 46.

Die Chronik des Jakob Twinger von Königshofen, in *Die Chroniken der oberrheinischen Städte: Strassburg*, ed. K. Hegel, 2 vols, Die Chroniken der deutschen Städte VIII–IX (Leipzig, 1870–1).

Die Chronik Erhards von Appenwiler 1439–71, in *Basler Chroniken*, III, ed. August Bernoulli, 4 vols (Leipzig, 1890).

'Ein Chronikmarchen an den historischen Tatsachen kontrolliert', in *Aus der Frühgeschichte der Syphilis*, ed. Karl Sudhoff, *Studien zur Geschichte der Medizin*, Heft 9 (Leipzig, 1912), 141–53.

Chronique de Jean le Bel, ed. Jules Viard and Eugène Déprez, 2 vols (Paris, 1904–5).

Chronique des Pays-Bas, de France, D'Angleterre et de Tournai (un ms de la bibliothèque de Bourgogne), in *Recueil des Chroniques de Flandre publié sous la direction de la Commission Royale d'histoire*, III, ed. J.-J. de Smet (Brussels, 1856), 115–569.

Chronique de Richard Lescot religieux de Saint-Denis (1328–1344) suive de la continuation de cette chronique (1344–1364), ed. Jean Lemoine, Société de l'histoire de France, CCLXXVIII (Paris, 1896).

Chronique des Pays-Bas, de France, D'Angleterre et de Tournai, in *Recueil des Chroniques de Flandre publié sous la direction de la Commission Royale d'histoire*, III, ed. J.-J. de Smet (Brussels, 1856).

Chronique du religieux de Saint-Denys, contenant le règne de Charles VI, 1380 à 1422, ed. M. L. Bellaguet, Collection des documents inédits, 6 vols (Paris, 1839–52).

Chronique et annales de Gilles le Muisit (1272–1352), ed. Henri Lemaître (Paris, 1906).

Chronique latine de Guillaume de Nangis de 1113 à 1300 avec les continuations de cette chronique de 1300 à 1368, II, ed. Hercule Géraud (Paris, 1843).

Chroniques des Ducs de Brabant, par Edmond de Dynter, ed. P. F. X. de Ram, 2 vols (Brussels, 1854).

Cortusii Patavini duo, sive Gulielmi et Albrigeti Cortusiorum. *Historia de Novitatibus Paduae, et Lombardiae ab anno MCCLVI usque ad MCCCLXIV*, in RIS, XII, ed. Ludovico Muratori (Milan, 1728).

Crinitus, Petrus. *De poetis latinis, lib V, in Aphrodisiacus*, 119.

Cronaca di Pisa di Ranieri Sardo, ed. Ottavio Banti, Fonti per la Storia d'Italia 99 (Rome, 1963).

La Cronaca ferrarese dello Zambotti, in Corradi, 'Nuovi documenti', 346–7.

Cronaca Senese attribuita ad Agnolo di Tura del Grasso detta La Cronaca Maggiore [A. 1300–1351], in *Cronache senesi*, ed. Alessandro Lisini and Fabio Iacometti, RIS 15/6.1 (Bologna, 1931–9).

Cronica della città di Perugia dal 1309 al 1491 nota col nome di Diario del Graziani [Pietro Angelo di Giovanni], ed. Francesco Bonaini, Ariodante Fabretti, and Filippo-Luigi Polidori, *Archivio Storico Italiano* XVI (1850).

Cronica del Racional de la Ciutat (1334–1417), in *Recull des Documents i estudis*, I, ii (Barcelona, 1921).

Cronica der Hilligen stat Coellen., in *Aphrodisiacus*, 54.

Cronica inedita di Giovanni da Parma Canonico di Trento, in Angelo Pezzana, *Storia della città di Parma* (Parma, 1937), Appendice, 50–79.

Cronica volgare di Anonimo Fiorentino dall'anno 1385 al 1409 già attribuita a Piero di Giovanni Minerbetti, ed. Elena Bellondi, in *RIS* 27/2 (Città di Castello, 1915–18).

Le Croniche di Giovanni Sercambi Lucchese, ed. Salvatore Bongi, 3 vols, Istituto Storico Italiano, Fonti per la Storia d'Italia 19–21 (Rome, 1892).

Cumanus, Marcellus. *Observationes Medicae*, in *Aphrodisiacus*, 52–4.

Cyprian. *De mortalitate*, in *Corpus Scriptorum ecclesiasticorum Latinorum*, III: *S. Thasci Caecili Cypriani opera omnia* (Vienna, 1868), pt 1, 297–314.

D'Amico, Arnaldo. 'AIDS, medaglia d'oro a Donat-Cattin', *La Republica*, 30 September 1993, 13.

Da Vigo, Giovanni. In Luisini, I, 386–92.

Da Vigo, Giovanni. *De apostemate virgae*, in *Aphrodisiacus*, 126.

Dalle Tuatte. *Historia di Bologna*, in Corradi, 'Nuovi documenti', 346.

de Cieça de Leon, Petrus. *Chronica del Peru* (1554), in *Aphrodisiacus*, 141–2.

De morbo Gallico Petrihaschardi insulani, medici chirurgi, Tractatus, in *Appendici*, ed. Luisini, II, 72.

De novo orbe in lingua Hispana in Ital. traducto, 1501, in *Aphrodisiacus*, 116–17.

de Rubeis, Jo. Fran. Bernardo Maria. *Monumenta Ecclesiae Aquilejensis* (Strasbourg, 1740).

de Zuccano, Leon Lunensis. *De Morbo Gallico, Ex methodo curandi febres, Tumoresque praeternaturam excerptum*, in *Appendici*, ed. Luisini, II, 48–50.

DeClure, Anita and Billy G. Smith, 'Wrestling the "Pale Faced Messenger": The Diary of Edward Garrigues during the 1798 Philadelphia Yellow Fever Epidemic', *Pennsylvania History*, 65 (1998): 243–68.

Dekker, Thomas. *The Wonderfull Yeare. 1603* (London, 1603).

[Demosthenes]. *Orations*, III: *Orations 21–26*, trans. J. H. Vince, LCL 299 (Cambridge, MA, 1935).

Diacius, *Tratado contro la enfermedad de las bubas, c.*1555, in *Aphrodisiacus*, 162–3.

I Diarii di Girolamo Priuli, 1494–1512, ed. Roberto Cessi, RIS 24/3 (Città di Castello, 1912).

Diaz, Ruy de Isla. *Tratado Ilamado de todos los Santos contra el mal de la ysla Española* (Seville: Dominico de Robertis, 1539).

Dio Cassius. *Roman History*, trans. E. Carey, 9 vols, LCL 176 (Cambridge, MA, 1925).

Dio Chrysostom, III. *Discourses, 31–36*, trans. J. E. Cohoon and H. Lamar Crosby, LCL 358 (Cambridge, 1940).

Dio Chrysostom, III. *Discourses*, IV: *37–60, On Concord with the Nicaeans*, trans. H. Lamar Crosby, LCL 376 (Cambridge, MA, 1946).

Diodorus Siculus. *The Library of History*, II: *Books 2.35–4.58*, trans. C. H. Oldfather, LCL 303 (Cambridge, MA, 1935).

Diodorus Siculus. *The Library of History*, III: *Books 4.59–8*, trans. C. H. Oldfather, LCL 340 (Cambridge, MA, 1939).

Diodorus Siculus. *The Library of History*, XII: *Books 33–40*, trans. Francis R. Walton, LCL 423 (Cambridge, MA, 1967).

Diogenes Laertius. *Lives of Eminent Philosophers*, trans. R. D. Hicks, LCL 184–5, 2 vols (Cambridge, MA, 1925).

Dionysius of Halicarnassus. *Roman Antiquities*, trans. Earnest Carey, LCL 319, 347, 357, 364, 372, 378, 388, 7 vols (Cambridge, 1937–50).

Dionysius of Halicarnassus. *The Ancient Orators 5. Thucydides*, trans. Stephen Usher, LCL 465 (Cambridge, MA, 1974).

Dollo, Corrado. *Peste e untori nella Sicilia Spagnola: Presupposti teorici e condizionamenti sociali*, ed. A. Giarrusso, M. A. Alaymo, F. Fedeli, F. Guerreri, and G. B. Hodierna (Naples, 1991).

Doyle, Sir Arthur Conan. *The Poison Belt* (London, 1913).

Ecclesia Spalatensis, in *Illyrici sacri*, t. III (Venice, 1765).

Engels, Frederick. *The Conditions of the Working Class in England*, trans. W. O. Henderson and W. H. Chaloner (Stanford, CA, 1958; German edn, 1845).

Epistolario di Coluccio Salutati, ed. Francesco Novati, Instituto Storico Italiano, Fonti per la Storia d'Italia 14–18, 4 vols (Rome, 1891–1911).

Euripides. *Dramatic Fragments*, VII, ed. Christopher Collard and Martin Cropp, LCL 506 (Cambridge, MA, 2009).

Europius. *Breviarium ab urbe condita*, ed. Joseph Hellegouarc'h, Collection des Universités de France (Paris, 1999).

Eusebius. *Ecclesiastical History*, II: *Books 6–10*, trans. J. E. L. Oulton, LCL 265 (Cambridge, MA, 1932).

Evagrius. *Ecclesiastical History of Evagrius Scholasticus*, trans. Michael Whitby, Translated Texts for Historians 33 (Liverpool, 2000).

Falloppio, Gabriele. *De Morbo Gallico* (Padua, 1564).

Falloppio, Gabriele. *De Morbo Gallico: Tractatus*, in Luisini, I, 661–720.

Fernel, Jean. *De luis venereare curatione perfectissima liber primio editio* (1579), in *Aphrodisiacus*, 142–3.

Fernel, Jean. *Ambiani de lue venera dialogus*, ex lib II, in Lusini, I, 524–8.

Ferrandi, Consalvo. *De Guaiacano Ligno, Tractatus Unus: De Ligno Sancti*, in Luisini, I, 308–9.

Ferrandi, Consalvo. *De ligno sancto*, in Luisini, I, 309.

Ferri, Alfonso. *De ligni sancti multiplici medicina, et vini exhibitione libri quatuor, quibus nunc primum additus est Syphilis; sive morbus Gallicus; omnia multo emendatiora quam antea* (Paris: apud Vivat Gaultherot, 1543).

Ferri, Alfonso. *De morbo Gallico, et ligni sancti natura, usque multiplici*, in Luisini, I, 347–85.

Ferrier, Auger. *De lue Hispanica sive morbo gallico* (Paris: Aegidium Gillium, 1564).

Fiochetto, Giovanni Francesco. *Trattato della Peste et Pestifero contagio di Torino* (Turin: G. G. Tisma, 1631).

Fiochetto, Giovanni Francesco. *Peste a Torino: La città durante il contagio*, ed. Massimo Centini and Sandy Furlini (Turin, 2010).

Fioravanti, Leonardo. *De' Capricci Medicinali* (Venice: Michele Bonibelli, 1595 [first published in Venice in 1564]).

Flanagan, Jane. 'South African Men Rape Babies as "Cure" for Aids', *Telegraph*, 11 November 2001.

Fontana, Alexander. *Morbo Gallico et ligno indico: Quaestiones*, in Luisini, I, 610–15.

Fornasini, Luigi. 'Intorno al cholera di Brescia: Observazioni del dottor Liugi Fornasini', *AUM*, 38, Fasc. 401 (mag, 1850): 225–90.

Fracantiani [Francanzani], Antonio. *De Morbo Gallico*, in Luisini, I, 721–34.

Fracastoro, Girolamo. *De Contagione et Contagiosos Morbis et eorum Curatione, Libri III*, ed. and trans. W. C. Wright (New York, 1930).

Fracastoro's Syphilis: Introduction, Text, Translation and Notes, ed. Geoffrey Eatough, ARCA Classical and Medieval Texts 12 (Liverpool, 1984).

Frammenti degli Annali di Sicilia, cited in Corradi, 'Nuovi documenti', 347.

Fréour, Le Docteur. 'Le choléra à Bordeaux', in Chevalier, *La première épidémie du XIXe siècle*, 109–20.

Fuschsius, Leonardus. *De Morbo Gallico*, in Luisini, I, 137–9.

Galar Y Beirdd: Marwnadau Plant/Poets' Grief: Medieval Welsh Elegies for Children, ed. and trans. Dafydd Johnston (Cardiff, 1993).

Galli, Antonio. *De ligno sancto non permiscendo, Opus*, in Luisini, I, 392–421.

Galli, Antonio. *De Ligno Sancto non permiscendo* (Paris: apud Simonem Colinaeum, 1540).

Gatacre, W. F. *Report on the Bubonic Plague, 1896–97* (Bombay, 1897).

Gatari, Galeazzo and Bartolomeo Gatari. *Cronaca Carrarese confrontata con la redazione di Andrea Gatari [AA. 1318–1407]*, ed. Antonio Medin and Guido Tolomei, vol. 1, RIS XVII/1 (Città di Castello, 1931).

Gesta archiepiscoporum Magdeburgensium, Continuatio I a. 1143–1367, in MGH, XIV, ed. Georg Waitz (Hanover, 1883).

Gigli, Giacinto. *Diario Romano (1608–1670)*, ed. Giuseppe Ricciotii (Rome, 1958).

Giovio, Paolo. *Historiarum Sui Temporis*, Book IV, in *Aphrodisiacus*, 125.

Giovio, Paolo. *Historiae Sui Temporis*, Lib. IIII, 79, in *Aphrodisiacus*, 125.

Giulini, Alessandro. 'Un diario secentesco inedito d'un notaio milanese (Pietro Antonio Calco, per gli anni 1632–38)', *Archivio Storico Lombardo*, 57 (1930): 466–82.

Gois, Damião de. *Chronica do feliccissimo rey dom Emanuel da gloriosa memoria...* (Lisbon, 1619).

Les Grandes Chroniques de France, 9: *Charles IV, Le Bel, Philippe VI de Valois*, ed. Jules Viard (Paris, 1937).

Il Grappa. *Cicalamenti del Grappa intorno al sonetto 'Poi che mia speme è lunga a venir troppo'. De ligni sancti multiplici medicina, et vini exhibitione libri quatuor, quibus nunc primum additus est Syphilis; sive morbus Gallicus...* (Mantua: Venturino Ruffinelli, 1545).

Great Britain Privy Council. *Papers Relative to the Disease called Cholera Spasmodica in India* (London, 1831).

Greek Iambic Poetry from the Seventh to Fifth Century BC, trans. Douglas E. Gerber, LCL 259 (Cambridge, MA, 1999).

Greek Mathematical Works, I: *Thales to Euclid*, trans. Ivor Thomas, LCL 335 (Cambridge, MA, 1939).

Gride Ducali provisioni, gratie et ragioni delle città di Modena (Modena: [Paolo Gadaldini], 1575).

Gruner, Christian Gothridus. *Aphrodisiacus sive De Lue Venerea in duas partes divisus... Aloysius Luisinus...* (Jena, 1789).

Gruner, Christian Gothridus. *De Morbo Gallico scriptores Medici et historici, partim inediti partim rari et notationibus aucti. Accedunt Morbu Gallico origines Maranicae* (Jena, 1793).

Gruner, Christian Gothridus. 'Morbi Gallici Origines Maranicae', *De Morbo Gallico scriptores*, xxv–vi.

Guicciardini, Francesco. *Storia d'Italia*, ed. Silvana Seidel Menchi, 3 vols (Turin, 1971).

Heraclitus: Homeric Problems, ed. and trans. Donald A. Russell and David Konstan (Atlanta, GA, 2005).

Herodian. *History of the Empire*, I: *Books 1–4*, ed. C. R. Whittaker, LCL 454 (Cambridge, MA, 1969).

Herodotus, *The Persian Wars*, trans. A. D. Godley, LCL 117, 120 (Cambridge, MA, 1920–5).

Hesiod. *Theogony. Works and Days. Testimonia*, trans. Glen W. Most, LCL 57 (Cambridge, MA, 2007).

Hippocrates of Cos. *Ancient Medicine. Airs, Waters, Places*, I, trans. W. H. S. Jones, LCL 147 (Cambridge, MA, 1923).

Hippocrates of Cos. *Epidemics 1 and 3*, I, trans. W. H. S. Jones, LCL 147 (Cambridge, MA, 1923).

Hirst, L. Fabian. *The Conquest of Plague: A Study of the Evolution of Epidemiology* (Oxford, 1953).

Historia Augusta, trans. David Magie, LCL 139–40, 263, 3 vols (Cambridge, MA, 1921–32).

Historia di Bologna del R.P.M. Cherubino Ghirardacci, ed. Albano Sorbelli, RIS, XXXIII/1 (Città di Castello, 1915).

Holmes, Oliver Wendell, 'Currents and Counter-Currents in Medical Science', *The American Journal of Medical Science*, 40 (1860): 462–74.

Holmes, Oliver Wendell, 'Reflections on his Annual Address' before the Massachusetts Medical Society, May 1860', in *American Journal of Medical Science*, 40 (1860): 474.

Homer, *Iliad*, I: *Books 1–12*, trans. A. T. Murray and William F. Wyatt, LCL 170 (Cambridge, MA, 1924).

Infessura, Stefano. *Diario della città di Roma*, cited in *Aphrodisiacus*, 38.

Ingrassia, Giovan Filippo. *Parte quinta di Giouan Filippo Ingrassia del pestifero, & contagioso morbo*...(Palermo: Giovan Mattheo Mayda, 1577).

'Jeddah', *Lancet*, 153 (6 May 1899): 1261–2.

Jew in the Medieval World: A Source Book, 315–1791, ed. Jacob Rader Marcus, 2nd edn (Cincinnati, OH, 1999).

The Jews in the Duchy of Milan, ed. Shlomo Simonsohn, 6 vols (Jerusalem, 1982).

Josephus. *The Life. Against Apion*, I., trans. H. St. J. Thackeray, LCL 186 (Cambridge, MA, 1926).

Josephus. *The Jewish War*, II: *Books 3–4*, trans. H. St. J. Thackeray, LCL 487 (Cambridge, MA, 1927).

Josephus. *The Jewish War*, III: *Books 5–7*, trans. H. St. J. Thackeray, LCL 210 (Cambridge, MA, 1928).

Josephus. *Jewish Antiquities*, I: *Books 1–3*, trans. H. St. J. Thackeray, LCL 242 (Cambridge, MA, 1930).

Josephus. *Jewish Antiquities*, III: *Books 7–8*, trans. Ralph Marcus, LCL 281 (Cambridge, MA, 1934).

Josephus. *Jewish Antiquities*, IV: *Books 9–11*, trans. Ralph Marcus, LCL 326 (Cambridge, MA, 1937).

Josephus. *Jewish Antiquities*, X: *Books 14–15*, trans. Ralph Marcus and Allen Wikgren, LCL 489 (Cambridge, MA, 1943).

Journal d'un bourgeois de Paris de 1405 à 1449, ed. Colette Beaune (Paris, 1990).

Keating, J. M. *History of the Yellow Fever: The Yellow Fever Epidemic of 1878, in Memphis, Tenn.* (Memphis, TN, 1879).

Kritovoulos of Imbros. *History of Mehmed the Conqueror*, trans. Charles Riggs (Princeton, NJ, 1954).

Lafaille, M. G. *Annales de la Ville de Toulouse depuis la réünion de la comté de Toulouse à la Couronne*, 2 vols (Toulouse: Guillaume-Louis Colomyez, 1687–1701).

Lampugnano, Agostino. *La Pestilenza seguita in Milano, l'anno 1630* (Milan: Carlo Ferrandi, 1634).

Langland, William. *Piers the Ploughman*, trans. J. F. Goodridge (Harmondsworth, 1959).

Lastri, Marco. *Ricerche sull'antica e moderna popolazione della città di Firenze* (Florence, 1785).

Latomus, Iohannis. *Acta aliquot vetustior in civitate Francofurtensi..., 793–1519*, in *Fontes rerum Germanicarum: Geschichtsquellen Deutschlands*, IV, ed. J. H. Böhmer (Stuttgart, 1868), 399–429.

Lattuada, Pietro Antonio. 'Cronaca inedita sulle peste di Milano del 1630', ed. Carlo Annoni in *L'Amico Cattolico*, 3 (1849): 281–94.

Legnani, Emilio Sioli. 'Cinque lettere inedite sulla peste di Milano del 1630' (BNCM, Misc Manz. C 148), Estratto da *La Rassegna della letteratura italiana*, Anno 68, nn. 2–3 (1964): 399–409.

Leo Africanus. *De totius Africae...*, in *Aphrodisiacus*, 125.

Leonicini Vincentini, Nicolai. *Librum de Epidemia, quam itali Morbum Gallicum vocant*, in Lusini, I, 14–35.

'Lettera, Mantova, 1534 da Roma al Duca di Mantova', in Corradi, 'Nuovi documenti', 335.

Libellus Iosephi Grunbebkii de mentulargra alias Morbo Gallico, in *Aphrodisiacus*, 63–9.

Libanius. *Oration: XIV: Upon Avenging Julian*, in *Selected Orations*, I, trans. A. F. Norman, LCL 451 (Cambridge, MA, 1969).

Le livre de Podio ou Chroniques d'Etienne Médicis, bourgeois du Puy, ed. Augustin Chassaing, 2 vols (Le Puy-en-Velay, 1869).

The Life of S. Bernardine of Siena, Minor Observantine (London, 1873).

Linturius, in *Aphrodisiacus*, 119–20.

Livy, *History of Rome*, I: Books 1–2, trans. B. O. Foster, LCL 114 (Cambridge, MA, 1919).

Livy. *History of Rome*, II: Books 3–4, trans. B. O. Foster, LCL 133 (Cambridge, MA, 1922).

Livy. *History of Rome*, III: Books 5–7, trans. B. O. Foster, LCL 172 (Cambridge, MA, 1924).

Livy. *History of Rome*, V: Books 21–2, trans. B. O. Foster, LCL 233 (Cambridge, MA, 1929).

Livy. *History of Rome*, XII: Books 40–2, trans. Evan T. Sage and Alfred C. Schlesinger, LCL 332 (Cambridge, MA, 1938).

Livy. *History of Rome*, VI: Books 23–5, trans. Frank Gardner Moore, LCL 355 (Cambridge, MA, 1940).

Livy. *History of Rome*, VII: Books 26–7, trans. Frank Gardner Moore, LCL 367 (Cambridge, MA, 1943).

Livy. *History of Rome, Summaries, Fragments, Julius Obsequens*, trans. Alfred C. Schlesinger, LCL 404 (Cambridge, MA, 1959).

[Livy], Julius Obsequens. *A Book of Prodigies after the 505th Year of Rome*, trans. Alfred C. Schlesinger, LCL 404 (Cambridge, MA, 1959).

London, Jack. *Scarlet Plague, London Magazine* (1912).

Lopez de Gomara, Franciscus. *Sacerdos Hispanis* (1519), in *Aphrodisiacus*, 129.

Lopez Pinna, Pedro. *Tratado de Morbo Gallico, en el qual se declara su origen, causas señales, pronosticos y curacion*, 2nd edn (Seville, 1719).

Lucan. *The Civil War*, trans. J. D. Duff, LCL 220 (Cambridge, MA, 1928).

Lucian. IV: *Alexander the False Prophet*, trans. A. M. Harmon, LCL 162 (Cambridge, MA, 1925).

Lucretius, *On the Nature of Things*, trans. W. H. D. Rouse, rev. M. F. Smith, LCL 181 (Cambridge, MA, 1924).

Luisini, Luigi (ed.), *De Morbo Gallico Petrihaschardi Insulano*, in *De Morbo Gallico omnia quae extant apud omnes medicos cuiuscunque nationis*, 2 vols (Venice: Apud Iordanum Zilettum, 1566–7).

Lupi, Giovanni Battista. *Storia della peste avvenuta nel Borgo di Busto Arsizio, 1630 (1632–42)*, ed. Franco Bertolli and Umberto Colombo (Busto Arsizio, 1990).

'Madeira', *Lancet*, 168 (29 December 1906): 1809–10.

Manardi, Giovanni. *Epistolae duae*, 1: *Eiusdem de ligno Indico*, in Luisini, I, 518.

Manetho, *History of Egypt and Other Works*, trans. W. G. Waddell, LCL 350 (Cambridge, MA, 1940).

Manzoni, Alessandro. *I promessi sposi*, ed. Salvatore Nigro (Milan, 2002).

Manzoni, Alessandro. *I promessi sposi storia della colonna infame*, intro. Silvano Nigro (Turin, 2012).

Marcha di Marco Battagli da Rimini [AA. 1212–1354], ed. Aldo Francesco Massèra, RIS 16/3 (Città di Castello, 1913).

Marcus Manilius. *Astronomica*, trans. G. P. Goold, LCL 469 (Cambridge, MA, 1977).

Marioni, P. A. *Peste in Milano nel 1630*, in Fabio Mutinelli, *Storia arcana ed aneddotica raccontata da Veneti ambasciatori*, 4 (Venice, 1855–8).

'Martin Pollichs von Mellerstadt erste Syphilisthesen aus dem Jahre 1496', in *Aus der Frühgeschichte der Syphilis*, ed. Karl Sudhoff, *Studien zur Geschichte der Medizin*, Heft 9 (Leipzig, 1912), 42–7.

Martines, Lauro. *An Italian Renaissance Sextet: Six Tales in Historical Context*, translations by Murtha Baca (New York, 1994).

Marx–Engels Collected Works, 50 vols (London, 1975–).

Mathias de Nuwenberg. *Chronica: Recensio B*, ed. A. Hofmeister, MGH: Scriptores rerum Germanicarum (Hanover, 1920–40).

Maynardi, Pietro. *Morbo Gallico, Tractatus Duo*, in Luisini, I, 336–40.

Mertens, Charles de. *An Account of the Plague Which Raged at Moscow, 1771* (London, 1799; first published in Latin, 1778).

Michele da Piazza. *Cronica*, ed. Antonino Giuffrida (Palermo, 1980).

Montani, Io. Baptistae. *Epistola: Pro generoso polono*, in Luisini, I, 495.

Montani, Io. Baptistae. *Tractatus etiam utilissimus de Morbo Gallico* (Venice: Bathassarem Constantinum, 1554).

Montius, Hieronymus. *Halosis Febrium* . . . (Lyon, 1563), in *Aphrodisiacus*, 163–6.

Montuus, Sebatianus. *De morbo gallico, Dialexion Medinalium libri duo* . . . (Lyon, 1537), in *Aphrodisiacus*, 139–40.

Morelli, Giovanni di Pagolo. *Ricordi*, in *Mercanti Scrittori: Ricordi nella Firenze tra Medioevo e Rinascimento*, ed. Vittore Branca (Milan, 1986).

Muratori, Ludovico. *Del Governo della peste, e delle maniere di guardarsene* (Milan, 1832; first edition, Modena, 1710).

'Notes from India', *Lancet*, 153 (16 April 1898): 1080–1.

'Notes from India', *Lancet*, 153 (1 April 1899a): 929–31.

'Notes from India', *Lancet*, 154 (23 September 1899b): 858–9.

'Notes from India: Riots at Kolhapur', *Lancet*, 154 (28 October 1899c): 1196–7.

'Notes from India', *Lancet*, 154 (23 December 1899d), 1766–7.

'Notes from India', *Lancet*, 155 (12 May 1900a): 1402.

'Notes from India', *Lancet*, 155 (26 May 1900b): 1548.

'Notes on India: The Cawmpore [sic] Plague Riots', *Lancet*, 155 (30 June 1900c): 911.

'Notes from India: Disturbances in the Punjab', *Lancet*, 156 (1 June 1901): 1571.

'Notes from India: Plague Riot in Patiala', *Lancet*, 157 (29 March 1902): 922.

'Notes from India', *Lancet*, 162 (28 November 1903): 1534.

Old Testament. New King James Version, Leviticus.

Oldoini, Stefano. 'Storia delle epidemie di colera avvenute nel Comune di Spezia durante gli anni 1884–85–86', *Annali universali di medicina e chirurgia*, 281, Fasc. 845.

'Gli Ordinamenti sanitari del Comune di Pistoai contro la pestilenza del 1348', ed. A. Chiappelli, *ASI*, ser 4, XX (1887): 8–22.

Orosius, Paulus. *The Seven Books of History Against the Pagans*, trans. Roy J. Deferrati (Washington, DC, 1964).

Orosius: Seven Books of History against the Pagans, trans. and ed. A. T. Fear, Translated Texts for Historians 54 (Liverpool, 2010).

'Our Risk in Cholera on the Continent', *Lancet*, 176 (10 September 1910): 836–7.

'The Outbreaks of Plague in Jeddah and Trebizond', *Lancet*, 168 (25 August 1906): 525–6.

Ovid. *Metamorphoses*, vol. 1, trans. F. J. Miller, rev. G. P. Goold, LCL 42 (Cambridge, MA, 1916).

Oviedo, Fernandez de. *Historia general y natural de las Indias*, 5 vols. Biblioteca de Autores Españoles, CXVII–CXXI (Madrid, 1992).

Paciudi, 'Missa Beati Jobi contra Morbum gallicum', in Corradi, 'Nuovi documenti', no. 18.

Papon, Jean Pierre. *De la peste ou époques mémorables de ce fléau et les moyens de s'en préserver*, 2 vols (Paris: Lavillette, 1800).

Paracelsius [Aureolus Theophrastus]. *De Morbo Gallico*, in *Aphrodisiacus*, 134–7.

Pausanias. *Description of Greece*, trans. W. H. S. Jones and H. A. Ormerod, LCL 93, 188, 272, 3 vols (Cambridge, MA, 1918, 1926, 1933).

Penni, Joannes. *Chroniche delle magnifiche et onorate Pompe*, in Corradi, 'Nuovi documenti', 371.

Pepere, (P.). 'Rapporto sul cholera a S. Giovanni a Teduccio nel 1865', *AUM*, 63, f. 597 (1867): 611–12.

La peste di Milano del 1630 del Padre Benedetto Cinquanta (1580–1640), in *Il teatro tragico italiano: Storia e testi del teatro tragico in Italia*, ed. Federico Doglio (Parma, 1960), 529–692.

Petronius. *Satyricon,* trans. Michael Heseltine, W. H. D. Rouse, revised by E. H. Warmington LCL 15 (Cambridge, MA, 1913).

Philo. I: *Allegorical Interpretation of Genesis* 2, 3, trans. F. H. Colson and G. H. Whitaker, LCL 226 (Cambridge, MA, 1929).

Philo. III: *On the Unchangeableness of God*, trans. F. H. Colson and G. H. Whittaker, LCL 247 (Cambridge, MA, 1930).

Philo. III: *Concerning Noah's Work as a Planter*, trans. F. H. Colson and G. H. Whittaker, LCL 247 (Cambridge, MA, 1930).

Philochorus: The Story of Athens: The Fragments of the Local Chronicles of Attika, ed. and trans. Phillip Harding (London, 2008).

Pinctor, Petrus. *Tractatus de morbo foedo et occulto . . .* , in *Aphrodisiacus*, 85–115.

Piorry, P. A. *Clinique médicale de l'Hôpital de la Pitié et de l'Hospice de la Salpétrière* (Paris, 1835).

'Plague in the Far East', *Lancet*, 176 (31 December 1910): 1909.

'Plague Riot in Seistan', *Lancet*, 167 (5 May 1906): 1286.

Pliny the Elder. *Natural History*, VII: *Books 24–27*, trans. W. H. S. Jones and A. C. Andrews, LCL 393 (Cambridge, MA, 1956).

Plutarch. *Lives*, I: *Theseus and Romulus*, trans. Bernadotte Perrin, LCL 46 (Cambridge, MA, 1914).

Plutarch. *Lives*, III: *Pericles and Fabius Maximus. Nicias and Crassus*, trans. Bernadotte Perrin, LCL 65 (Cambridge, MA, 1916).

Plutarch. *Lives*, IV: *Alcibiades and Coriolanus*, trans. Bernadotte Perrin, LCL 80 (Cambridge, MA, 1916).

Plutarch. *Lives*, VII: *Demosthenes and Cicero. Alexander and Caesar*, trans. Bernadotte Perrin, LCL 99 (Cambridge, MA, 1919).

Plutarch. *Moralia*, II, trans. Frank Cole Babbitt, LCL 222 (Cambridge, MA, 1928).

Plutarch. *Moralia*, IV: *Roman Questions. Greek Questions. Greek and Roman Parallel Stories*, trans. Frank Cole Babbitt, LCL 305 (Cambridge, MA, 1936).

Plutarch. *Moralia*, V: *The Obsolescence of Oracles*, trans. Frank Cole Babbitt, LCL 306 (Cambridge, MA, 1936).

Plutarch. *Moralia*, XII: *Whether Land or Sea Animals Are Cleverer*, trans. Harold Cherniss and W. C. Helmbold, LCL 406 (Cambridge, MA, 1957).

Porter, Katherine Anne. *Pale Horse, Pale Rider*, in *Pale Horse, Pale Rider: Three Short Novels* (New York, 1964, 1st edn, 1936).

Processo agli untori: Milano 1630: Cronaca e atti giuriziari in edizione integrale, ed. Giuseppe Farinelli and Ermanno Paccagnini (Milan, 1988).

Procopius, *History of the Wars*, I: *Books 1–2 (Persian War)*, trans. H. B. Dewing, LCL 48 (Cambridge, MA, 1914); II: *Books 5–6.15 (Gothic War)*, trans. H. B. Dewing, LCL 107 (Cambridge, MA, 1916).

Prudentius. Vol. 2: *Crowns of Martyrdom*, trans. H. J. Thomson, LCL 398 (Cambridge, MA, 1953).

Pucci, Antonio. 'Come in questo quadro delle crudeltà della pestilenza', in *Storia Letteraria d'Italia*, ed. Natalino Sapegno (Milan, 1948).

Pseudo-Dionysius of Tel-Mahre: Chronicle, Part III, transl. Witold Witakowsk, Translated Texts for Historians, 22 (Liverpool, 1997).

Quinn, Reverend Denis Alphonsus. *Heroes and Heroines of Memphis or Reminisces of the epidemics... of 1873, 1878 and 1879* (Providence, RI, 1887).

[Quintilian], *The Lesser Declamations*, II, trans. E. R. Shackleton Bailey, LCL 501 (Cambridge, MA 2006).

Quintus Curtius, *History of Alexander*, II: *Books 6–10*, trans. J. C. Rolfe, LCL 369 (Cambridge, MA, 1946).

Raymond of Capua, *The Life of St Catherine of Siena*, trans. George Lamb (London, 1960).

Remains of Old Latin, II: Pacuvius, *Tragedies*, trans. E. H. Warmington, LCL 314 (Cambridge, MA, 1936).

Remede tres salutaire contre le mal françois (Nîmes: Guido Malignan, 1591).

'La Repubblica di Lucca: Provissioni... alla difesa delle meretrici, 1552 e 1534', in Corradi, 'Nuovi documenti', XLVI, 376.

Ripamonti, Giuseppe. *La Peste di Milano del 1630*, ed. Francesco Cusani (Milan, 1841).

Ripamonti, Giuseppe. *La Peste di Milano del 1630: De peste quae fuit anno MDCXXX libri V*, ed. Cesare Reposi, trans. Stefano Corsi (Milan, 2009).

Rocznik Miechowski, 880–96, and 947–1434, ed. A. Bielowski, in *Monumenta Poloniae historica* [series I], 2 (Lvov, 1872).

Rogers, Sir Leonard. 'Cholera Incidence in India in Relation to Rainfall, Absolute Humidity and Pilgrimages: Inoculation of Pilgrims as a Preventive Measure', *Transactions of the Royal Society of Tropical Medicine and Hygiene*, 38 (1944): 73–94.

Rondelet, Guillaume. *Methodus curandorum omnium morborum corporis humani in tres libros distincta. [...] De morbo Gallico...* (Paris: Apud Carolum Macaeum... 1574).

Rondeletti, Guilelmus. *De Morbo Gallico*, in *Appendici*, ed. Luisini, II, 77–93.

Rostinio [also Rostini, Rossettini, and Rositini], Pietro. *Trattato del Mal Francese...: raccolto da quanti n'hanno scritto, e in particolar dal Brasavola...* (Venice: Giorgio de' Cavalli 1565).

Rubys, Claude. *Discours sur la contagion de peste qui a esté ceste presente annee en la ville de Lyon* (Lyon: Par Jean d'Ogerolles, 1577).

Rudio, Eustachio. *De morbo Gallico Libri quinque* (Venice: Apud Damianum Zenarium, 1604).

Sacchi, G. 'Relazione della commissione sanitaria di Milano sul cholera-morbus nell'anno 1855', *Annali universali di statistica economia pubblica*, 6, f. 16 (1855): 445–6.

Sanuto, Marino. *Vitæ Ducum Venetorum italice scriptæ ab origine urbis, sive ab Anno CCCXXI usque ad Annum MCCCCXCIII*, in RIS, XXII (Milan, 1733).

Schellig, Konrad. *Consilium breve contra malas pustulas*, in *Aphrodisiacus*, 41.

Schivenoglia, Andrea. *Cronaca di Mantova dal 1445 al 1484*, ed. Carlo d'Arco (Mantua, 1857).

'The Seistan Plague Riot', *Lancet*, 167 (26 May 1906): 1506–7.

Serao, Matilde. *Il Ventre di Napoli*, 2nd edn (Naples, 1906).

Shapter, Thomas. *History of the Cholera in Exeter* in 1832 (London, 1849; reprinted, 1971).

Shrimpton, Charles and Lionel Smith. *Cholera: Its Seat, Nature, and Treatment* (London, 1866).

Sigismondo dei Conti da Foligno. *Le Storie de' suoi tempi dal 1475 al 1510*, trans. D. Zanelli and F. Calabro, 2 vols (Rome, 1883).

Somaglia, Carlo Girolamo Cavatio della. *Alleggiamento dello stato di Milano per Le imposte e loro ripartimenti* (Milan: Reg. Duc. Corte, Gio. Battista e Giulio Cesare Malatesta, 1653).

Sophocles. I: *Ajax, Electra, Oedipus Tyrannus*, trans. Hugh Lloyd-Jones, LCL 20 (Cambridge, MA, 1994).

Sozomen. *The Ecclesiastical History…a History of the Church, from A.D. 324 to A.D. 440*, trans. E. Walford (London, 1855).

Spaccini, Giovan Battista. *Cronaca di Modena anni 1630–1636*, ed. Rolando Bussi and Carlo Giovannini, Materiali per la storia di Modena: Medievale e Moderna, XIX, 2 vols (Modena, 2008).

The Statistical Accounts of Scotland: Accounts of 1834–45, XV [Edina, online edition].

Stefani, Marchionne di Coppo. *Cronica fiorentina*, ed. Niccolò Rodolico, RIS, XXX/1 (Città di Castello, 1903).

Storia della città di Parma continuata da Angelo Pezzana, 1: *1346–1400*, ed. P. Ireneo Affò (Parma, 1837).

Storie Pistoresi [MCCC–MCCCXLVIII]. Ed. Silvio Adrasto Barbi, RIS, 11/5 (Città di Castello, 1907).

Stumpf, Iannes. *Löblicher Eydgenossenschafft Chronik* (Zurich, 1548).

Suau, Jean. *Traitez contenans la pure et vraye doctrine de la peste & de la Coqueluche, Les impostures Spagyriques & plusieurs abus de la Medecine, Chirurgie, & Pharmacie, tres doctes & tres-utiles* (Paris: Didier Millot, 1586).

Suetonius. *Lives of the Caesars*, trans. J. C. Rolfe, LCL 31 and 38 (Cambridge, MA, 1914).

Symphorianus Champerius. *De lichen seu mentagra, sive pudendagra, quam nostri Neapolitanum morbum vocant, Itali vero Gallicum*, in *Aphrodisiacus*, 128–9.

Ein Syphilis-Consilium von Doktor med. Thomas von Hochberg aus dem Jahre 1503, in *Studien zur Geschichte der Medizin*, Heft 9: *Karl Sudhoff, Aus der Frühgeschichte der Syphilis* (Leipzig, 1912), 137–40.

Tacitus. *Histories*, III: *Books 4–5*, trans. Clifford H. Moore and John E. Jackson, LCL 249 (Cambridge, MA, 1931).

Tadino, Alessandro. *Raguaglio dell'origine et giornali successi della Gran Peste: Contagiosa, Venefica & Malefica seguita nella cittdi Milano & suo Ducato dall'anno 1629 sino all'anno 1632…* (Milan: Per Filippo Ghisolfi, 1653, first published in 1648).

Taylor, John. *The Fearfull Summer, or London's Calamitie* (Oxford, 1625).

Theodosius. *Medicinales Espistolae LXVIII* (1553), in *Aphrodisiacus*, 140–1.

Thomas Philologus. *Mali Glaeci Sanandi, Vini Ligni, & aquae: Unctionis, Ceroti, Suffumigii, Praecipitati, ac Regliquorum modi omnes* (Venice: Ioan. Ant. Nicolinis de Sabio, 1538).

Thucydides. *History of the Peloponnesian War*, I: *Books I and II*, trans. C. Forster Smith, LCL 108 (Cambridge, MA, 1919).

Tomitano, Bernardino. *De Morbo Gallico*, in Luisini, II, 58–75.

Torella. *De pudendagra: tractatus unus*, in Luisini, I, 421–9.

Torella. *De dolore in pudendagra, Dialogus*, in Lusini, I, 429–53.

Torella. *De Ulceribus in Pugendagra*, in Luisini, I, 453–69.

Torella. *Adversus Pudendagram*, in Luisini, I, 469–76.

'Le Triomphe de très haulte et puissante dame Verolle, royne dy puy d'Amours, nouvellement composé par l'inventeur des menus plaisirs honnestes', in *Recueil de poesies françoises des XVe et XVIe siècles*, ed. M. Anatole de Montaiglon (Paris, 1856).

Türr, Stefania. 'Un'eroina della Guerra', *La Madre Italiana: Rivista Mensile* (October 1918), 439–41.

UNAIDS Gap Report. Available online at <http://www.unaids.org/sites/default/files/media_asset/UNAIDS_Gap_report_en>.

Usque, Samuel. *Consolação ás Tribulações de Israel* (Ferrara, 1553).

Valerius Maximus. *Memorable Doings and Sayings*, I: *Books 1–5*, trans. D. R. Shackleton Bailey, LCL 492 (Cambridge, MA, 2000).

van Reygersbergen, Johan. *Cronijck van Zeelandt*, 2nd edn, corrected by Marcus van Boxhorn (Middleberg, 1644; 1st edn, 1551).

Vergesaci, Antonio Chalmetei. *Liber, ex Enchiridio ipsius Chirurgico excerptus*, in Luisini, II, appendice, 1–8.

Villalba, Joaquin de. *Epidemiologia española, ó historia cronológica de las pestes…*, 2 vols (Madrid, 1803).

Villani, Matteo. *Cronica con la continuazione di Filippo Villani*, ed. Giuseppe Porta, 2 vols (Parma, 1995).

Virgil, *Aeneid: Books 1–6*, trans. H. Rushton Fairclough and G. P. Goold, LCL 63 (Cambridge, MA, 1999).

Visconti, Filippo. *Commentarius de peste quae anno domini MXCXXX Mediolani saeviit*, in *Archivio Storico Italiano*, ed. F. Polidori, I, Appendice IX (1842–3): 487–514.

Vochs, Ioannes. *De pestilentia anni presentis* (1507), in *Aphrodisiacus*, 120–1.

Von Hutten, Ulrich. *De guaiaici medicina et morbo gallico liber unus* (Mainz: cum priuilegio Caesareo Sexenni, 1519).

Vvendelini, Hick de Brackenav. *De Morbo Gallico, Opus*, in *Aphrodisiacus*, 268–96.

'Was sagen die altesten gedruckten französischen Chroniken von der Franzosenkrankheit bsw. vom "Mal de Naples"? Das "Remede contre la grosse verolle" von Lyon, 1501', in *Aus der Frühgeschichte der Syphilis*, ed. Karl Sudhoff, *Studien zur Geschichte der Medizin*, Heft 9 (Leipzig, 1912), 154–8.

Weiss, Ernst. *Georg Letham: Physician and Murderer* (Vienna, 1931 [2010]).

Welkenhuysen, Andries. 'La Peste en Avignon (1348) décrite par un témoin oculaire, Louis Sanctus de Beringen (édition critique, traduction, éléments de commentaire)', in *Pascua Mediaevalia: Studies voor Prof. J. M. De Smet*, ed. R. Lievensm, E. Van Mingroot, and W. Verbeke (Leuven, 1983).

Wells, H. G. *The War of the Worlds* (London, 1898).

Die Weltchronik des Mönchs Albert, 1273/77–1454/56, ed. Rolf Sprandel, MGH, Scriptores rerum Germanicarum in usum scholarum, new ser., XVII (Munich, 1994).

Wilkinson, Major E. *Report on Plague and Inoculation in the Punjab from Oct. 1st to Sept. 30 1901* (Lahore, 1903).

SECONDARY SOURCES

Aberth, John. *Plagues in World History* (Lanham, MD, 2011).

Abu-Lughod, Janet L. *Race, Space, and Riots in Chicago, New York, and Los Angeles* (Oxford, 2009).

Ackerknecht, Erwin H. 'Anticontagionism between 1821 and 1867: The Fielding H. Garrison Lecture', *BHM*, 22 (1948): 462–93.

Ackerknecht, Erwin H. *History and Geography of the Most Important Diseases* (New York, 1965).

Ackerknecht, Erwin H. *Medicine and Ethnology: Selected Essays*, ed. H. H. Walser and H. M. Koelbing (Baltimore, MD, 1971).

Adam-Smith, Derek and Fiona Goss. 'Opportunity Lost: HIV/AIDS, Disability and Legislation', in *AIDS: Activism and Alliances*, 25–40.

Aggleton, Peter. Series Editor's Preface to Social Aspects of AIDS series, in Altman, *Power and Community*, vii.

Aggleton, Peter, Peter Davies, and Graham Hart (eds.). *AIDS: Activism and Alliances* (London, 1997).

Aggleton, Peter, Peter Davies, and Graham Hart (eds.). *Families and Communities Responding to AIDS,* Social Aspects of AIDS Series (London, 1999).

Alcamo, Edward. *AIDS in the Modern World* (Malden, MA, 2002).

Alcamo, Edward. 'Smallpox in Colonial Latin America', in *Encyclopedia of Pestilence, Pandemics, and Plagues,* II, 659–62.

Alchon, Suzanne Austin. *A Pest in the Land: New World Epidemics in a Global Perspective* (Albuquerque, NM, 2003).

Alexander, John T. *Bubonic Plague in Early Modern Russia: Public Health & Urban Disaster* (Baltimore, MD, 1980).

Alfani, Guido. *Il Grand Tour dei Cavalieri dell'Apocalisse: L'Italia del 'lungo Cinquecento' (1494–1629)* (Venice, 2010).

Alfani, Guido. 'The Famine of the 1590s in Northern Italy: The Analysis of the Greatest "System Shock" in the Sixteenth Century', *Histoire & Mesure,* 26 (2011): 17–50.

Alfani, Guido and Samuel K. Cohn, Jr. 'Nonantola 1630: Anatomia di una pestilenza e meccanismi del contagio (con riflessioni a partire dalle epidemie milanesi della prima Età Moderna)', *Popolazione e Storia,* 8 (2007): 99–138.

Alfani, Guido and Alessia Melegaro. *Pandemie d'Italia: Dalla peste nera all'influenza suina: l'impatto sulla società* (Milan, 2010).

Alonge, R. 'Campani, Niccolò', *Dizionario Biografico degli Italiani,* 17 (Rome, 1974), 404–6.

Altman, Dennis. *AIDS in the Mind of America: The Social, Political, and Psychological Impact of a New Epidemic* (Garden City, NY, 1986).

Altman, Dennis. 'Gays Testify on Homophobic Violence', *The Advocate,* 11 November 1986.

Altman, Dennis. *Power and Community: Organizational and Cultural Responses to AIDS* (London, 1994).

Altman, Dennis. 'Legitimation through Disaster: AIDS and the Gay Movement', in *AIDS: The Burdens of History,* ed. Elizabeth Fee and Daniel M. Fox (Berkeley, 1988), 301–15.

Altman, Dennis et al. 'Men Who Have Sex with Men: Stigma and Discrimination', *Lancet,* 380/9839 (28 July–3 August 2012): 439–45.

Amelang, James S. *A Journal of the Plague Year: The Diary of the Barcelona Tanner Miquel Parets 1651* (New York, 1991).

Andrews, Margaret W. 'Epidemics and Public Health: Influenza in Vancouver, 1918–1919', *British Columbia Studies,* 34 (1977): 21–44.

Annuario Generale dei communi e delle frazioni d'Italia (Turin, 1985).

Archambeau, Nicole. 'Healing Options during the Plague: Survivor Stories from a Fourteenth-Century Canonization Inquest', *BMH,* 85 (2011): 531–59.

Arnold, David. 'Smallpox and Colonial Medicine in Nineteenth-Century India', in *Imperial Medicine and Indigenous Societies,* ed. David Arnold (Manchester, 1988).

Arnold, David. *Colonizing the Body: State Medicine and Epidemic Disease in Nineteenth-Century India* (Berkeley, 1993).

Arnold, David. 'The Rise of Western Medicine in India', *Lancet,* 348 (19 October 1996): 1075–8.

Arnold, Klaus. 'Pest—Geißler—Judenmorde: Das Beispiel Würzburg', in *Strukturen der Gesellschaft im Mittelalter: Interdisziplinäre Mediävistik in Würzburg,* ed. Dieter Rödel and Joachim Schneider (Wiesbaden, 1996), 358–69.

Arrizabalaga, Jon. 'Medical Responses to the "French Disease" in Europe at the Turn of the Sixteenth Century', in *Sins of the Flesh: Responding to Sexual Disease in Early Modern Europe,* ed. Kevin Siena (Toronto, 2005), 33–55.

Arrizabalaga, Jon, John Henderson, and Roger French. *The Great Pox: The French Disease in Renaissance Europe* (New Haven, CT, 1997).

Avrich, Paul. *Russian Rebels 1600–1800* (New York, 1972).

Baehrel, René. 'Epidémie et terreur: histoire et sociologie', *Annales historiques de la Révolution française*, 23 (1951): 113–22.

Baehrel, René. 'La haine de classe en temps d'épidémie', *Annales: E.S.C.*, 7 (1952): 351–60.

Bailey, Gauvin et al. *Hope and Healing: Painting in Italy in a Time of Plague, 1500–1800* (Worcester, MA, 2005).

Baker, Thomas H. 'Yellow Jack: The Yellow Fever Epidemic of 1878 in Memphis, Tennessee', *BMH*, 42 (1968): 241–64.

Baldwin, Peter. *Contagion and the State in Europe, 1830–1930* (Cambridge, 1999).

Baldwin, Peter. *Disease and Democracy: The Industrialized World Faces AIDS* (Berkeley, 2005).

Barber, Malcolm. 'Lepers, Jews and Moslems: The Plot to Overthrow Christendom in 1321', *History*, 66 (1981): 1–17.

Bardot, J.-P., P. Bourdelais, P. Guillaume, F. Lebrun, and C. Quétel (eds.). *Peurs et terreurs face à la contagion* (Paris, 1988).

Bar-Kochva, Bezalel. *The Image of the Jews in Greek Literature: The Hellenistic Period* (Berkeley, 2010).

Baron, Salo. *A Social and Religious History of the Jews*, XIII: *Inquisition, Renaissance, and Reformation*, 2nd edn (New York, 1969).

Barrett, Ron. 'The 1994 Plague in Western India: Human Ecology and the Risks of Misattribution', in *Terrorism, War, or Disease? Unraveling the Use of Biological Weapons*, ed. Anne Clunan, Peter Lavoy, and Susan Martin (Stanford, CA, 2008), 49–71.

Barry, John M. *The Great Influenza: The Story of the Deadliest Pandemic in History*, 2nd edn (New York, 2005).

Bayer, Ronald. 'The Dependent Center: The First Decade of the AIDS Epidemic in New York City', in *Hives of Sickness*, 131–50.

Baylies, Carolyn. 'Community-Based Research on AIDS in the Context of Global Inequalities—Making a Virtue of Necessity?', in *HIV and AIDS in Africa: Beyond Epidemiology*, ed. Ezekiel Kalipeni, Susan Craddock, Josephus R. Oppong, and Jauati Ghosh (Malden, MA, 2004), 229–39.

Beauvieux, Fleur. 'Expériences ordinaires de la peste: La société marseillaise en temps d'épidémie (1720–1724)', thèse dirigée par Jean Boutier, École des Hautes Études en Sciences Sociales, Centre Norbert Élias (2017).

Bellickfeb, Pam. 'Red Cross Faces Attacks at Ebola Victims' Funerals', *New York Times*, 12 February 2015.

Benadusi, Giovanna. *A Provincial Elite in Early Modern Tuscany: Family and Power in the Creation of the State* (Baltimore, MD, 1996).

Benedict, Carol. *Bubonic Plague in Nineteenth Century China* (Stanford, CA, 1996).

Bercé, Yves-Marie. *Le chaudron et la lancette* (Paris, 1984).

Bercé, Yves-Marie. *Revolt and Revolution in Early Modern Europe: An Essay on the History of Political Violence*, trans. Joseph Bergin (Manchester, 1987 [1980]).

Bercé, Yves-Marie. 'Les semeurs de peste', in *La vie, la mort, la foi, le temps: Mélanges offerts à Pierre Chaunu*, ed. Jean-Pierre Bardet and Madeleine Foisil (Paris, 1993), 85–94.

Berco, Cristian. 'Syphilis, Sex, and Marriage in Early Modern Spain', *Journal of Early Modern History*, 15 (2011): 223–53.

Berridge, Virginia. 'AIDS: History and Contemporary History', in *The Time of AIDS: Social Analysis, Theory, and Method*, ed. Gilbert Herdt and Shirley Lindenbaum (Newbury

Park, CA, 1992), 41–64; and introduction to *AIDS and Contemporary History*, ed. Virginia Berridge and Philip Strong (Cambridge, 1993), 1–14.

Bertolli, Franco and Umberto Colombo. 'Capitoli introduttivi', in Lupi, *Storia della Peste*.

Bewell, Alan. *Romanticism and Colonial Disease* (Baltimore, MD, 2000).

Bilson, Geoffrey. *A Darkened House: Cholera in Nineteenth-Century Canada* (Toronto, 1980).

Biographie universelle (Michaud) ancienne et moderne, new edn, 45 vols (Paris, 1843–65).

Biraben, J.-N. *Les hommes et la peste en France et dans les pays européens et méditerranéens*, II: *Les hommes face à la peste*, 2 vols, Civilisations et sociétés 36 (Paris, 1975–6).

Black, David. *The Plague Years: A Chronicle of AIDS, The Epidemic of Our Times* (New York, 1986).

Blasucci, Antonio. 'Colomba, da Rieti, beata, 1467–1501', *BS*, IV, cols 101–3.

Bliss, Michael. *Plague: A Story of Smallpox in Montreal* (Toronto, 1991).

Bloch, Iwan. 'The History of Syphilis', in *A System of Syphilis in Six Volumes*, ed. D'Arcy Power and J. Keogh Murphy (London, 1908–10), 3–19.

Bloch, Marc. *Les caractères originaux de l'histoire rurale française*, 2nd edn (Paris, 1955).

Bloom, Khaled J. *The Mississippi Valley's Great Yellow Fever Epidemic of 1878* (Baton Rouge, LA, 1993).

Blume, Stuart. 'Anti-Vaccination Movements and their Interpretations', *Social Science & Medicine*, 62 (2006): 628–42.

Boeckl, Christine M. *Images of Leprosy: Disease, Religion, and Politics in European Art* (Kirksville, MO, 2011).

Bollea, Luigi. 'Untori piemontesi e untori milanesi nella peste manzoniana del 1630', *Bollettino Storico Bibliografico Subalpino*, 27 (1925): 3–19.

Bollet, Alfred Jay. *Plagues & Poxes: The Impact of Human History on Epidemic Disease*, 2nd edn (New York, 2004).

Bonderup, Gerda. *Cholera-Morbo'er og Danmark: Billeder til det 19. arhundredes samfunds-og kulturhistorie* (Aarhus, 1994).

Bootsma, Martin and Neil Ferguson. 'The Effect of Public Health Measures on the 1918 Influenza Pandemic in U.S. Cities', *PNAS*, 104/18 (1 May 2007): 7588–93.

Bornstein, Daniel E. *The Bianchi of 1399: Popular Devotion in Late Medieval Italy* (Ithaca, NY, 1993).

Bourdelais, Patrice and Jean-Yves Raulot. *Une Peur Bleue: Histoire du choléra en France 1832–1854* (Paris, 1987).

Bowsky, William. 'The Impact of the Black Death upon Sienese Government and Society', *Speculum*, 39 (1964): 1–34.

Bowsky, William. 'The Medieval Commune and Internal Violence: Police Power and Public safety in Siena, 1287–1355', *American Historical Review*, 73 (1967): 1–18.

Brading, D. A. *The First America: The Spanish Monarchy, Creole Patriots, and the Liberal State 1492–1867* (Cambridge, 1991), 31–44.

Braid, Robert. '"Et non ultra": politiques royales du travail en Europe Occidentale au XIVe siècle', *Bibliothèque de l'École des Chartes*, 161 (2003): 437–91.

Braid, Robert. 'Peste, prolétaires et politiques: la législation du travail et les politiques économiques en angleterre aux XIIIeme et XIVeme siècles'. PhD, Université Paris, 2 vols (Paris 7, 2008).

Brandt, A. M. *No Magic Bullet: A Social History of Venereal Disease in the U.S. since 1880* (New York, 1985; revised edition, 1987).

Brandt, A. M. 'AIDS: From Social History to Social Policy', in *AIDS: The Burdens of History*, ed. Elizabeth Fee and Daniel M. Fox (Berkeley, 1988), 147–71.

Brandt, A. M. 'How AIDS Invented Global Health', *New England Journal of Medicine*, 368/23 (6 June 2013): 2149–52.

Brandt, A. M. 'Aids and Metaphor: Toward the Social Meaning of Epidemic Disease', in *Time of Plague*, 91–110.

Brandt, A. M. 'Plagues and Peoples: the AIDS Epidemic', in *No Magic Bullet*, 183–204.

Braudel, Fernand and Frank Spooner, 'Prices in Europe from 1450 to 1750', in *The Cambridge Economic History of Europe*, vol. VI, ed. E. E. Rich and C. H. Wilson (Cambridge, 1967), 374–486.

Bresalier, Michael. 'Uses of a Pandemic: Forging the Identities of Influenza and Virus Research in Interwar Britain', *SHM*, 25 (2011): 400–24.

Breuer, Mordechai. 'The "Black Death" and Antisemitism', in *Antisemitism through the Ages*, ed. Shmuel Almog and trans. Nathan H. Reisner (Exeter, 1988), 139–51.

Briese, Olaf. *Angst in den Zeiten der Cholera*, 4 vols (Berlin, 2003).

Briggs, Charles L. 'Theorizing Modernity Conspiratorially: Science, Scale, and the Political Economy of Public Discourse in Explanations of a Cholera Epidemic', *American Ethnologist*, 31 (2004): 164–87.

Bristow, Nancy K. *American Pandemic: The Lost Worlds of the 1918 Influenza Epidemic* (Oxford, 2012).

Bristow, Nancy K. ' "You Can't Do Anything for Influenza": Doctors, Nurses and the Power of Gender during the Influenza Pandemic in the United States', in *The Spanish Influenza Pandemic of 1918–19*, 58–69.

Bujra, Janet M. and Carolyn Baylies. 'Solidarity and Stress: Gender and Local Mobilization in Tanzania and Zambia', in *Families and Communities Responding to AIDS*, 35–52.

Burgard, Friedhelm et al. (eds.). *Hochfinanz im Westen des Reiches, 1150–1500* (Trier, 1996).

Burnet, Frank MacFarlane and Ellen Clark. *Influenza* (Melbourne, 1942).

Burnett, Kirstin. 'Race, Disease, and Public Violence: Smallpox and the (Un)Making of Calgary's Chinatown, 1892', *SHM*, 25 (2012): 362–79.

Burnham, John. *How Superstition Won and Science Lost: Popularizing Science and Health in the United States* (New Brunswick, NJ, 1987).

Burrell, Sean. 'The Irish Cholera Epidemic of 1831–2: Riots, Catholicism and the Wake', in *Cholera and Conflict*, 224–67.

Butler's Lives of the Saints, rev. Paul Burns et al., 12 vols (Tunbridge Wells, 1995–2000).

Byrne, J. P. (ed.). *Encyclopedia of Pestilence, Pandemics, and Plagues*, 2 vols (Westport, CT, 2008).

Cady, Diane. 'Linguistic Dis-ease: Foreign Language as Sexual Disease in Early Modern England', in *Sins of the Flesh: Responding to Sexual Disease in Early Modern Europe*, ed. Kevin Siena (Toronto, 2005), 159–86.

Calvi, Giulia. 'The Florentine Plague of 1630–33: Social Behaviour and Symbolic Action', in *Maladies et société (XIIe–XVIIIe siècles): Actes du colloque de Bielefeld novembre 1986*, ed. Neithard Bulst and Robert Delort (Paris, 1989), 327–36.

Cameron, Alan. *Circus Factions: Blues and Greens at Rome and Byzantium* (Oxford, 1976).

Cameron, Charles Alexander. *History of the Royal College of Surgeons in Ireland* (Dublin, 1886).

Cantù, Cesare. *Sulla storia Lombarda del secolo XVII: Ragionamenti...per commento agli Promessi sposi*, 5th edn (Lugano, 1833).

Caraffa, Filippo (ed.). *Bibliotheca sanctorum*. Istituto Giovanni XXIII nella Pontificia Universita lateranense (Rome, 1961–87) [hereafter *BS*].

Carmichael, Ann G. *Plague and the Poor in Renaissance Florence* (Cambridge, 1986).

Carmichael, Ann G. and A. M. Silverstein. 'Smallpox in Europe before the Seventeenth Century: Virulent Killer or Benign Disease?', *Journal of the History of Medical and Allied Sciences*, 42 (1987): 147–68.

Carrigan, Jo Ann. 'Yellow Fever: Scourge of the South', in Joann P. Krieg, *Epidemics in the Modern World* (New York, 1992), 55–78.

Carrigan, Jo Ann. *The Saffron Scourge: A History of Yellow Fever in Louisiana, 1796–1905* (Lafayette, LA, 1994).

Casper, Virginia. 'AIDS: A Psychosocial Perspective', in *The Social Dimensions of AIDS: Method and Theory*, ed. Douglas A. Feldman and Thomas M. Johnson (New York, 1986), 197–209.

Cassiano da Langasco, Mecatti. 'Gerardo, beato', *BS*, IX, 257–8.

Castiglione Trovato, Carmela, 'Introduzione' to Michele Amari, *Descrizione del cholera di Sicilia* (Naples, 1990).

Catanach, Ian. 'Fatalism? Indian Responses to Plague and Other Crises', *Asian Profile*, 12 (1984): 183–92.

Catanach, Ian. 'Poona Politicians and the Plague', *South Asia*, 7 (1984): 1–18.

Catanach, Ian. 'Plague and the Tensions of Empire: India 1896–1918', in *Imperial Medicine and Indigenous Societies*, ed. David Arnold (Manchester, 1988), 149–71.

Chandavarkar, Rajnarayan. 'Plague Panic and Epidemic Politics in India, 1896–1914', in *Epidemics and Ideas*, 203–40; reprinted in Chandavarkar, *Imperial Power and Popular Politics: Class, Resistance and the State in India, c. 1850–1950* (Cambridge, 1998), ch. 7.

Chase, Marilyn. *The Barbary Plague: The Black Death in San Francisco* (New York, 2003).

Chevalier, Louis (ed.), *La première épidémie du XIXe siècle* (La Roche-sur-Yon, 1958).

Cipolla, Carlo. *Faith, Reason, and the Plague: A Tuscan Story of the Seventeenth Century*, trans. Muriel Kittel (Brighton, 1977).

Clark, Fiona. 'Gaps Remain in Russia's Response to HIV/AIDS', *Lancet*, 388/10047 (27 August 2016): 857–8.

Clarke, Graeme. 'Third-Century Christianity', in *Cambridge Ancient History*, XII: *The Crisis of Empire, CE 193–337*, ed. A. K. Bowman, P. Garnsey, and A. Cameron, 2nd edn (Cambridge, 2005), 589–671.

Clemens, John D., et al. 'Cholera', *Lancet*, 390 (23 September 2017): 1539–49.

Codero, Franco. *La Fabbrica della peste* (Bari, 1984).

Cogan, Jeanne and Gregory Herek, 'Stigma', in *Encyclopedia of AIDS*, 466–7.

Cohn, Jr., Samuel K. *The Black Death Transformed: Disease and Culture in Early Renaissance Europe* (London, 2002).

Cohn, Jr., Samuel K. *Lust for Liberty: The Politics of Social Revolt in Medieval Europe, 1200–1425* (Cambridge, MA, 2006).

Cohn, Jr., Samuel K. 'After the Black Death: Labour Legislation and Attitudes towards Labour in Late-Medieval Western Europe', *Economic History Review*, 60/3 (2007): 457–85.

Cohn, Jr., Samuel K. 'The Black Death and the Burning of Jews', *Past & Present*, 196 (August 2007): 3–36.

Cohn, Jr., Samuel K. 'Changing Pathology of Plague', in *XLI Settimana di Studi: Le interazioni fra economia e ambiente biologico nell'Europa preindustriale, Secc. XIII–XVIII (Prato, 26–30 aprile 2009)*, ed. Simonetta Cavaciocchi (Florence, 2010), 33–56.

Cohn, Jr., Samuel K. *Cultures of Plague: Medical Thinking at the End of the Renaissance* (Oxford, 2010).

Cohn, Jr., Samuel K. 'Review of Shona Kelly Wray, *Communities and Crisis*', *Speculum*, 86 (2011): 1136–8.

Cohn, Jr., Samuel K. *Popular Protest in Late Medieval English Towns* (Cambridge, 2013).

Cohn, Jr., Samuel K. 'Cholera Riots: A Class Struggle We May Not Like', *Social History*, 42/2 (May 2017): 1–19.

Cohn, Jr., Samuel K. and Guido Alfani. 'Households and Plague in Early Modern Italy', *Journal of Interdisciplinary History*, 38 (2007): 177–205.

Cohn, Jr., Samuel K. and Ruth Kutalek, 'Historical Parallels, Ebola and Cholera: Understanding Community Distrust and Social Violence with Epidemics', *PLOS: Current Outbreaks* (26 January 2016), 8 pp.

Colgrove, J. K. 'Between Persuasion and Compulsion: Smallpox Control in Brooklyn and New York, 1894-1902', *BHM*, 78 (2004): 349–78.

Collier, Richard. *The Plague of the Spanish Lady: The Influenza Pandemic of 1918–1919* (London, 1974).

Commager, Jr., H. S. 'Lucretius' Interpretation of the Plague', *Harvard Studies in Classical Philology*, 62 (1957): 105–18.

Conner, Susan P. 'The Pox in Eighteenth-Century France', in *The Secret Malady*, 15–33.

Connolly, S. J. 'The "Blessed Turf": Cholera and Popular Panic in Ireland, June 1832', *Irish Historical Studies*, 23 (1983): 214–32.

Cook, S. F. 'The Smallpox Epidemic of 1797 in Mexico', *BHM*, 7 (1939): 739–69.

Corbin, Alain. 'La grande peur de la syphilis', in *Peurs et terreurs face à la contagion*, 328–48.

Corbin, Alain. *Women for Hire: Prostitution and Sexuality in France after 1850*, trans. Alan Sheridan (Cambridge, MA, 1990).

Corradi, Alfonso. *Annali delle epidemie occorse in Italia dalle prime memorie fino al 1850*, 5 vols (Bologna, 1865–94).

Corradi, Alfonso. 'Nuovi documenti per la storia delle malattie veneree in Italia dalla fine del quattrocento alla metà del cinquecento', *Annali universali di medicina e chirurgia*, 269 (1884).

Cosmacini, Giorgio. *Medicina e sanità in Italia nel ventesimo secolo: dalla 'Spagnola' alla II guerra mondiale* (Bari, 1989).

Cottignoli, Alfredo. 'Il Trattato e l'inchiesta: Peste e unti dal Muratori al Manzoni', in *Il Buon Uso della Paura: Per una introduzione allo studio del trattato muratoriano 'Del Governo della Peste'* (Florence, 1990), 65–73.

Craddock, Susan. *City of Plagues: Disease, Poverty, and Deviance in San Francisco* (Minneapolis, MN, 2000).

Crawford, E. Margaret (ed.). *The Hungry Stream: Essays on Emigration and Famine* (Belfast, 1997).

Crawford, E. Margaret. 'Typhus in Nineteenth-Century Ireland', in *Medicine, Disease and the State in Ireland, 1650–1940*, ed. Greta Jones and Elizabeth Malcolm (Cork, 1999), 121–37.

Creighton, Charles. *History of Epidemics in Britain*, ed. D. E. C. Eversley, 2 vols (London, 1965; original, Cambridge, 1891–4).

Crosby, Alfred W. 'Smallpox', in *The Cambridge World History of Human Disease*, ed. Kenneth F. Kiple (Cambridge, 1993), 1008–13.

Crosby, Alfred W. 'Smallpox: "There Never Was a Cure"', in *Plague, Pox & Pestilence*, ed. Kenneth F. Kiple (London, 1997), 74–9.

Crosby, Alfred W. *America's Forgotten Pandemic: The Influenza of 1918*, 2nd edn (Cambridge, 2003).

Crosby, Alfred W. 'Hawaiian Depopulation as a Model for the Amerindian Experience', in *Epidemics and Ideas*, 175–201.

Crosby, Molly C. *The American Plague: The Untold Story of Yellow Fever* (New York, 2006).

Cueto, Marco. *The Return of Epidemics: Health and Society in Peru during the Twentieth Century* (Farnham, 2001).

Cueto, Marco. 'Stigma and Blame during an Epidemic: Cholera in Peru, 1991', in *Disease in the History of Modern Latin America: From Malaria to AIDS*, ed. D. Armus (Durham, NC, 2003), 268–89.

Dadrian, V. N. 'The Role of Turkish Physicians in the World War I Genocide of Ottoman Armenians', *Holocaust and Genocide Studies*, 1 (1986): 169–92.

Dadrian, V. N. *History of the Armenian Genocide* (Providence, RI, 1995).

Davidson, Roger and Lesley A. Hall (eds.). *Sex, Sin, and Suffering: Venereal Disease and European Society since 1870* (London, 2001).

Davis, Ryan A. *The Spanish Flu: Narrative and Cultural Identity in Spain, 1918* (Basingstoke, 2013).

de Kruif, Paul. *Microbe Hunters* (London, 1927).

de Waal, Alex. *AIDS and Power: Why there is No Political Crisis—Yet* (London, 2006).

Deacon, Harriet, Leana Uys, and Rakgadi Mohlahlane, 'HIV and Stigma in South Africa', in *HIV/AIDS in South Africa: 25 Years On*, 105–21.

Delaporte, François. *Disease and Civilization*, trans. A. Goldhammer (Cambridge, 1986).

della Perutta, Franco. *Mazzini e i revoluzionari italiani: Il 'partito d'azione' 1830–1845* (Milan, 1974).

della Perutta, Franco. *Società e classi popolari nell'Italia dell' 800* (Milan, 1985).

Delumeau, Jean. *Vie économique et sociale de Rome dans la seconde moitié du XVIe siècle*, 2 vols (Paris, 1957–9).

Delumeau, Jean. *Rassurer et protéger: Le sentiment de securité dans l'Occident d'autrefois* (Paris, 1989).

Demaitre, Luke E. *Leprosy in Premodern Medicine: A Malady of the Whole Body* (Baltimore, MD, 2007).

Dewey, Frank L. 'Thomas Jefferson's Law Practice: The Norfolk Anti-Inoculation Riots', *The Virginia Magazine of History and Biography*, 91 (1983): 39–53.

Dineur, Monique and Charles Engrand, 'Le choléra à Lille', *La première épidémie du XIXe siècle*, 47–95.

Doka, Kenneth J. *AIDS, Fear, and Society: Challenging the Dreaded Disease* (London, 1997).

Dolan, Claire. *La notaire, la famille et la ville (Aix-en-Provence à la fin du XVIe siècle)* (Toulouse, 1998).

Douglas, Paul. 'Wages and Hours of Labour in 1919', *Journal of Political Economy*, 29 (1921): 78–80.

Drummond, A. 'Rome in the Fifth Century: The Social and Economic Framework', *The Cambridge Ancient History*, VII: *The Rise of Rome to 220 B.C.*, ed. F. W. Walbank, A. E. Austin, M. W. Frederiksen, and R. M. Ogilvie, 2nd edn (Cambridge, 1989), 113–71.

Duffy, John. 'Smallpox and the Indians in the American Colonies', *BHM*, 25 (1951): 324–41.

Duffy, John. *Epidemics in Colonial America* (Port Washington, NY, 1953).

Duffy, John. *Sword of Pestilence: The New Orleans Yellow Fever Epidemic of 1853* (Baton Rouge, LA, 1966).

Duffy, John. 'Social Impact of Disease in the Late Nineteenth Century', *Bulletin of the New York Academy of Medicine*, 47 (1971): 797–810.

Duncan-Jones, R. P. 'The Impact of the Antonine Plague', *Journal of Roman Archaeology*, 9 (1996): 108–36.

Durey, Michael. *The Return of the Plague: British Society and the Cholera 1831–2* (Dublin, 1979).

Dutton, Paul E. *Charlemagne's Moustache and Other Cultural Clusters of a Dark Age* (Basingstoke, 2004).

Eamon, William. 'Cannibalism and Contagion: Framing Syphilis in Counter-Reformation Italy', *Early Science and Medicine*, 3 (1998): 1–31.

Echenberg, Myron. *Black Death, White Medicine: Bubonic Plague and the Politics of Public Health in Colonial Senegal, 1914–45* (Portsmouth, NH, 2002).

Echenberg, Myron. *Plague Ports: The Global Urban Impact of Bubonic Plague, 1894–1901* (New York, 2007).

Echenberg, Myron. *Africa in the Time of Cholera: A History of Pandemics from 1817 to the Present* (Cambridge, 2011).

Echenberg, Myron. 'Cholera: Seventh Pandemic, 1961–Present', *Encyclopedia of Pestilence, Pandemics, and Plagues*, I, 114–17.

Echeverri, Beatriz. 'Spanish Influenza Seen from Spain', in *The Spanish Influenza Pandemic of 1918–19*, 173–90, 283–5.

Edward, Lee. *Goldwater: The Man Who Made a Revolution* (Washington, DC, 1995).

Edwards, Mark. 'AIDS Policy Communities in Australia', *AIDS: Activism and Alliances*, 41–58.

El-Bushra, Judy. 'How Should We Understand Sexual Violence and HIV and AIDS in Conflict Contexts?', in *The Fourth Wave*, 245–68.

Ellis, John H. 'Businessmen and Public Health in the Urban South during the Nineteenth Century: New Orleans, Memphis, and Atlanta', part 2, *BMH*, 44 (1970): 197–212.

Emery, Richard W. 'The Black Death of 1348 in Perpignan', *Speculum*, 42 (1967): 611–23.

Emias, Richard. 'Yellow Fever in North American to 1810', in *Encyclopedia of Pestilence, Pandemics, and Plagues*, II, 791–4.

Engelmann, Lukas. 'Photographing AIDS: On Capturing a Disease in Pictures of People with AIDS', *BMH*, 90 (2016): 250–78.

Esch, Arnold. 'Processi medioevali per la cononizzazione di Santa Francesca Romana (1440–1451)', in *La canonizzazione di Santa Francesca Romana: Santità, cultura e istituzioni a Roma tra medioevo ed età moderna. Atti del Convegno internazionale, Roma, 19–21 novembre 2009*, ed. Alessandra Bartolomei Romagnoli and Giorgio Picasso (Florence, 2013), 39–51.

Evans, Richard J. *Death in Hamburg: Society and Politics in the Cholera Years 1830–1910* (Oxford, 1987).

Evans, Richard J. 'Epidemics and Revolutions: Cholera in Nineteenth-Century Europe', in *Epidemics and Ideas*, 149–73.

Evesley, David. 'L'Angleterre', in *La première épidémie du XIXe siècle*, 157–88.

Fabricius, Johannes. *Syphilis in Shakespeare's England* (London, 1994).

Fairhead, James. 'Understanding Social Resistance to Ebola Response in Guinea' (2015), <http://www.ebola-anthropology.net/evidence/1269/>, last accessed 16 September 2015.

Fanning, Patricia J. *Influenza and Inequality: One Town's Tragic Response to the Great Epidemic of 1918* (Amherst, MA, 2010).

Farinelli, Giuseppe. 'Atti del processo agli untori: Ricostruzione e trascrizione integrale, cronologia, note esplicative e filologiche', in *Processo agli untori*, 147–82.

Farmer, Paul. *Pathologies of Power: Health, Human Rights, and the New War on the Poor* (Berkeley, 2003).

Farmer, Paul. *AIDS and Accusation: Haiti and the Geography of Blame*, 2nd edn (Berkeley, 2006).

Farmer, Paul, with J. S. Mukherjee, *Haiti after the Earthquake* (New York, 2011).

Fee, Elizabeth and Daniel M. Fox, 'Introduction', in *AIDS: The Burdens of History*, ed. Elizabeth Fee and Daniel M. Fox (Berkeley, 1988).

Feldman, Jamie L. *Plague Doctors: Responding to the AIDS Epidemic in France and America* (Westport, CT, 1995).

Fenn, Elizabeth A. *Pox Americana: The Great Smallpox Epidemic of 1775–82* (New York, 2001).

Fineberg, Harvey V. 'The Social Dimension of AIDS', *Scientific American*, 259 (October, 1988): 106–12.

Foa, Anna. 'The New and the Old: The Spread of Syphilis (1494-1530)', *Sex and Gender in Historical Perpective*, ed. Edward Muir and Guido Ruggiero (Baltimore, MD, 1990), 26–45.

Foa, Anna. *The Jews of Europe after the Black Death*, trans. Andrea Grover (Berkeley, 2000).

Foege, William H. 'Plague: Perceptions of Risk and Social Responses', in *Time of Plague*, 9–20.

Foley, Caitriona. *The Last Irish Plague: The Great Flu Epidemic in Ireland 1918–19* (Dublin, 2011).

Fontenrose, Joseph. *The Delphic Oracle: Its Responses and Operations with a Catalogue of Responses* (Berkeley, 1978).

Fouz-Hernández, Santiago. 'Queer in Spain: Identity without Limits', in *Queer in Europe: Contemporary Case Studies*, ed. Lisa Downing and Robert Gillett (Farnham, 2011), 189–202.

Fox, Daniel M. 'AIDS and the American Health Polity: The History and Prospects of a Crisis of Authority', in *AIDS: The Public Context of an Epidemic* ed. Ronald Bayer, Daniel M. Fox, and David P. Willis, *The Milbank Quarterly*, 64, Supplement 1 (Cambridge, 1986): 7–33.

Fox, Renee C., Linda H. Aiken, and Carla M. Messikomer, 'The Culture of Caring: AIDS and the Nursing Profession', in *A Disease of Society*, 119–49.

Furdell, Elizabeth Lane. *The Royal Doctors 1485–1714: Medical Personnel at the Tudor and Stuart Courts* (Rochester, NY, 2001).

Galishoff, Stuart. 'Newark and the Great Influenza Pandemic of 1918', *BHM*, 43 (1969): 246–58.

Gall, G. E. C. et al., 'Quarantine as a Public Health Measure against an Emerging Infectious Disease: Syphilis in Zurich at the Dawn of the Modern Era (1496–1585)', *GMS Hygiene and Infection Control*, 11 (2016): 1–10.

Gallagher, Nancy. *Egypt's Other Wars: Epidemics and the Politics of Public Health* (Syracuse, NY, 1990).

Gallo, Robert C. and Luc Montagnier. 'The Chronology of AIDS Research', *Nature*, 326 (8 April 1987): 435–6.

Gallo, Robert C. and Luc Montagnier. 'AIDS in 1988', *Scientific American*, 259, 4 (October 1988): 25–32.

Gamsa, Mark. 'The Epidemic of Pneumonic Plague in Manchuria, 1910–1911', *Past and Present*, 190 (2006): 147–83.

García, Mario. *Desert Immigrants: The Mexicans of El Paso, 1880–1920* (New Haven, CT, 1981).

Garnsey, Peter. *Famine and Food Supply in the Graeco-Roman World: Responses to Risk and Crisis* (Cambridge, 1988).

Garrison, Fielding H. 'The Destruction of the Quarantine Station on Staten Island in 1858', *Bulletin of the New York Academy of Medicine*, 2 (1926): 1–4; reprinted, *Journal of Urban Health*, 76 (1999): 380–3.

Gibbs, Frederick. 'Poison Libels and Epidemic Disease', in *Encyclopedia of Pestilence, Pandemics, and Plagues*, II, 544–6.

Gill, Geoffrey and Michael Holland, 'Conclusion: The Cholera Riots in Context', in *Cholera and Conflict*, 331–41.

Gill, Geoffrey, Sean Burrell, and Jody Brown. 'Fear and Frustration—the Liverpool Cholera Riots of 1832', *Lancet*, 358/9277 (21 July 2001), 233–7.

Gilman, Sander. 'AIDS and Syphilis: The Iconography of Disease', *October*, 43 (1987): 87–107.

Ginzburg, Carlo. 'Deciphering the Sabbath', in *Early Modern European Witchcraft: Centres and Peripheries*, ed. B. Ankarloo and G. Henningsen (Oxford, 1990), 121–38.

'Global Epidemics and the Impact of Cholera', WHO website: Health Topics: Cholera (2013).

Goldstein, Richard. 'The Implicated and the Immune Responses to AIDS in the Arts and Popular Culture', in *A Disease of Society*, 17–42.

Gomme, A. W., K. J. Dover, and A. Andrews. *A Historical Commentary on Thucydides: The Ten Years' War*, 5 vols (Oxford, 1956–81).

Goodman, Bryna. *Native Place, City, and Nation: Regional Networks and Identities in Shanghai, 1853–1937* (Berkeley, 1995).

Gostin, Larry. 'The AIDS Litigation Project: A National Review of Court and Human Rights Commission Decisions on Discrimination', in *AIDS: The Making of a Chronic Disease*, ed. Elizabeth Fee and Daniel M. Fox (Berkeley, 1992), 144–69.

Graus, František. *Pest—Geissler—Judenmorde: Das 14. Jahrhundert als Krisenzeit* (Göttingen, 1987).

The Great Irish Famine of 1845–1846: A Collection of Leading Articles, Letters, and Parliamentary and other Public Statements (London, 1880).

Greslou, Nicolas. *La Peste en Savoie (Aux XVIe et XVIIe Siècles)*, Mémories et Documents publiés par la Société d'Histoire et d'Archéologie, LXXXV (Chambéry, 1973), 129–33.

Griffith, Sally F. '"A Total Dissolution of the Bonds of Society": Community Death and Regeneration in Mathew Carey's *Short Account of the Malignant Fever*', in *A Melancholy Scene of Devastation*, 45–59.

Grmek, Mirko D. *Diseases in the Ancient World*, trans. M. Muellner and L. Muellner (Baltimore, MD, 1983).

Grmek, Mirko D. *Histoire di sida: Début et origine d'une pandémie actuelle*, new edition (Paris, 1990).

Gruskin, Sofia. 'Tackling Violence and HIV/AIDS: Global Health Imperatives', *American Journal of Public Health*, 101 (2011): 968.

Guarinieri, Mauro and Lital Hollander, 'From Denver to Dublin: The Role of Civil Society in HIV Treatment and Control', in *HIV/AIDS in Europe*, 86–100.

Guerchberg, Séraphine. 'La controverse sur les prétendus semeurs de la "Peste Noire"', *Revue des études juives*, 108 (1948): 3–40.

Guida d'Italia del Touring Club Italiano: Toscana (Milan, 1974).

Guiral, Pierre. 'Le choléra à Marseille', in *La première épidémie du XIXe siècle*, 121–40.

Gussow, Zachary. *Leprosy, Racism, and Public Health: Social Policy in Chronic Disease Control* (Boulder, CO, 1989).

Gussow, Zachary and George S. Tracy. 'Stigma and the Leprosy Phenomenon: The Social History of a Disease in the Nineteenth and Twentieth Centuries', *BHM*, 44 (1970): 425–49.

Hamlin, Christopher. 'Predisposing Causes and Public Health in Early Nineteenth-Century Medical Thought', *SHM*, 5 (1992): 43–70.

Hamlin, Christopher. *Cholera: The Biography* (Oxford, 2009).

Hamonet, Marie-Annick. *Les épidémies de typhus dans le Royaume-Uni au XIXe siècle*, Université de la Sorbonne nouvelle, Paris III (Paris, 1996).

Harden, Victoria. *AIDS at 30: A History* (Washington, DC, 2012).

Harden, Victoria. 'AIDS in the U.S.', *Encyclopedia of Pestilence*, I, 7–13.

Harden, Victoria. 'Smallpox', *Encyclopedia of Pestilence, Pandemics, and Plagues*, II, 647–50.

Hardiman, David. 'The 1918 Influenza Epidemic and the Adivasis of Western India', *SHM*, 25 (2012): 644–64.

Hardiman, Sue. *The 1832 Cholera Epidemic and its Impact on the City of Bristol*, Bristol Branch of the Historical Association, n. 114 (Bristol, 2005).

Hardy, Ann. 'Urban Famine or Urban Crisis? Typhus in the Victorian City', *Medical History*, 32 (1988): 401–25

Hardy, Ann. *The Epidemic Streets: Infectious Disease and the Rise of Preventive Medicine, 1856–1900* (Oxford, 1993).

Harper, Kristin N. 'Pandemics and the Passages to Late Antiquity: Rethinking the Plague of c. 249–270 Described by Cyprian', *Journal of Roman Archaeology*, 28 (2015): 223–60.

Harris, Edward M. 'The Family, the Community and Murder: The Role of Pollution in Athenian Homicide Law', *Public and Private in Ancient Mediterranean Law and Religion*, ed. Clifford Ando and Jörg Rüpke (Berlin, 2015), 11–35.

Harrison, Mark. *Public Health in British India: Anglo-Indian Preventive Medicine 1859–1914* (Cambridge, 1994).

Hart, Angie. 'Men Who Buy Heterosexual Sex in Spain', in *Culture and Sexual Risk: Anthropological Perspectives on AIDS*, ed. Han ten Brummelhuis and Gilbert Herdt (Amsterdam, 1995), 135–54.

Hatcher, John. 'England in the Aftermath of the Black Death', *Past & Present*, 144 (1994): 3–35.

Hatchett, Richard, Carter Mecher, and Marc Lipsitch, 'Public Health Interventions and Epidemic Intensity during the 1918 Influenza Pandemic', *PNAS*, 104/18 (1 May 2007): 7582–7.

Haverkamp, Alfred. 'Die Judenverfolgungen zur Zeit des Schwarzen Todes im Gesellschaftsgefüge deutscher Städte', in *Zur Geschichte der Juden im Deutschland des späten Mittelalters und der frühen Neuzeit*, ed. Alfred Haverkamp (Stuttgart, 1981), 27–93.

Hays, J. N. *The Burdens of Disease: Epidemics and Human Response in Western History* (New Brunswick, NJ, 1998).

Hayton, Darin. 'Joseph Grünpeck's Astrological Explanation of the French Disease', in *Responding to Sexual Disease in Early Modern Europe*, ed. Kevin Siena (Toronto, 2005), 241–74.

Heaphy, Brian, Jeffrey Weeks, and Catherine Donovan. 'Narratives of Care, Love and Commitment: AIDS/HIV and Non-Heterosexual Family Formations', in *Families and Communities Responding to AIDS*, 67–82.

Henderson, John. 'The Black Death in Florence: Medical and Communal Responses', in *Death in Towns: Urban Responses to the Dying and the Dead, 1000–1600*, ed. S. Bassett (Leicester, 1992), 136–50.

Henderson, John. 'Coping with Epidemics in Renaissance Italy: Plague and the Great Pox', in *The Fifteenth Century*, XII: *Society in an Age of Plague*, ed. Linda Clarke and Carole Rawcliffe (Woodbridge, 2013), 175–94.

Henderson, John. 'Epidemics in Renaissance Florence: Medical Theory and Government Response', in *Maladies et société (XIIe –XVIIIe siècles): Actes du colloque de Bielefeld novembre 1986*, ed. Neithard Bulst and Robert Delort (Paris, 1989), 165–86.

Henderson, John. 'Fracastoro, Mal Francese e la cura con il Legno Santo', in *Girolamo Fracastoro: Fra medicina, filosofia e scienze della natura*, ed. A. Pastore and E. Peruzzi (Florence, 2006), 73–89.

Henderson, Patrick. 'Smallpox and Patriotism', *The Virginia Magazine of History and Biography*, 73 (1965): 413–24.

Henry, Patrick J. *Sligo: Medical Care in the Past 1800–1965* (Dublin, 1995).

Hentschnell, Roze. 'Fracastoro, Mal Francese e la cura con il Legno Santo', in *Girolamo Fracastoro: Fra medicina, filosofia e scienze della natura*, ed. A. Pastore and E. Peruzzi (Florence, 2006), 73–89.

Hentschnell, Roze. 'Luxury and Lechery: Hunting the French Pox in Early Modern England', in *Sins of the Flesh: Responding to Sexual Disease in Early Modern Europe*, ed. Kevin Siena (Toronto, 2005), 133–54.

Henze, Charlotte E. *Disease, Health Care and Government in Late Imperial Russia: Life and Death on the Volga, 1823–1914* (London, 2011).

Herring, D. Ann and Alan C. Swedlund (eds.). *Plagues and Epidemics: Infected Spaces Past and Present* (Oxford, 2010).

Hewlett, Mary. 'The French Connection: Syphilis and Sodomy in Late-Renaissance Lucca', in *Sins of the Flesh: Responding to Sexual Disease in Early Modern Europe*, ed. Kevin Siena (Toronto, 2005), 239–60.

Hildreth, Martha L. 'The Influenza Epidemic of 1918–1919 in France: Contemporary Concepts of Aetiology, Therapy, and Prevention', *SHM*, 4 (1991): 277–94.

Holland, Michael. 'Resurrectionists, Anatomy Act and Child Farming', in *Cholera and Conflict*, 204–23.

Holland, Michael. Geoffrey Gill, and Sean Burrell (eds.). *Cholera and Conflict: 19th Century Cholera in Britain and its Social Consequences* (London, 2009).

Honigsbaum, Mark. *Living with Enza: The Forgotten Story of Britain and the Great Flu Pandemic of 1918* (London, 2009).

Honigsbaum, Mark. 'The Great Dread: Cultural and Psychological Impacts and Responses to the "Russian" Influenza in the United Kingdom, 1889–1893', *SHM*, 23 (2010): 299–319.

Honigsbaum, Mark. *A History of the Great Influenza Pandemics: Death, Panic and Hysteria, 1830–1920* (London, 2014).

Hooper, Finley. *Roman Realities* (London, 1968).

Hopkins, Donald R. *The Greatest Killer: Smallpox in History* (Chicago, 2002).

Hornblower, Simon. *A Commentary of Thucydides*, 3 vols (Oxford, 1991–2008).

Hughes, Dennis D. *Human Sacrifice in Ancient Greece* (London, 1991).

Humphreys, Margaret. *Yellow Fever and the South* (New Brunswick, NJ, 1992).

Humphreys, Margaret. 'No Safe Place: Disease and Panic in American History', *American Literary History*, 14 (2002): 848–9.

Humphreys, Margaret. 'A Stranger to Our Camps: Typhus in American History', *BHM*, 80 (2006): 269–90.

Humphreys, Margaret. 'Appendix II: Yellow Fever since 1793: History and Historiography', in *A Melancholy Scene of Devastation*, 183–98.

Humphries, Mark O. 'A Pandemic Prelude: The 1889–91 Influenza Pandemic in Canada', in idem, *The Last Plague: Spanish Influenza and the Politics of Public Health in Canada* (Toronto, 2013), 58–67.

Humphries, Mark O. *A History of the Great Influenza Pandemics: Death, Panic and Hysteria, 1830–1920* (London, 2014).

Hyde, Sandra Teresa. *Eating Spring Rice: The Cultural Politics of AIDS in Southwest China* (Berkeley, 2007).

Iliffe, John. *The African AIDS Epidemic* (Oxford, 2006).

Irwin, Julia. 'Scapegoats and Epidemic Disease', in *Encyclopedia of Pestilence*, II, 618–20.

Isseroff, Ami. 'Lisbon Massacre', *Zionism and Israel:Encyclopedia and Dictionary, Zionism and Israel on the Web*, 31 March 2009.

James, Gregory. *The Chinese Labour Camps (1916–1920)* (Hong Kong, 2013).

Jenks, Stuart. 'Judenverschuldung und Verfolgung von Juden im 14. Jahrhundert: Franken bis 1349', *Vierteljahrschrift für Sozial- und Wirtschaftsgeschichte*, 65 (1978): 309–56.

Jillings, Karen. 'Plague, Pox and the Physician in Aberdeen, 1495–1516', *Journal of the Royal College of Physicians, Edinburgh*, 40 (2010): 70–6.

John-Langba, Johannes. 'HIV, Sexual Violence and Exploitation during Post-Conflict Transitions: The Case of Sierra Leone', in *The Fourth Wave*, 103–16.

Johnson, Niall. *Britain and the 1918–19 Influenza Pandemic: A Dark Epilogue* (London, 2006).

Johnson, Niall. 'The Over-Shadowed Killer: Influenza in Britain, 1918–19', in *The Spanish Influenza Pandemic of 1918–19*, 132–45 and 275–80.

Johnson, Niall and Jürgen Mueller. 'Updating the Accounts: Global Mortality of the 1918–1920 "Spanish" Influenza Pandemic', *BHM*, 76 (2002): 105–15.

Jones, Esyllt W. *Influenza 1918: Disease, Death, and Struggle in Winnipeg*, Studies in Gender and History (Toronto, 2007).

Jones, Pamela. 'San Carlo Borromeo and the Plague Imagery in Milan and Rome', in *Hope and Healing*, 65–96.

Jütte, Robert. 'Syphilis and Confinement: Hospitals in Early Modern Germany', in *Institutions of Confinement: Hospitals, Asylums, and Prisons in Western Europe and North America, 1500–1950*, ed. Norbert Finzsch and Robert Jütte (Cambridge 1996), 97–115.

Kaiser, Hilmar. 'Genocide at the Twilight of the Ottoman Empire', in *The Oxford Handbook of Genocide Studies*, ed. Donald Bloxham and A. Dirk Moses (Oxford, 2010), 365–89.

Karras, Ruth. *Common Women: Prostitution and Sexuality in Medieval England* (New York, 1996).

Kelton, Paul. *Cherokee Medicine, Colonial Germs: An Indigenous Nation's Fight against Smallpox, 1518–1824* (Norman, OK, 2015).

Kidambi, Prashant. *The Making of an Indian Metropolis: Colonial Governance and Public Culture in Bombay, 1890–1920* (Aldershot, 2007).

Kinealy, Christine. *The Great Irish Famine: Impact, Ideology and Rebellion* (Basingstoke, 2002).

King, Helen. 'Comparative Perspectives on Medicine and Religion in the Ancient World', in *Religion, Health and Suffering*, ed. John R. Hinnells and Roy Porter (London, 1999), 276–94.

King, Martina. *Das Mikrobielle in der Literatur und Kultur der Moderne: Zur Wissensgeschichte eines und ephemeren Gegenstandes 1880–1930* (Habilitation, Bern, 2015; forthcoming Berlin, 2018).

Kisch, Guido. *The Jews in Medieval Germany: A Study of their Legal and Social Status* (Chicago, 1949).

Klein, Ira. 'Plague, Policy and Popular Unrest in British India', *Modern Asian Studies*, 22 (1988): 723–55.

Klot, Jennifer F. and Vinh-Kim Nguyen (eds.). *The Fourth Wave: Violence, Gender, Culture & HIV in the 21st Century* (Paris, 2011).

Kobasa, Suzanne C. Ouellette. 'AIDS Volunteering Links to the Post and Future Prospects', in *A Disease of Society*, 172–88.

Korosak, Bruno. 'Bernardino da Siena', *BS*, II, cols 1294–1321.

Kraut, Alan M. *Silent Travellers: Germs, Genes, and the 'Immigrant Menace'* (New York, 1994).

Kraut, Alan M. 'Plagues and Prejudice: Nativism's Construction of Disease in Nineteenth-and Twentieth-Century New York City', in *Hives of Sickness*, 65–94.

Kudlick, Catherine J. *Cholera in Post-Revolutionary Paris: A Cultural History* (Berkeley, 1996).

Kumhera, Glenn. *The Benefits of Peace: Private Peacemaking in Late Medieval Italy: Private Peacemaking in Late Medieval Italy* (Leiden, 2017).

Langer, William L. 'The Black Death', *Scientific American*, 210 (1964): 114–21.

Langford, Christopher. 'Did the 1918–19 Influenza Pandemic Originate in China?', *Population and Development Review*, 31 (2005): 473–505.

Lapsansky, Phillip. ' "Abigail, a Negress": The Role and Legacy of African Americans in the Yellow Fever Epidemic', in *A Melancholy Scene of Devastation*, 61–78.

Lay, Shawn. *War, Revolution and the Klu Klux Klan: A Study of Intolerance in a Border City* (El Paso, TX, 1985).

Leavitt, Judith Walzer. 'Politics and Public Health: Smallpox in Milwaukee, 1894–1895', in *Sickness and Health in America: Readings in the History of Medicine and Public Health*, ed. Judith Walzer Leavitt and Ronald L. Numbers (Madison, WI, 1978), 403–13; first published in *BHM*, 50 (1976): 553–68.

Leavitt, Judith Walzer. *The Healthiest City: Milwaukee and the Politics of Health Reform* (Princeton, NJ, 1982).

Leavitt, Judith Walzer. *Typhoid Mary: Captive to the Public's Health* (Boston, MA, 1996).

Levack, Brian P. *The Witch-Hunt in Early Modern Europe*, 3rd edn (Harlow, 2006).

Levine, Carol. 'AIDS and Changing Concepts of Family', in *A Disease of Society*, 45–70.

Little, Lester (ed.). *Plague and the End of Antiquity: The Pandemic of 541–750* (Cambridge, 2007).

Littman, R. J. and M. L. Littman, 'Galen and the Antonine Plague', *The American Journal of Philology*, 94 (1973): 243–55.

Littré, E. 'Les semeurs de peste', in *Médicine et médicins des Grandes Epidémies*, 3rd edn (Paris, 1875): 492–509.

Lloyd, G. E. R. *In the Grip of Disease: Studies in the Greek Imagination* (Oxford, 2003).

Longrigg, James. 'Epidemic, Ideas and Classical Athenian Society', in *Epidemics and Ideas*, 21–44.

Lorenzo, Maria Pia. *Colera sovversive: Le rivolte di Verbicaro (1855 e 1911)* (Salerno, 1990).

Low, R. Bruce. 'The Incidence of Small-Pox throughout the World in Recent Years', *Reports to the Local Government Board on Public Health and Medical Subjects*, no. 117 (London, 1918).

Luckingham, Bradford. *Epidemic in the Southwest 1918–1919*, Southwestern Studies 72 (El Paso, TX, 1984).

Luzio, Alessandro and Rodolfo Renier, 'Contributo alla storia del malfrancese ne' costumi e nella letteratura italiana del secolo XVI', *Giornale storico della letteratura italiana*, 5/3 (1885): 408–32.

Lynteris, Christos. 'Epidemics as Events and as Crises: Comparing Two Plague Outbreaks in Manchuria (1910–11 and 1920–21)', *Cambridge Anthropology*, 32 (2014): 62–76.

Mack, Arien (ed.). *Time of Plague: The History and Social Consequences of Lethal Epidemic Disease* (New York, 1991).

McDuff, Laura. 'The 1832 Liverpool Cholera Riots', in *Cholera and Conflict*, 95–107.

McGinnis, Janice P. Dicken. 'The Impact of Epidemic Influenza: Canada, 1918–1919', in *Medicine in Canadian Society: Historical Perspectives*, ed. S. E. D. Shortt (Montreal, 1980), 447–77.

McGough, Laura J. *Gender, Sexuality, and Syphilis in Early Modern Venice: The Disease that Came to Stay* (Basingstoke, 2010).

McGough, Laura J. 'Quarantining Beauty: The French Disease in Early Modern Venice', in *Sins of the Flesh: Responding to Sexual Disease in Early Modern Europe*, ed. Kevin Siena (Toronto, 2005), 211–39.

McGrew, Roderick E. *Russia and the Cholera 1823–32* (Madison, WI, 1965).

McLean, David. *Public Health and Politics in the Age of Reform: Cholera, the State and the Royal Navy in Victorian Britain* (London, 2006).

McNeill, J. R. *Mosquito Empires: Ecology and War in the Greater Caribbean 1620–1914* (Cambridge, 2010).

Maier, Pauline. *From Resistance to Revolution: Colonial Radicals and the Development of American Opposition to Britain, 1765–1776* (London, 1972).

Mallet, Michael and Christine Shaw, *The Italian Wars, 1494–1559: War, State, and Society in Early Modern Europe* (Harlow, 2012).

Marshall, Louise. 'Manipulating the Sacred: Image and Plague in Renaissance Italy', *Renaissance Quarterly*, 47/3 (1994): 485–532.

Martines, Lauro. *Furies: War in Europe 1450–1700* (New York, 2013).

Matic, Sdran. 'Twenty-Five Years of HIV/AIDS in Europe', in *HIV/AIDS in Europe*, 1–14.

Matic, Srdan, Jeffery V. Lazarus, and Martin C. Donoghoe (eds.). *HIV/AIDS in Europe: Moving from Death Sentence to Chronic Disease Management* (Copenhagen, 2006).

Mayer, Kenneth, Olive Shisanna, and Chris Beyrer. 'AIDS 2016: From Aspiration to Implementation', *Lancet*, 387/10037 (18 June 2106): 2484–5.

Mbali, Mandisa. *South African AIDS Activism and Global Health Politics* (Basingstoke, 2013).

Meerloo, Joost A. M. *Patterns of Panic* (New York, 1950).

Mentgen, Gerd. 'Herausragende jüdische Finanziers im mittelalterlichen Straßburg', in *Hochfinanz im Westen des Reiches*, 75–100.

Merians, Linda E. (ed.). *The Secret Malady: Venereal Disease in Eighteenth-Century Britain and France* (Lexington, KY, 1996).

Merians, Linda E. 'The London Lock Hospital and the Lock Asylum for Women', in *The Secret Malady*, 128–45.

Messina, Anna Lucia Forti. 'L'Italia dell'Ottocento di fronte al Colera', *Storia d'Italia: Annali 7: Malattia e medicina*, ed. Franco della Perutta (Turin, 1984), 429–94.

Michael, Pamela and Steven Thompson. *Public Health in Wales, 1800–2000: A Brief History* (Cardiff, 2012).

Mohr, James. *Plague and Fire: Battling Black Death and the 1900 Burning of Honolulu's Chinatown* (Oxford, 2005).

Molina, Natalia. *How Race Is Made in America: Immigration, Citizenship, and the Historical Power of Racial Scripts* (Berkeley, 2014).

Monter, William. 'Witchcraft in Geneva, 1537–1662', *Journal of Modern History*, 43 (1971): 179–204.

Monter, William. *Witchcraft in France and Switzerland: The Borderlands during the Reformation* (Ithaca, NY, 1976).

Moore, R. I. *The Formation of a Persecuting Society: Power and Deviance in Western Europe, 950–1250* (Oxford, 1987).

Morabito, Giuseppe. 'Angelo da Gerusalemme o da Licata, santo', *BS*, I, 1240–3.

Morelli, Carlo. 'Pietro Betti, *Sul cholera asiatico che contristò la Toscana*: Annalisi bibliografica', in *AUM*, 24, f. 480 (1857): 608–45.

Morris, R. J. *Cholera 1832: The Social Response to an Epidemic* (London, 1976).

Müller, Jörge R. '*Erez gererah*—"Land of Persecution": Pogroms against the Jews in the *regnum Teutonicum* from c. 1280 to 1350', in *The Jews of Europe in the Middle Ages (Tenth* to Fifteenth Centuries): *Proceedings of the International Symposium, Speyer, 20–25 October 2002*, ed. Christoph Cluse (Turnhout, 2004), 245–60.

Mutreja, A. et al. 'Evidence for Several Waves of Global Transmission in the Seventh Cholera Pandemic', *Nature*, 477/7365 (24 August 2011): 462–5.

Naphy, William G. *Plagues, Poisons and Potions: Plague-Spreading Conspiracies in the Western Alps c. 1530–1640* (Manchester, 2002).

Napier, A. David. *Foreign Bodies: Performance, Art, and Symbolic Anthropology* (Berkeley, 1992).

Napier, A. David. *Masks, Transformation, and Paradox* (Berkeley, 1986).

Naruszewicz, Pietro. 'Cunegonda (Kinga, Kunga)', *BS*, IV, 460–1.

Nash, Gary B. *Forging Freedom: The Formation of Philadelphia's Black Community, 1720–1840* (Cambridge, 1988).

Nathan, C. J. *Plague Prevention and Politics in Manchuria 1910–1931* (Cambridge, MA, 1967).

Nelkin, Dorothy and Sander Gilman. 'Placing Blame for Devastating Disease', *Social Research*, 55 (1988): 362–78, reprinted in *Time of Plague* (1991).

Nelkin, Dorothy and Stephen Hilgartner. 'Disputed Dimensions of Risk: A Public School Controversy over AIDS', in *AIDS: The Public Context of an Epidemic*, ed. Ronald Bayer, Daniel M. Fox, and David P. Willis, *The Milbank Quarterly*, 64, Supplement 1 (Cambridge, 1986): 118–42.

Nelkin, Dorothy, David P. Willis, and Scott V. Parris (eds.). *A Disease of Society: Cultural and Institutional Responses to AIDS* (Cambridge, 1991).

Netchkina, M. V., K. V. Sivkov, and A. L. Sidorov. 'La Russie', in *La première épidémie du XIXe siècle*, 143–55.

Newman, Ruth. 'Salisbury in the Age of Cholera: "We Mustn't Frighten the Readers"', in *Cholera and Conflict*, 124–41.

Ngalamulume, Kalala. 'Smallpox and Social Control in Colonial Saint-Louis-du-Senegal, 1850–1916', in *HIV/AIDS, Illness, and African Well-Being*, ed. Toyin Falola and Mathew H. Heaton (Rochester, NY, 2007), 62–78.

Nguyen, Vinh-Kim. *The Republic of Therapy: Triage and Sovereignty in West Africa's Time of AIDS* (Durham, NC, 2010).

Nicolini, Fausto. *Peste e untori nei 'Promessi Sposi' e nella realtà storica*, Biblioteca di cultura moderna, n. 305 (Bari, 1937).

Nicolini, Fausto. 'Parte III: La Peste 1629–1632', in *Storia di Milano*, X, ed. G. Treccani degli Alfieri, (Milan, 1957), 497–557.

Nohl, Johannes. *The Black Death: A Chronicle of the Plague Compiled from Contemporary Sources*, trans. C. H. Clarke (London, 1926; originally, Potsdam, 1924).

Norberg, Kathryn. 'From Courtesan to Prostitute: Mercenary Sex and Venereal Disease 1730–1802', in *The Secret Malady*, 34–50.

Noymer, Andrew. 'Epidemics and Time: Influenza and Tuberculosis during and after the 1918–1919 Pandemic', in *Plagues and Epidemics*, 137–52.

Nutton, Vivian. 'Medicine', in *The Cambridge Ancient History*, XI: *The High Empire*, AD 70–192, ed. A. K. Bowman, Peter Garnsey, and Dominic Rathbone, 2nd edn (Cambridge, 2000), 943–65.

Nutton, Vivian. *Ancient Medicine* (New York, 2004).

Ó Gráda, Cormac. *Ireland's Great Famine: Interdisciplinary Perspective* (Dublin, 2005).

Oldstone, Michael. *Viruses, Plagues, and History*, 2nd edn (Oxford, 2010).

Origo, Iris. *The World of San Bernardino* (New York, 1962).

Paccagnini, Ermanno. 'Cronaca di un contagio', in *Processo algi untori*, 9–143.

Pagden, Anthony. 'The Challenge of the New', in *The Oxford Handbook of the Atlantic World c.1450–c.1850*, ed. Nicholas Canny and Philip Morgan (Oxford, 2011), 449–62.

Palmer, Robert C. *English Law in the Age of the Black Death, 1348–1381: A Transformation of Governance and Law* (Chapel Hill, NC, 1993).

Parker, Geoffrey. *Global Crisis: War, Climate Change and Catastrophe in the Seventeenth Century* (New Haven, CT, 2013).

Parker, Richard and Peter Aggleton, 'HIV and AIDS-Related Stigma and Discrimination: A Conceptual Framework and Implications for Action', *Social Science & Medicine*, 57 (2003): 13–24.

'Parliamentary Intelligence'. *Lancet*, 155 (5 May 1900): 1333.

Pastore, Alessandro. *Crimine e giustizia in tempo di Peste nell'Europa moderna* (Bari, 1991).

Patterson, K. David. 'Cholera Diffusion in Russia, 1823–1923', *Social Science Medicine*, 38 (1994): 1171–91.

Patton, Cindy. *Sex and Germs: The Politics of AIDS* (Boston, MA, 1985).

Patton, Cindy. *Globalizing AIDS* (Minneapolis, MN, 2002).

Patton, Cindy. *Inventing AIDS* (New York, 1990).

Peckham, Robert. 'Symptoms of Empire: Cholera in Southeast Asia, 1820–1850', in *Routledge History of Disease*, ed. Mark Jackson (London, 2017), 183–201.

Pelling, Margaret. *Cholera, Fever and English Medicine 1825–1865* (Oxford, 1978).

Penn, Simon and Christopher Dyer. 'Wages and Earnings in Late Medieval England: Evidence from the Enforcement of the Labour Laws', *Economic History Review*, 2nd ser., 43 (1990): 356–76.

Pepin, Jacques. *The Origins of AIDS* (Cambridge, 2011).

Pernick, Martin S. 'Politics, Parties, and Pestilence: Epidemic Yellow Fever in Philadelphia and the Rise of the First Party System', in *Sickness and Health in America: Readings in the History of Medicine and Public Health*, ed. Judith Walzer Leavitt and Ronald L. Numbers (Madison, WI, 1978), 241–56.

Phillips, Howard. *'Black October': The Impact of the Spanish Influenza Epidemic of 1918 on South Africa* (Pretoria, 1990).

Phillips, Howard. 'HIV/AIDS in the Context of South Africa's Epidemic History', in *AIDS and South Africa: The Social Expression of a Pandemic*, ed. Kyle D. Kauffman and David L. Lindauer (Basingstoke, 2004), 31–47.

Phillips, Howard. 'Second Opinion: The Recent Wave of "Spanish" Flu Historiography', *SHM*, 27 (2014): 789–808.

Phillips, Howard and David Killingray (eds.). *The Spanish Influenza Pandemic of 1918–19: New Perspectives* (London, 2003).

Picasso, Giorgio. 'Introduzione', in *La canonizzazione di Santa Francesca Romana: Santità, cultura e istituzioni a Roma tra medioevo ed età moderna. Atti del Convegno internazionale, Roma, 19–21 novembre 2009*, ed. Alessandra Bartolomei Romagnoli and Giorgio Picasso (Florence, 2013), xix–xxvii.

Pierce, John R. and Jim Writer. *Yellow Jack: How Yellow Fever Ravaged America and Walter Reed Discovered Its Deadly Secrets* (Hoboken, NJ, 2005).

Pieri, Dino. *Lo Zingaro Maledetto: Colera e società nella Romagna dell'ottocento* (Bologna, 1985).

Pierluigi, Patriarca. *Gli anni del colera, i giorni della 'Spagnola': La Valtellina di fronte ai due ultimi grandi flagelli epidemici dell'umanità* (Sondrio, 2003).

Piot, Peter. *No Time to Lose: A Life in Pursuit of Deadly Viruses* (New York, 2012).

Plague Manual: Epidemiology, Distribution, Surveillance and Control (Geneva: WHO, 1999).

Platt, Jerome, Maurice Jones, and Arleen Platt. *The Whitewash Brigade: The Hong Kong Plague of 1894* (London, 1998).

Poirier, Richard. 'AIDS and Traditions of Homophobia', in *Time of Plague*, 139–67.

Polidori. 'Avvertimento', in Visconti, *Commentarius de peste*, 489–90.

Pollitzer, Robert. *Plague* (Geneva, 1954).

Poos, Lawrence. 'The Social Context of Statute of Labourers Enforcement', *Law & History Review*, 27 (1983), 27–52.

Porter, Dorothy and Roy Porter. 'The Enforcement of Health: The British Debate', in *AIDS: The Burdens of History*, ed. Elizabeth Fee and Daniel M. Fox (Berkeley, 1988), 97–120.

Porter, Roy. 'The Case of Consumption', in *Understanding Catastrophe*, ed. J. Bourriau (Cambridge, 1992), 179–203.

Powell, J. H. *Bring Out Your Dead: The Great Plague of Yellow Fever in Philadelphia in 1793* (Philadelphia, 1949); new edn by Kenneth R. Foster, Mary F. Jenkins, and Anna Coxe Toogood (Philadelphia, PA, 1993).

Preto, Paolo. *Peste e società a Venezia in 1576* (Vicenza, 1978).

Preto, Paolo. *Epidemia, paura e politica nell'Italia moderna* (Bari, 1987).

Preto, Paolo. 'Le grandi pesti dell'età moderna 1575–77 e 1630–31', in *Venezia e la peste 1348/1797* (Venice, 1979), 123–6.

Price, Polly J. 'A Legislative History of the Shotgun Quarantine', *Emory Legal Studies Research Paper* No. 15-352 (5 August 2015): 1–72.

Prinzing, Friedrich. *Epidemics Resulting from Wars*, ed. Harald Westergaard (Oxford, 1916).

Proksch, J. K. *Die Geschichte der venerischen Krankheiten: Eine Studie*, 2 vols (Bonn, 1895).

Pullan, Brian. 'Plague and Perceptions of the Poor in Early Modern Italy', in *Epidemics and Idea*, 101–23.

Quétel, Claude. *History of Syphilis*, trans. Judith Braddock and Brian Pike (Cambridge, 1990).

Quiney, Linda J. 'Borrowed Halos: Canadian Teachers as Voluntary Aid Detachment Nurses during the Great War', *Historical Studies in Education*, 15 (2003): 78–99.

Quiney, Linda J. '"Rendering Valuable Service": The Politics of Nursing during the 1918–19 Influenza Crisis', in *Epidemic Encounters: Influenza, Society, and Culture in Canada, 1918–20*, ed. Magda Fahrni and Esyllt W. Jones (Vancouver, 2012), 48–69.

Quinn, Tom. *Flu: A Social History of Influenza* (London, 2008).

Raimond-Waarts, Loes L. and Catrien Santing. 'Sex: A Cardinal's Sin: Punished by Syphilis in Renaissance Rome', *Leidschrift: Historisch Tijdschrift*, 25 (2010): 169–82.

Ramanna, Mridula. 'Coping with the Influenza Pandemic: The Bombay Experience', in *The Spanish Influenza Pandemic of 1918–19*, 86–98 and 268–71.

Ranger, Terence and Paul Slack. *Epidemics and Ideas: Essays on the Historical Perception of Pestilence* (Cambridge, 1992).

Rawcliffe, Carole. *Leprosy in Medieval England* (Woodbridge, 2006).

Rawcliffe, Carole. *Urban Bodies: Communal Health in Late Medieval English Towns and Cities* (Woodbridge, 2013).

Rawlinson, H. G. 'Early Contacts between India and Europe', in *A Cultural History of India*, ed. A. L. Basham (Oxford, 1975), 421–41.

Reeds, Karen. 'Smallpox in Colonial North America', in *Encyclopedia of Pestilence, Pandemics, and Plagues*, II, 663–7.

Repossi, Cesare. 'Cronologia della vita di Giuseppe Ripamonti', in Ripamonti, *La Peste di Milano del 1630*, lxxxii–xcvii.

Rice, Geoffrey W. 'Australia and New Zealand in the 1918–19 Influence Epidemic', in *Occasional Papers on Medical History, Australia*, IV: *New Perspectives of the History of Medicine*, ed. H. Attwood, R. Gillespie, and M. Lewis (Sydney, 1989), 67–74.

Rice, Geoffrey W. *Black November: The 1918 Influenza Pandemic in New Zealand*, 2nd edn (Canterbury, 2005).

Richardson, Ruth. *Death, Dissection and the Destitute*, 2nd edn (London, 1988).

Risse, Guenter B. 'Revolt against Quarantine: Community Responses to the 1916 Polio Epidemic, Oyster Bay, New York', *Transactions and Studies of the College of Physicians of Philadelphia*, 14 (1992): 23–50.

Risse, Guenter B. *Plague, Fear, and Politics in San Francisco's Chinatown* (Baltimore, MD, 2012).

Robertson, R. G. *Rotting Face: Smallpox and the American Indian* (Caldwell, ID, 2001).

Robins, Natalie. *Copeland's Cure: Homeopathy and the War between Conventional and Alternative Medicine* (New York, 2005).

Robins, Steven. *From Revolution to Rights in South Africa: Social Movements, NGOs and Popular Politics after Apartheid* (Rochester, NY, 2008).

Rodgers, Naomi. 'A Disease of Cleanliness: Polio in New York City, 1900–1990', in *Hives of Sickness: Public Health and Epidemics in New York City*, ed. David Rosner (New Brunswick, NJ, 1995), 115–30.

Rodrígucz Ocaña, Esteban. *El cólera de 1834 en Granada: Enfermeda catatófica y crisis social* (Granada, 1983).

Roe, Michael. 'Cumpston, John Howard Lidgett (1880–1954)', in *Australian Dictionary of Biography* (Melbourne, 1981).

Rogaski, Ruth. *Hygenic Modernity: Meanings of Health and Disease in Treaty-Port China* (Berkeley, 2004).

Rohleder, Poul et al. (eds.). *HIV/AIDS in South Africa: 25 Years On: Psychosocial Perspectives* (Berlin, 2009).

Roland, Charles G. *Courage under Siege: Starvation, Disease, and Death in the Warsaw Ghetto* (New York, 1992).

Rollet, Catherine and Agnès Sauriac. 'Épidémies ct mentalités: Le choléra de 1832 en Seine-et-Oise', *Annales: E.S.C.*, 29/4 (1974): 935–66.

Rosenberg, Charles E. *The Cholera Years: The United States in 1832, 1849, and 1866* (Chicago, 1962).

Rosenberg, Charles E. 'What Is an Epidemic? AIDS in Historical Perspective', *Daedelus*, 118, (1989): 1–17.

Rosner, David (ed.). *Hives of Sickness: Public Health and Epidemics in New York City* (New Brunswick, NJ, 1995).

Ross, Richard S., III. *Contagion in Prussia, 1831: The Cholera Epidemic and the Threat of the Polish Uprising* (Jefferson, NC, 2015).

Rossiaud, Jacques. *Medieval Prostitution*, trans. Lydia Cochrane (New York, 1988).

Roth, Cecil. *The History of the Jews of Italy* (Philadelphia, PA, 1946).

Roth, Mitchel Philip. 'The Western Cholera Trail: Studies in the Urban Response to Epidemic Disease in the Trans-Mississippi West, 1848–1850', PhD dissertation, University of California at Santa Barbara, 1993.

Roucaud, Joseph. *La peste à Toulouse des origines au dix-huitième siècle: Thèse pour le doctorat en médecine* (Toulouse, 1918).

Rousey, Dennis C. 'Yellow Fever and Black Policemen in Memphis: A Post-Reconstruction Anomaly', *Journal of Southern History*, 51 (1985): 357–74.

Ruffie, Jacques. 'SIDA et civilisations', in *SIDA: Epidémies et sociétés, 20 et 21 juin 1987* (Lyon, 1987), 85–7.

Rushing, William A. *The AIDS Epidemic: Social Dimensions of an Infectious Disease* (Boulder, CO, 1995).

Russo, Salvatore (ed.). *I moti del 1837 a Siracusa e la Sicilia degli anni trenta* (Caltanissetta, 1987).

Rütten, Thomas. 'Cholera in Thomas Mann's *Death in Venice*', *Gesnerus*, 66 (2009): 229–57.

Sabatier, Renée. *Blaming Others: Prejudice, Race and Worldwide AIDS* (London, 1988).

Salomé, Karine. 'Le massacre des "empoisonneurs" à Paris au temps du choléra (1832)', *Revue historique*, 673 (2015): 103–24.

Sannazzaro, Giovanni Battista. 'Note sull'immagine agiografia della Milano di San Carlo Borromeo', in *Florence and Milan: Comparisons and Relations*, II, ed. G. H. Smyth and G. C. Garfagnini, 2 vols (Florence, 1989), 33–47.

Sansone, Alfonso. *Gli Avvenimenti del 1837 in Sicilia (con documenti…)* (Palermo, 1890).

Sarkar, Aditya. 'The Tie that Snapped: Bubonic Plague and Mill Labour in Bombay, 1896–1898', *International Revue of Social History*, 59 (2014): 181–214.

Satya, Laman D. *Medicine, Disease and Ecology in Colonial India: The Deccan Plateau in the 19th Century* (New Delhi, 2008).

Scheidel, Walter. 'Germs for Rome', *Rome the Cosmopolis*, ed. Catharine Edwards and Greg Woolf (Cambridge, 2003), 158–76.

Schoepf, Brooke Grundfest. 'Culture, Sex Research and AIDS Prevention in Africa', in *Culture and Sexual Risk: Anthropological Perspectives on AIDS*, ed. Han ten Brummelhuis and Gilbert Herdt (Amsterdam, 1995), 29–51.

Serra, Girolamo. *La storia della antica Liguria e di Genova*, 4 vols (Turin, 1834).

Shah, Nayan. *Contagious Divides: Epidemics and Race in San Francisco's Chinatown* (Berkeley, 2001).

Shah, Sonia. *Pandemic: Tracking Contagions from Cholera to Ebola and Beyond* (New York, 2016).

Sherman, Irwin W. *The Power of Plagues* (Washington, DC, 2006).

Shilts, Randy. *And the Band Played On: Politics, People, and the AIDS Epidemic* (New York, 1987).

Siena, Kevin. *Venereal Disease, Hospitals and the Urban Poor: London's 'Foul Wards,' 1600–1800* (Rochester, NY, 2004).

Silverman, Mervyn. 'The Plague of Our Time: Societal Responses to AIDS', in *Encyclopedia of AIDS*, 27–8.

Simmons, Brian J., et al. 'Smallpox: 12000 Years from Plague to Eradication: A Dermatogic Ailment Shaping the Face of Society', *JAMA Dermatology*, 151/5 (May 2015): 482.

Simonetti, Nicola and Mimma Sangiorgi. *Il colera in Puglia dal 1831 ai giorni nostri* (Fasano, 2003).

Siraisi, Nancy. *History, Medicine, and the Traditions of Renaissance Learning* (Ann Arbor, MI, 2007).

Slack, Paul. *The Impact of Plague in Tudor and Stuart England* (London, 1985).

Slack, Paul. 'Responses to Plague in Early Modern Europe: The Implications of Public Health', *Social Research*, 55/3 (1988): 433–53.

Sloeck, Jean. 'Aedes aegypti Mosquitoes in the Americas: A Review of their Interactions with the Human Population', *Social Science and Medicine*, 23 (1986): 249–57.

Smail, Daniel Lord. 'Accommodating Plague in Medieval Marseille', *Continuity and Change*, 11 (1996): 11–41.

Small, Neil. 'Suffering in Silence? Public Visibility, Private Secrets and the Social Construction of AIDS', in *AIDS: Activism and Alliances*, 15–24.

Smelser, Neil. *The Theory of Collective Behaviour* (London, 1962; reprinted, 1998).

Smith, Billy G. *Ship of Death: A Voyage That Change the Atlantic World* (New Haven, CT, 2013).

Smith, Billy G. 'Comment: Disease and Community', in *A Melancholy Scene of Devastation*, 147–62.

Smith, F. B. 'The Russian Influenza in the United Kingdom, 1889–1994', *SHM*, 8 (1995): 55–73.

Smith, Raymond A. (ed.). *Encyclopedia of AIDS: A Social, Political, Cultural, and Scientific Record of the HIV Epidemic* (Chicago, 1998).

Snowden, Frank M. *Naples in the Time of Cholera 1884–1911* (Cambridge, 1995).

Solomon, Tom. 'Hong Kong, 1894: The Role of James A. Lowson in the Controversial Discovery of the Plague Bacillus', *Lancet*, 350 (5 July 1997): 59–62.

Sontag, Susan. *Aids and its Metaphors* (New York, 1988).

Sontag, Susan. *Illness as Metaphor, and AIDS and its Metaphors* (London, 1991).

Soyer, François. 'The Massacre of the New Christians of Lisbon in 1506: A New Eyewitness Account', *Cadernos de Estudos Sefarditas*, 7 (2007): 221–43.

Stannard, Jerry. 'Diseases of Western Antiquity', in *The Cambridge World History of Human Disease*, ed. Kenneth F. Kiple, 2 vols (Cambridge, 1993).

Starr, Issac. 'Influenza in 1918: Recollections of the Epidemic in Philadelphia', *Annals of Internal Medicine*, 85 (1976): 516–18.

Stathakopoulos, Dionysios Ch. *Famine and Pestilence in the Late Roman and Early Byzantine Empire: A Systematic Survey of Subsistence Crises and Epidemics* (Aldershot, 2004).

Stathakopoulos, Dionysios Ch. 'Plagues of the Roman Empire', in *Encyclopedia of Pestilence*, II, 536–8.

Stein, Claudia. *Negotiating the French Pox in Early Modern Germany* (Farnham, 2009).

Stobbe, Otto. *Die Juden in Deutschland während des Mittelalters in politicher, socialer und rechticher Beziehung* (Braunschweig, 1866; reprinted Amsterdam, 1968).

Stöver, Heino and Rick Lines. 'Silence Still = Death: 25 Years of HIV/AIDS in Prisons', in *HIV/AIDS in Europe*, 67–85.

Strachan, Hew. *The First World War: A New Illustrated History* (London, 2003).

Strong, Philip. 'Epidemic Psychology: A Model', *Sociology of Health and Illness*, 12/3 (1990): 249–59.

Sudhoff, Karl. 'Die ersten Maßnahmen der Stadt Nürnberg gegen die Syphilis in den Jahren 1496 und 1497', *Archiv für Dermatologie und Syphilis*, 118 (1913): 1–30.

Sullivan, R. J. 'Cholera and Colonialism in the Philippines, 1899–1903', in *Disease, Medicine, and Empire: Perspectives on Western Medicine and the Experience of European Expansion*, ed. Roy Macleod and Milton Lewis (London, 1988), 284–300.

Summers, W. C. *The Great Manchurian Plague of 1910–1911: The Geopolitics of an Epidemic Disease* (New Haven, CT, 2012).

Swedlund, Alan C. 'Everyday Mortality in the Time of Plague: Ordinary People in Massachusetts before and during the 1918 Influenza Epidemic', in *Plagues and Epidemics*, 153–78.

Swenson, Robert M. 'Plagues, History, and AIDS', *American Scholar*, 57 (1988): 183–200.

Syme, Ronald. 'Livy and Augustus', *Harvard Studies in Classical Philology*, 64 (1959): 27–87.

Taksa, Lucy. 'The Masked Disease: Oral History, Memory and the Influenza Pandemic 1918–19', in *Memory & History in Twentieth-Century Australia*, ed. Kate Darian-Smith and Paula Hamilton (Melbourne, 1994), 77–91.

Taubenberger, Jeffrey K., Johna V. Hultin, and David M. Morens. 'Discovery and Characterization of the 1918 Pandemic Influenza Virus in Historical Context', *PMC* (22 May 2008).

Terry-Fritsch, Allie. 'Introduction', in *Beholding Violence in Medieval and Early Modern Europe*, ed. Terry-Fritsch (Farnham, 2012), 24–6.

Thomas, Keith. *Religion and the Decline of Magic* (New York, 1971).

Toch, Michael. 'Geld und Kredit in einer spätmittelalterlichen Landschaft: Zu einem unbeachteten hebraïschen Schuldenregister aus Niederbayern (1329–1332)', *Deutsches Archiv für Erforschung des Mittelalters*, 38 (1982), 499–550.

Toch, Michael. 'Between Impotence and Power—the Jews in the Economy and Polity of Medieval Europe', in *Poteri economici e poteri politici, secc. XIII–XVIII: atti della 'trentesima settimana di studi', 27 aprile–1 maggio 1998*, ed. Simonetta Cavaciocchi (Florence, 1999), 221–43.

Tognotti, Eugenia. *La 'Spagnola' in Italia: Storia dell'influenza che fece temere la fine del mondo (1918–19)* (Milan, 2002).

Tognotti, Eugenia. 'Scientific Triumphalism and Learning from Facts: Bacteriology and the "Spanish Flu" Challenge of 1918', *SHM*, 16 (2003), 97–110.

Tomes, Nancy. *The Gospel of Germs: Men, Women, and the Microbe in American Life* (Cambridge, MA, 1998).

Tomič, Zlata Blažina and Vedsna Blažina. *Expelling the Plague: The Health Office and the Implementation of Quarantine in Dubrovnik 1377–1533* (Montreal, 2015).

Tomkins, Sandra. 'The Failure of Expertise: Public Health Policy in Britain during the 1918–19 Influenza Epidemic', *SHM*, 5 (1992): 435–54.

Tomkins, Sandra.'The Influenza Epidemic in Western Samoa', *Journal of Pacific History*, 27 (1992): 181–97.

Toner, J. M. 'History of Inoculation in Massachusetts', *Massachusetts Medical Society*, 2/1–3 (1856): 151–204.

Touati, François-Olivier. *Maladie et société au Moyen Age: La lèpre, les lépreux et les léproseries dans la province ecclésiastique de Sens jusqu'au milieu du XIVe siècle*, Bibliothèque du Moyen Age, no. 11 (Brussels, 1998).

Tractenberg, Joshua. *The Devil and the Jews: The Medieval Conception of the Jew and its Relation to Modern Antisemitism* (New Haven, CT, 1943).

Treichler, Paula A. *How to Have Theory in an Epidemic: Cultural Chronicles of AIDS* (Durham, NC, 1999).

Trexler, R. C. 'Florentine Religious Experience: The Sacred Image', *Studies in the Renaissance*, 19 (1972): 7–41.

Tuckel, Peter, et al. 'The Diffusion of the Influenza Pandemic of 1918 in Hartford, Connecticut', *Social Science History*, 30/2 (2006): 167–96.

Tuells, J. 'La "Revolta da vacina" en Río (1904): Resistencia violent a la ley de vacunacíon obligatoria contra la viruela propuesta por Oswaldo Cruz', *Vacunas*, 20/4 (2009): 140–7.

Twigg, Graham. *Bubonic Plague: A Much Misunderstood Disease* (Ascot, 2013).

Vaccaro, Emanziana. 'Francesca Anna-Francesca Romana', *BS*, V, cols 1011–28.

van de Pol, Lotte. *The Burgher and the Whore: Prostitution in Early Modern Amsterdam*, trans. Liz Waters (Oxford, 2011).

van der Horst, Pieter W. 'From Liberation to Expulsion: The Exodus in the Earliest Jewish-Pagan Polemics', in *Israel's Exodus in Transdisciplinary Perspective: Text, Archaeology, Culture Geoscience*, Quantitative Methods in the Humanities and Social Sciences (Heidelberg, 2015), 389–94.

Varlik, Nükhet. *Plague and Empire in the Early Modern World: The Ottoman Experience, 1347–1600* (Cambridge, 2015).

Vauchez, André. 'San Rocco', *BS*, XI, cols 264–73.

Vaughan, Megan. 'Slavery, Smallpox, and Revolution: 1792 in Ile de France (Mauritius)', *SHM*, 13 (2000): 411–28.

Vetro, Carmello. 'Società, medici e terapie nel colera del 1837', in *Malattie terapie e istitutzioni sanitare in Sicilia* (Palermo, 1985), 189–213.

Vidalenc, Jean. 'Les départements normands', in *La première épidémie du XIXe siècle*, 99–108.

Vincent, Bernard. 'Le cholera en Espagne au XIXe siècle', in *Peurs et terreurs face à la contagion*, 43–55.

Voitgländer, Nico and Hans-Joachim Voth. 'Persecution Perpetuated: The Medieval Origins of Anti-Semitic Violence in Nazi Germany', *Quarterly Journal of Economics*, 127 (2012): 1339–92.

Voltmer, Ernst. 'Zur Geschichte der Juden im spätmittelalterlichen Speyer', in *Zur Geschichte der Juden im Deutschland des späten Mittelalters und der frühen Neuzeit*, ed. Alfred Haverkamp (Stuttgart, 1981), 94–121.

Walkowitz, Judith R. *Prostitution and Victorian Society: Women, Class, and the State* (Cambridge, 1980).

Wanrooij, Bruno P. F. ' "The Thorns of Love": Sexuality, Syphilis and Social Control in Modern Italy', in *Sex, Sin, and Suffering*, 137–59.

Wasserstein, Bernard. *Barbarism and Civilization: A History of Europe in Our Time* (Oxford, 2007).

Watson, William. 'The Sisters of Charity, the 1832 Cholera Epidemic in Philadelphia and Duffy's Cut', *U.S. Catholic Historian*, 27 (2009): 1–16.

Wear, Andrew. 'Fear, Anxiety, and the Plague in Early Modern England: Religion and Medical Responses', in *Religion, Health and Suffering*, ed. John R. Hinnells and Roy Porter (London, 1999), 339–63.

Weeks, Jeffrey. 'AIDS and the Regulation of Sexuality', in *AIDS and Contemporary History*, ed. Virginia Berridge and Philip Strong (Cambridge, 1993), 17–36.

Weindling, Paul J. *Epidemics and Genocide in Eastern Europe 1890–1945* (Oxford, 2000).

Wenzlhuemer, Ronald. *Connecting the Nineteenth-Century World: The Telegraph and Globalization* (Cambridge, 2013).

Willrich, Michael. *Pox: An American History* (New York, 2011).

Winslow, Ola Elizabeth. *A Destroying Angel: The Conquest of Smallpox in Colonial Boston* (Boston, MA, 1974).

Witte, Wilfried. *Erklärungsnotstand: Die Grippe-Epiedmie 1918–1920 in Deutschland unter besonderer Berücksichtung Badens* (Herbolzheim, 2006).

Witte, Wilfried. 'The Plague that Was Not Allowed to Happen: German Medicine and the Influenza Pandemic of 1918–19 in Baden', in *The Spanish Influenza Pandemic of 1918–19*, 49–57.

Wooten, David. *Bad Medicine: Doctors Doing Harm since Hippocrates* (Oxford, 2006).

Worcester, Thomas. 'Saint Roch vs. Plague, Famine, and Fear', in *Hope and Healing*, 153–75.

Worth Estes, J. and Billy G. Smith (eds.). *A Melancholy Scene of Devastation: The Public Response to the 1793 Philadelphia Yellow Fever Epidemic* (Philadelphia, PA, 1997).

Wray, Shona Kelly. *Communities and Crisis: Bologna during the Black Death*, The Medieval Mediterranean: Peoples, Economies and Cultures, 400–1500, no. 83 (Leiden and Boston, MA, 2009).

Wrightson, Keith. *Ralph Tailor's Summer: A Scrivener, his City, and the Plague* (New Haven, CT, 2011).

Wu Lien-Teh (G. L. Tuck). 'First Report of the North Manchurian Plague Prevention Service', *Journal of Hygiene*, 13 (1913–14): 237–90.

Wu Lien-Teh (G. L. Tuck). *A Treatise on Pneumonic Plague* (Geneva, 1926).

Wu Lien-Teh (G. L. Tuck). 'Historical Aspects', in Wu Lien-Teh, J. W. H. Chun, Robert Pollitzer, and C. Y. Wu, *Plague: A Manual for Medical and Public Health Workers* (Shanghai Station, 1936).

Wu Lien-Teh (G. L. Tuck). *Plague Fighter: The Autobiography of a Modern Chinese Physician* (Cambridge, 1959).

Yerushalmi, Yosef Hayim. *The Lisbon Massacre of 1506 and the Royal Image in the 'Shebet Yehudah'* (Cincinnati, OH, 1976).

Zaccarini, Matteo. 'The Return of Theseus to Athens: A Case Study in Layered Tradition and Reception', *Histos*, 9 (2015): 174–98.

Zanrè, Domenico. 'French Diseases and Italian Responses: Representations of the *mal francese* in the literature of Cinquecento Tuscany', in *Sins of the Flesh: Responding to Sexual Disease in Early Modern Europe*, ed. Kevin Siena (Toronto, 2005), 187–206.

Zavitziano, Spiridion C. and Dr Mally. 'Turkey: A Case of Plague in Trieste', in *Public Health Reports (1896–1970)*, 14 (1899): 2214–15.

Zeheter, Michael. *Epidemics, Empire, and Environments: Cholera in Madras and Quebec City 1818–1910* (Pittsburgh, PA, 2015).

Ziwes, Franz-Josef. 'Zum jüdischen Kapitalmarkt im spätmittelalterlichen Koblenz', in *Hochfinanz im Westen des Reiches*, 49–74.

Index

Printed and bound by CPI Group (UK) Ltd, Croydon, CR0 4YY